Autism: A Clinical Approach

Autism: A Clinical Approach

Edited by Paul Hiddleston

AMERICAN
MEDICAL PUBLISHERS
www.americanmedicalpublishers.com

American Medical Publishers,
41 Flatbush Avenue,
1st Floor, New York,
NY 11217, USA

Visit us on the World Wide Web at:
www.americanmedicalpublishers.com

ISBN: 978-1-63927-281-5

Cataloging-in-Publication Data

Autism : a clinical approach / edited by Paul Hiddleston.
p. cm.
Includes bibliographical references and index.
ISBN 978-1-63927-281-5
1. Autism. 2. Autism--Treatment. I. Hiddleston, Paul.
RC553.A88 A88 2022
616.858 82--dc23

Table of Contents

Preface

Autism is a development disorder in which an individual experiences difficulty in social interaction and communication. Individuals with autism often exhibit restricted and repetitive behavior. Such signs develop slowly but usually become visible by the age of three. Asperger syndrome, autism and pervasive developmental disorder constitute the larger set of autism spectrum disorder. In autism, information processing in the brain is altered with the reorganization of nerve cells and their synapses. During pregnancy, infections with rubella, exposure to toxins including alcohol, cocaine, air pollution, pesticides and valproic acid, autoimmune diseases and fetal growth restriction can become risks for autism. Children with autism may require support even after reaching adulthood. Speech therapy and behavioral interventions early in life can improve social and communication skills. This book aims to shed light on some of the unexplored aspects of autism and the recent researches in this medical condition. Different approaches, evaluations, methodologies and advanced studies on autism have been included in this book. It is a complete source of knowledge on the present status of our understanding of autism.

The researches compiled throughout the book are authentic and of high quality, combining several disciplines and from very diverse regions from around the world. Drawing on the contributions of many researchers from diverse countries, the book's objective is to provide the readers with the latest achievements in the area of research. This book will surely be a source of knowledge to all interested and researching the field.

In the end, I would like to express my deep sense of gratitude to all the authors for meeting the set deadlines in completing and submitting their research chapters. I would also like to thank the publisher for the support offered to us throughout the course of the book. Finally, I extend my sincere thanks to my family for being a constant source of inspiration and encouragement.

Editor

1

Intact priors for gaze direction in adults with high-functioning autism spectrum conditions

Philip J. Pell[1], Isabelle Mareschal[2], Andrew J. Calder[1^], Elisabeth A. H. von dem Hagen[1,4], Colin W.G. Clifford[5], Simon Baron-Cohen[3] and Michael P. Ewbank[1,6*]

Abstract

Background: Autism Spectrum Conditions (ASC) are associated with a range of perceptual atypicalities, including abnormalities in gaze processing. Pellicano and Burr (Trends Cogn Sci 16(10):504-10, 2012) have argued that these atypicalities might be explained within a Bayesian framework, in which perception represents the combination of sensory information with prior knowledge. They propose that the Bayesian priors of individuals with ASC might be attenuated, such that their perception is less reliant on prior knowledge than neurotypical individuals. An important tenet of Bayesian decision theory is that increased uncertainty about incoming sensory information will lead to a greater influence of the prior on perception. Consistent with this, Mareschal et al. (Curr Biol 23(8):717-21, 2013) showed that when noise is added to the eyes of a face (increasing uncertainty about gaze direction), gaze is more likely to be perceived as direct.

Methods: We adopted the same paradigm as Mareschal et al. to determine whether the influence of a prior on gaze perception is reduced in neurotypical participants with high numbers of autistic traits (experiment 1) and in individuals with a clinical diagnosis of ASC (experiment 2). Participants were presented with synthetic faces and asked to make a judgement about the relative gaze directions of the faces. Uncertainty about gaze direction was manipulated by adding noise to the eyes of a face.

Results: Consistent with previous work, in both experiment 1 and experiment 2, participants showed a bias towards perceiving gaze as direct under conditions of uncertainty. However, there was no evidence that the magnitude of this bias was reduced either in the ASC group or in neurotypical controls with a high number of autistic traits.

Conclusions: Our findings challenge the attenuated priors theory of perception in ASC (Trends Cogn Sci 16(10):504-10, 2012) and related proposals (Trends Cogn Sci 17(1):1, 2013, Front Hum Neurosci 8:302, 2014), and suggest priors for gaze direction are intact in high-functioning ASC.

Keywords: Autism, Bayesian priors, Gaze perception, Autistic traits, Uncertainty

* Correspondence: michael.ewbank@mrc-cbu.cam.ac.uk
^Deceased
[1]Medical Research Council, Cognition and Brain Sciences Unit, Cambridge, UK
[6]MRC Cognition and Brain Sciences Unit, 15 Chaucer Road, Cambridge CB2 7EF, UK
Full list of author information is available at the end of the article

Background

Autism Spectrum Conditions (ASC) are characterised by impairments in social communication and social interaction, alongside restricted, repetitive patterns of behaviour and unusually narrow interests, and difficulty adjusting to unexpected change [1]. Research indicates that individuals with ASC often show sensory and perceptual atypicalities, including both hyper- and hypo-sensory sensitivity [2], reduced perception of coherent motion, superior processing of embedded figures and, in some instances, reduced susceptibility to visual illusions [3]. Atypicalities in the perception of social stimuli include difficulties in the processing of facial identity [4] and eye gaze [5], although recent work has found evidence of typical response patterns in ASC in other areas of social perception [6, 7].

Pellicano and Burr [8] have argued that perceptual atypicalities found in ASC might be explained within a Bayesian decision framework. According to the Bayesian decision models of perception, our perceptual system generates the most probable interpretation of the environment by combining sensory information with prior expectations. Pellicano and Burr propose that the priors of individuals with ASC might be attenuated ('hypo-priors') such that previous experience will have less influence on perception. In this sense, they suggest that individuals with ASC can be considered as perceiving the world more 'accurately' than neurotypical controls (although see [9] for an alternative interpretation wherein 'hypo-priors' could lead to less accurate perception) and that attenuated priors are consistent with evidence of superior visual perception in ASC [10–12]. In a similar approach, Lawson et al. [13] explain perceptual atypicalities in ASC within the neural instantiation of Bayesian inference—predictive coding [14]— (see also Friston et al., [15]), and suggest that perceptual atypicalities in ASC can be explained as aberrant encoding of precision, i.e. an imbalance between sensory evidence and prior beliefs, with greater weight being applied to sensory evidence.

If priors are atypical in ASC, this should manifest in differences in perceptual phenomena that emerge as a consequence of previous visual experience. Perceptual adaptation is a clear form of experience-dependent plasticity, which, within a Bayesian framework, is driven by a mismatch between sensory experience and prior expectations leading to a change in perception [16]. Consistent with the attenuated priors theory of perception in ASC, perceptual aftereffects for both facial identity and eye gaze have been shown to be reduced in children and adolescents with ASC [17, 18]. However, more recent work found no evidence of reduced facial aftereffects in adults with ASC [19–21]. At a neural level, repetition of a stimulus leads to habituation (a reduction in neural activity), and a study by Kleinhans et al. [22] found that individuals with ASC showed attenuated habituation of the amygdala to repeated presentations of faces.

Visual illusions have also been cited as an example of how priors are used to formulate the most likely interpretation of noisy or ambiguous sensory input [23]). In accordance with the attenuated priors theory, individuals with ASC show reduced susceptibility to visual illusions (e.g. Happé [24]), although the reliability of this effect has been challenged [3]. An important tenet of Bayesian decision theory is that increased uncertainty about incoming sensory information will lead to an increased influence of prior expectations on perception. Mareschal et al. [25] showed that when noise is added to the eyes of a face (thus increasing uncertainty about gaze direction), gaze is more likely to be perceived as direct (and see also [26]). This suggests that humans have a prior expectation that eye gaze is directed towards them.

The aim of this study was to test the attenuated priors theory of perception in ASC in a visual social perception task by determining: (1) whether the influence of a prior on gaze perception is reduced in individuals with a high number of autistic traits, relative to those with a low number of autistic traits, within a neurotypical sample (experiment 1) and (2) whether individuals with a formal diagnosis of ASC show evidence of reduced influence of gaze priors relative to age and IQ-matched controls (experiment 2). One proposal is that ASC is an extreme end of a normal distribution [27, 28] that extends into the neurotypical population (and see also Ruzich et al. [29] for a systematic review of autistic traits in the non-clinical population). Moreover, individual differences in autistic traits have been shown to predict performance in neurotypical and clinical populations on a number of tasks that are impaired in ASC, including reading others' mental states [30], face recognition [31], and gaze processing [32]. Recent work has also shown that repetition suppression to faces and non-faces in occipitotemporal cortex is diminished as a function of increasing autistic traits in a neurotypical population [33]. Thus, investigating the effect of autistic traits in neurotypical participants provides a complementary approach to the study of individuals with a clinical diagnosis of ASC.

Following Mareschal et al. [25], we predicted that the neurotypical groups would show evidence of a prior for direct gaze. However, if this effect is diminished in participants with greater numbers of autistic traits, and also significantly weaker in the ASC group relative to controls, this would provide support for the attenuated priors theory of perception in ASC. In a modification to the original paradigm, we calibrated the noise contrast for each participant based on their performance on a baseline gaze discrimination task. This enabled us to equate the effectiveness of the noise across participants; thus, if gaze priors are similar for the control and ASC group, then the absence of a difference in gaze priors is unlikely to be explained by differences in sensory noise. To our knowledge, this study represents the first direct test of the theory of attenuated priors in ASC in high-level social perception.

Experiment 1

Methods

Participants

Thirty-four participants (18 female) completed the experiment. All were right-handed and had normal or corrected to normal vision. Participants completed the Autism Spectrum Quotient (AQ), a 50-item validated measure of autistic traits that is suitable for use in neurotypical and clinical populations [27], and the Social Responsiveness Scale (SRS) (SRS-second edition), a quantitative measure for identifying ASC symptoms in neurotypical and clinical adult populations [34]. Participants were assigned to either a low or high AQ group using a median split of total AQ score (median = 13.5) (see Table 1 for participant information for each group). Previous work found that 79 % of individuals with high-functioning autism/Asperger syndrome scored above 32 on the AQ [27]; however, the AQ is not a diagnostic measure [27] and no participants had a clinical diagnosis of an ASC. Similarly, a total raw score above 67 on the SRS is associated with 'deficiencies in reciprocal social interaction,' but SRS scores alone are not diagnostic of an ASC. The study was approved by the Cambridge Psychology Research Ethics Committee (CPREC.2013.57). All volunteers were naive to the aims and objectives of the experiment, provided written informed consent and were paid for participating.

Stimuli

Stimulus generation, stimulus presentation and response recording were controlled by MATLAB (Mathworks Ltd) and PsychToolbox run on a Dell Optiplex 745 computer. Stimuli were viewed at a distance of 57 cm and displayed on a calibrated Dell P791 CRT monitor (1024 × 768, 75 Hz) driven by the computer's built-in ATI Radeon X1300 Pro graphics card. Grayscale synthetic neutral faces, subtending, on average, 15.1° × 11.2° visual angle, were created using Daz software (http://www.daz3d.com/). The deviation of each eye was independently controlled with MATLAB procedures, giving precision down to the nearest pixel for horizontal eye rotations. Eight grayscale faces (four female) were used in the mixed gaze discrimination task. Fractal noise (1/f amplitude spectrum) was added to the eyes in noise conditions, and the contrast between pupil and sclera varied according to performance on the baseline gaze discrimination task (see below).

Procedure

Baseline noise threshold To equate performance across participants, noise was added to the eyes of computer-generated faces and participants were asked to judge whether the gaze in a forward facing head (15°) was to their left or to their right. A Psi Bayesian adaptive procedure was employed which estimates the choice of the next trial stimulus level based on the responses to all the

Table 1 Demographics for participants in experiment 1 and experiment 2

	Experiment 1			Experiment 2		
	Low AQ	High AQ	Comparison	Control	ASC	Comparison
N	17	17		11	11	
Sex (n male to n female)	8:9	8:9		9:2	9:2	
Age (years)						
Mean (SD)	25.19 (4.72)	29.65 (8.82)	$p = .07$	32.27 (7.17)	32 (9.23)	$p = .94$
Range	19–36	21–40		22–44	18–45	
AQ						
Mean (SD)	7.75 (2.57)	23.24 (4.8)	$p < .001$	12.17 (4.73)	40.73 (5.68)	$p < .001$
Range	2–11	16–30		4–19	30–48	
SRS						
Mean (SD)	25.5 (12.37)	57.35 (21.8)	$p < .001$	36.2 (25.59)	109 (23.43)	$p < .001$
Range	8–50	21–105		11–81	60–133	
Full-scale IQ						
Mean (SD)	N/A	N/A		127.18 (10)	126.45 (13.62)	$p = .89$
Range	N/A	N/A		113–141	99–143	

SRS scores represent raw total score
N/A not available

previous trials. The procedure optimises the stimulus placement, while being more robust to changes in slope, and therefore is well-suited to test clinical populations. It converges at the end of 30 trials on the pupil/sclera contrast level leading to 80.3 % correct discrimination [35]. Participants were given instructions on the task and then completed four runs of 30 trials back to back. The median noise threshold from the four runs was used in the mixed gaze discrimination task.

Mixed gaze discrimination

Observers discriminated the direction of gaze between two same identity faces in a two-interval forced-choice task (Fig. 1). One was the 'test' face with a fixed gaze deviation (9° left or 9° right) and the other was a 'comparator' face with an offset (−20°, −10°, −5°, −2°, 2°, 5°, 10°, 20°) added to the fixed test deviation, and the observer's task was to indicate whether the direction of gaze of the face in the second interval was averted to the left or to the right compared to the direction of gaze of the face in the first interval. Noise was added to the eyes of one of the two faces at the noise contrast determined in the baseline noise threshold task. The noisy face occurred with equal frequency in the two intervals, and noise was added either to the 'test' or 'comparator' with equal occurrence. Each offset level was sampled 12 times in a run, and a logistic function was fit to the data to obtain an estimate of the gaze offset producing 50 % right responses ('bias'). After a short practice (15 trials from the first run), two runs were performed back-to-back with a short break in between. The order of test deviations (−9 vs. 9) was counterbalanced within AQ groups.

Results

Following Mareschal et al. [25], linear fits were made through bias scores at the two test deviations (−9° and 9°). The direct gaze bias identified by Mareschal et al. [25] is characterised by a significant difference in the slopes of the fits, depending on whether noise was added to the test or to the comparator, with more positive slopes for the comparator noise condition and more negative slopes for the test noise condition. To test for this effect and potential effects of autistic traits, slopes were entered into a 2 × 2 ANCOVA with noise condition (test, comparator) as a within-participants factor and AQ group (high AQ, Low AQ) as a between-participants factor. Threshold (individual thresholds from the baseline noise threshold task) was included as a covariate to examine whether the relationship between slope and threshold differs across noise conditions.

The ANCOVA revealed a significant main effect of noise condition ($F(1, 31) = 11.27$, $p = .002$, $\eta_p^2 = .27$), but no effect of AQ group ($F(1, 31) = 2.23$, $p = .15$) and, crucially, no significant interaction between noise condition and AQ group ($F(1, 31) < 1$, $p = .89$) (Fig. 2a, b). These results indicate that slopes in the comparator noise condition are significantly more positive than in the test noise condition, consistent with a bias towards perceiving uncertain gaze directions as direct (see also Fig. 2c, d for a summary of individual participants' slopes). However, there was no evidence that the magnitude of this effect is modulated by autistic traits. The ANCOVA also revealed an effect of threshold ($F(1, 31) = 4.58$, $p = .04$, $\eta_p^2 = .13$) and a significant interaction between threshold and noise condition ($F(1, 30) = 7.44$, $p = .01$, $\eta_p^2 = .14$). To further explore this finding, separate Person's correlations were used to examine the relationship between threshold and slope in each noise condition. There was a significant negative relationship between slope and threshold in the comparator noise condition $r = -.47$, $p = .005$ (as threshold decreases, comparator noise slope becomes more positive), and a trend towards a positive relationship in the test noise condition $r = .31$, $p = .07$ (as threshold decreases, test noise slopes becomes more negative). These results indicate that the strength of the direct gaze bias (as signified by increasingly positive comparator noise slopes or increasingly negative test noise slopes) increases as stimulus noise increases, consistent with a Bayesian decision framework. Importantly, the average gaze discrimination thresholds did not differ between the AQ groups (low AQ = .202, high AQ = .201) $t(32) < 1$, $p = .99$) indicating that effective noise is well-matched across groups.

As the mean age of the high AQ group was marginally greater than the low AQ group, we performed an additional ANCOVA including age as a covariate of no interest. Again, this revealed a significant main effect of noise condition ($F(1, 30) = 4.26$, $p = .049$, $\eta_p^2 = .13$), no effect of AQ group ($F(1, 30) = 1.35$, $p = .26$) and no significant interaction between noise condition and AQ group ($F(1, 30) < 1$, $p = .98$).

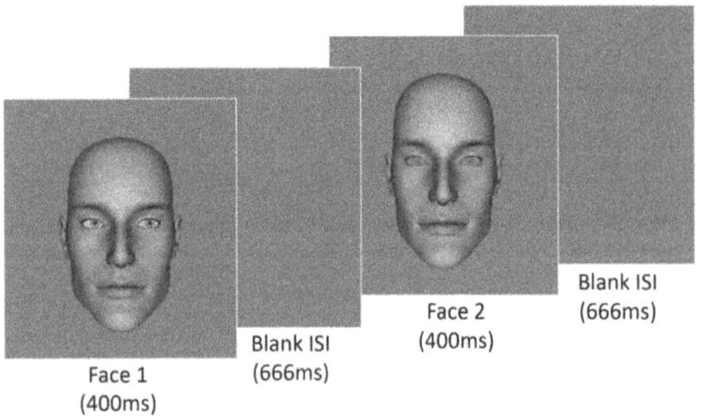

Fig. 1 Experimental procedure showing a sample trial (with noise added to the second face) used in experiments 1 and 2. The same identity face was presented twice, and participants were required to indicate the direction of gaze in the second interval relative to the first

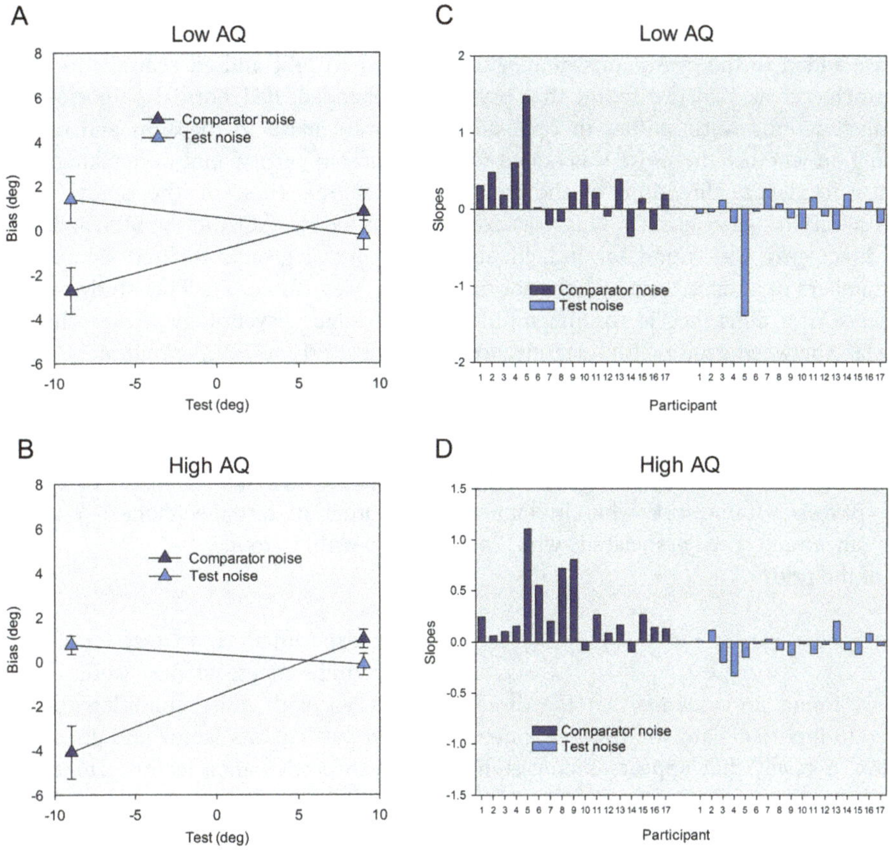

Fig. 2 Experiment 1. Average bias scores for (**a**) the low AQ group and (**b**) the high AQ group when the test contained noise (*filled diamonds*) and when the comparator contained noise (*crossed diamonds*) at each test deviations −9° and 9°. Individual slopes of the biases for all participants in the (**c**) low AQ group and (**d**) the high AQ group when the test contained noise (*filled bars*) and when the comparator contained noise (*crossed bars*)

Inspection of Fig. 2c reveals that one participant (P5) in the low AQ group showed a particularly large bias. To investigate whether the results for this individual have a disproportionate effect on the overall results of the ANCOVA, this test was repeated without P5. All significant effects found in the previous analysis remained significant ($p < .05$), and again, we found no significant interaction between noise condition and AQ group ($F(1, 30) = 2.35$, $p = .14$). Finally, Pearson's correlation analysis revealed no evidence of a significant relationship between total SRS scores and slopes for each noise condition, whether or not P5 was included in the analysis ($r < .17, p > .36$).

Bayesian analysis

Statistical tests using Bayes factors (BF) were conducted to quantify the strength of the evidence for the null hypothesis (no difference between groups) versus the alternative (low AQ > high AQ). It is important to conduct Bayesian analysis as studies claiming no difference between groups typically rely on null hypothesis significance testing to imply the null hypothesis is true, without quantifying the degree to which the evidence supports the null hypothesis. As a point of reference: BF_{10} of 1–3 indicates weak/anecdotal evidence for the alternative hypothesis; BF_{10} of 3–10 corresponds to positive/substantial support for the alternative hypothesis and BF_{10} >10 indicates positive/strong evidence for the alternative hypothesis [36, 37]. Using JASP (https://jasp-stats.org) [38], a Bayesian independent *t* tests was conducted, with default prior scales for each experiment, comparing difference scores (noise > comparator) between groups. The results revealed 'substantial' evidence in favour of the null hypothesis ($BF_{10} = 3.3$).

Discussion

Previous research suggests that humans have a prior expectation that gaze is directed towards them [25]. The purpose of this experiment was to test whether the strength of this effect is influenced by individual variation in autistic traits in a neurotypical sample. Participants completed a short baseline noise threshold task to determine the contrast level (in the context of fractal noise) required to discriminate the left from the right gaze at 80.3 % correct performance levels. In a subsequent mixed discrimination task, they had to compare the gaze direction of a face with noise added to the eye region (tailored to their contrast threshold) with that of a face with no noise added to the eyes. Consistent with the results of Mareschal et al. [25], we found that psychometric response functions were shifted in opposite directions depending on whether the noise was added to the test face (with a fixed gaze direction) or the comparator face (with a varying gaze offset). This bias towards perceiving direct gaze was found for individuals with high or low numbers of autistic traits. Furthermore, there was no evidence of a difference in the magnitude of the direct gaze bias between groups. Importantly, we found no difference in the overall threshold across groups indicating that these results cannot be explained in terms of differences in sensitivity to noise. Moreover, direct gaze bias was negatively correlated with threshold, which supports a Bayesian framework wherein higher noise (i.e. higher uncertainty) is associated with increased influence of the prior.

Experiment 2

Background

In experiment 1, we found no evidence that the direct gaze prior is related to increasing autistic traits in a neurotypical population, a result that appears inconsistent with the attenuated priors theory of perception in ASC. However, it is possible that attenuated priors are only a characteristic of individuals with clinical diagnosis of an ASC or that any attenuation of priors in neurotypical individuals is too small or inconsistent to be detected with our paradigm. To address this potential limitation, in experiment 2, we used the same paradigm with a group of individuals with a diagnosis of high-functioning autism (ASC) and a group of neurotypical controls matched on IQ, age and sex. If ASC is associated with attenuated priors, then the ASC group should show a smaller bias towards perceiving gaze as direct relative to controls.

Methods

Participants

For the neurotypical control group, 11 participants (2 females, mean age 32.27) were recruited from the MRC CBU volunteer panel. All were right-handed and had an AQ <20 (see Table 1). The ASC group consisted of 11 volunteers (2 females, mean age 32) recruited via the Cambridge Autism Research Centre. All had written confirmation of an independent diagnosis of an ASC (high-functioning autism or Asperger syndrome) by a qualified clinician using DSM-IV criteria [39]. In addition, six had a confirmed diagnosis using the Adult Asperger Assessment (AAA) [40] and two using the Autism Diagnostic Observation Schedule (ADOS) [41]. Individuals with any other current psychiatric diagnosis (other than ASC in the ASC group) were excluded from the study. All participants completed the Wechsler Abbreviated Scale of Intelligence – second edition (WASI-II) [42] and all scored >99. All participants were right-handed, had normal or corrected to normal vision and were naive to the aims and objectives of the experiment. No participants were taking psychotropic medication at the time of the study. All participants also completed the AQ and the SRS, and as expected, the ASC and control groups differed significantly on both measures (see Table 1). The study was approved by the Cambridge Psychology Research Ethics Committee (CPREC.2013.57). All volunteers provided written informed consent and were paid for participating.

Procedure

The procedure was identical to that of experiment 1. The order of test deviations (−9 vs. 9) was counterbalanced within groups.

Results

As in experiment 1, to test for a direct gaze bias and group differences, slopes were entered into a 2×2 ANCOVA with noise condition (test, comparator) as a within-participants factor and group (ASC, control) as a between-participants factor. Threshold (baseline noise threshold) was included as a covariate. The results revealed a main effect of noise condition ($F(1, 19) = 20.26$, $p < .001$, $\eta_p^2 = .27$), but no effect of group ($F(1, 19) < 1$, $p = .52$) and crucially, no interaction between noise condition and group ($F(1, 19) = 1.768$, $p = .20$) (Fig. 3a, b) (see also Fig. 3c, d for a summary of individual participants' slopes). The main effect of threshold was not significant ($F(1, 19) < 1$, $p = .38$), but as in experiment 1, there was a significant interaction between threshold and noise condition ($F(1, 19) = 11.50$, $p = .003$, $\eta_p^2 = .38$). Again, the relationship between slope and threshold was negative in the comparator noise condition ($r = -.54$, $p = .009$) and positive in the test noise condition ($r = .50$, $p = .018$). Thresholds did not differ significantly between groups (ASC = .25, control = .23) ($t(20) < 1$, $p = .37$).

Finally, a Pearson's correlation analysis revealed no evidence of a significant relationship between total SRS score and slopes in the comparator or test noise condition ($r < .16$, $p > .48$). In summary, the results of experiment 2 indicate that participants show a bias towards perceiving direct gaze in conditions of uncertainty. However, we found no evidence of any difference in this bias between neurotypical controls and individuals with ASC.

Bayesian analysis

A Bayesian independent t tests comparing difference scores (noise > comparator) between groups revealed substantial evidence in favour of the null hypothesis ($BF_{10} = 3.8$) (i.e. no difference between groups).

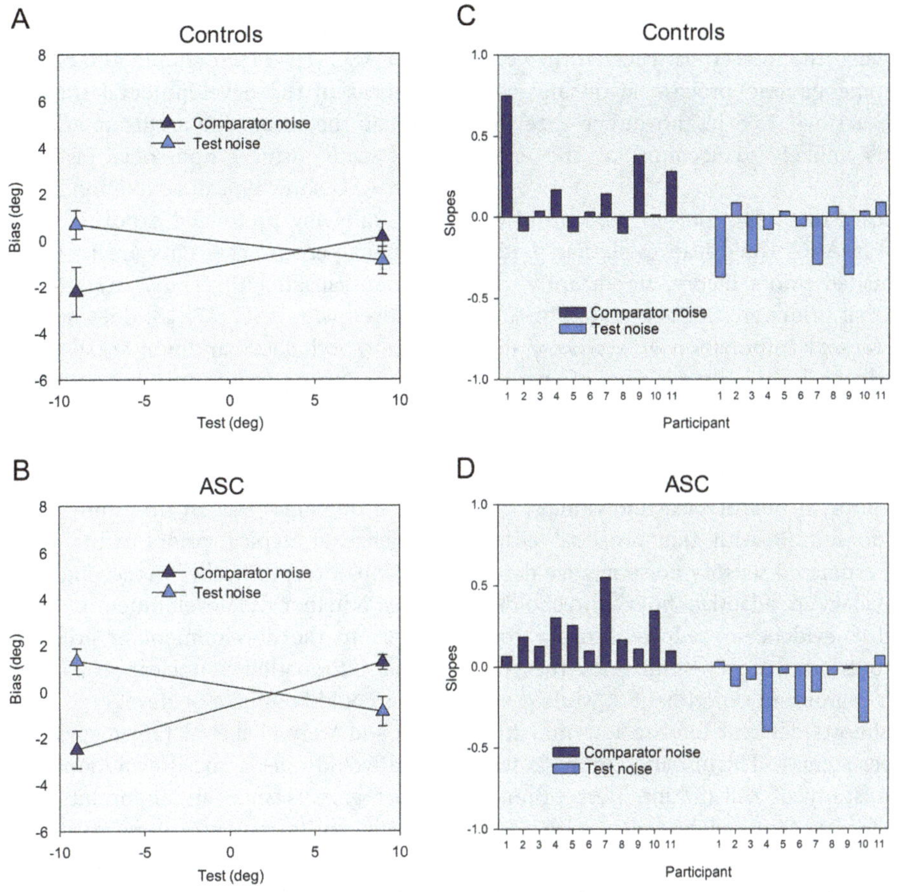

Fig. 3 Experiment 2. Average bias scores data for (**a**) the control group and (**b**) the ASC group when the test contained noise (*filled diamonds*) and when the comparator contained noise (*crossed diamonds*) at each test deviations −9° and 9°. Individual slopes of the biases for all participants in the (**c**) control group and (**d**) the ASC group when the test contained noise (*filled bars*) and when the comparator contained noise (*crossed bars*)

General discussion

In two separate experiments, we used a gaze discrimination paradigm to investigate whether priors for direct gaze are diminished in neurotypical individuals with high numbers of autistic traits and in individuals with a clinical diagnosis of high-functioning ASC. In experiment 1, neurotypical individuals showed evidence of a bias towards perceiving gaze as direct under conditions of uncertainty (viewing eyes through noise), consistent with a prior for direct gaze [25]. However, we found no evidence that the strength of the direct gaze bias is reduced in individuals with high numbers of autistic traits. Experiment 2 compared the strength of the direct gaze bias between individuals with ASC and matched neurotypical controls. Both control and ASC groups showed evidence of a direct gaze bias, and the magnitude of this effect did not differ between groups. To our knowledge, this is the first study to empirically test the theory of attenuated priors in ASC [8] in high-level social perceptual processing. Our results support the proposal that humans have a bias towards perceiving gaze as direct [25, 26] but suggest that priors for gaze direction are not diminished in adults with high-functioning ASC.

In both experiments, we found an interaction between threshold and noise condition, reflecting an increase in the magnitude of the direct gaze bias with an increase in stimulus noise. This result accords with a Bayesian framework where increased uncertainty is associated with increased influence of the prior. Furthermore, there was no evidence that sensitivity to noise differed between groups, indicating that an equivalent influence of priors on perception in ASC is unlikely to result from a combination of hypo-priors and increased sensory uncertainty.

One alternative explanation for the findings of this experiment, and previous studies on the direct gaze bias, is that the perceptual shift towards direct gaze reflects a generalised tendency to perceive objects as being centred (in this case, centring the iris in the sclera) rather than a specific prior towards direct gaze. In a previous study, Mareschal et al. [26] addressed this by performing a comparable discrimination task using a grey circle placed within a larger white circle. In contrast with the gaze results, there was only a weak and non-significant bias towards viewing the object as centred ($p > 0.3$). Thus, although some generic process favouring symmetry might have a small role in the direct gaze bias found here, this is unlikely to account for the entire effect.

Brock [43] proposed that a 'bottom-up' account of enhanced perception in ASC would lead to similar predictions as the attenuated priors theory. Importantly, this account proposes that priors are not attenuated in ASC. Rather, incoming sensory information is less noisy than in neurotypical individuals (i.e. the variance of the sensory observation is narrower) [43]. With less uncertainty about the noisy sensory observation, the prior has less influence on perception even though its variance is equivalent to the prior in neurotypical individuals. Our current findings do not fit with this proposal either. Moreover, we also estimated sensory noise in gaze detection judgements using an adaptive noise thresholding task. This revealed no evidence of reduced sensory noise in ASC as thresholds were highly similar for the ASC and matched control group in experiment 2, while group thresholds were almost identical for the low and high AQ groups in experiment 1. This finding contrasts with those of a recent study of self-motion perception in ASC [44] that found that adolescents with ASC showed increased sensitivity to visual noise. One possible explanation for this apparent difference is that any increased sensitivity to visual noise in ASC may be less apparent in the context of higher-level stimuli, such as faces, compared to lower-level stimuli such as moving dots.

Zaidel et al. [44] also found evidence for reduced use of priors in adolescents with ASC, a result that accords with the attenuated priors theory of perception in ASC. However, their study specifically investigated the use of recently acquired priors, suggesting that evidence of a difference in the use of prior information between the two studies may be a consequence of differences in the developmental acquisition of priors and/or atypicalities in the rapid acquisition of priors [45]. Similarly, individuals with ASC might possess priors that exert a similar influence to those of neurotypical individuals (as found here) but that develop differently or are applied with less flexibility. One proposal is that autistic atypicalities are a consequence of overly constrained priors, leading to 'overfitted' and non-generalizable predictions [46, 47] (and see also Qian and Lipkin's [48] learning theory style of ASC). Thus, the developmental trajectory of the direct gaze prior could differ for neurotypical individuals and those with ASC (e.g. steeper acquisition in neurotypical individuals) but eventually converge in adulthood. Differences in the development of priors might also explain why diminished adaptation aftereffects for faces in children with ASC [17, 18] are not found in adults with ASC [19–21]. It should also be noted that while differences in the developmental trajectory of priors may explain the absence of an group effect in our study, a recent study, using a non-social task, found that children with ASC show typical adaptation of perceptual causality (i.e. following prolonged exposure to causal events, subsequent perceptual events are more likely to be judged as non-causal) [49]. Thus, any attenuation of priors in children with ASC [17, 18] does not appear to be generalise to both social and non-social domains.

Given the significant heterogeneity of symptoms across individuals with ASC, it is also possible that attenuated priors are only found in a subset of individuals within the autistic spectrum or in specific behavioural domains [50]. In this study, we failed to find any evidence of atypical priors in the domain of social perception, or specifically, perceiving the direction of eye gaze. Whether the development of a prior for direct gaze differs to the development of priors for other types of social information is unclear. For example, a direct gaze prior could be innate or develop in infancy. Baron-Cohen [51] and Mareschal et al. [25] suggest a bias towards direct gaze would offer a social/evolutionary advantage because direct gaze is such an important social cue that often signals an imminent interaction (e.g. attack or prosocial approach). Assuming that gaze is direct when one is unsure would represent a safer strategy than trying to calculate the precise gaze direction [52, 53]. Future work will be needed to determine whether ASC is associated with specific differences in the acquisition and use of newly learned priors and to what extent any differences generalise across both social and non-social domains.

It should be noted that participants with ASC in this study were all high-functioning, with both the ASC and control groups having a high average IQ. It is not known if these findings would generalise to individuals with lower-functioning ASC. In addition, 'standard' assessments were not available for all participants included in experiment 2. Despite these caveats, it is important to note that the behavioural atypicalities reported by individuals in our sample (social or otherwise) were sufficient to cause problems in everyday life and lead to significant distress; otherwise, they would not have a clinical diagnosis. This indicates that the presence of typical priors (in at least one domain) does not necessarily signify typical social functioning. Indeed, we found no evidence that the strength of the direct gaze bias is related to the number of self-reported autistic traits on the SRS, a measure of the extent of autistic social impairment [34]. Moreover, despite evidence indicating atypical social perception in ASC, there are a number of studies reporting typical social perception in ASC, including orientating towards facial stimuli and interpreting other people's actions perception [6, 7]. An alternative reason for the lack of significant group differences in experiment 2 is due to the small sample size used. However, Bayesian analyses revealed substantial evidence in favour of the null hypothesis for experiment 2. Thus, even with a smaller sample size in experiment 2, evidence indicates that both studies show substantial evidence in favour of the null hypothesis, i.e. no difference between groups. Taken together, both experiments indicate that the influence of priors on perception does not differ between groups on the basis of autistic traits or on a clinical diagnosis of high-functioning ASC. However, future studies would benefit not only from larger sample sizes but also by including more representative (i.e. lower IQ) and better characterised samples of the autistic population.

Finally, atypical gaze processing is considered a core symptom of ASC, and numerous studies report atypicalities in gaze processing in ASC, such as reduced attention to the eyes [54], differences in following another's gaze [55] and difficulty in inferring mental states from the eyes [30]. Although any task involving eye gaze contains a strong 'social' component, it should be emphasised that the thresholding and gaze priors tasks required participants to make a perceptual discrimination of gaze direction ('is the second face looking to the left or the right of the first?'), rather than asking them to make an explicit social judgement (e.g. an evaluation of how the gaze relates to them, or inferring the mental states of the face). Thus, intact performance on this task does not imply typical performance on tasks that relate to understanding the communicative intent and emotional significance signalled by direct gaze. Moreover, our results can only speak to the role of perceptual priors in the domain of visual social perception, and further studies will be needed to test the hypo-priors theory using less 'social' tasks. It is important to note, however, that Pellicano and Burr [8] make no distinction in the use of perceptual priors between social and non-social stimuli or between different sensory modalities.

Conclusions

In summary, we found that participants show a bias towards perceiving gaze as direct under conditions of uncertainty, replicating findings by Mareschal et al. [25]. Importantly, however, we found no evidence that the strength of this bias is reduced in neurotypical individuals with high numbers of autistic traits or in individuals with a diagnosis of ASC. These results challenge the attenuated priors theory of ASC [8] and suggest no apparent atypicalities in the use of prior information in gaze perception in adults with high-functioning ASC.

Abbreviations

AAA: Adult Asperger Assessment; ADOS: Autism Diagnostic Observation Schedule; AQ: Autism Spectrum Quotient; ASC: Autism Spectrum Conditions; SRS: Social Responsiveness Scale; WASI-II: Wechsler Abbreviated Scale of Intelligence – second edition.

Competing interests

The authors declare that they have no competing interests.

Authors' contributions

PP, IM, AC, EvdH, SBC and ME helped to conceive and design the study. PP was responsible for the participant recruitment, data collection and statistical analysis. ME performed the ADOS assessments. PP, IM and ME contributed to the interpretation of the results. PP, IM, EvdH, CC, SBC and ME drafted the manuscript. SBC provided the access to the ASC sample. All authors read and approved the final manuscript with the exception of AC (deceased).

Acknowledgements

We are grateful to Thomas Powell for his help with the data collection and ADOS assessments in the early stages of this project. This research was supported by the UK Medical Research Council under project code MC-A060-5PQ50 (Andrew J. Calder). IM was supported by a Leverhulme Trust Project Grant. CC was supported by an Australian Research Council Future Fellowship. SBC was supported by the MRC, the Wellcome Trust and the Autism Research Trust during the period of this work. The research was also supported by the National Institute for Health Research (NIHR) Collaboration for Leadership in Applied Health Research and Care East of England at Cambridgeshire and Peterborough NHS Foundation Trust. The views expressed are those of the author(s) and not necessarily those of the NHS, the NIHR or the Department of Health. This paper is dedicated to the memory of Andy Calder (1965–2013).

Author details

[1]Medical Research Council, Cognition and Brain Sciences Unit, Cambridge, UK. [2]School of Biological and Chemical Sciences, Psychology Department, Queen Mary University of London, London, UK. [3]Autism Research Centre, Department of Psychiatry, University of Cambridge, Cambridge, UK. [4]School of Psychology, Cardiff University, Cardiff, UK. [5]School of Psychology, UNSW Australia, Sydney, NSW, Australia. [6]MRC Cognition and Brain Sciences Unit, 15 Chaucer Road, Cambridge CB2 7EF, UK.

References

1. American Psychiatric Association. Diagnostic and statistical manual of mental disorders. 5th ed. Arlington: American Psychiatric Publishing; 2013. doi:10.1176/appi.books.9780890425596.
2. Marco EJ, Hinkley LB, Hill SS, Nagarajan SS. Sensory processing in autism: a review of neurophysiologic findings. Pediatr Res. 2011;69(5 Pt 2):48R–54R. doi:10.1203/PDR.0b013e3182130c54.
3. Simmons DR, Robertson AE, McKay LS, Toal E, McAleer P, Pollick FE. Vision in autism spectrum disorders. Vis Res. 2009;49(22):2705–39. doi:10.1016/j.visres.2009.08.005.
4. Weigelt S, Koldewyn K, Kanwisher N. Face identity recognition in autism spectrum disorders: a review of behavioral studies. Neurosci Biobehav Rev. 2012;36(3):1060–84. doi:10.1007/s11065-010-9138-6.
5. Leekam S, BaronCohen S, Perrett D, Milders M, Brown S. Eye-direction detection: A dissociation between geometric and joint attention skills in autism. Brit J Dev Psychol. 1997;15:77–95. doi:10.1111/j.2044-835X.1997.tb00726.x.
6. Shah P, Gaule A, Bird G, Cook R. Robust orienting to protofacial stimuli in autism. Curr Biol. 2013;23(24):R1087–8. doi:10.1016/j.cub.2013.10.034.
7. Cusack JP, Williams JH, Neri P. Action perception is intact in autism spectrum disorder. J Neurosci. 2015;35(5):1849–57. doi:10.1523/JNEUROSCI.4133-13.2015.
8. Pellicano E, Burr D. When the world becomes 'too real': a Bayesian explanation of autistic perception. Trends Cogn Sci. 2012;16(10):504–10. doi:10.1016/j.tics.2012.08.009.
9. Teufel C, Subramaniam N, Fletcher PC. The role of priors in Bayesian models of perception. Front Comput Neurosci. 2013;7:25. doi:10.3389/fncom.2013.00025.

10. Jolliffe T, Baron-Cohen S. Are people with autism and Asperger syndrome faster than normal on the Embedded Figures Test? J Child Psychol Psychiatry. 1997;38(5):527–34.
11. Plaisted K, O'Riordan M, Baron-Cohen S. Enhanced visual search for a conjunctive target in autism: a research note. J Child Psychol Psychiatry. 1998;39(5):777–83.
12. Plaisted K, O'Riordan M, Baron-Cohen S. Enhanced discrimination of novel, highly similar stimuli by adults with autism during a perceptual learning task. J Child Psychol Psychiatry. 1998;39(5):765–75.
13. Lawson RP, Rees G, Friston KJ. An aberrant precision account of autism. Front Hum Neurosci. 2014;8:302. doi:10.3389/fnhum.2014.00302.
14. Friston K. A theory of cortical responses. Philos Trans R Soc Lond. 2005; 360(1456):815–36. doi:10.1098/rstb.2005.1622.
15. Friston KJ, Lawson R, Frith CD. On hyperpriors and hypopriors: comment on Pellicano and Burr. Trends Cogn Sci. 2013;17(1):1. doi:10.1016/j.tics.2012.11.003.
16. Kleinschmidt DF, Jaeger TF. Robust speech perception: recognize the familiar, generalize to the similar, and adapt to the novel. Psychol Rev. 2015; 122(2):148–203. doi:10.1037/a0038695.
17. Pellicano E, Jeffery L, Burr D, Rhodes G. Abnormal adaptive face-coding mechanisms in children with autism spectrum disorder. Curr Biol. 2007; 17(17):1508–12. doi:10.1016/j.cub.2007.07.065.
18. Pellicano E, Rhodes G, Calder AJ. Reduced gaze aftereffects are related to difficulties categorising gaze direction in children with autism. Neuropsychologia. 2013;51(8):1504–9. doi:10.1016/j.neuropsychologia.2013.03.021.
19. Cook R, Brewer R, Shah P, Bird G. Intact facial adaptation in autistic adults. Autism Res. 2014;7(4):481–90. doi:10.1002/aur.1381.
20. Walsh JA, Maurer D, Vida MD, Rhodes G, Jeffery L, Rutherford MD. Norm-based coding of facial identity in adults with autism spectrum disorder. Vis Res. 2015;108:33–40. doi:10.1016/j.visres.2014.11.018.
21. Walsh JA, Vida MD, Morrisey MN, Rutherford MD. Adults with autism spectrum disorder show evidence of figural aftereffects with male and female faces. Vis Res. 2015;115(Pt A):104–12. doi:10.1016/j.visres.2015.08.010.
22. Kleinhans NM, Johnson LC, Richards T, Mahurin R, Greenson J, Dawson G, et al. Reduced neural habituation in the amygdala and social impairments in autism spectrum disorders. Am J Psychiatry. 2009;166(4):467–75. doi:10.1176/appi.ajp.2008.07101681.
23. Geisler WS, Kersten D. Illusions, perception and Bayes. Nat Neurosci. 2002; 5(6):508–10. doi:10.1038/nn0602-508.
24. Happé FG. Studying weak central coherence at low levels: children with autism do not succumb to visual illusions. A research note. J Child Psychol Psychiatry. 1996;37(7):873–7.
25. Mareschal I, Calder AJ, Clifford CW. Humans have an expectation that gaze is directed toward them. Curr Biol. 2013;23(8):717–21. doi:10.1016/j.cub.2013.03.030.
26. Mareschal I, Otsuka Y, Clifford CW. A generalized tendency toward direct gaze with uncertainty. J Vis. 2014;14(12). doi:10.1167/14.12.27.
27. Baron-Cohen S, Wheelwright S, Skinner R, Martin J, Clubley E. The autism-spectrum quotient (AQ): evidence from Asperger syndrome/high-functioning autism, males and females, scientists and mathematicians. J Autism Dev Disord. 2001;31(1):5–17. doi:10.1023/A:1005653411471.
28. Happé F, Ronald A, Plomin R. Time to give up on a single explanation for autism. Nat Neurosci. 2006;9(10):1218–20. doi:10.1038/nn1770.
29. Ruzich E, Allison C, Smith P, Watson P, Auyeung B, Ring H, et al. Measuring autistic traits in the general population: a systematic review of the Autism-Spectrum Quotient (AQ) in a nonclinical population sample of 6,900 typical adult males and females. Mol Autism. 2015;6:2. doi:10.1186/2040-2392-6-2.
30. Baron-Cohen S, Wheelwright S, Hill J, Raste Y, Plumb I. The "Reading the Mind in the Eyes" Test revised version: a study with normal adults, and adults with Asperger syndrome or high-functioning autism. J Child Psychol Psychiatry. 2001;42(2):241–51. doi:10.1017/S0021963001006643.
31. Rhodes G, Jeffery L, Taylor L, Ewing L. Autistic traits are linked to reduced adaptive coding of face identity and selectively poorer face recognition in men but not women. Neuropsychologia. 2013;51(13):2702–8. doi:10.1016/j.neuropsychologia.2013.08.016.
32. Bayliss AP, Tipper SP. Gaze and arrow cueing of attention reveals individual differences along the autism spectrum as a function of target context. Br J Psychol. 2005;96(Pt 1):95–114. doi:10.1348/000712604X15626.
33. Ewbank MP, Rhodes G, von dem Hagen EA, Powell TE, Bright N, Stoyanova RS et al. Repetition Suppression in Ventral Visual Cortex Is Diminished as a Function of Increasing Autistic Traits. Cereb Cortex. 2014. doi:10.1093/cercor/bhu149.
34. Constantino J, Gruber C. The Social Responsiveness Scale. Los Angeles: Western Psychological Services; 2005.
35. Kontsevich LL, Tyler CW. Bayesian adaptive estimation of psychometric slope and threshold. Vis Res. 1999;39(16):2729–37. doi:10.1016/S0042-6989(98)00285-5.
36. Kass RE, Raftery AE. Bayes Factors. J Am Stat Assoc. 1995;90(430):773–95. doi: 10.1080/01621459.1995.10476572.
37. Jeffreys H. Theory of probability. Oxford: University Press; 1961.
38. Love J, Selker R, Marsman M, Jamil T, Dropmann D, Verhagen AJ, et al. JASP (Version 0.7). 2015.
39. American Psychiatric Association. Diagnostic and statistical manual of mental disorders: DSM- IV. 4th ed. Washington, DC: American Psychiatric Association; 2000. doi:10.1176/appi.books.9780890423349.
40. Baron-Cohen S, Wheelwright S, Robinson J, Woodbury-Smith M. The Adult Asperger Assessment (AAA): a diagnostic method. J Autism Dev Disord. 2005;35(6):807–19. doi:10.1007/s10803-005-0026-5.
41. Lord C, Risi S, Lambrecht L, Cook EH, Leventhal BL, DiLavore PC, et al. The Autism Diagnostic Observation Schedule-Generic: A standard measure of social and communication deficits associated with the spectrum of autism. J Autism Dev Disord. 2000;30(3):205–23. doi:10.1023/A:1005592401947.
42. Weschler D, Corporation TP. WASI -II : Wechsler abbreviated scale of intelligence – second edition. San Antonio: Psychological Corporation; 2011.
43. Brock J. Alternative Bayesian accounts of autistic perception: comment on Pellicano and Burr. Trends Cogn Sci. 2012;16(12):573–4. doi:10.1016/j.tics.2012.10.005.
44. Zaidel A, Goin-Kochel RP, Angelaki DE. Self-motion perception in autism is compromised by visual noise but integrated optimally across multiple senses. Proc Natl Acad Sci U S A. 2015;112(20):6461–6. doi:10.1073/pnas.1506582112.
45. Series P, Seitz AR. Learning what to expect (in visual perception). Front Hum Neurosci. 2013;7:668. doi:10.3389/fnhum.2013.00668.
46. Van de Cruys S, De-Wit L, Evers K, Boets B, Wagemans J. Weak priors versus overfitting of predictions in autism: Reply to Pellicano and Burr (TICS, 2012). I-Perception. 2013;4(2):95–7. doi:10.1068/I0580ic.
47. Van de Cruys S, Evers K, Van der Hallen R, Van Eylen L, Boets B, de-Wit L, et al. Precise minds in uncertain worlds: predictive coding in autism. Psychol Rev. 2014;121(4):649–75. doi:10.1037/a0037665.
48. Qian N, Lipkin RM. A learning-style theory for understanding autistic behaviors. Front Hum Neurosci. 2011;5:77. doi:10.3389/fnhum.2011.00077.
49. Karaminis T, Turi M, Neil L, Badcock NA, Burr D, Pellicano E. Atypicalities in perceptual adaptation in autism do not extend to perceptual causality. PLoS One. 2015;10(3):e0120439. doi:10.1371/journal.pone.0120439.
50. Brock J. Combining the old and the new: Bayesian and predictive coding accounts of autistic cognition. The Psychologist. 2014;27:750–3.
51. Baron-Cohen S. Mindblindness: An essay on autism and theory of mind. Cambridge: MIT Press; 1995.
52. Clifford CW, Mareschal I, Otsuka Y, Watson TL. A Bayesian approach to person perception. Conscious Cogn. 2015. doi:10.1016/j.concog.2015.03.015.
53. Langton SR, Honeyman H, Tessler E. The influence of head contour and nose angle on the perception of eye-gaze direction. Percept Psychophys. 2004;66(5):752–71. doi:10.3758/BF03194970.
54. Jones W, Klin A. Attention to eyes is present but in decline in 2-6-month-old infants later diagnosed with autism. Nature. 2013;504(7480):427–31. doi: 10.1038/nature12715.
55. Nation K, Penny S. Sensitivity to eye gaze in autism: is it normal? Is it automatic? Is it social? Dev Psychopathol. 2008;20(1):79–97. doi:10.1017/S0954579408000047.

2

Cytokine levels and associations with symptom severity in male and female children with autism spectrum disorder

Anne Masi[1], Edmond J. Breen[2], Gail A. Alvares[3,4], Nicholas Glozier[1], Ian B. Hickie[1], Anna Hunt[3], Jennie Hui[5,6,7], John Beilby[5,6], David Ravine[5,6], John Wray[8], Andrew J. O. Whitehouse[3,4] and Adam J. Guastella[1*]

Abstract

Background: Autism spectrum disorders (ASDs) are complex, pervasive, and heterogeneous neurodevelopmental conditions with varying trajectories, significant male bias and largely unknown etiology. However, an understanding of the biological mechanisms driving pathophysiology is evolving. Immune system aberrations, as identified through cytokine profiles, are believed to have a role in ASD. Altered cytokine levels may facilitate identification of ASD subtypes as well as provide biological markers of response to effective treatments. Research exploring the relationship between cytokine profiles and ASD symptoms is, however, in its infancy. The objective of this study was to explore relationships between cytokine levels and the severity of ASD and other clinical traits.

Methods: Multiplex assay techniques were used to measure levels of 27 cytokines in plasma samples from a cohort of 144 children diagnosed with ASD.

Results: Overall, results showed a significant negative association between platelet-derived growth factor (PDGF)-BB, and the severity of ASD symptoms. Furthermore, a significant interaction with sex suggested a different immune profile for females compared to males. ASD symptom severity was negatively associated with levels of 4 cytokines, IL-1β, IL-8, MIP-1β, and VEGF, in females, but not in males.

Conclusions: Results of the present study suggest that an altered cytokine response or profile is associated with the severity of ASD-related symptoms, with sex a potential modifier of this relationship. Further research in larger populations which recognizes the importance of sex comparisons and longitudinal assessments are now required to extend and further describe the role of the immune system in ASD.

Keywords: Autism spectrum disorder, Cytokine, Behavior, Pediatric, Severity

Background

Autism spectrum disorders (ASDs) are complex, pervasive, and heterogeneous neurodevelopmental disorders of primarily unknown etiology and pathogenesis. Recent epidemiological studies estimate prevalence to be as high as 1 in 68 [1]. Diagnosis is currently based on clinical observation of behavioral features, defined as persistent deficits in social communication and interaction, and restricted, repetitive patterns of behavior, interests or activities; severity classifications are based on required levels of support [2]. While ASD is considered a lifelong condition [3], developmental trajectories vary significantly [4] with a range of prognoses [5]. Sex is believed to have an important role in development, with significantly more males diagnosed with ASD (4:1) [6] and different characteristic phenotypes presenting for females [7]. Many genes have been proposed to converge on common pathways affecting neuronal and synaptic homeostasis [8]. Environmental factors may also play a role in etiology through, for example, the impact of maternal immune activation or antibodies on a developing brain or by impacting a susceptible physiology [9–11]. This complex etiology, manifesting as vast

* Correspondence: adam.guastella@sydney.edu.au
[1]Autism Clinic for Translational Research, Brain and Mind Centre, Central Clinical School, Sydney Medical School, University of Sydney, 100 Mallett Street, Camperdown, New South Wales 2050, Australia
Full list of author information is available at the end of the article

clinical heterogeneity, has been a catalyst for investigations aiming to characterize potential biological subtypes of ASD.

Immune system alterations related to immunogenetics, maternal immune activation, and a family history of autoimmune disorders, suggests a relationship between ASD and the immune system [12]. Accumulating evidence of alterations in central and peripheral immune system functioning supports the proposal that there is a subgroup of individuals with ASD who have some form of immune system dysregulation [11]. Previous work has highlighted significantly altered peripheral levels of primarily pro-inflammatory cytokines in ASD compared to healthy controls [13]. Levels of both pro-inflammatory and anti-inflammatory cytokines and chemokines have been associated with the severity of aberrant behavior and more impaired developmental and adaptive function [14–16]. However, numerous differences in immune function have been identified in ASD, suggesting that these aberrations may be due to reduced immune system regulation rather than a dominance of one type of inflammatory response signal [11].

Despite extensive immunological evidence suggesting immune system aberrations in ASD, further research is required to clarify the relationship between immune profiles and ASD symptoms [12]. Such investigations may further knowledge about potentially useful biomarkers for ASD and the severity of symptoms, and provide clues for potential causative relationships and factors that might characterize subgroups of ASD. The pathophysiological significance of commonly identified comorbidities in ASD, such as gastrointestinal dysfunction and sleep disorder, with respect to the identified immune system aberrations, is also unknown [17–19]. While understanding the influence of sex has been a recent research priority [20], partially because of the higher ratio of ASD diagnosis of males [21], to date, there has been limited investigation of potential sex differences in immunological profiles [22]. Sex-specific immunological aberrations have been described in a rodent model, with females exhibiting attenuation of induced behavioral and immunological alterations compared to males [23]. Therefore, there is a need to characterize the relationship between immune system dysfunction, specifically cytokine alterations, and severity of ASD symptoms, including disordered sleep and gastrointestinal dysfunction, between males and females.

The present study utilized a large, well-characterized repository of biological samples and multiplex assay techniques to investigate the relationship between cytokine levels and symptom severity of ASD. Cytokine profiles were investigated in relation to clinical traits, including variability in social functioning, sleep problems, and gastrointestinal dysfunction, along with the role of sex.

Methods

Participants

Participants (113 males, 31 females) were part of the Western Australian Autism Biological Registry (WAABR), located at the Telethon Kids Institute in Perth, Western Australia [24]. Ethics approval was granted by the Human Ethics Committee at Princess Margaret Hospital for Children in Perth, Western Australia. Informed consent was provided by the primary caregiver. Participants were recruited during the period January 2011 to March 2013 through newspaper advertisements and via flyers distributed among local service providers and clinicians. Children with a DSM-IV clinical diagnosis of autistic disorder, Asperger's syndrome, or pervasive developmental disorder—not otherwise specified—were included in the study. Diagnosis in Western Australia mandates a consensus diagnosis following a multidisciplinary assessment by a pediatrician, clinical psychologist, and speech-language pathologist [25]. The Autism Diagnostic Observation Schedule-Generic (ADOS-G) was administered to each participant [26]. The ADOS-G is a semi-structured assessment using simple activities and questions to elicit and observe the communicative, social, and stereotyped behaviors relevant to the diagnosis of ASD. Research-accredited professionals administered the ADOS-G to all participants. Each participant's ADOS-G raw scores and total score was converted to the updated ADOS-2 calibrated severity score [27–29], as this score is less influenced by child characteristics than raw totals. ADOS diagnostic classification was based on a range of severity scores, where 1 reflects minimal to no evidence of autism spectrum-related symptoms, and 10 represents a high severity of autism spectrum-related symptoms. Based on the level of autism-related symptoms and comparison scores, participants were categorized as mild/moderate or severe, as per established procedures [30]. Calibrated domain scores for social-communication and restricted and repetitive behavior were also derived [31]. A primary caregiver completed a questionnaire about family history, including details of previously diagnosed comorbidities and gastrointestinal problems (classified as present or absent), the Social Responsiveness Scale (SRS) [32], and the Children's Sleep Habits Questionnaire (CSHQ) [33]. The SRS is a 65-item questionnaire which measures social behavior, language, and repetitive behavior/restricted interests. Higher total score indicates higher severity of social impairment of ASD. The CSHQ is a 33-item questionnaire assessing the frequency of common sleep problems in children with higher scores indicating more disordered sleep. All participants followed the same schedule of assessments, with specimen collection occurring immediately following the ADOS-G assessment.

Blood sample collection procedure

Peripheral blood (non-fasting) was collected into anticoagulant treated tubes (EDTA, 4 ml vacutainer, K2E, 7.2 mg, BD). The tube was inverted immediately after collection to mix the EDTA with the blood as per standard procedure. Samples were centrifuged for 10 min at 3500 rpm at room temperature in an Eppendorf 5810R centrifuge. The harvested plasma was stored at – 80 °C, and the analysis was conducted on the day of the first thawing of samples. The samples were defrosted on ice and a 100 μl aliquot was supplied for the multiplex assays.

Cytokine analysis

Cytokine analysis was conducted using a magnetic bead-based multiplex assay system, which facilitated the detection and quantification of multiple cytokines from a single sample of plasma. A human cytokine 27-plex assay (Bio-Plex Pro Human Cytokine 27-plex #M500KCAFOY) simultaneously quantified levels of 27 cytokines (eotaxin, fibroblast growth factor (FGF) basic, granulocyte colony-stimulating factor (G-CSF), granulocyte–macrophage colony-stimulating factor (GM-CSF), interferon (IFN)-γ, interleukin (IL)-1β, IL1 receptor antagonist (IL-1ra), IL-2, IL-4, IL-5, IL-6, IL-7, IL-8, IL-9, IL-10, IL-12p70, IL-13, IL-15, IL-17, interferon gamma-induced protein (IP)-10, monocyte chemotactic protein (MCP)-1, macrophage inflammatory protein (MIP)-1α, MIP-1β, platelet-derived growth factor (PDGF)-BB, regulated on activation normal T cell expressed and secreted (RANTES), tumor necrosis factor (TNF)-α and vascular endothelial growth factor (VEGF)). All standards, reagents, and samples were prepared according to the manufacturer's instructions (Bio-Plex® Multiplex System, Bio-Plex Pro™ Human Cytokine, Chemokine and Growth Factor Assays; Bio-Rad Laboratories Pty., Ltd. Hercules, CA, USA). The plates were analyzed using a multiplexing diagnostic instrument (LUMINEX®200™; Luminex Corp.), and fluorescent data for each cytokine was extracted using the manufacturers software (xPONENT for LX200 3.1.971.0; Luminex Corp.). Blood samples for the 144 participants were analyzed blinded to participant's severity of ASD and all other characteristics including sex. Samples were spread across two plates and two runs (one plate per run). One sample was excluded from cytokine estimations due to misclassification. Standards and blanks were analyzed in duplicate and two duplicate plasma samples were analyzed on each plate to allow an assessment of assay uniformity.

Cytokine level values calculated from participant plasma samples can be lower than the associated lowest cytokine standard or blank. Participant cytokine expression values lower than the associated blanks and standards are considered a result of different matrix effects in plasma and the diluent used in blanks and standards [34] or possibly due to the fact that the actual analytes used with the standards are constructed using recombinant proteins that may differ from natively expressed analytes found in the biological samples [35]. Therefore, a background correction procedure for estimating cytokine levels was used [36, 37]. The correction procedure assumes that any non-specific binding occurring in the blank and standards are nullified by matrix effects in the test samples. Output from the formula was a corrected subject median fluorescence value for each cytokine. Fluorescence values were used as, unlike concentrations, there are no missing values, a level of detection (LOD) does not need to be specified, and low signals can be analyzed which adds more statistical power for testing differences in analyte expression levels. See Additional file 2 for further information. The best matching standard was the standard that had the observed median fluorescence value closest to the median of the subjects for that cytokine. The fluorescence value for the associated best matched standard was used to estimate the expected concentration of that standard using back calculation [38]. Several models were tested to estimate the expected concentrations for the best matched standard for each cytokine (Additional file 1: Table S1). Using correlations between expected and estimated concentration for best matched standards, and associated correlations (R^2), estimates according to a third order polynomial fit to the log-log transformation of the expected concentrations and fluorescence values yields the best fit standards compared to unweighted 4 parameter logistic (4PL) and 5PL curve fits (Additional file 2: Figure S1). Consequently, this method was used to predict the participant cytokine levels.

As different plates contained different groups of participants, a normalization procedure was developed to address any potential differences in cytokine levels between the two runs. The log2 of fluorescence values were modeled for run and cytokine interaction, taking in to account the level of each cytokine on each plate. The residuals from the model hold the differences in cytokine levels due to any explanatory variable, which was not cofounded with run differences. Additional file 1: Figure S2 illustrates the effect of the run normalization procedure.

Statistical analysis

Descriptive statistics were calculated for participant characteristics. Missing values were imputed using the multiple imputation by chained equations (MICE) method (Additional file 1: Table S2) [39, 40]. A variable clustering procedure was used to identify homogeneous clusters of variables and eliminate variables conveying similar information [41]. Multinomial logistic regression was undertaken to assess that each plate was balanced with respect to cofactors, or participant characteristics, across runs [42]. All statistical tests were done using R version 3.2.3 (2015-12-10). Type 3 ANOVA tests were done using ANOVA from the car package [43]. Interaction tests were done using test interactions routine from the phia package [44]. Wilcoxon two sample and signed-rank tests were done using the R's Wilcox test from the coin package [45]. Multiple test corrections were done via the Holm method [46]. Cytokine correlations were obtained using Spearman's rank correlation. The network visualization of the Spearman's rank correlation matrix between cytokine levels were obtained using R's graphing package qgraph version 1.3.3 [47]. qgraph is a visualization tool and a tool for applying network analysis from data for estimating network structures, where the network can be weighted (correlations) or unweighted and undirected. Here, each node represents a cytokine and each edge the correlation between the connecting nodes. For example, qgraph can draw a correlation network, not just as circular network but where strongly correlated nodes are drawn near each other [48]. Generally, correlation networks are drawn fully connected, i.e., showing all non-zero edges between nodes, and when the number of nodes is large this can often make the network hard to interpret. One solution, using model selection to estimate the best graph structure, is to remove edges, set them to zero, with weak correlations using a user specified threshold. Depending on how this is done, the centrality of the network can also be affected. However, thresholding does not consider how removal of these edges changes relationships (correlations) within the network, or how well the network explains the data. An alternative approach and a well-established method for simultaneously estimating parameters and performing model selection on a correlation network, as done here, is to employ LASSO, using the R glasso package [49]. These network models were selected using penalized maximum likelihood solution in which the likelihood is penalized for the sum of absolute parameter estimates using LASSO [50], via qgraph, which can be used to estimate a network that minimizes the Extended Bayesian Information Criterium (EBIC) [51].

Table 1 Participant clinical characteristics

	Total	Male	Female
N	144	113	31
Age (years)			
Mean	8.16	7.96	9.53
SD	4.21	4.05	4.79
Range	2.08–18.25	2.83–18	2.25–18.25
BMI (kg/m2)			
Mean	18.34	16.74	21.12
SD	4.63	2.05	7.09
Range	12.26–46.96	13.50–21.74	13.45–46.96
Head circumference (cm)			
Mean	53.86	53.67	54.20
SD	3.01	2.21	3.46
Range	46–62	49.5–59	46–61
ADOS module			
Module 1	35	28	7
Module 2	58	49	9
Module 3	42	31	11
Module 4	9	6	3
Severity (ADOS comparison score)			
Median	6	6	6
Range	1–10	1–10	1–9
Severity of symptoms			
Mild/moderate	85	68	17
Severe	59	45	14
SRS			
Mean	88.18	86.43	97.27
SD	15.71	11.09	19.11
Range	44–126	64–106	44–126
Sleep scores			
Median	12.5	53	56
Range	1–31	46–78	46–72
GI symptoms			
Absent	85	65	20
Present	59	47	11

Abbreviations: *BMI* body mass index, *ADOS* autism diagnostic observation schedule, *SRS* social responsiveness scale, *GI* gastrointestinal

Results

Samples for this analysis were collected from 144 participants, aged between 2 and 18 (mean 8.2 SD ± 4.2). Sex distribution was 78% male and 22% female. Eighty-three percent of participants identified as Caucasian. Additional demographic and clinical characteristics of participants are presented in Table 1. The variable clustering procedure resulted in the inclusion of six variables in the reduced set: age, sex, gastrointestinal symptoms, severity of ASD, sleep score, and SRS total score (Table 1). Assessment of covariate balance with respect to the two different plates or runs identified a run difference only due to sex ($p = 0.042$) (Additional file 1: Table S3).

Descriptive statistics for cytokine levels in plasma samples are shown in Table 2. Significance analysis of mixed

Table 2 Cytokine median fluorescence values and ranges

Cytokine	Range	Median	IQR
Basic FGF	37–150	71	60–85.5
Eotaxin	35–392	94	67.25–151.5
G-CSF	26–189	57.5	45.5–80.5
GM-CSF	60–1128	406	279.5–550.25
IFN-γ	17–164	43.5	33–61.75
IL-10	31–333.5	77	61–96
IL-12p70	32.5–346	66	48–89.75
IL-13	25.5–598	81	60–133
IL-15	25–427	97	72–130.25
IL-17A	40–222.5	90.5	76.5–105.25
IL-1β	19–541	57	39–96.25
IL-1RA	19–719	52	40–68.5
IL-2	35–563.5	85	70–102
IL-4	20–158	45.5	35–61.25
IL-5	15–136.5	28	22–39
IL-6	26–402.5	48	41–66.5
IL-7	17–157	28.5	24–37
IL-8	26–1716	97	62.25–224.5
IL-9	74–1397	138	113.5–166.75
IP-10	56–2275	371.5	200.25–659.5
MCP-1	41.5–331.5	91	75.25–123
MIP-1α	33–193	75	59.75–93.5
MIP-1β	101.5–2070.5	449	275.5–698.25
PDGF-BB	221–7644.5	1382.5	715.25–2542.75
RANTES	3842–17,915	12,039	8658.5–14,675
TNF-α	19–185	32.5	26–42
VEGF	71.5–941.5	157	110–207.5

IQR (interquartile range). IQR is based on dividing a data set into quartiles Q1, Q2, and Q3 that divides a rank-ordered data set into four equal parts. IQR = Q3-Q1
Abbreviations: *Basic FGF* basic fibroblast growth factor, *G-CSF* granulocyte colony-stimulating factor, *GM-CSF* granulocyte macrophage colony-stimulating factor, *IFN-γ* interferon-γ, *IL* interleukin,*IL.1RA* IL-1 receptor antagonist, *IP-10* interferon gamma-inducible protein 10, *MCP-1* monocyte chemotactic protein-1, *MIP-1α* macrophage inflammatory protein-1α, *MIP-1β* macrophage inflammatory protein-1β, *PDG* platelet derived growth factor-BB, *RANTES* regulated on activation, normal T cell expressed and secreted, *TNF-α* tumor necrosis factor-α, *VEGF* vascular endothelial growth factor

effect modeling identified an interaction in cytokine levels with respect to two clinical covariates: age ($p < 0.001$) and the severity of ASD ($p = 0.02$; Table 3, Additional file 2: Table S4). There was no interaction between cytokine levels and remaining clinical variables (SRS, sleep, and gastrointestinal symptoms) or a significant main effect. The effect of sex was also investigated to determine if the interaction between cytokine expression and covariates were due to sex differences. Statistically significant effects in females were identified for interactions between cytokine levels and age ($p = 0.03$), severity of presentation ($p < 0.001$), and SRS score ($p = 0.04$), while in males there was a statistically significant effect between cytokine levels and age ($p < 0.001$; Table 3). Significance for the interaction effects with respect to age, severity, and SRS were then investigated for males and females. Reduced levels of IL-1β ($p < 0.001$), IL-8 ($p < 0.001$), MIP-1β ($p = 0.006$), PDGF-BB ($p = 0.005$), and VEGF ($p = 0.03$) were associated with increased severity of autism in females (Table 4). Reduced levels of PDGF-BB ($p = 0.03$) were associated with increased severity of autistic symptomatology in males (Table 4). With the exception of IL-15, cytokine levels appear to decrease with respect to increasing severity (Table 4). Higher levels of IL-8 ($p = 0.03$) were associated with higher scores on the SRS in females. Increased levels of IL-15 ($p = 0.04$) and reduced levels of IL-8 ($p = 0.005$) and MIP-1β ($p = 0.009$) were associated with increasing age in males, while reduced levels of IP-10 ($p = 0.001$) was associated with increasing age in females (Table 4).

Correlations between the levels of each of the 27 cytokines were analyzed (Additional file 1: Figures S3 and S4), with Spearman's (ρ) correlations above 0.80 highlighted (Additional file 1: Tables S5-S7). A network visualization of the Spearman's rank correlation matrix between cytokine expression values was created and also optimized for networks separated for sex (Fig. 1, Additional file 1: Figure S5). In the optimal graph networks, visual inspection suggests different network topologies for males and females.

Discussion

To our knowledge, this study consists of the largest cohort of male and female ASD children to date investigating the relationship between clinical traits of ASD and cytokine levels. Overall, results show evidence of a significant association between decreased cytokine levels and increasing severity of ASD-related symptoms. In particular, decreased levels of the growth factor PDGF-BB were associated with increased severity of ASD-related symptoms. Results also suggested cytokine expression was moderated by the sex of participants. Exploratory analysis showed that decreased levels of an additional four cytokines (IL-1β, IL-8, MIP-1β, and VEGF) were associated with increased severity of presentation in females only. Additionally, increased levels of IL-8 were associated with greater caregiver reported social difficulties. An interaction effect for age was identified across both males and females, although there were different cytokines interacting with age in males and females. Increasing age in males was associated with higher levels of IL-15, and reduced levels of IL-8 and MIP-1β, while increasing age in females was associated

Table 3 Significance analysis of interaction effects in cytokine levels and clinical covariates

	Combined sex			Males			Females		
Effect	Chisq	Df	Pr(>Chisq)	Chisq	Df	Pr(>Chisq)	Chisq	Df	Pr(>Chisq)
(Intercept)	387.78	1	< 0.001	239.73	1	< 0.001	105.51	1	< 0.001
Severity	3.28	1	0.07	1.48	1	0.22	0.88	1	0.35
Age	0.01	1	0.91	0.12	1	0.73	0.44	1	0.51
SRS	0.13	1	0.72	0.06	1	0.81	1.35	1	0.25
Sleep	0.08	1	0.78	0.23	1	0.63	0.38	1	0.54
GI	0.53	1	0.47	0.96	1	0.33	0.25	1	0.62
Analyte	1079.27	26	< 0.001	787.12	26	< 0.001	247.60	26	< 0.001
Severity:analyte	43.64	26	0.02	16.42	26	0.93	71.10	26	< 0.001
Age:analyte	75.23	26	< 0.001	60.36	26	< 0.001	41.61	26	0.03
SRS:analyte	10.96	26	1.00	19.09	26	0.83	40.28	26	0.04
Sleep:analyte	17.09	26	0.91	12.47	26	0.99	28.20	26	0.35
GI:analyte	9.65	26	1.00	13.11	26	0.98	23.97	26	0.58

Analysis of deviance tables (type III Wald chi-square tests) for the statistical model: mY~(severity + age + sex + SRS + sleep + GI)*Analyte + (1|ID). Where mY represents the normalized log2 of the fluorescence responses with respect to run (Additional file 1: Figure S2)

with lower levels of IP-10. There were no associations between the other quantitative clinical traits, sleep behavior or gastrointestinal symptoms, and cytokine levels.

Previous studies have reported associations between levels of various cytokines and aberrant behaviors. For example, higher expression of cytokines, including IL-1β, IL-6, IL-8, and IL-12p40 were associated with more impaired stereotyped patterns of behavior [15] while increased levels of the chemokines MCP-1, RANTES, and eotaxin were associated with worsening behavioral symptoms and cognitive and adaptive ability [14]. Further, lower concentration levels of transforming growth factor beta1 (TGFβ1), a regulatory cytokine, has previously been associated with worsening behavior symptoms and lower adaptive behaviors [52]. These findings are in line with a heightened inflammatory state associated with the severity of autism-related symptoms, a cytokine profile similar to that previously identified in participants with ASD compared to healthy controls [13]. In the present study, higher levels of IL-8, which is involved in the recruitment of predominantly neutrophils to settings of tissue inflammation, were associated with higher severity of social impairments in females only. Our remaining findings revealed primarily decreased levels of significant cytokines associated with increased severity of autism-related symptoms, suggesting an altered cytokine profile may be associated with severity of autism-related symptoms. Unlike the possibility of a negative correlation of levels of PDGF-BB with severity of ASD in males and females identified in this study, a positive association between serum levels of PDGF-BB and worsening stereotyped patterns of behavior has previously been identified in a smaller male only cohort [53]. PDGF-BB has been found to be upregulated in healthy children between ages 7 to 17 compared to younger children and adults [54]. PDGF-BB has a complex profile, with PDGF-BB signaling implicated in development and a range of diseases through numerous roles and pathways [55]. Overall, with the exception of IL-15, a pro-inflammatory cytokine considered to be a central factor in the pathogenesis of celiac disease [56], cytokine levels appeared to decrease with respect to increasing symptom severity. However, for most of these cytokines, these differences did not reach significance at the individual cytokine level.

The association of reduced levels of IL-1β, IL-8, MIP-1β, and VEGF, with higher severity levels of ASD in females suggests sex differences in cytokine expression in children with ASD. This was also supported by the exploratory optimal network visualization graphs of cytokine correlations for males and females. Results from recent DNA analysis suggests that females could be more resilient to genetic insults due to carrying more extreme neurodevelopmental-related genetic mutations than males with the same symptoms [57]. Further investigation, particularly with larger female cohorts of ASD that use repeated testing over time, are now required to further support a potential sex-specific biology underlying different cytokine profiles between males and females with ASD. Our results also suggest that age appears to play an important moderating role in these effects; in males, an overall decline in cytokine levels was associated with increasing age. However, this effect was more mixed in females with only about half of the cytokine levels declining with older age. The physiological changes occurring during the onset of puberty and beyond may contribute to the variations of cytokine levels with age and sex. Age-related changes in cytokine

Table 4 Adjusted slope for Age, Severity and SRS

	Age				Severity				SRS			
	Male		Female		Male		Female		Male		Female	
Analyte	Slope	Pr(>Chisq)	Slope	Pr(>Chisq)	Slope	Pr(>Chisq)	Slope	Pr(>Chisq)	Slope	Pr(>Chisq)	Slope	Pr(>Chisq)
Basic FGF	−0.01	0.89	0.00	0.98	−0.04	0.39	−0.06	0.37	0.00	0.97	0.00	0.97
Eotaxin	−0.03	0.16	−0.02	0.77	−0.06	0.13	−0.11	0.07	0.00	0.97	−0.01	0.85
G-CSF	0.02	0.48	0.04	0.55	−0.03	0.48	−0.03	0.68	0.01	0.96	0.00	0.97
GM-CSF	−0.01	0.85	0.02	0.85	−0.01	0.89	−0.01	0.87	0.01	0.96	0.00	0.98
IFN-γ	−0.02	0.77	0.00	0.98	−0.04	0.34	−0.07	0.35	0.00	0.97	−0.01	0.97
IL-10	−0.03	0.16	−0.02	0.85	−0.01	0.89	−0.08	0.22	−0.01	0.90	−0.01	0.97
IL-12p70	−0.04	0.07	0.00	0.98	−0.02	0.68	−0.12	0.05	−0.01	0.88	0.00	0.97
IL-13	0.01	0.77	−0.01	0.89	−0.01	0.75	−0.05	0.44	0.00	0.97	−0.01	0.70
IL-15	0.04	0.04*	0.04	0.48	0.00	0.96	0.04	0.54	0.00	0.97	0.00	0.97
IL-17A	−0.02	0.77	0.00	0.99	−0.03	0.48	−0.04	0.54	0.00	0.97	0.00	0.97
IL-1β	−0.02	0.72	0.02	0.85	−0.06	0.15	−0.20	< 0.001*	−0.01	0.88	0.01	0.85
IL-1RA	−0.01	0.85	0.02	0.77	−0.04	0.35	−0.08	0.22	0.00	0.97	0.00	0.97
IL-2	0.00	0.98	0.01	0.87	0.00	1.00	−0.04	0.57	0.00	0.97	0.00	0.97
IL-4	0.00	0.98	0.01	0.87	−0.04	0.37	−0.07	0.31	0.00	0.97	0.00	0.97
IL-5	−0.02	0.77	0.00	0.98	−0.05	0.22	−0.06	0.39	0.00	0.97	−0.01	0.85
IL-6	−0.01	0.84	0.02	0.85	−0.04	0.39	−0.06	0.39	0.00	0.97	0.00	0.97
IL-7	0.00	0.95	0.01	0.98	−0.04	0.34	−0.06	0.35	0.00	0.97	0.00	0.97
IL-8	−0.06	0.01*	0.02	0.77	−0.05	0.22	−0.29	< 0.001*	0.00	0.97	0.02	0.03*
IL-9	−0.01	0.85	0.00	0.98	−0.01	0.74	0.00	1.00	−0.01	0.90	0.00	0.97
IP-10	−0.04	0.09	−0.10	0.001*	−0.05	0.22	−0.02	0.74	−0.01	0.80	−0.02	0.21
MCP-1	0.01	0.91	0.02	0.84	−0.03	0.48	−0.05	0.48	0.00	0.97	0.00	0.97
MIP-1α	−0.01	0.84	−0.01	0.89	−0.03	0.48	−0.03	0.60	0.00	0.97	0.00	0.97
MIP-1β	−0.05	0.01*	−0.03	0.63	−0.01	0.75	−0.16	0.01*	−0.01	0.85	0.01	0.97
PDGF-BB	−0.04	0.08	−0.02	0.85	−0.08	0.03*	−0.16	0.01*	−0.01	0.80	0.01	0.85
RANTES	−0.01	0.88	0.01	0.87	−0.02	0.54	−0.09	0.20	0.00	0.97	0.01	0.85
TNF-α	−0.02	0.72	0.00	0.99	−0.05	0.22	−0.05	0.44	0.00	0.97	0.00	0.97
VEGF	−0.04	0.09	0.01	0.98	−0.03	0.48	−0.13	0.03*	0.00	0.97	0.00	0.97

Chisq tests: *p* value adjustment method: false discovery rate

Abbreviations: *Basic.FGF* basic fibroblast growth factor, *G.CSF* granulocyte colony-stimulating factor, *GM* granulocyte macrophage colony-stimulating factor, *IFN. γ* interferon-γ, *IL* interleukin, *IL.1β* IL-1 beta, IL.1RA, IL-1 receptor antagonist, *IP* interferon gamma-inducible protein 10, *MCP.1* monocyte chemotactic protein-1, *MIP.1α* macrophage inflammatory protein-1α, *MIP.1β* macrophage inflammatory protein-1β, *PDGF.BB* Platelet derived growth factor-BB, *RANTES* regulated on activation, normal T cell expressed and secreted, *TNF. α* tumor necrosis factor-α, *VEGF* vascular endothelial growth factor. * indicates significant difference at $P <$ 0.05 or better

expression in healthy children have been described elsewhere [54, 58, 59], although there is limited age-matched reference data of cytokine expression that can assist with more specific interpretation of these findings.

The results of the present study suggest that an altered cytokine response could be associated with severity of presentation, particularly in females. These results do not corroborate with some previous work that has identified associations between increased levels of pro-inflammatory cytokines and behavioral impairments in ASD, and are also not consistent with peripheral immune system abnormalities in ASD manifesting only as a pro-inflammatory bias [60]. The elucidation of possible neural circuitry mechanisms that are impacted by an aberrant peripheral immune system resulting in downstream changes in behavior are imperative. Evidence from investigations involving a rodent model deficient in adaptive immunity suggest that social deficits may result from impaired circuitry homeostasis derived from dysfunctional immunity [61], supporting the importance of this type of research in ASDs. The heterogeneity in ASD substantially increases the complexity associated with the identification of either markers of a pathological state that manifest in a

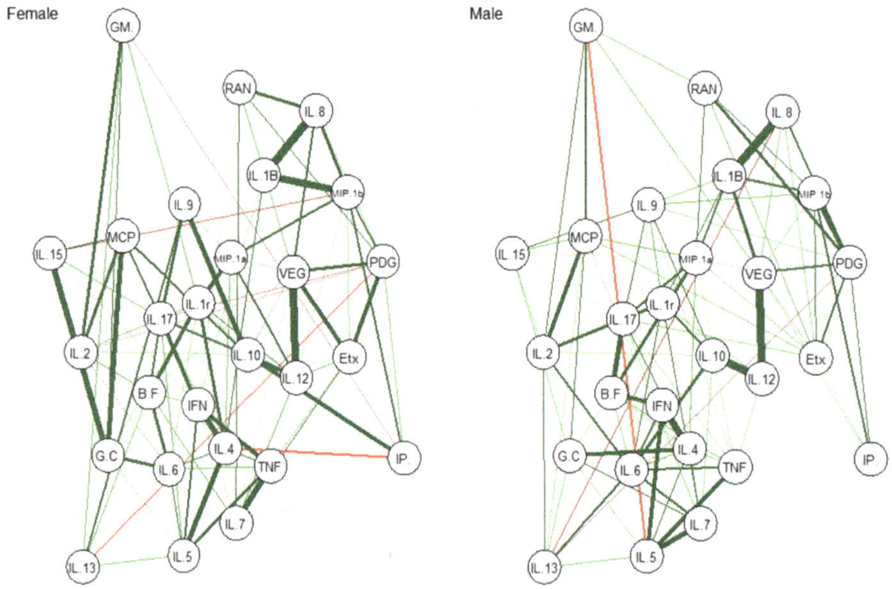

Fig. 1 Optimal network graphs representing cytokine correlations separated for sex. Each node represents a cytokine, and each edge represents a Spearman's correlation between two cytokines. Green edges indicate positive correlations and red edges represent negative correlations. The width of the edge corresponds to the absolute value of the correlation: the higher the correlation, the thicker and more saturated is the edge. Node abbreviations: B.F basic fibroblast growth factor, Etx eotaxin, G.C granulocyte colony-stimulating factor, GM granulocyte macrophage colony-stimulating factor, IFN interferon-gamma, IL interleukin, IL.1B 1 beta, IL.1r IL-1 receptor antagonist, IL.12 IL-12p70, IL.17 IL-17A, IP interferon gamma-inducible protein 10, MCP monocyte chemotactic protein-1, MIP.1a macrophage inflammatory protein-1 alpha, MIP.1b macrophage inflammatory protein-1 beta, PDG platelet-derived growth factor-BB, RAN regulated on activation, normal T cell expressed and secreted, TNF tumor necrosis factor-alpha, VEG vascular endothelial growth factor

subgroup of ASD or biomarkers of response to treatment that are specific and sensitive enough to be consistent measures of change.

The objective of this study was to utilize a well characterized cohort to establish if there is a relationship between cytokine levels and symptom severity of ASD and other clinical traits, including variability in social functioning, sleep problems, and gastrointestinal dysfunction. The levels of cytokines were analyzed using fluorescent data. There is a need for consensus in the literature about the use of absolute or fluorescent levels, and the treatment of concentrations obtained below the sensitivity LOD when presenting cytokine data. The use of absolute values has been more common in past autism research [14, 15]; however, the use of fluorescent levels is also an acceptable method [36]. While the concurrent analysis of a control group would have highlighted any cytokine differences between the ASD cohort and healthy controls, these differences have previously been well established [13] and would not facilitate the identification of potential relationships between the immune system aberrations and severity in ASD. The elucidation of these latter relationships have greater potential to contribute to knowledge about the relationship between symptoms and immune function in autism. Control groups typically vary widely on many characteristics beyond autism symptoms and their use in understanding the immune circuitry underpinning autism profiles may be debated. This cohort reflects the ratio of approximately four affected males to one affected female in the general population; however, larger cohorts of females are required to replicate and extend the sex-related findings. Furthermore, the duplication of samples across plates would have clarified the run difference that was linked to sex. The assessment of the severity of ASD-related symptoms undertaken using the ADOS was conducted by one assessor, strengthening the reliability of diagnoses and evaluations of severity. Additionally, ADOS assessments were conducted on the day of blood draw, therefore cytokine expression levels were relevant to that time point. While the ADOS-2 calibrated severity metric was approximated using a large sample [27], it is not representative of a population distribution of ADOS scores. Diagnostic and assessment measures, such as the ADOS, used in the ASD population are primarily behaviorally defined. There is a growing body of evidence implicating comorbid psychopathology and medical conditions in ASD [62–64], highlighting the importance of comprehensive characterization of participants, particularly with respect to the assessment and reporting of all medical and mental health comorbidities. It is possible that there were participants with an undiagnosed comorbidity, allergies or concurrent illness at the time of blood draw that may elevate risk of immune system dysfunction and peripheral upregulation or downregulation of cytokines. Additionally, describing the onset of symptoms is important as previous research has suggested that regression may be associated with elevated cytokine expression [15].

Conclusions

The present study highlights the importance of an interdisciplinary approach to address the complexity of an autism presentation [65], particularly with respect to the pathological significance of immune system abnormalities. Longitudinal investigations in large cohorts with comprehensive, clinically relevant comprehensive biological data relating to medical comorbidities found in ASD, such as sleep disorders, and gastrointestinal and immune dysfunction, and controlling for variables that continually interact with the immune system, such as age, pubertal status, infections, and allergies, are required in order to thoroughly characterize the mechanisms of action behind these types of results. Further work is required to extend these findings to determine whether cytokines can be employed as either a sensitive marker of a pathological state-related to a subgroup in ASD or as a biomarker of response to treatment.

Abbreviations

ADOS: Autism diagnostic observation schedule; ADOS-G: ADOS-Generic; ASD: Autism spectrum disorder; BMI: Body mass index; CSHQ: Children's Sleep Habits Questionnaire; DSM: Diagnostic and Statistical Manual of Mental Disorders; EBIC: Extended Bayesian Information Criterium; FGF: Fibroblast growth factor; G-CSF: Granulocyte colony-stimulating factor; GI: Gastrointestinal; GM-CSF: Granulocyte–macrophage colony-stimulating factor; IFN: Interferon; IL: Interleukin; IL-1ra: IL1 receptor antagonist; IP: Interferon gamma induced protein; IQR: Interquartile range; LOD: Level of detection; MCP: Monocyte chemotactic protein; MICE: Multiple imputation by chained equations; MIP: Macrophage inflammatory protein; PDGF: Platelet-derived growth factor; PL: Parameter logistic; RANTES: Regulated on activation normal T cell expressed and secreted; SRS: Social Responsiveness Scale; TNF: Tumor necrosis factor; VEGF: Vascular endothelial growth factor

Acknowledgements

The authors gratefully acknowledge the families who have contributed to the WAABR. We thank PathWest Laboratory Medicine WA for facilitating collection and access to blood samples, Irma Larma and the Centre for Microscopy, Characterization and Analysis, The University of Western Australia for facilitating multiplex analysis of plasma samples, and Dr. Kirsty Short for her comments on the manuscript. This research was partially supported by a NHMRC project grants (1043664; 1125449) and a Sydney University near-miss grant to Guastella. Author Guastella is funded by a NHMRC Career Development Fellowship (APP1061922). Author Whitehouse is supported by a Senior Research Fellowship (#1077966) from the National Health and Medical Research Council. Author Alvares is funded by the Cooperative Research Centre for Living with Autism (Autism CRC), established and supported under the Australian Government's Cooperative Research Centres Program.

Funding

This research was partially supported by a NHMRC project grant (1043664) to Guastella and Whitehouse. The funding body had no role in the design of the study and collection, analysis and interpretation of data or in writing of the manuscript.

Authors' contributions

AM contributed to study conception and design, conducted the experiment, assisted with the statistical design, collected, analyzed, and interpreted the data, prepared and critically revised the manuscript, and was responsible for final content. EB assisted with the statistical design, data analysis and interpretation and the preparation of the manuscript. GA collected and interpreted the data, revised the manuscript for intellectual content, and was responsible for final content. NG reviewed data analysis procedures, interpreted data, and revised the manuscript for intellectual content. IBH interpreted data and revised the manuscript for intellectual content. AH collected data and revised the manuscript for intellectual content. JH, JB, DR, and JW established the data collection protocols, interpreted the data and critically appraised the manuscript. AJOW established the data collection protocols, collected and interpreted data, and revised the manuscript for intellectual content. AJG contributed to the study conception and design, interpreted the data and critically revised the manuscript for intellectual content. All authors read and approved the final manuscript.

Competing interests

Author IBH is a Commissioner in Australia's new National Mental Health Commission from 2012. He is the Co-Director, Health and Policy at the Brain and Mind Centre which operates two early-intervention youth services under contract to headspace. IBH has led a range of community-based and pharmaceutical industry-supported depression awareness and education and training programs. He has led projects for health professionals and the community supported by governmental, community agency, and pharmaceutical industry partners (Wyeth, Eli Lily, Servier, Pfizer, AstraZeneca) for the identification and management of depression and anxiety. He has received honoraria for presentations of his own work at educational seminars supported by a number of non-government organizations and the pharmaceutical industry (including Servier, Pfizer, AstraZeneca, and Eli Lilly). He is a member of the Medical Advisory Panel for Medibank Private and also a Board Member of Psychosis Australia Trust. He leads an investigator-initiated study of the effects of agomelatine on circadian parameters (supported in part by Servier) and has participated in a multicenter clinical trial of the effects of agomelatine on sleep architecture in depression and a Servier-supported study of major depression and sleep disturbance in primary care settings.
The remaining authors declare they have no competing interests.

Author details

[1]Autism Clinic for Translational Research, Brain and Mind Centre, Central Clinical School, Sydney Medical School, University of Sydney, 100 Mallett Street, Camperdown, New South Wales 2050, Australia. [2]Australian Proteome Analysis Facility, Macquarie University, Sydney, Australia. [3]Telethon Kids Institute, University of Western Australia, Perth, Western Australia, Australia. [4]Cooperative Research Centre for Living with Autism (Autism CRC), Long Pocket, Brisbane, Queensland, Australia. [5]Pathwest Laboratory Medicine WA, Nedlands, Western Australia, Australia. [6]School of Pathology and Laboratory Medicine, University of Western Australia, Perth, Western Australia, Australia. [7]School of Population Health, University of Western Australia, Perth, Western Australia, Australia. [8]School of Pediatrics and Child Health, University of Western Australia, Perth, Western Australia, Australia

References

1. CDC. Prevalence of autism spectrum disorder among children aged 8 years—autism and developmental disabilities monitoring network, 11 sites, United States, 2010. Morbidity and Mortality Weekly Report: Surveillance Summaries. 2014;63:1–14.
2. American Psychiatric Association. Diagnostic and statistical manual of mental disorders. 5th ed. Washington, DC: American Psychiatric Press; 2013.
3. Howlin P, Goode S, Hutton J, Rutter M. Adult outcome for children with autism. J Child Psychol Psychiatry. 2004;45:212–29.

4. Szatmari P, Georgiades S, Duku E, et al. Developmental trajectories of symptom severity and adaptive functioning in an inception cohort of preschool children with autism spectrum disorder. JAMA Psychiatry. 2015; 72:276–83.
5. Fein D, Barton M, Eigsti IM, Kelley E, Naigles L, Schultz RT, Stevens M, Helt M, Orinstein A, Rosenthal M. Optimal outcome in individuals with a history of autism. J Child Psychol Psychiatry. 2013;54:195–205.
6. Werling DM, Geschwind DH. Sex differences in autism spectrum disorders. Curr Opin Neurol. 2013;26:146–53.
7. Kirkovski M, Enticott PG, Fitzgerald PB. A review of the role of female gender in autism spectrum disorders. J Autism Dev Disord. 2013;43: 2584–603.
8. Huguet G, Ey E, Bourgeron T. The genetic landscapes of autism spectrum disorders. Annu Rev Genomics Hum Genet. 2013;14:191–213.
9. Herbert MR. Contributions of the environment and environmentally vulnerable physiology to autism spectrum disorders. Curr Opin Neurol. 2010;23:103–10.
10. Croen LA, Braunschweig D, Haapanen L, Yoshida CK, Fireman B, Grether JK, Kharrazi M, Hansen RL, Ashwood P, Van de Water J. Maternal mid-pregnancy autoantibodies to fetal brain protein: the early markers for autism study. Biol Psychiatry 2008; 64:583-588.
11. Mead J, Ashwood P. Evidence supporting an altered immune response in ASD. Immunol Lett. 2015;163:49–55.
12. Gesundheit B, Rosenzweig JP, Naor D, Lerer B, Zachor DA, Procházka V, Melamed M, Kristt DA, Steinberg A, Shulman C, et al. Immunological and autoimmune considerations of autism Spectrum disorders. J Autoimmun. 2013;44:1–7.
13. Masi A, Quintana DS, Glozier N, Lloyd AR, Hickie IB, Guastella AJ. Cytokine aberrations in autism spectrum disorder: a systematic review and meta-analysis. Mol Psychiatry. 2015;20:440–6.
14. Ashwood P, Krakowiak P, Hertz-Picciotto I, Hansen R, Pessah IN, Van de Water J. Associations of impaired behaviors with elevated plasma chemokines in autism spectrum disorders. J Neuroimmunol. 2011b;232:196–9.
15. Ashwood P, Krakowiak P, Hertz-Picciotto I, Hansen R, Pessah I, Van de Water J. Elevated plasma cytokines in autism spectrum disorders provide evidence of immune dysfunction and are associated with impaired behavioral outcome. Brain Behav Immun. 2011a;25:40–5.
16. Napolioni V, Ober-Reynolds B, Szelinger S, Corneveaux JJ, Pawlowski T, Ober-Reynolds S, Kirwan J, Persico AM, Melmed RD, Craig DW, et al. Plasma cytokine profiling in sibling pairs discordant for autism spectrum disorder. J Neuroinflammation. 2013;10:38.
17. Veatch OJ, Maxwell-Horn AC, Malow BA. Sleep in autism Spectrum disorders. Curr Sleep Med Rep. 2015;1:131–40.
18. McElhanon BO, McCracken C, Karpen S, Sharp WG. Gastrointestinal symptoms in autism spectrum disorder: a meta-analysis. Pediatrics. 2014;133:872–83.
19. Mannion A, Leader G, Healy O. An investigation of comorbid psychological disorders, sleep problems, gastrointestinal symptoms and epilepsy in children and adolescents with autism Spectrum disorder. Res Autism Spectr Disord. 2013a;7:35–42.
20. Halladay AK, Bishop S, Constantino JN, Daniels AM, Koenig K, Palmer K, Messinger D, Pelphrey K, Sanders SJ, Singer AT, et al. Sex and gender differences in autism spectrum disorder: summarizing evidence gaps and identifying emerging areas of priority. Mol Autism. 2015;6:1–5.
21. Fombonne E. Epidemiology of pervasive developmental disorders. Pediatr Res. 2009;65:591–8.
22. Manzardo AM, Henkhaus R, Dhillon S, Butler MG. Plasma cytokine levels in children with autistic disorder and unrelated siblings. Int J Dev Neurosci. 2012;30:121–7.
23. Schneider T, Roman A, Basta-Kaim A, Kubera M, Budziszewska B, Schneider K, Przewlocki R. Gender-specific behavioral and immunological alterations in an animal model of autism induced by prenatal exposure to valproic acid. Psychoneuroendocrinology. 2008;33:728–40.
24. Taylor LJ, Maybery MT, Wray J, Ravine D, Hunt A, Whitehouse AJO. Are there differences in the behavioural phenotypes of autism Spectrum disorder probands from simplex and multiplex families? Res Autism Spectr Disord. 2015;11:56–62.
25. Lord C, Petkova E, Hus V, Gan W, Lu F, Martin D, Ousley O, Guy L, Bernier R, et al. A multisite study of the clinical diagnosis of different autism spectrum disorders. Arch Gen Psychiatry. 2012;69:306–13.
26. Lord C, Risi S, Lambrecht L, Cook EH Jr, Leventhal BL, DiLavore PC, Pickles A, Rutter M. The autism diagnostic observation schedule-generic: a standard measure of social and communication deficits associated with the spectrum of autism. J Autism Dev Disord. 2000;30:205–23.
27. Gotham K, Pickles A, Lord C. Standardizing ADOS scores for a measure of severity in autism spectrum disorders. J Autism Dev Disord. 2009;39:693–705.
28. Hus V, Lord C. The autism diagnostic observation schedule, module 4: revised algorithm and standardized severity scores. J Autism Dev Disord. 2014a;44:1996–2012.
29. Shumway S, Farmer C, Thurm A, Joseph L, Black D, Golden C. The ADOS calibrated severity score: relationship to phenotypic variables and stability over time. Autism Res. 2012;5:267–76.
30. Lord C, Rutter M, Di Lavore P, Risi S, Gotham K, Bishop S. Autism diagnostic observation schedule, second edition (ADOS-2). Los Angeles: Western Psychological Services; 2012.
31. Hus V, Gotham K, Lord C. Standardizing ADOS domain scores: separating severity of social affect and restricted and repetitive behaviors. J Autism Dev Disord. 2014b;44:2400–12.
32. Constantino J, Davis S, Todd R, Schindler M, Gross M, Brophy S, Metzger L, Shoushtari C, Splinter R, Reich W. Validation of a brief quantitative measure of autistic traits: comparison of the social responsiveness scale with the autism diagnostic interview-revised. J Autism Dev Disord. 2003;33:427–33.
33. Owens JA, Spirito A, McGuinn M. The Children's sleep habits questionnaire (CSHQ): psychometric properties of a survey instrument for school-aged children. Sleep. 2000;23:1043–52.
34. Rosenberg-Hasson Y, Hansmann L, Liedtke M, Herschmann I, Maecker HT. Effects of serum and plasma matrices on multiplex immunoassays. Immunol Res. 2014;58:224–33.
35. Wadhwa M, Mire-Sluis A, Thorpe R. Standardization and calibration of cytokine immunoassays. Revue de l'ACOMEN. 1999;5
36. Breen EJ, Polaskova V, Khan A. Bead-based multiplex immuno-assays for cytokines, chemokines, growth factors and other analytes: median fluorescence intensities versus their derived absolute concentration values for statistical analysis. Cytokine. 2015;71:188–98.
37. Breen EJ, Tan W, Khan A. The statistical value of raw fluorescence signal in Luminex xMAP based multiplex immunoassays. Sci Rep. 2016;6:26996.
38. Davis D, Zhang A, Torrence J, Emily D. Selection of standards for bio-Plex cytokine assays. In: Tech note 2900: bio-Rad 2900.
39. Azur MJ, Stuart EA, Frangakis C, Leaf PJ. Multiple imputation by chained equations: what is it and how does it work? Int J Methods Psychiatr Res. 2011;20:40–9.
40. van Buuren S, Groothuis-Oudshoorn K. Mice: multivariate imputation by chained equations in R. Journal of statistical software. 2011; 45.
41. Chavent M, Kuentz-Simonet V, Liquet B, Saracco J. ClustOfVar: an R package for the clustering of variables. J Stat Softw. 2012;50:1–16. http://www.jstatsoft.org/v50/i13/
42. Venables WN, Ripley BD. Modern applied statistics with S. New York: Springer; 2002.
43. Fox J, Weisberg S. An {R} companion to applied regression. 2nd ed. Thousand Oaks: Sage; 2011.
44. phia: Post-Hoc Interaction Analysis. R package. http://CRAN.R-project.org/package=phia.
45. Hothorn T, Hornik K, van de Wiel MA, Achim Z. Implementing a class of permutation tests: the coin package. J Stat Softw. 2008;28:1–23.
46. Holm S. A simple sequentially Rejective multiple test procedure. Scand J Stat. 1979;6:65–70.
47. Epskamp S, Cramer AOJ, Waldorp LJ, Schmittmann VD, Borsboom D. Qgraph: network visualizations of relationships in psychometric data. J Stat Softw. 2012;48:1–18.
48. Fruchterman T, Reingold E. Graph drawing by force-directed placement. Software: Practice and Experience. 1991;21:1129–64.
49. Meinshausen N, Bühlmann P. High-dimensional graphs and variable selection with the lasso. Ann Stat. 2006:1436–62.
50. Friedman J, Hastie T, Tibshirani R. Sparse inverse covariance estimation with the graphical lasso. Biostatistics. 2008;9:432–41.
51. van Borkulo CD, Borsboom D, Epskamp S, Blanken TF, Boschloo L, Schoevers RA, Waldorp LJ. A new method for constructing networks from binary data. Sci Rep 2014; 4:5918.

53. Kajizuka M, Miyachi T, Matsuzaki H, Iwata K, Shinmura C, Suzuki K, Suda S, Tsuchiya KJ, Matsumoto K, Iwata Y, et al. Serum levels of platelet-derived growth factor BB homodimers are increased in male children with autism. Prog Neuro-Psychopharmacol Biol Psychiatry. 2010;34:154–8.
54. Kleiner G, Marcuzzi A, Zanin V, Monasta L, Zauli G. Cytokine levels in the serum of healthy subjects. Mediat Inflamm. 2013;2013:6.
55. Andrae J, Gallini R, Betsholtz C. Role of platelet-derived growth factors in physiology and medicine. Genes Dev. 2008;22:1276–312.
56. Benahmed M, Meresse B, Arnulf B, Barbe U, Mention JJ, Verkarre V, Allez M, Cellier C, Hermine O. Cerf–Bensussan N. Inhibition of TGF-β signaling by IL-15: a new role for IL-15 in the loss of immune homeostasis in celiac disease. Gastroenterology. 2007;132:994–1008.
57. Jacquemont S, Coe BP, Hersch M, Duyzend MH, Krumm N, Bergmann S, Beckmann JS, Rosenfeld JA, Eichler EE. A higher mutational burden in females supports a "female protective model" in neurodevelopmental disorders. Am J Hum Genet. 2014,94.415–25.
58. Hartel C, Adam N, Strunk T, Temming P, Muller-Steinhardt M, Schultz C. Cytokine responses correlate differentially with age in infancy and early childhood. Clin Exp Immunol. 2005;142:446–53.
59. Chang W-S, Kim E-J, Lim Y-M, Yoon D, Son J-Y, Park J-W, Hong S-J, Cho S-H, Lee J-S. Age-related changes in immunological factors and their relevance in allergic disease development during childhood. Allergy Asthma Immunol Res. 2016;8:338–45.
60. Rose D, Ashwood P. Potential cytokine biomarkers in autism spectrum disorders. Biomark Med. 2014;8:1171–81.
61. Filiano AJ, Xu Y, Tustison NJ, Marsh RL, Baker W, Smirnov I, Overall CC, Gadani SP, Turner SD, Weng Z, et al. Unexpected role of interferon-γ in regulating neuronal connectivity and social behaviour. Nature. 2016;535:425–9.
62. Brereton AV, Tonge BJ, Einfeld SL. Psychopathology in children and adolescents with autism compared to young people with intellectual disability. J Autism Dev Disord. 2006;36:863–70.
63. Bauman ML. Medical comorbidities in autism: challenges to diagnosis and treatment. Neurotherapeutics. 7:320–7.
64. Matson JL, Nebel-Schwalm MS. Comorbid psychopathology with autism spectrum disorder in children: an overview. Res Dev Disabil. 2007;28:341–52.
65. Aldinger KA, Lane CJ, Veenstra-VanderWeele J, Levitt P. Patterns of risk for multiple co-occurring medical conditions replicate across distinct cohorts of children with autism Spectrum disorder. Autism Res. 2015;8:771–81.

3

Early development of infants with neurofibromatosis type 1

Anna May Kolesnik[1†], Emily Jane Harrison Jones[1*†], Shruti Garg[2], Jonathan Green[2], Tony Charman[3], Mark Henry Johnson[1] and the EDEN-BASIS Team+

Abstract

Background: Prospective studies of infants at familial risk for autism spectrum disorder (ASD) have yielded insights into the earliest signs of the disorder but represent heterogeneous samples of unclear aetiology. Complementing this approach by studying cohorts of infants with monogenic syndromes associated with high rates of ASD offers the opportunity to elucidate the factors that lead to ASD.

Methods: We present the first report from a prospective study of ten 10-month-old infants with neurofibromatosis type 1 (NF1), a monogenic disorder with high prevalence of ASD or ASD symptomatology. We compared data from infants with NF1 to a large cohort of infants at familial risk for ASD, separated by outcome at age 3 of ASD (n = 34), atypical development (n = 44), or typical development (n = 89), and low-risk controls (n = 75). Domains assessed at 10 months by parent report and examiner observation include cognitive and adaptive function, sensory processing, social engagement, and temperament.

Results: Infants with NF1 showed striking impairments in motor functioning relative to low-risk infants; this pattern was seen in infants with later ASD from the familial cohort (HR-ASD). Both infants with NF1 and the HR-ASD group showed communication delays relative to low-risk infants.

Conclusions: Ten-month-old infants with NF1 show a range of developmental difficulties that were particularly striking in motor and communication domains. As with HR-ASD infants, social skills at this age were not notably impaired. This is some of the first information on early neurodevelopment in NF1. Strong inferences are limited by the sample size, but the findings suggest implications for early comparative developmental science and highlight motor functioning as an important domain to inform the development of relevant animal models. The findings have clinical implications in indicating an important focus for early surveillance and remediation in this early diagnosed genetic disorder.

Keywords: NF1, Infant, Translational neurodevelopment, Autism, Prospective longitudinal, Adaptive functioning, Cognition, Sensory processing, Social engagement, Development

Background

Autism spectrum disorder (ASD) is a neurodevelopmental disorder that affects social communication and flexible behaviour in up to 1.5% of the population [1]. Identifying causal paths that link genetic and environmental risk factors to later behaviour is a critical target for the field, because of the potential to yield new routes to intervention. Symptoms of ASD likely emerge through a complex developmental cascade of interactions between genetics, the brain, cognition, behaviour, and the child's interaction with their environment [2]. ASD can be reliably diagnosed by ages 2 to 3[3], and risk factors act predominately prenatally [4, 5]. Thus, a focus on early brain development is critical to differentiating putative causal paths from compensatory, adaptive, or secondary cascading effects of early symptoms [6]. Linking those causal paths to specific neurobiological systems is critical to developing new pharmacological treatments to complement existing behavioural therapies [7].

* Correspondence: e.jones@bbk.ac.uk
†Equal contributors
[1]Centre for Brain and Cognitive Development and Department of Psychology, Birkbeck, University of London, Malet Street, London WC1E 7HX, UK
Full list of author information is available at the end of the article

Prospective longitudinal studies of infants with older siblings with ASD have yielded significant insights into its earliest features in this group [2]. In the first year of life, behavioural differences in infants with later ASD are difficult to detect and may be most common in sensory and motor functioning [8, 9]. For example, 6-month-old infants with later ASD are more likely to show poor head control [10] and infants at familial risk as a group show poor postural control [11] and more limited reaching and grasping skills [12]. In contrast, social communication appears relatively typical in the first 6 months [8, 13], although neurocognitive measures reveal subtle vulnerabilities in social engagement [14], response to eye gaze [15], and declining interest in eyes [16]. By the end of the first year, clear differences are present in a range of ASD-related behavioural phenotypes, including poorer language and communication skills [8], reduced joint attention [17], diminishing social interest [13], and the emergence of unusual interests in objects [18]. Measures like the Autism Observational Scale for Infants begin to show reasonable sensitivity to ASD outcome at this time [19, 20], although diagnosis is still difficult until the second or third year of life [3]. Thus, it appears that clear delays in ASD-relevant domains emerge over the first year of life but may be preceded by alterations in early brain development that affect lower-level sensorimotor systems.

The unclear aetiology of ASD in infants at polygenic familial risk makes it difficult to translate such insights to animal models, which are mainly based on single gene knock-out approaches. This in turn limits our ability to tie insights to particular neurobiological systems or pathways and to generate new pharmacological treatment strategies. A complementary way to study the emergence of ASD that may facilitate translational insights is to test infants with defined genetic syndromes associated with a heightened incidence of ASD. Examples of conditions that can be potentially identified in early development, carry a high risk of ASD, and have been successfully modelled in animals include fragile X syndrome, tuberous sclerosis complex, and neurofibromatosis type 1 (NF1). One challenge to this approach is that these conditions are rare. Identified genetic syndromes only account for a small proportion of cases of ASD, and thus, the generalisability of mechanisms observed in particular disorders remain unclear [21, 22]. Thus, the optimal strategy may be to establish which antecedent biomarkers observed in studies of infants at familial risk are also present in infants with genetic syndromes. In this way, we can identify generalised causal paths that are likely widely applicable but that can also be more carefully probed at the molecular and neurobiological levels.

Prospective studies of infants with NF1 provide an important complementary approach in this context. In contrast to other monogenic syndromes, NF1 is not complicated by severe intellectual disability or seizures. NF1 is the most common autosomal-dominant single-gene condition associated with increased risk for neurodevelopmental disorders, with birth incidence of 1:2700 [23]. Fifty percent of the cases are inherited, while the rest are de novo cases due to spontaneous mutation of the NF1 gene located on chromosome 17q11.2, which encodes for the protein neurofibromin. Although well known for its cutaneous manifestations, the main challenges experienced by people with NF1 are cognitive, social, and behavioural. The overall IQ is in the low-average range, although specific learning impairments are common [24]. There is a high prevalence of ASD in NF1, with rates of 25% full ASD and 20% with partial ASD symptoms in the pediatric NF1 population [25]. The phenotypic profile of ASD in NF1 is also broadly similar to idiopathic ASD [26], making insights from NF1 more likely to generalise to understanding ASD more broadly.

The downstream molecular consequences of impaired NF1 function have been well characterised in NF1 knock-out mouse models [27]. Impaired disinhibition of the Ras/MAP kinase pathway leads to changes in synaptic proteins, GABA/glutamate disequilibrium, and impairments in synaptic function [28]. Further, abnormalities in cyclic AMP and dopamine homeostasis underlie the attention system abnormalities in NF1 [29]. The social learning and attention impairments characteristic of ASD have been recapitulated in NF1 knock-outs [28, 30]. Targeted treatments such as lovastatin [31] and lamotrigine [32] reverse the NF1-associated cognitive impairments in knock-out models, but translational clinical trials in humans have so far had mixed results [33]. A major impediment for clinical trials is the lack of sensitive outcome measures on which to target treatment and a poor understanding of neurodevelopmental trajectories in children with NF1. Longitudinal studies mapping the developmental trajectories of children with NF1 will allow inferences about causal mechanisms as well as identify candidate biomarkers for future intervention studies. Treatments targeted in the prodromal period (before behavioural symptoms of ASD and ADHD emerge) could prevent or ameliorate the later emergence of symptoms [34].

Diagnosis of NF1 is made on clinical assessment using the National Institute of Health clinical consensus criteria. Since 50% of the cases are inherited, NF1 can be diagnosed in infancy using cord blood mutation testing or on clinical assessment. The comparison of developmental levels between infants with NF1 and infants with older siblings with ASD (defined on familial risk status) is thus putatively less confounded by ascertainment bias than for other comparable syndromes. Unless there are parental concerns, most infants with NF1 do not receive routine developmental monitoring. To our knowledge, this is the first study to report the developmental profile of NF1 in infancy.

Present study

To understand early developmental profiles and the emergence of behaviours related to ASD in infants with NF1, we recently launched a prospective longitudinal study of this population. Our projected group size will be 30 infants with data on a rich battery of behavioural and neurocognitive measures at 5, 10, 14, 24, and 36 months; this report represents the first ten infants with data at 10 months enrolled in the study. This is a particularly interesting age, because it appears to mark the beginning of the emergence of behavioural signs of ASD in infants at familial risk [2]. The present study had two goals: first, to determine what developmental areas might be affected by the NF1 mutation in early development, and second, to examine whether infants with NF1 show profiles that resemble those of infants who develop ASD through other risk pathways. To do this, we compared the developmental profiles of infants with NF1 to those of a larger group of infants at high familial risk for ASD with different developmental outcomes at age 3 (typical development, ASD, or other atypical developmental profiles), in addition to a sample of low-risk typically developing infants. Taken together, our study provides the first evidence of the profile of developmental difficulties in infants with NF1 and their similarities and differences to profiles observed in infants at familial risk for ASD.

Methods

Participants

Participants described in this case series include ten 10-month-old children (4 male; 6 female) with an NF1 diagnosis through the Early Development in Neurofibromatosis Type 1 (EDEN) research project. NF1 is a rare disorder, with a birth incidence of approximately one in 2700 births in the UK per year [37]. Thus, our recruitment methods aimed to maximise the representativeness of our sample within the context of the rarity of the disorder. Participants were recruited via local and regional genetic centers (Manchester, Leeds, Newcastle, Southampton) and via advertisements placed in the NF charities' social media webpages. The study has R&D approval for recruitment across all specialist genetic centers across the UK. The study information was offered to eligible participants at routine clinical appointments. Within the general population, NF1 is approximately 50% familial and 50% sporadic [35].Our sample consists primarily of familial cases (8/10) because they are typically identified earlier in development through cord blood testing. Of note, our previous behavioural phenotyping studies have shown no differences between familial and de novo cases [26].

All of the participants who had inherited NF1 were confirmed via molecular testing of cord blood samples (n = 8) or clinical diagnosis based on NIH consensus criteria (n = 2) [36]. Six of the infants had at least one older sibling. Behavioural and cognitive profiles of these infants were compared to a large corpus of data from the British Autism Study of Infant Siblings (BASIS, phases 1 and 2; http://basisnetwork.org). These children either had a family history of ASD and went onto receive a diagnosis at 36 months (HR-ASD, n = 34, 8F), had other indications of atypical development (such as high scores on ASD-related symptom measures or poor cognitive development; HR-Atyp, n = 43, 20F), or were typically developing (HR-no ASD, n = 89, 44F); or were 'low-risk' controls, i.e. had no family history of ASD (LR, n = 72, 37F). ASD diagnoses were made at age 3 years for research purposes only through expert clinical judgment based on all available clinical and behavioural assessments (including gold-standard ADOS and ADI measures) collected at 24 and 36 months (for details, see Additional file 1). The study was approved by the National Research Ethics Service London Central Ethical Committee and conducted in accordance with the Declaration of Helsinki (1964). As the study is ongoing, it is not yet possible to estimate how many of the children with NF1 will go on to receive an ASD diagnosis.

Procedures

Informed consent was obtained from all families. All assessments took place at the Centre for Brain and Cognitive Development, Birkbeck, London. Behavioural measures described below were administered as part of a more extensive experimental protocol; for summary, see Additional file 1: Table S1.

Cognitive and adaptive skills

Cognitive ability was assessed through the Mullen Scales of Early Learning (M) administered according to the manual [37]. This is an observational measure that assesses gross and fine motor skills, expressive and receptive language, and visual reception. We report t scores per subdomain (M = 50, SD = 10), based on the US norms. Adaptive skills were assessed using the Vineland Adaptive Behavior Scale Parent Survey (VABS; [38]) form, a parent-report questionnaire that assesses socialisation, communication, motor behaviour, and daily living skills. We report standard scores per domain (M = 100, SD = 15) based on the US norms.

ASD symptoms

The Autism Observation Scale for Infants (AOSI; [39, 40]) is a 19-item interactive play schedule and was administered to five of the infants. It is designed to monitor early signs of ASD and measure aspects of visual attention, social communication, and development of sensory and motor skills. Absence/presence of behaviours is rated 0–3, where 0 signifies normal function, and higher values suggests increasing deviation from the normal behaviour expected at the age of assessment. Total scores range from 0–50 [19, 41].

Temperament

Parents completed the Infant Behavior Questionnaire (IBQ [42]), a parent-report measure that comprises 14 subscales grouped into three overarching factors labelled Surgency (the child's tendency to show excitement, positive affect, and approach), Negative Affect (the child's tendency to cry, be avoidant, or otherwise fussy), and Effortful Control (the child's ability to regulate their mood and behaviour) [42, 43]. Parents of infants at high familial risk for ASD completed the original form of the IBQ-R [44]; parents of infants with NF1 completed the short form [42]. For comparability between cohorts, we rescored the long form of the IBQ-R by only selecting items also included on the short form.

Sensory processing

Parents completed the Infant/Toddler Sensory Profile (ITSP [45]). This questionnaire produces scores in four quadrants that reflect the child's responsiveness to different types of sensory experiences. Sensation Seeking (generating higher sensory input for oneself) and Low Registration (noticing fewer sensory cues) encompass high-threshold responses. Sensory Sensitivity and Sensation Avoiding reflect low-threshold responses and are combined into a low-threshold quadrant score (detecting more sensory input than others, with negative affect and low self-regulation). Further, the scale includes five sensory processing scores for different processing systems (e.g. visual, auditory, tactile). Norms are available, and score ranges for typical performance or probable or definite differences are provided per subscale.

Examiner-rated behaviour

Levels of social engagement (SE) were examined through consensus coding of six different aspects of infant behaviour, including social affect, temperament, and vocalising; researchers used a 7-point Likert Scale at the end of the testing day ([46]; see Additional file 1).

Analytic strategy

We first present case vignettes for each infant. For measures with available norms (Mullen, VABS, and ITSP), we interpret scores as below average (< – 1SD) or low (< – 2SD) based on common convention using terminology specific to each measure. Sensory behaviours measured through the ITSP were rated as either probably more/less than others if one standard deviation away from the mean and definitely more/less than others when the score is two standard deviations away; note that cut-off scores vary per subdomain for this measure [45]. We also report qualitative summaries of non-standardised measures (IBQ, SE). However, it is important to note that all measures were administered in a research, not clinical context, and thus should not be considered diagnostic.

Second, we compared the performance of infants with NF1 at a group level with our other cohorts (HR-TD, HR-Atyp, HR-ASD, and LR) using ANCOVA with age as a covariate.

Results

Case summaries

Acronyms are used to identify the source of information provided about their level of cognitive/sensory development (e.g. IBQ, VABS). Descriptive data and scores are presented in Additional file 1: Tables S2, S3, S4, S5, and S6.

Case 1: male, diagnosis of NF1, at 10 months

Significant delays in gross motor skills (M, VABS), for example, he was not able to move from sitting to hands and knees, roll over, or pull up from supine to a sitting position. Fine motor abilities were below average for the age group, as he demonstrated a partial pincer grasp but could not take blocks in/out of a container or bang them together (M). Cognitive skills were within the average range (M). Infant demonstrated object permanence, appropriate use of objects, and understanding inhibitory commands. Expressive language was below average and consisted of voluntary babbling and consonant sounds, with no first words or jabbering with inflection (M); receptive language was adequate, but he had difficulty understanding verbal requests and questions from the examiner (M). Broader communication skills were moderately low (VABS). Social skills were a relative strength and judged at age-expected levels (VABS). Examiners reported moderate levels of eye contact and attentiveness, but relatively low levels of shared affect (SE). He showed altered sensory processing across all domains relative to age-appropriate norms (particularly auditory, vestibular, and oral processing); this mainly reflected more registration of sensory stimuli and a low threshold for noticing sensory changes (ITSP). By parent report of temperament, surgency, negative affect, and effortful control were all within one standard deviation of average values in the low-risk sample (IBQ).

Case 2: male, diagnosis of NF1, at 11 months

Gross motor skills were within the normal range by examiner observation (M), and he had strong fine motor skills (M); he had mastered balance and control of the upper/lower extremities and was gaining upright mobility. However, his overall adaptive motor skills were rated lower than average by parent report (e.g. sitting and crawling behaviours occurred lower relative to the age-matched population norm). Cognitive skills were a relative strength—he achieved object permanence and demonstrated early spatial awareness and visual memory (M). Communication skills were relatively poor, specifically in receptive language; he was able to understand simple verbal input (e.g. response to own name or familiar names/words) but failed to give a toy in response to a request and a gesture or identify an object after hearing it named (M). Expressive language was in the average range, marked by presence of first word, as well as communication of intentions through jargon combined with gestures. By parent report, his everyday communication behaviour was relatively strong, as were his social skills (e.g. responding to parent with vocalisation, engaging in games of 'peek-a-boo'; VABS). Examiners reported frequency of eye contact, shared affect, and social responsiveness (SE). Temperamentally, his surgency and negative affect were within the normal range (though he showed high activity levels in the lab SE), but he showed relatively lower levels of effortful control than low-risk infants (IBQ). Sensory processing was considered typical for most domains, though he showed probably altered auditory processing and definitely less sensation seeking than other infants (ITSP).

Case 3: male, diagnosis of NF1, at 11 months (*)
Gross motor skills were very low (unable to sit independently), and fine motor skills were below average (M): he was able to grasp and manipulate objects, as well as display a partial pincer grasp, but was not able to use both hands together when playing with an object or turn pages in a book. Parent report suggests his use of motor skills in everyday life was adequate but gross motor skills were poorer than fine motor skills (VABS). He had marked difficulty in controlling motor behaviour, although no atypical motor/sensory behaviours specifically related to ASD were noted (AOSI). Cognitive skills were in the low-average range (M); he showed object permanence and began associating objects with functions but was unable to open/close a book or pay attention to pictures. Expressive language skills were very low; he did not babble or produce consonant sounds during the assessment (M). Receptive language was also below average; he was able to give a toy on request, but only when it was accompanied by a gesture, and was not able to understand simple questions from the experimenter (M). During the AOSI, he showed no social babbling. However, by parent report, his communication skills at home were adequate (VABS) and his social skills were strong (VABS). During the day, the child was rated as moderately socially responsive, with moderate eye contact and shared affect (SE), but he showed clearly atypical eye contact, reciprocal smiling, and social interest when probed (AOSI). Temperament was parent-rated as comparable to other groups for surgency and negative affect, but effortful control was lower than in low-risk controls (> – 1SD) (IBQ); examiners also rated him as moderately negative and quite active (SE). Sensory ratings indicated altered visual processing, and definitely 'less' low registration (meaning he was less likely to fail to notice sensory stimuli in the environment).

Case 4: male, diagnosis of NF1, at 12 months
Gross motor skills were very low for his age group (M, VABS). He was unable to pull up on furniture or get into a sitting position from hands and knees (M). Fine motor abilities were age-appropriate—he was able to use both hands to manipulate an object and displayed finer coordination of movement (M). Cognitive scores were a relative strength; he obtained object permanence and early spatial awareness and could associate an object and its function (M). Expressive language was very low—he was unable to voluntarily babble or produce any consonant sounds (M). He also showed below-average receptive language ability and was unable to identify an object or respond to a verbal request (M). By parent report, his communication skills were just in the average range. Daily living and social skills were adequate (VABS); examiners also rated his eye contact, affect, and social responsiveness as frequency (SE). Surgency and effortful control were within one standard deviation of the typical range (IBQ), and examiners rated his temperament as very positive (SE); however, by parent report, he showed elevated negativity relative to low-risk controls (IBQ). Sensory sensitivity was within the typical range for all scores, apart from probably altered sensitivity to vestibular sensations (items include needs support for sitting, enjoying physical play, and resists having head tipped back).

Case 5: female, diagnosis of NF1, at 9 months (*)
Gross motor skills were below average in the lab (M) and low in everyday contexts (VABS). Fine motor skills were below average; she was able to use a partial pincer grip, but not both hands together, or turn pages in a book sequentially (M). During the AOSI, she showed marked difficulty controlling motor behaviour, as well as atypical sensory and motor behaviours (AOSI). Cognitive skills were very delayed, with partial object tracking, no object permanence, and failure to associate objects with functions (M). However, by parent report, her daily living skills were typical (VABS). Communication skills were delayed (VABS); during testing, her receptive language skills were rated as below average, while expressive language was a relative strength and age-appropriate, with voluntary babbling and production of several words (M). Everyday social skills were below average (VABS); however, during the testing day, the child maintained relatively frequent eye contact and shared affect with the experimenter (SE)

and showed good social skills on the AOSI. Temperamentally, her surgency (e.g. expression of pleasure) and negativity were within expected levels but effortful control was rated lower than low-risk controls (< – 1SD; IBQ). The child showed pervasive atypicalities in the sensory domain, with atypical auditory, visual, tactile, and oral sensory behaviours; these were likely related to more low registration (reduced attention towards environmental cues; ITSP).

Case 6: female, diagnosis of NF1, at 10 months

Gross motor abilities were at floor level in the lab (M), equivalent to a 3 month old (M). Child was able to bear weight on forearms and hold her head steady in a supported seated position but was not able to roll over or grasp fingers and pull up from a supine into a sitting position. However, she performed at an 'above average' level on fine motor skills (M); adaptive fine motor skills were low but in the average range (VABS), showing evidence of the development of more precise coordination of movement. Visual reception skills were age-appropriate, for example, she achieved object permanence and was able to associate objects with functions (M). Expressive language was within the average range; she produced varied and controlled vocalisations and was able to say one recognisable word (M); receptive language skills were below average (M). Parent ratings also indicated moderately low communication abilities (VABS) but relatively strong social skills. During the testing day, she showed frequent eye contact, moderate shared affect, and social responsiveness. Temperamentally, she was rated during the testing day as showing a highly positive temperament though with low attentiveness (SE), and by parent report, surgency, negativity, and effortful control scores were within the average range of control groups (IBQ). Finally, she showed no overt atypicalities in sensory behaviours across all domains (ITSP).

Case 7: female, diagnosis of NF1, at 10 months (*)

Gross motor skills and adaptive motor behaviours were below average for the age range, but fine motor skills were typical (M, VABS) and she showed no motor atypicalities on the AOSI. She had good cognitive ability, including object permanence, early spatial awareness and visual memory (M). Language skills were poor, with low expressive language; she showed voluntary babbling and production of consonants but was unable to vocalise two-syllable sounds or produce first words as expected for the age group (M). She showed very poor receptive language (the 5-month level); she did not respond to her name or understand simple verbal input. Adaptive communication skills were considered strong by parent report (VABS). Social skills in everyday contexts were also typical by parent report (VABS); during testing, she showed frequent eye contact, moderate shared affect, and social responsiveness but became distressed when without her parents. She showed some evidence of diminished social responsiveness to an unfamiliar examiner when promoted (A). Temperamentally, surgency and effortful control were low (< – 1SD) and negative affect was high (> + 2SD) relative to typical controls, although was rated as relatively active and attentive (SE). Sensory responses were altered for auditory and visual domains, likely because she is more likely to notice less sensory cues from the immediate environment (ITSP).

Case 8: female, diagnosis of NF1, at 10 months (*)

Gross motor functioning was poor; she was unable to pull herself to stand or move from sitting position to hands and knees (M); this was accompanied by atypical motor control and behaviours, such as hand waving (AOSI). She also showed poor fine motor skills and was unable to manipulate objects or demonstrate a pincer grasp (M); adaptive motor function was also rated low by parents (VABS). Cognitive skills were below average (although an area of relative strength), with partial object permanence (M), and poor disengagement (AOSI). Language skills were also significantly delayed in both expressive and receptive domains (M) and in everyday contexts (VABS). She was unable to voluntarily babble or produce consonant sounds and showed absent responses to sound or voice/face of the experimenter (M). Social skills in an everyday context were also delayed (VABS). In the lab, she showed moderate to poor eye contact but poor shared affect and social responsiveness (AOSI; SE). Temperamentally, her levels of surgency were relatively low (> – 1SD), as was her effortful control (IBQ). During the testing day, she showed low attentiveness and activity level (SE). Parent-rated reports indicated atypical sensory behaviours across auditory and visual/vestibular and oral sensory domains, mainly related to higher levels of failing to notice sensory stimuli as well as a higher likelihood to have a low threshold for distress reactions (ITSP).

Case 9: female, diagnosis of NF1, at 11 months

Gross motor function was poor; she could sit independently but was not able to walk with one hand held or stand up independently (M). Fine motor skills were typical, including using both hands together and coordinated movements (M); composite motor skills in an everyday context were low to average (VABS). Cognitive skills were below average—she was able to show object permanence and appropriate use of objects but failed to pay attention to pictures shown by experimenter (M). Expressive language skills were very low, with no voluntary babbling or consonant sounds (M). Receptive language was just below average, including giving a toy in response to a verbal request and understanding actions (i.e. waving goodbye or clapping). Overall adaptive communication was rated as adequate (VABS). Social skills were also rated as adequate (VABS), and during the day, she showed frequent eye contact, shared affect, and generally positive temperament (SE). Temperamentally, she showed low surgency and negative affect (< 1SD) relative to low-risk controls; effortful control was high (> 1SD). In the sensory domain, she showed a broadly typical profile, with altered visual processing, probably less likelihood of failing to notice sensory stimuli and probably more sensation seeking (ITSP).

Case 10: female, diagnosis of NF1, at 11 months (*)

Gross motor abilities were low, though she was able to sit independently and turn to reach a toy placed on the side (M). Fine motor skills were also below average, including a partial pincer grasp and object manipulation; however, she was unable to use both hands together or turn pages in a book (M). Adaptive motor skills at home were in the normal range by parent report (VABS), but she showed atypical motor control and behaviours during interaction with an examiner (AOSI). Her visual reception skills were low-average, though she understood object permanence and simple problem solving (M). Expressive language was below average; she is able to babble voluntarily but could not produce consonant sounds and first words or engage in a gesture/language game such as 'peek-a-boo' (M). She was functioning at a very low range on receptive language; she did not respond to own name or understand simple verbal input (M). Adaptive communication skills were moderately low by parent report (VABS). Social skills were within the typical range; in the lab, she showed relatively frequent eye contact, but limited shared affect and social responsiveness and social babbling (SE, AOSI). Temperamentally, she showed relatively high levels of negative affect (> 2SD), low effortful control (< 2SD), and high surgency (> 1SD) (IBQ). Sensory behaviours were within the typical range (ITSP).

Group analysis

Motor skills

There was a significant main effect of group on motor (Vineland Motor and Mullen Fine and Gross Motor) skills ($F(12{,}624.7) = 6.36$, $p < .001$, $\eta^2 = 0.097$; with age covaried $F(12{,}622.043) = 5.86$, $p < .001$, $\eta^2 = 0.090$). This reflected differences across Gross Motor ($F(4{,}238) = 10.16$, $p < .001$, $\eta^2 = 0.15$) and Fine Motor subscales of the Mullen ($F(4{,}238) = 6.28$, $p < .001$, $\eta^2 = 0.096$) and adaptive Motor skills on the VABS ($F(4{,}238) = 9.28$, $p < .001$, $\eta^2 = 0.14$; see Figs. 1 and 2). Bonferroni-corrected pairwise comparisons revealed that infants with NF1 showed significantly lower scores on Gross Motor skills on the Mullen relative to all four comparison groups (all $ps < .01$). Infants with NF1 showed significantly lower Fine Motor scores than the LR ($p = 0.006$) and HR-no ASD group ($p = 0.009$) but not the HR-Atyp ($p = 0.5$) or HR-ASD ($p = 1$) groups. On the VABS Motor domain, they showed lower scores than LR ($p = 0.003$) and marginally the HR-no ASD ($p = .009$) group but were comparable to the HR-Atyp ($p = 1$) and HR-ASD group ($p = 0.93$). The HR-ASD group also showed significantly lower scores than the LR group for the VABS motor domain ($p = 0.033$), Mullen fine motor skills ($p = 0.012$), and marginally Mullen gross motor scores ($p = 0.099$). Thus, both infants with NF1 and the HR-ASD group showed significantly poorer motor skills than low-risk infants.

Cognitive skills

There was a significant main effect of group on cognitive (Mullen visual reception and VABS Daily Living) skills ($F(8{,}474) = 2.99$, $p = 0.003$, $\eta^2 = 0.048$; with age covaried ($F(8{,}472) = 3.08$, $p = 0.002$, $\eta^2 = 0.05$). This group effect was seen for both Visual Reception ($F(4{,}238) = 4.22$, $p = 0.003$, $\eta^2 = 0.066$) and Daily Living scales ($F(4{,}238) = 2.78$, $p = 0.028$, $\eta^2 = 0.045$; see Figs. 1 and 2). Bonferroni-corrected pairwise comparisons revealed that infants with NF1 showed significantly lower Visual Reception scores than the LR group ($p = 0.022$), marginally lower than the HR-no ASD group ($p = 0.11$) but not the HR-Atyp ($p = 1$) or HR-ASD ($p = 1$) groups. Daily Living Skills were comparable to all other groups ($p = 1$). The HR-ASD group showed significantly lower scores for Daily Living Skills than the LR group ($p = 0.033$); this was not the case for Visual Reception ($p = 0.3$). Inspection of the means in Fig. 2 indicates that infants with NF1 showed comparable values to the HR-ASD group; thus, the absence of clear group differences may be related to the smaller size of that group.

Language

There was a significant main effect of group on language (Mullen Expressive and Receptive Language and VABS Communication) skills ($F(12{,}624.7) = 5.25$, $p < 0.001$, $\eta^2 = 0.081$; with age covaried ($F(12{,}622.043) = 5.82$, $p < 0.001$, $\eta^2 = 0.090$). This reflected differences across Receptive Language ($F(4{,}238)= 7.42$, $p < 0.001$, $\eta^2 = 0.11$), Expressive Language ($F(4{,}238) = 6.03$, $p < 0.001$, $\eta^2 = 0.09$), and adaptive Communication ($F(4{,}238) = 6.02$, $p < 0.001$, $\eta^2 = 0.092$; see Figs. 1 and 2). Bonferroni-corrected pairwise comparisons revealed that infants with NF1 showed significantly lower scores for Receptive Language than low-risk infants ($p = 0.001$) and the HR-TD ($p < 0.001$) and HR-Atyp ($p = 0.007$) groups but not the HR-ASD ($p = 0.17$) groups. For expressive language, infants with NF1 showed significantly lower scores than all other groups ($ps \leq 0.001$). For Vineland Communication scores, the NF1 group

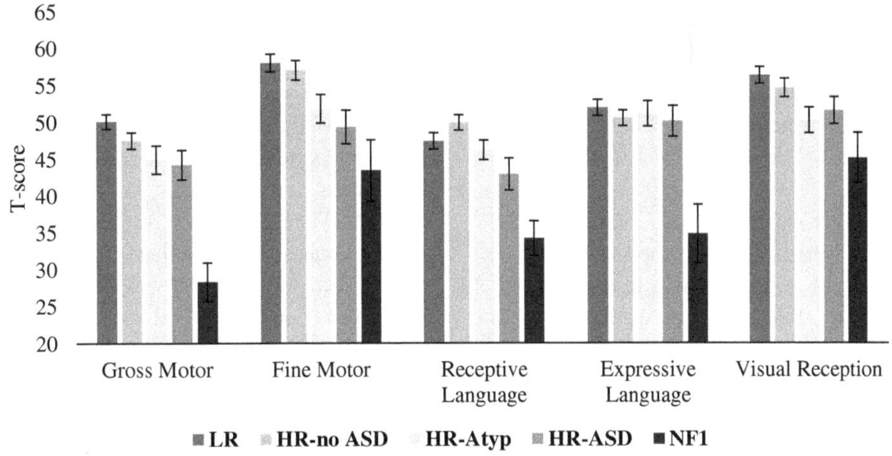

Fig. 1 Average standard scores for the subscales of the Mullen Scale of Early Learning from groups of infants with LR (low familial risk of ASD), HR-no ASD (high familial risk with later typical development), HR-Atyp (high familial risk with other atypical developmental profiles), HR-ASD (high familial risk with later ASD outcome), and infants with NF1. Error bars are ± 1 SE

showed significantly lower scores than LR infants only ($p = 0.025$; other groups $ps > 0.3$). The HR-ASD group showed significantly lower scores than the HR-no ASD group for receptive language ($p = 0.007$) than the LR group for VABS Communication ($p = 0.025$); other comparisons were not significant ($ps > 0.3$). Thus, both infants with NF1 and the HR-ASD group showed lower communication scores than LR infants.

Social functioning

There were no significant group differences in Vineland socialisation scores ($F(4,239) = 2.063$, $p = 0.086$, $\eta^2 = 0.033$). We did not compute statistical comparisons for the AOSI, since only five infants with NF1 completed it, but the distribution of scores within the NF1 group appeared similar to those for the HR-ASD group (Fig. 3).

Temperament

There were no significant group differences on the IBQ ($F(12,622.043) = 1.25$, $p - 0.24$, $\eta^2 = 0.021$).

Discussion

We present the first developmental profiles of infants with NF1 and compare them to a large cohort of infants at familial risk with later ASD. Our initial report was designed to address two questions. First, what are the developmental challenges experienced by infants with NF1? Second, how do those

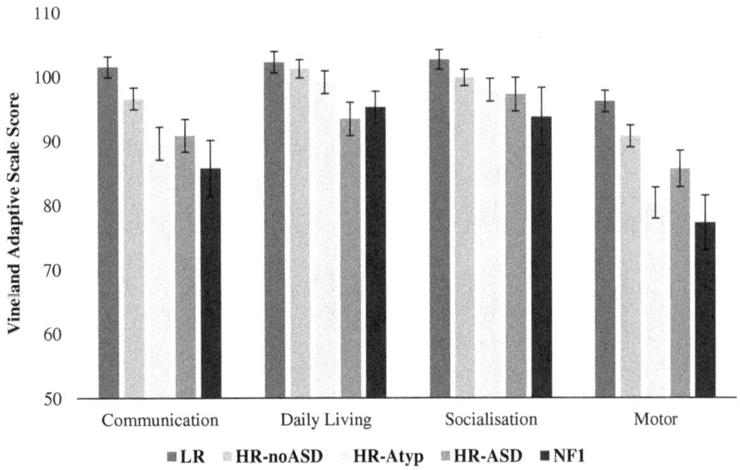

Fig. 2 Average standard scores for the subscales of the Vineland Adaptive Behavior Scale from groups of infants with LR (low familial risk of ASD), HR-no ASD (high familial risk with later typical development), HR-Atyp (high familial risk with other atypical developmental profiles), HR-ASD (high familial risk with later ASD outcome), and infants with NF1. Error bars are ± 1 SE

challenges compare to infants with other familial routes to ASD? Findings reveal developmental delays across multiple domains that show some intriguing similarities to the pattern of difficulties seen in infants with familial risk routes to ASD.

Developmental difficulties experienced by infants with NF1

Infants with NF1 showed broad developmental difficulties across a number of cognitive and motor domains. The most consistently affected areas were motor and communication skills, for which delays relative to low-risk infants were observed across both the Mullen and the Vineland. In addition, seven of the ten infants showed atypical scores on at least one domain of sensory responsivity, though the nature of the atypicality was heterogeneous. Similar developmental problems are observed in other genetic disorders linked to ASD, like Fragile X (FXS). For example, Hogan and colleagues report a case series of eight infants with FXS followed from 9 to 24 months of age, half of whom later met criteria for ASD [43]. Many infants showed relatively high levels of emergent autism-like behaviours on the Autism Observational Scale for Infants (AOSI), particularly those with a later outcome of autism. By the end of the first year, cognitive and adaptive deficits were seen in almost all infants and did not appear to differ by autism diagnosis. Thus, early developmental delays may be a common feature in infants with genetic syndromes linked to ASD.

Recent research has shown that the NF1 gene mutation confers a general vulnerability for cognitive difficulties in the preschool period. A study of 40 children with NF1 aged 3–6 years found weaker cognitive abilities on all subscales of the Differential Ability Scales compared to controls matched for age and socioeconomic status [47]. At least a third of preschool children with NF1 have difficulties with expressive and receptive language skills as well as phonological awareness [48]. A cross-sectional study of 39 toddlers with NF1 aged 21–30 months assessed using Bayley Scales of Infant Development, Wechsler preschool scale of intelligence, and parental measures of behaviour found poorer cognitive, motor, and language development in the NF1 group compared to age-matched controls [49]. Cognitive development was in the low to average range, 1 SD lower than controls, with below-average motor development in a third of the cohort. Further, parental responses indicated delayed receptive and expressive language development in over 70% of the NF1 cohort. Our current data indicates that these delays observed in preschoolers are present from at least 10 months of age and appear to be more pronounced in infancy. Longitudinal follow-up of our current cohort will be required to determine whether delays partially resolve over time.

Clinical information suggests low rates of identification of other co-occurring neurodevelopmental conditions within children with NF1, with substantial 'diagnostic overshadowing' in ascribing cognitive and behavioural problems to the NF1 diagnosis alone [25]. Diagnostic delays limit effectiveness of interventions, with life-long impacts on social and occupational functioning [50, 51]. There is an urgent need to develop early assessment and intervention approaches for ASD in NF1 that could significantly improve developmental outcomes for children. Our work indicates that developmental delays are apparent from at least 10 months of age, and so, early intervention may be particularly critical. Early

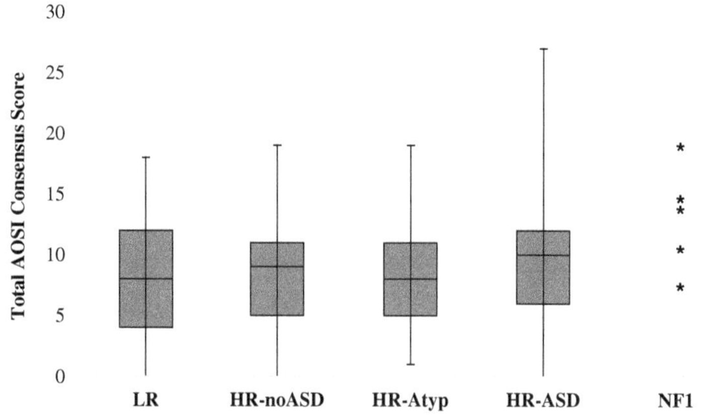

Fig. 3 Box-and-whisker plots showing the distribution of total scores on the Autism Observation Scale for Infants (mean, lower and upper quartile, and whiskers show full range). No statistical comparisons were carried out as the sample size for NF1 was too small. Asterisks (*) depict the individual scores from the NF1 sample. Of note, this task was added to the protocol later in the study and so was only completed by five infants

interventions are not routinely provided; current guidelines recommend developmental assessment in order to support additional needs on starting school [52].

NF1 and familial routes to ASD

Some elements of the developmental profile of infants with NF1 were similar to those seen in infants with familial routes to ASD. On the Vineland Adaptive Behavior Scales, socialisation profiles did not significantly differ between infants with NF1, infants with later ASD from familial risk cohorts, and low-risk infants. Further, infants with NF1 were rated as having relatively typical profiles of social engagement during the lab visit. Our rating scale was adapted from one used within infants with later ASD [46], and here too, infants were rated as relatively engaged at this age, with scores declining across the second year. It would be important to see whether infants with NF1 display the same profile of emerging social difficulties with age. At the group level on the Vineland, children with later ASD from our comparison samples showed the worst performance in motor skills and the best in socialisation and daily living, with communication skills at an intermediate level; the group means for children with NF1 show the same pattern albeit with more pronounced motor difficulties (see also [8] for no differences in socialisation at 12 months in infants at high familial risk for ASD). Longitudinal follow-up will be required to determine whether a similar profile is seen in the subgroup of infants with NF1 who develop later ASD. Nonetheless, our work suggests that relatively unaffected social functioning at the behavioural level at 10 months may be a shared phenotype between infants with both genetic and familial routes to ASD.

At the group level, developmental difficulties in infants with NF1 were generally more pronounced across all domains than in our comparison samples at familial risk of ASD, including those who went on to have an ASD outcome. This may be associated with the generally low likelihood of intellectual disability in samples of infants at familial risk relative to the broader population of children with ASD [2]. Interestingly, cognitive outcomes for children with NF1 tend to be better than for other neurodevelopmental conditions, so it will be important to determine whether over time many children catch up (to a degree) with their peers. Nonetheless, reports that the earliest behavioural signs related to later ASD are in motor skill (e.g. head lag) and sensory functioning [8–10] is somewhat consistent with the motor delays and atypical sensory responsivity we observed in infants with NF1. One important next step is to understand whether these early motor delays have cascading effects on later functioning and whether they can be related to observations in animal models of NF1. Interestingly, there is preclinical evidence of a role of the NF1 gene in skeletal development and growth [53] and normal muscle function [54]; further work should establish whether this contributes to the delays in gross motor skills seen in our infant cohorts.

Our children with later ASD from the familial risk group showed comparable profiles on the Mullen and Vineland. In contrast, children with NF1 generally showed more impairment on the Mullen than the Vineland. Interpreting these effects is difficult because of differences in the way the measures are administered. Possibly, parents of children with NF1 are less likely to recognise developmental difficulties. Further, some infants with NF1 did not have older siblings ($n = 4$) and this may affect how parents judge their early development. Another potential limitation is that we made group-based comparisons to a historical cohort of data (in order to present data on autism outcome) collected by different teams at the same site. Any differences between measure administration by different examiners would affect Mullen scores but not the Vineland or IBQ, because identical parent report forms were used across cohorts. Taken together, the consistent identification of motor and communication delays across both the Mullen and Vineland scales (despite their different limitations) gives particular confidence to these findings.

Clinical implications

This initial case series is too preliminary for any definitive clinical implication, but it should alert the clinical community. Identification and early surveillance will often concentrate initially on the clinical genetic and neurocutaneous aspects. Our findings indicate an important focus for early developmental assessment and appropriate remediation in newly diagnosed NF1 infants.

Limitations and future directions

Data collection for our project is still ongoing, and we do not yet know which of the infants with NF1 will later meet criteria for ASD or show elements of the broader ASD phenotype. Outcomes for children with genetic syndromes are highly heterogeneous [21]. ASD is not present in every child with NF1; many also develop other co-occurring conditions like epilepsy, intellectual disability, or severe attention problems. Thus, longitudinal prospective studies that can tease out predictors of these different outcomes are required. However, studying children with NF1 as a group (rather than dividing the group into those with and without ASD outcome) is the closest comparison to animal modelling approaches (which typically contrast NF1 knock-outs with wildtype). Given the rarity of NF1, our sample size is also relatively small, consistent with other recent reports on infants with rare disorders [43], [55]. Although our recruitment methods were designed to increase the likelihood that our cases would be representative of the broader population with NF1 (by recruiting through all UK genetic clinics), this remains a potential limitation to the generalisability of our conclusions and indicates the importance of continuing to build larger samples in this field. Because there are no previous reports from prospective studies of infants with NF1, it is impossible to determine the extent to which our sample is representative of the broader population of infants with NF1 in terms of ability level and outcome. Planned longitudinal follow-up in toddlerhood will be necessary to address this question. One potential difference is that within the general population, 50% of cases of NF1 are familial and 50% are sporadic [35]. Within our sample, 8/10 cases were familial and two infants had a de novo mutation identified postnatally through clinical presentation (usually the presence of café au lait spots). This imbalance is because familial NF1 is detected much earlier in development (through cord blood testing). Consistent with previous reports in older children [26] there did not appear to be anything clearly different about these two infants, though further work with larger samples is required to investigate this question fully. Further, it is important to note that in the present study there was remarkable consistency in the domains most affected across individual infants. For example, motor skills were delayed in almost all infants. Our findings are consistent with the proposal that infants with genetic syndromes may show somewhat more consistent profiles than infants with other routes to ASD, providing one way to constrain heterogeneity. Further, the observation of motor delays supports preclinical observations of a critical role for NF1 in musculoskeletal development [54]. Other limitations were that our comparison infants were slightly younger than infants with NF1, but we controlled for age in all analyses. Further, we did not have contextual data on the ITSP and social engagement scales from other cohorts, and thus, the interpretability of these measures is limited to the qualitative case reports.

Conclusions

At 10 months, infants with NF1 in the present study showed delays in motor and communication functioning, with milder difficulties in visual reception. Seven out of ten infants showed atypicality in at least one domain of sensory function. In contrast, temperament and social engagement appear relatively typical. This profile shares some similarity with infants from familial risk samples who develop ASD, where very early behavioural difficulties are typically observed in sensory and motor domains (rather than social functioning). Our work introduces a new route to establishing a translational developmental neuroscience of ASD. Prospective longitudinal studies of infants with neurofibromatosis hold great promise for illuminating the neurodevelopmental systems that mediate between genetic risk and later behavioural symptoms. Our findings reveal a distinct profile of early impairment that will be of substantial interest to work on animal models of ASD. Further, our work indicates the critical importance of careful developmental monitoring of infants with NF1. Early delays should be identified and appropriate intervention provided.

Abbreviations

AOSI: Autism Observational Scale for Infants; ASD: Autism spectrum disorder; IBQ: Infant Behavior Questionnaire Short Form; ITSP: Infant/Toddler Sensory Profile; Mullen: Mullen Scales of Early Learning; NF1: Neurofibromatosis type 1; Vineland: Vineland Adaptive Behavior Scales

Acknowledgements

We would like to thank the families who have participated in our research. +The EDEN-BASIS team includes Simon Baron-Cohen, Jannath Begum-Ali, Patrick Bolton, Celeste Cheung, Leila Dafner, Kim Davies, Mayada Elsabbagh, Janice Fernandes, Laurel Fish, Isobel Gammer, Marian Greensmith, Teodora Gliga, Sarah Kalwarowsky, Michelle Liew, Greg Pasco, Andrew Pickles, Helena Ribeiro, Erica Salomone, Chloe Taylor, Leslie Tucker, and Sam Wass, the *NF1 Clinical consortium: Manchester NF1 service* Emma Burkitt-Wright, D Gareth Evans, Grace Vassallo, Judith Eelloo, Siobhan West, Elizabeth Howard, Eileen Hupton, Sue Huson, Lauren Lewis, and Karen Tricker, the *Yorkshire Regional NF1 service* Angus Dobbie, Ruth Drimer, and Saghira Malik Sharif, the *Southampton Clinical Genetics Service* Diane Baralle and Carolyn Redman, the *West Midlands Regional Clinical Genetics Unit* Saba Sharif and Carolyn Symth, the *Edinburgh Genetic Service* Wayne Lam, the *Sheffield NF1 clinic* Alyson Bradbury, Neil Harrower, and Oliver Quarrell, the *Newcastle NF1 service* Helen Bethell, Rachel Jones, Susan Musson, Catherine Prem, and Miranda Splitt, the *Sunderland NF1 clinic* Karen Horridge, the *Wirral University Hospitals NF1 clinic* Christine Steiger, and the Service User collaborator Carly Jim. We would also like to thank the NF charities Neuro Foundation & Childhood Tumour Trust.

Funding

This work was supported by Action Medical Research (GN2385), GOSH Children's Charity and The Baily Thomas Charitable Fund, an MRC Programme grant no. G0701484 (MR/K021389/1), the BASIS funding consortium led by Autistica, a grant from the European Community's Horizon 2020 Program under grant agreement no. 642990 (Brainview), and the Innovative Medicines Initiative Joint Undertaking under grant agreement no. 115300, resources of which are composed of financial contribution from the European Union's Seventh Framework Programme (FP7/2007–2013) and of EFPIA companies' in kind contribution.

Authors' contributions

EJ, AK, and SG wrote the manuscript; AK and members of the B-ES team under the supervision of EJ, MHJ and TC collected and processed the data; AK and EJ analysed the data; SG and JG led recruitment for infants with NF1 with members of the B-ES team; EJ, SG, JG, and MHJ conceived of the study, MHJ and TC led the BASIS program; all authors edited the manuscript. All authors read and approved the final manuscript.

Competing interests

The authors declare that they have no competing interests.

Author details

[1]Centre for Brain and Cognitive Development and Department of Psychology, Birkbeck, University of London, Malet Street, London WC1E 7HX, UK. [2]Neuroscience & Experimental Psychology, Manchester Academic Health Science Centre, University of Manchester and Royal Manchester Children's Hospital, Central Manchester University Hospitals NHS Foundation, [3]

Manchester, UK. Department of Psychology, Institute of Psychiatry, Psychology & Neuroscience, King's College London, London, UK.

References

1. Baird G, et al. Prevalence of disorders of the autism spectrum in a population cohort of children in South Thames: the Special Needs and Autism Project (SNAP). Lancet. 2006;368(9531):210–5.
2. Jones EJH, Gliga T, Bedford R, Charman T, Johnson MH. Developmental pathways to autism: a review of prospective studies of infants at risk. Neurosci Biobehav Rev. 2014;39:1–33.
3. Ozonoff S, et al. Diagnostic stability in young children at risk for autism spectrum disorder: a baby siblings research consortium study. J Child Psychol Psychiatry. 2015;56(9):988–98.
4. Sanders SJ. First glimpses of the neurobiology of autism spectrum disorder. Curr Opin Genet Dev. 2015;33:80–92.
5. Hornig M, et al. Prenatal fever and autism risk. Mol Psychiatry. 2017;(00):1-8.
6. Johnson MH, Jones EJH, Gliga T. Brain adaptation and alternative developmental trajectories. Dev Psychopathol. 2015;27(2):425–42.
7. Loth E, Spooren W, Murphy DG. New treatment targets for autism spectrum disorders: EU-AIMS. Lancet Psychiatry. 2014;1(6):413–5.
8. Estes A, et al. Behavioral, cognitive, and adaptive development in infants with autism spectrum disorder in the first 2 years of life. J Neurodev Disord. 2015;7(1):1–10.
9. Clifford SM, Hudry K, Elsabbagh M, Charman T, Johnson MH. Temperament in the first 2 years of life in infants at high-risk for autism spectrum disorders. J Autism Dev Disord. 2013;43(3):673–86.
10. Flanagan JE, Landa R, Bhat A, Bauman M. Head lag in infants at risk for autism: a preliminary study. Am J Occup Ther. 2012;66(5):577–85.
11. Nickel LR, Thatcher AR, Keller F, Wozniak RH, Iverson JM. Posture development in infants at heightened vs. low risk for autism spectrum disorders. Infancy Off J Int Soc Infant Stud. 2013;18(5):639–61.
12. Libertus K, Sheperd KA, Ross SW, Landa RJ. Limited fine motor and grasping skills in 6-month-old infants at high risk for autism. Child Dev. 2014;85(6):2218–31.
13. Ozonoff S, et al. A prospective study of the emergence of early behavioral signs of autism. J Am Acad Child Adolesc Psychiatry. Mar. 2010;49(3):256–266.e2.
14. Jones EJH, et al. Reduced engagement with social stimuli in 6-month-old infants with later autism spectrum disorder: a longitudinal prospective study of infants at high familial risk. J Neurodev Disord. 2016;8:7.
15. Elsabbagh M, et al. Infant neural sensitivity to dynamic eye gaze is associated with later emerging autism. Curr Biol. 2012;22(4):338–42.
16. Jones W, Klin A. Attention to eyes is present but in decline in 2-6-month-old infants later diagnosed with autism. Nature. 2013;504(7480): 427–31.
17. Macari SL, Campbell D, Gengoux GW, Saulnier CA, Klin AJ, Chawarska K. Predicting developmental status from 12 to 24 months in infants at risk for autism spectrum disorder: a preliminary report. J Autism Dev Disord. 2012;42(12):2636–47.
18. Ozonoff S, Macari S, Young GS, Goldring S, Thompson M, Rogers SJ. Atypical object exploration at 12 months of age is associated with autism in a prospective sample. Autism Int J Res Pract. 2008;12(5):457–72.
19. Zwaigenbaum L, Bryson S, Rogers T, Roberts W, Brian J, Szatmari P. Behavioral manifestations of autism in the first year of life. Int J Dev Neurosci Off J Int Soc Dev Neurosci. 2005;23(2–3):143–52.
20. Gammer I, et al. Behavioural markers for autism in infancy: scores on the Autism Observational Scale for infants in a prospective study of at-risk siblings. Infant Behav. Dev. 2015;38:107–15.
21. Richards C, Jones C, Groves L, Moss J, Oliver C. Prevalence of autism spectrum disorder phenomenology in genetic disorders: a systematic review and meta-analysis. Lancet Psychiatry. 2015;2(10):909–16.
22. Reddy KS. Cytogenetic abnormalities and fragile-X syndrome in autism spectrum disorder. BMC Med Genet. 2005;6:3.
23. Evans DG, et al. Birth incidence and prevalence of tumor-prone syndromes: estimates from a UK family genetic register service. Am J Med Genet A. 2010;152A(2):327–32.
24. Lehtonen A, et al. Cognition in children with neurofibromatosis type 1: data from a population-based study. Dev Med Child Neurol. 2015;57(7):645–51.
25. Garg S, et al. Neurofibromatosis type 1 and autism spectrum disorder. Pediatrics. 2013;132(6):e1642–8.
26. Garg S, et al. Autism spectrum disorder profile in neurofibromatosis type I. J Autism Dev Disord. 2015;45(6):1649–57.
27. Costa RM, et al. Mechanism for the learning deficits in a mouse model of neurofibromatosis type 1. Nature. 2002;415(6871):526–30.
28. Molosh AI, et al. Social learning and amygdala disruptions in Nf1 mice are rescued by blocking p21-activated kinase. Nat Neurosci. 2014;17(11): 1583–90.
29. Diggs-Andrews KA, Tokuda K, Izumi Y, Zorumski CF, Wozniak DF, Gutmann DH. Dopamine deficiency underlies learning deficits in neurofibromatosis-1 mice. Ann Neurol. 2013;73(2):309–15.
30. Diggs-Andrews KA, Gutmann DH. Modeling cognitive dysfunction in neurofibromatosis-1. Trends Neurosci. 2013;36(4):237.
31. Li W, et al. The HMG-CoA reductase inhibitor lovastatin reverses the learning and attention deficits in a mouse model of neurofibromatosis type 1. Curr Biol CB. 2005;15(21):1961–7.
32. Omrani A, et al. HCN channels are a novel therapeutic target for cognitive dysfunction in Neurofibromatosis type 1. Mol Psychiatry. 2015; 20(11):1311–21.
33. van der Vaart T, et al. Simvastatin for cognitive deficits and behavioural problems in patients with neurofibromatosis type 1 (NF1-SIMCODA): a randomised, placebo-controlled trial. Lancet Neurol. 2013;12(11):1076–83.
34. Green J, et al. Randomised trial of a parent-mediated intervention for infants at high risk for autism: longitudinal outcomes to age 3 years. J Child Psychol Psychiatry. 2017; https://doi.org/10.1111/jcpp.12728.
35. Littler M, Morton NE. Segregation analysis of peripheral neurofibromatosis (NF1). J Med Genet. 1990;27(5):307–10.
36. Office of Medical Applications of Research, National Institutes of Health. Neurofibromatosis. Conference statement. National Institutes of Health Consensus Development Conference. Arch Neurol. 1988;45(5):575–8.
37. Mullen EM. Mullen scales of early learning. MN: AGS Circle Pines; 1995.
38. Sparrow SS. Vineland Adaptive Behavior Scales. In: Kreutzer JS, DeLuca J, Caplan B, editors. Encyclopedia of clinical neuropsychology. NY: Springer; 2011. p. 2618–21.
39. Bryson SE, Zwaigenbaum L. Autism Observation Scale for Infants. In: Patel VB, Preedy VR, Martin CR, editors. Comprehensive guide to autism. New York: Springer; 2014. p. 299–310.
40. Brian J, et al. Clinical assessment of autism in high-risk 18-month-olds. Autism. 2008;12(5):433–56.
41. Bryson SE, Zwaigenbaum L, McDermott C, Rombough V, Brian J. The Autism Observation Scale for Infants: scale development and reliability data. J Autism Dev Disord. 2008;38(4):731–8.
42. Putnam SP, Helbig AL, Gartstein MA, Rothbart MK, Leerkes E. Development and assessment of short and very short forms of the infant behavior questionnaire-revised. J Pers Assess. 2014;96(4):445–58.
43. Hogan AL, Caravella KE, Ezell J, Rague L, Hills K, Roberts JE. Autism spectrum disorder symptoms in infants with fragile X syndrome: a prospective case series. J Autism Dev Disord. 2017;47(6):1628–44.
44. Gartstein MA, Rothbart MK. Studying infant temperament via the revised infant behavior questionnaire. Infant Behav Dev. 2003;26(1):64–86.
45. Dunn W, Daniels DB. Initial development of the infant/toddler sensory profile. J Early Interv. 2002;25(1):27–41.
46. Ozonoff S, et al. A prospective study of the emergence of early behavioral signs of autism. J Am Acad Child Adolesc Psychiatry. 2010; 49(3):256–266.e2.
47. Klein-Tasman BP, et al. Cognitive and psychosocial phenotype of young children with neurofibromatosis 1. J Int Neuropsychol Soc JINS. 2014;20(1).88–98.
48. Brei NG, Klein-Tasman BP, Schwarz GN, Casnar CL. Language in young children with neurofibromatosis-1: relations to functional communication, attention, and social functioning. Res Dev Disabil. 2014;35(10):2495–504.
49. Lorenzo J, Barton B, Acosta MT, North K. Mental, motor, and language development of toddlers with neurofibromatosis type 1. J Pediatr. 2011;158(4):660–5.
50. Hummelvoll G, Antonsen KM. Young adults' experience of living with neurofibromatosis type 1. J Genet Couns. 2013;22(2):188–99.

50. Hummelvoll G, Antonsen KM. Young adults' experience of living with neurofibromatosis type 1. J Genet Couns. 2013;22(2):188–99.
51. Pride NA, Crawford H, Payne JM, North KN. Social functioning in adults with neurofibromatosis type 1. Res Dev Disabil. 2013;34(10):3393–9.
52. Ferner RE, et al. Guidelines for the diagnosis and management of individuals with neurofibromatosis 1. J Med Genet. 2007;44(2):81.
53. Kolanczyk M, et al. Multiple roles for neurofibromin in skeletal development and growth. Hum Mol Genet. 2007;16(8):874–86.
54. Sullivan K, et al. NF1 is a critical regulator of muscle development and metabolism. Hum Mol Genet. 2014;23(5):1250–9.
55. McDonald NM, et al. Early autism symptoms in infants with tuberous sclerosis complex. Autism Res Off J Int Soc Autism Res. 2017. (e-print ahead of publication). doi:10.1002/aur.1846.

4

Effect of epilepsy on autism symptoms in Angelman syndrome

Kristin A. Bakke[1*], Patricia Howlin[2,3], Lars Retterstøl[4], Øivind J. Kanavin[5], Arvid Heiberg[4] and Terje Nærland[1,6]

Abstract

Background: Autism spectrum disorder and epilepsy often co-occur; however, the extent to which the association between autism symptoms and epilepsy is due to shared aetiology or to the direct effects of seizures is a topic of ongoing debate. Angelman syndrome (AS) is presented as a suitable disease model to explore this association.

Methods: Data from medical records and questionnaires were used to examine the association between age of epilepsy onset, autism symptoms, genetic aberration and communication level. Forty-eight participants had genetically verified AS (median age 14.5 years; range 1–57 years). A measure of autism symptoms (the Social Communication Questionnaire; SCQ) was completed for 38 individuals aged ≥ 4 years. Genetic cause was subgrouped into deletion and other genetic aberrations of the 15q11-q13 area. The number of signs used to communicate (< 20 sign and ≥ 20 signs) was used as a measure of nonverbal communication.

Results: Mean age of epilepsy onset was 3.0 years (range 3 months–7.8 years). Mean SCQ score for individuals without epilepsy was 13.6 (SD = 6.7) and with epilepsy 17.0 (SD = 5.6; $p = 0.17$); 58% used fewer than 20 signs to communicate. There were no age differences between groups according to presence of epilepsy, level of nonverbal communication or type of genetic aberration. SCQ scores were higher in individuals with the deletion than in those with other genetic aberrations (18.7 vs 10.8 $p = 0.008$) and higher in the group who used < 20 signs to communicate (19.4 vs 14.1 $p = 0.007$). Age of epilepsy onset was correlated with SCQ ($r = -0.61$, $p < 0.001$). Multiple regression showed that age of seizure onset was significantly related to SCQ score ($\beta = -0.90$; $p = 0.006$), even when the type of genetic abnormality was controlled ($R^2 = 0.53$; $F = 10.7$; $p = 0.001$).

Conclusions: The study provides support for the notion that seizures themselves contribute more to autism symptoms than expected from the underlying genetic pathology alone. The study demonstrates how a rare genetic syndrome such as Angelman syndrome may be used to study the relation between epilepsy and autism symptomatology.

Keywords: Angelman syndrome, Autism spectrum disorder, Epilepsy, Epileptic encephalopathy, Seizure onset

Background

Angelman syndrome (AS) is a neurodevelopmental disorder caused by an absent or non-functioning maternal allele of chromosome 15q11-q13 [1]. The typical AS phenotype is characterized by intellectual disability (ID), lack of speech, hyperactivity, ataxic gait, microcephaly, sleep disturbances, frequent laughter/smiling and an apparently happy demeanour [1–4]. ID ranges from moderate to profound, with most individuals functioning in the severe to profound range [5, 6]. Epilepsy occurs in 80% or more of cases [2, 7], usually involving multiple seizure types and starting in early childhood [7, 8]. High rates of autistic symptoms are also reported [9–11], with prevalence estimates of autism spectrum disorder (ASD) ranging from 24 to 81% [6, 10]. AS can be due to *UBE3A* mutations, uniparental disomy and imprinting defects [1, 12], but deletions are the predominant cause and are found in 68–75% of patients. Deletions are also associated with more severe AS-phenotype, and co-deletion of $GABA_A$-receptor genes (*GABRB3*, *GABRA5* and *GABRG3*) located adjacent to *UBE3A* gene is suggested as a possible explanation for this [1]. Dysfunction of *GABRB3* is highly associated with both epilepsy and autism symptoms [13, 14].

* Correspondence: kristinb@ous-hf.no
[1]NevSom, Department of Rare Disorders, Oslo University Hospital, Oslo, Norway
Full list of author information is available at the end of the article

A strong association between autism symptoms, epilepsy and ID has been found in a number of other genetic syndromes, such as fragile X and tuberous sclerosis complex (TSC), as well as in AS [6, 10]. It is evident, too, that the negative effect of seizures is particularly strong during infancy and early childhood [15–18]. Thus, onset of seizures during the first year of life is associated with increased prevalence and severity of ID and ASD and increased prevalence of brain abnormalities [19, 20]. However, there is a continuing debate [21–24] as to whether autism symptoms, epilepsy and ID are independent comorbidities [15, 16, 21, 25–27], whether they are all outcomes of the same underlying pathophysiological/genetic mechanisms [17, 21, 25, 28], or whether the epilepsy itself contributes to more severe cognitive and behavioural impairments than might be expected from the underlying pathology alone [15, 17, 29, 30], i.e. a so-called encephalopathic effect [30].

There are several reasons why AS offers a suitable disease model to investigate the association between epilepsy, ID and autism symptoms. Firstly, the rate of epilepsy in AS (> 80%) is as high as or higher than other genetic disorders in which epilepsy and autism commonly co-occur (e.g. TSC [80–90%]; fragile X syndrome [10–20%]) [29, 31, 32]. Secondly, epilepsy in AS tends to start in very early childhood. Seizures are also often treatment-resistant and refractory epilepsy has been shown to be an important predictor of autism symptoms [33]. Thirdly, unlike genetic conditions such as TSC, in which the numbers and location of tubers are associated with autism symptoms [17, 34], there are no specific structural brain abnormalities in AS that are known to affect the phenotype. Fourthly, knowledge of the specific genetic defects that cause AS makes it possible to evaluate the degree to which the association between epilepsy and autism symptoms is a result of the underlying genetic abnormality and to assess the independent contribution of seizures on level of autism symptoms.

The aims of the current study were to describe epilepsy characteristics and then investigate the relationship between epilepsy, autism symptoms, communication level and genetic cause in individuals with AS. Based on previous research on other populations with childhood epilepsy including TSC [18, 33, 35–37], we hypothesized that age of onset of epilepsy would be related to the number of autism symptoms in AS independent of the effect of the specific genetic abnormality.

Methods

The study was approved by the regional ethics committee in Norway (REK 2014/1880).

Recruitment procedures

From the records of the Frambu Resource Centre for Rare Disorders in Norway and the Norwegian Angelman Association, 115 individuals with AS were identified. Letters were sent to the parents/guardians of these individuals, and they were asked to complete two questionnaires: the Social Communication Questionnaire (SCQ), which measures autism symptoms [38], and a study-specific questionnaire assessing epilepsy, medication and developmental parameters. Written informed consent was given by all parents/guardians allowing the researchers access to medical records from all hospitals in Norway (Fig. 1).

Measures

Clinical information on epilepsy and genetic abnormality

Participants' medical records were used to collect information regarding epilepsy and the nature of the genetic abnormality. Information on age of epilepsy onset, type of seizure and treatment with anti-epileptic drugs was recorded when available. Medical records were not comprehensive for all individuals, and formal seizure classification was not always performed.

Genetic data were also variable. When information was available, the genetic abnormality was dichotomised into 'deletion' or 'other' (i.e. uniparental disomy, imprinting defects and point mutations).

Autism symptoms

The lifetime version of SCQ was used to assess the number of autism symptoms [38]. The SCQ contains 40 items scored 0 or 1 and was designed to screen for a possible diagnosis of autism in individuals aged 4 years and older and with a mental age above 2 years [38]. It has also frequently been used to measure autistic-type symptoms in individuals with genetic syndromes including those with AS [9, 11]. We did not classify participants as meeting/not meeting the suggested cut-off scores for autism or ASD (≥ 22 and ≥ 15, respectively [38]) since the validity of these criteria has not been established for individuals with genetic disorders associated with severe ID. Nevertheless, SCQ has often been used as the screening tool in samples with low IQ [39, 40].

Communication level

Information about level of development was particularly variable and often very limited. Although many parents reported that they had previously been told their child had severe to profound intellectual disability (in 7 cases, the description was of 'moderate' disability), formal test results were rarely recorded, and hence, the validity of these categories was unknown. Although there were no adequate data on IQ/developmental level, we did have data on communication level. Signing was the major mean of communication for most of the participants; the majority had no use of words and no one used more than 20 words. Categorical ratings of 'use of signs' (< 20 and 20–100 and > 100) were used to divide individuals

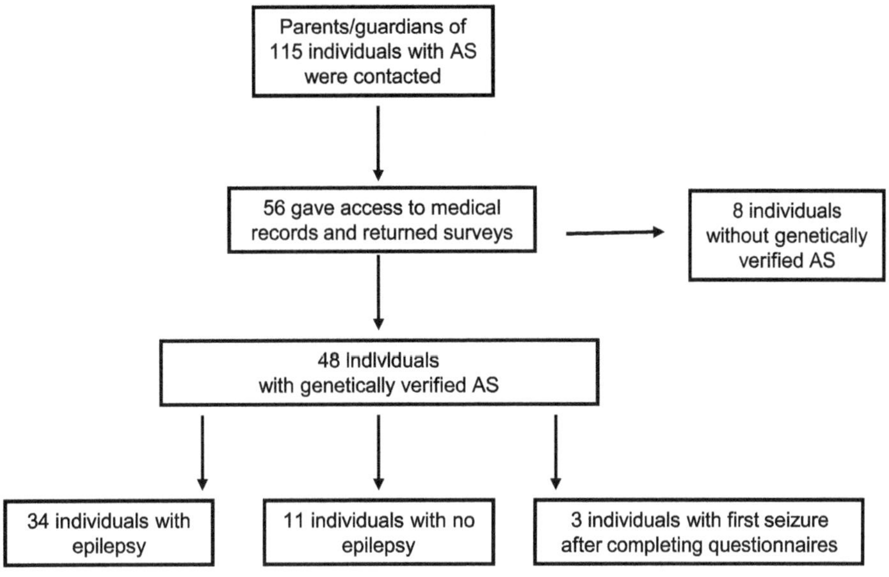

Fig. 1 Recruitment

into two groups; those using fewer than 20 signs to communicate and those with more than 20 signs.

Participants

Inclusion criteria

For the descriptive part of the study ('Epilepsy characteristics'), individuals were included if their parents/guardians gave their consent to participation/access to medical records and if their son/daughter had a genetically verified diagnosis of AS. For the second part of the study ('Relation between epilepsy and autism symptoms, nonverbal communication level and genetic aberration'), individuals were required to be at least 4 years of age (i.e. minimum age for the SCQ).

Parents/guardians of 56 out of the 115 individuals identified from the records (49%) consented to participate; 48 of these individuals (age range 1–57 years; median 14 years 6 months) had a genetically verified AS diagnosis. At the time of questionnaire completion (see Fig. 1), medical records confirmed that 34 individuals had epilepsy and 11 individuals did not. Three boys (aged 1, 1, and 4 years, respectively) subsequently developed seizures; hence, the 4-year-old was included in the no-epilepsy group in the part 2 of the study. SCQ questionnaires were completed for 38 of 40 individuals aged 4 years or older (SCQ was not completed for two participants aged 57 and 40 years). See Table 1 for participants' characteristics.

Statistical analysis

Associations between quantitative measures were analyzed by parametric statistics in SPSS (t test, Pearson's r). Due to small sample size, Mann-Whitney U test was used when comparing SCQ in subgroups with/without epilepsy and when comparing SCQ and age of epilepsy onset in subgroups with/without deletion. Fisher's exact test was used for categorical data. Due to small and unequal sample sizes, Hedges' g was used for effect sizes. Normality of residuals was checked using visual inspection of *P-P* plots. Multiple regression analysis was conducted to assess the impact of 'age at epilepsy onset'and 'type of genetic aberration' on SCQ scores. Due to the combination of dichotomous and continuous covariates, we report the standardized coefficients (β). To correct for multiple comparisons, a significance level of $p \leq 0.01$ was chosen; Bonferroni 'rule of thumb' was used to determine appropriate p level ($p = 0.05/5 = 0.01$).

Table 1 Characteristics of participants with Angelman syndrome in parts 1 and 2 of study

	Age	Gender	Genetics
Part 1: Epilepsy characteristics (n=48)	Range: 1–57 years Mean: 17.1 years Median: 14.5 years	Male: 30 Female: 18	Deletion: 26 (16 males) UPD: 4 (2 males) Imprinting: 3 (1 male) Mutation: 2 (1 male) Unknown: 13 (10 males)
Part 2: Relation between epilepsy and autism symptoms, nonverbal communication level and genetic aberration (n=40)	Range: 1–57 years Mean: 20.2 years Median: 19.1 years	Male: 30 Female: 15	Deletion: 26 (16 males) UPD: 2 (2 males) Imprinting: 2 (1 male) Mutation: 2 (1 male) Unknown: 12 (9 males)

Results

Part 1: epilepsy characteristics

Age of first seizure ranged from 3 months to 7 years 10 months (mean 3 years 0 months, SD 2 years 2 months). Four individuals had their initial seizure during the first year of life; 11 developed epilepsy during the second year. The number and type of seizures varied among individuals and varied over time in the same individuals. Two individuals (aged 38 and 27 years) had been diagnosed with Lennox-Gastaut syndrome. One individual had only 'atypical absence seizures', and all others had seizures with 'jerks' or 'convulsions'. More than one seizure type was recorded in 33 individuals. Seizures resembling generalized tonic-clonic seizures (sometimes described as generalized convulsions) were reported in 29 individuals. Seizures resembling atypical absence seizures were seen in 17 individuals, myoclonic seizures in 10 and atonic seizures in 13. Focal seizures were seen in four individuals. Sixteen individuals had their first seizure during a febrile episode, and 10 participants were reported to have epileptic seizures that were aggravated by fever. EEGs were recorded repeatedly in several participants, and findings were typical of those reported in AS [2]. When EEGs were recorded prior to first seizure, delta waves but no epileptiform activity were often reported. More epileptiform discharges in EEGs were recorded during periods of seizure aggravation. Seizures were commonly reported to be resistant to anti-epileptic drugs and drug resistance was particularly marked before 6 years of age, and 21 individuals had received benzodiazepine as emergency treatment. Three individuals had been treated with only one anti-epileptic drug, and all others had tried two or more anti-epileptic drugs. Valproate was the most frequently prescribed anti-epileptic drug (31 participants), followed by nitrazepam (18) and clonazepam (16).

Part 2: the relation between epilepsy and autism symptoms, nonverbal communication level and genetic aberration

Mean SCQ was 16.3 (SD = 5.9 range: 0–27). SCQ scores were higher in individuals with epilepsy ($n = 31$) than in those without ($n = 7$), but the difference was not significant (see Table 2). SCQ and age were not correlated ($p = 0.12$). Level of nonverbal communication did not differ between individuals with and without epilepsy; 19 of 33 (58%) with epilepsy and 4 of 7 (57%) (exact $p = 1.000$) without epilepsy used fewer than 20 signs to communicate. Individuals with the deletion were more likely to be in the group using < 20 signs to communicate than individuals with other genetic aberrations (exact $p = 0.022$).

Within the epilepsy group, age of epilepsy onset was lower among individuals using < 20 signs to communicate. Individuals with the deletion had significantly higher SCQ scores and lower age at epilepsy onset than individuals with other genetic aberrations. There were no differences in age between groups (see Table 2 for details).

Age at epilepsy onset was highly correlated with SCQ score ($r = -0.61$, $p = 0.0004$). A linear regression was conducted with SCQ as the dependent variable and age at seizure onset and type of genetic abnormality as the covariates (forced entry). Age at onset of seizures had an independent contribution when entering the type of genetic aberration as a covariate. The type of genetic aberration did not have an independent contribution in this model (see Table 3 and Fig. 2). As a supplementary analysis, we included level of nonverbal communication as a third covariate. Age of epilepsy onset was significant also in this model ($\beta = -0.81$, $p = 0.007$).

Discussion

This study explored the relationship between age of epilepsy onset, autism symptomatology, type of genetic aberration and nonverbal communication level in a Norwegian sample of individuals with AS. Among the 56 individuals with AS identified from the available databases, 48 (86%) had genetically verified AS. This is in line with other reports noting that no genetic abnormality can be identified in 10–15% of individuals with AS [4]. Other clinical findings were similar to those of previous studies of AS. Thus, deletions were the most common genetic cause identified [1, 4]. With regard to epilepsy, the prevalence in this study was 77%, somewhat lower than the rates of ≥ 80% commonly reported [4, 7, 8, 41]. However, our sample included several very young participants who may not yet have had their first seizure. We also excluded individuals in whom the cause of AS was unknown and there is some indication

Table 2 SCQ scores and age at onset of epilepsy according to communication level and genetic aberration

	Epilepsy ($N = 31$)	No epilepsy ($N = 7$)		Epilepsy and level of nonverbal communication ($n = 31$)			Epilepsy and type of genetic aberration ($n = 23$)		
			p value [Hedges' *g*]	< 20 signs ($n = 17$)	≥ 20 signs ($n = 14$)	*p* value [Hedges' *g*]	Deletion ($n = 18$)	Other genetic aberration ($n = 5$)	*p* value [Hedges' *g*]
SCQ mean (SD)	17.0 (5.6)	13.6 (6.7)	0.354 [0.59]	19.4 (4.4)	14.1 (5.7)	0.007 [1.05]	18.7 (5.0)	10.8 (6.6)	0.007 [1.48]
Age at onset of epilepsy mean (SD)	36.6 months (26.0)	na	na	30.2 months (18.5)	44.4 months (32.1)	0.160 [0.56]	25.2 months (13.7)	79.0 months (19.3)	< 0.001 [3.60]
Age (SD)	20.0 years (9.7)	13.0 years (9.6)	0.170 [0.72]	21.4 years (10.6)	18.2 years (8.6)	0.57 [0.33]	16.6 years (5.2)	17.4 years (9.5)	0.104 [0.13]

SCQ Social Communication Questionnaire score, *na* not applicable

Table 3 Statistical results of regression model with SCQ as dependent outcome

Covariate	Standardized coefficients β	p	Unstandardized coefficients B	Standard error	95% confidence interval
Model with two covariates $R^2 = 0.53$; $F = 10, 7$; $p = 0.001$					
Age at epilepsy onset	− 0.90	0.006	− 0.21	0.07	− 0.35/− 0.07
Genetic aberration	− 0.22	0.45	− 3.24	4.23	− 12.01/5.61

that individuals with AS of unknown cause may have the highest prevalence of seizures [7]. Epilepsy characteristics with early-onset epilepsy, multiple seizure types, a tendency to have seizures during febrile episodes and commonly treatment-resistant seizures, particularly in early childhood, are also in line with the findings reported by others [2, 7, 8, 41, 42], and the use of anti-epileptic drugs is comparable to other studies [7, 8, 41].

The main focus of the study was the association between age of epilepsy onset and extent of autism symptomatology when type of genetic abnormality was controlled for. Our findings from this study of individuals with AS provide support for the notion that seizures themselves contribute more to autism symptoms than might be expected from the underlying pathology alone [15–17, 21]. As anticipated, individuals with a deletion of 15q11-q13 had substantially more autism symptoms than individuals with other genetic aberrations ($g = 1.48$). However, when entered into a regression model with epilepsy onset, genetic aberration made no significant contribution to the number of autism symptoms reported. Although the lack of an independent effect of type of genetic aberration is likely due to the low number of causes other than deletion, it should be noted that the slope of the regression lines is similar for both genetic subgroups, thus supporting the importance of age at seizure onset across the sample. These findings from AS parallel evidence from studies in other rare disorders such as TSC; although both early seizures and encephalopathy are highly associated with type of genetic abnormality, early seizures may contribute to a worsening of developmental outcome [17, 43]. Similarly, from fragile X syndrome, research indicates that males with the FMR1 premutation are more likely to have ASD and ID if seizures occur in childhood [29, 44].

Although individuals with epilepsy had more autism symptoms than those without epilepsy, and despite a moderate to large effect size, this difference was not significant [15]. This may be due to the rarity of non-epilepsy cases among individuals with AS and hence the very small size of the no-epilepsy group. However, the findings also point towards the importance of viewing epilepsy as a spectrum disorder rather than a dichotomy [15]. Hence, the comorbidity between autism symptoms and epilepsy may be related both to the underlying pathology and to the effect of seizures. The high risk of ASD in populations with early-onset epilepsy has been used to support the encephalopathy hypothesis, i.e. that seizures may cause ASD [16, 25]. Others have argued against this because the relationship is bi-directional and individuals with ASD are at increased risk of future epilepsy and seizures may occur in adolescence or

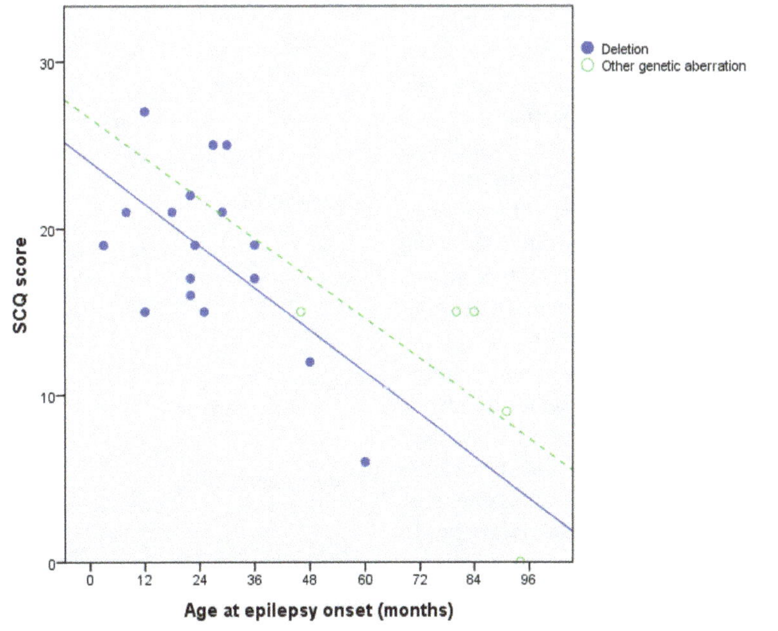

Fig. 2 Scatterplot of age at onset of epilepsy and SCQ. Fit-lines are shown according to the type of genetic abnormality

adulthood [21, 22, 45, 46]. This study highlights the importance of considering the additive effects of the underlying genetic aetiology and seizures contributing to autism symptoms in AS, which may be relevant also for other conditions [15, 29]. The encephalopathic effect may be greater when seizures start early. Early-life seizures may result in molecular changes which impact neural network structure, and the hippocampal region may be of particular importance. Molecular changes may also influence the expression of genes involved in autism symptoms and genetic syndromes such as *GABRB3*, *FMR1*, *TSC1* and *TSC2* [16, 29]. Moreover, research suggests that effects of seizures on $GABA_A$-receptor expression are age-dependent, a finding that further supports the notion that early seizures are particularly harmful [16].

There was no difference in the level of nonverbal communication between the epilepsy group and no–epilepsy group. Age of first seizure however, was associated with nonverbal communication ($g = 0.56$) and individuals with the lowest level of nonverbal communication had earlier seizure onset than those who used more signs to communicate. A number of other studies has found that earlier age of seizure onset is associated with poorer cognitive outcome [18, 33, 35–37, 47, 48]. Our study did not include a measure of development, only a measure of nonverbal communication. However, supplemental analysis showed that age of epilepsy remained significant also when nonverbal communication was entered as a covariate. This suggests that the number of autism symptoms was not explained only by the level of nonverbal communication.

Although the findings of this exploratory study have potentially important implications for understanding the complex links between autism symptoms and epilepsy, there are a number of limitations that must be taken into account in the interpretation of the data. Firstly, the sample size was small and the age of participants was very wide, ranging from infancy to adulthood. In addition, we did not have data on the level of ID, only an estimate of nonverbal communication was available. There were also few individuals with a genetic cause other than the 15q11 deletion, and we lacked data on size of deletions. Furthermore, information from medical records was often incomplete and formal seizure classification, except for tonic-clonic seizures, was rarely performed. Hence, some individuals may have had more types and higher frequency of seizures than reported (particularly those of short duration or less severe such as absences and myoclonic seizures). Finally, there was no clinical assessment of autism, and rather than a categorical distinction between ASD/non-ASD, we focused on the frequency of autism symptoms as measured by the SCQ. While this avoided the problems of misdiagnosing ASD in a population with severe developmental delay, it is well established that the number of autism symptoms is highly related to severity of ID [11]. Thus, high rates of autism symptoms were to be expected in this sample of individuals with AS [9, 10]. The severity of ID in AS is the main limitation when using this disorder as a disease model for studying the relation between autism symptoms and epilepsy.

It is clear that information from a larger sample of individuals with AS, with a larger range of genetic causes other than deletions, and detailed information on developmental level is needed to increase confidence in the current findings. More details of the genetic aberration, such as size and exact break points of the deletions, are also needed. Finally, further studies in this area should investigate which autism symptoms are particularly vulnerable to early seizures and which are less affected. Such knowledge may be of relevance for better understanding of the biology of ASD.

Conclusions

This study provides support for the notion that, in individuals with AS, seizures themselves contribute more to autism symptoms than expected from the underlying genetic pathology. This study demonstrates how a rare condition may illuminate core issues in research on developmental disorders. Individuals with Angelman syndrome show limited variation in genetic aetiology, and the condition is therefore a suitable one in which to investigate the relation between epilepsy and autism symptoms.

Abbreviations

AS: Angelman syndrome; ASD: Autism spectrum disorder; ID: Intellectual disability; SCQ: Social Communication Questionnaire; TSC: Tuberous sclerosis complex

Acknowledgements

We are thankful to the participants in the study and the Norwegian Angelman Society. We are thankful to Bjørg Hoem for sending out the questionnaires. This study is part of the BUPgen study group and the research network NeuroDevelop.

Funding

This study was funded by NevSom, University Hospital of Oslo.

Authors' contributions

KAB, ØJK, AH and TN planned and designed the study. KAB collected the clinical information from the medical records, and LR and AH collected the genetic data. KAB, PH and TN analysed the data and interpreted the results. KAB wrote the first draft of the manuscript. All authors contributed to the manuscript and have read and approved the final manuscript.

Competing interests
The authors declare that they have no competing interests.

Author details
[1]NevSom, Department of Rare Disorders, Oslo University Hospital, Oslo, Norway. [2]Institute of Psychiatry, Psychology and Neuroscience, King's College London, London, UK. [3]Faculty of Health Sciences, University of Sydney, Sydney, NSW, Australia. [4]Department of Medical Genetics, Oslo University Hospital, Oslo, Norway. [5]Frambu National Resource Center for Rare Disorders, Siggerud, Norway. [6]NORMENT, Institute of Clinical Medicine, University of Oslo, Oslo, Norway.

References

1. Buiting K, Williams C, Horsthemke B. Angelman syndrome—insights into a rare neurogenetic disorder. Nat Rev Neurol. 2016;12:584–93.
2. Thibert RL, Larson AM, Hsieh DT, Raby AR, Thiele EA. Neurologic manifestations of Angelman syndrome. Pediatr Neurol. 2013;48:271–9.
3. Pelc K, Cheron G, Dan B. Behavior and neuropsychiatric manifestations in Angelman syndrome. Neuropsychiatr Dis Treat. 2008;4:577–84.
4. Dagli AI, Mueller J, Williams CA. Angelman syndrome. In.: GeneReviews[Internet]; 2015.
5. Peters SU, Goddard-Finegold J, Beaudet AL, Madduri N, Turcich M, Bacino CA. Cognitive and adaptive behavior profiles of children with Angelman syndrome. Am J Med Genet A. 2004;128:110–3.
6. Moss J, Howlin P. Autism spectrum disorders in genetic syndromes: implications for diagnosis, intervention and understanding the wider autism spectrum disorder population. J Intellect Disabil Res. 2009;53:852–73.
7. Thibert RL, Conant KD, Braun EK, Bruno P, Said RR, Nespeca MP, et al. Epilepsy in Angelman syndrome: a questionnaire-based assessment of the natural history and current treatment options. Epilepsia. 2009;50:2369–76.
8. Fiumara A, Pittalà A, Cocuzza M, Sorge G. Epilepsy in patients with Angelman syndrome. Ital J Pediatr. 2010;36:31.
9. Moss J, Howlin P, Hastings RP, Beaumont S, Griffith GM, Petty J, et al. Social behavior and characteristics of autism spectrum disorder in Angelman, Cornelia de Lange, and cri du chat syndromes. Am J Intellect Dev Disabil. 2013;118:262–83.
10. Richards C, Jones C, Groves L, Moss J, Oliver C. Prevalence of autism spectrum disorder phenomenology in genetic disorders: a systematic review and meta-analysis. Lancet Psychiatry. 2015;2:909–16.
11. Moss J, Howlin P, Oliver C. The assessment and presentation of autism spectrum disorder and associated characteristics in individuals with severe intellectual disability and genetic syndromes. In: Burack J, Hodapp R, Iarocci G, Zigler E, (Eds). The Oxford Handbook of Intellectual Disability and Development. New York: Oxford University Press; 2011. pp. 275–302.
12. Gentile JK, Tan WH, Horowitz LT, Bacino CA, Skinner SA, Barbieri-Welge R, et al. A neurodevelopmental survey of Angelman syndrome with genotype-phenotype correlations. J Dev Behav Pediatr. 2010;31:592–601.
13. Frye RE, Casanova MF, Fatemi SH, Folsom TD, Reutiman TJ, Brown GL, et al. Neuropathological mechanisms of seizures in autism spectrum disorder. Front Neurosci. 2016;10:192.
14. Tanaka M, DeLorey TM, Delgado-Escueta A, Olsen RW. GABRB3, epilepsy, and neurodevelopment. In: Noebels JL, Avoli M, Rogawski MA, Olsen RW, Delgado-Escueta AV, editors. Jasper's basic mechanisms of the epilepsies. [Internet]. Bethesda (MD): National Center for Biotechnology Information (US); 2012.
15. Jensen FE. Epilepsy as a spectrum disorder: implications from novel clinical and basic neuroscience. Epilepsia. 2011;52:1–6.
16. Brooks-Kayal A. Molecular mechanisms of cognitive and behavioral comorbidities of epilepsy in children. Epilepsia. 2011;52:13–20.
17. Curatolo P, Aronica E, Jansen A, Jansen F, Kotulska K, Lagae L, et al. Early onset epileptic encephalopathy or genetically determined encephalopathy with early onset epilepsy? Lessons learned from TSC. Eur Journal Paediatr Neurol. 2016;20:203–11.
18. Capal JK, Bernardino-Cuesta B, Horn PS, Murray D, Byars AW, Bing NM, et al. Influence of seizures on early development in tuberous sclerosis complex. Epilepsy Behav. 2017;70:245 52.
19. Saemundsen E, Ludvigsson P, Hilmarsdottir I, Rafnsson V. Autism spectrum disorders in children with seizures in the first year of life—a population-based study. Epilepsia. 2007;48:1724–30.
20. Saemundsen E, Ludvigsson P, Rafnsson V. Risk of autism spectrum disorders after infantile spasms: a population-based study nested in a cohort with seizures in the first year of life. Epilepsia. 2008;49:1865–70.
21. Scott RC, Tuchman R. Epilepsy and autism spectrum disorders. Relatively related Neurology. 2016;87:130–1.
22. Sundelin HE, Larsson H, Lichtenstein P, Almqvist C, Hultman CM, Tomson T, et al. Autism and epilepsy: a population-based nationwide cohort study. Neurology. 2016;87:192–7.
23. Sundelin HE, Ludvigsson JF. Author response: autism and epilepsy: a population-based nationwide cohort study. Neurology. 2017;88:110.
24. Sethi NK. Letter re: autism and epilepsy. A population-based nationwide cohort study. Neurology. 2017;88:110.
25. Jeste SS, Tuchman R. Autism spectrum disorder and epilepsy: two sides of the same coin? J Child Neurol. 2015;30:1963–71.
26. Casanova EL, Sharp JL, Chakraborty H, Sumi NS, Casanova MF. Genes with high penetrance for syndromic and non-syndromic autism typically function within the nucleus and regulate gene expression. Mol Autism. 2016;7:18.
27. Berg AT, Plioplys S. Epilepsy and autism: is there a special relationship? Epilepsy Behav. 2012;23:193–8.
28. Amiet C, Gourfinkel-An I, Laurent C, Bodeau N, Génin B, Leguern E, et al. Does epilepsy in multiplex autism pedigrees define a different subgroup in terms of clinical characteristics and genetic risk? Mol Autism. 2013;4:47.
29. Hagerman RJ. Epilepsy drives autism in neurodevelopmental disorders. Dev Med Child Neurol. 2013;55:101–2.
30. Berg AT, Berkovic SF, Brodie MJ, Buchhalter J, Cross JH, Van Emde BW, et al. Revised terminology and concepts for organization of seizures and epilepsies: report of the ILAE Commission on Classification and Terminology, 2005–2009. Epilepsia. 2010;51:676–85.
31. Saxena A, Sampson JR. Epilepsy in tuberous sclerosis: phenotypes, mechanisms, and treatments. Semin Neurol. 2015;35:269–76.
32. Hagerman PJ, Stafstrom CE. Origins of epilepsy in fragile X syndrome. Epilepsy Curr. 2009;9:108–12.
33. van Eeghen AM, Pulsifer MB, Merker VL, Neumeyer AM, van Eeghen EE, Thibert RL, et al. Understanding relationships between autism, intelligence, and epilepsy: a cross-disorder approach. Dev Med Child Neurol. 2013;55:146–53.
34. Bolton PF, Griffiths PD. Association of tuberous sclerosis of temporal lobes with autism and atypical autism. Lancet. 1997;349:392–5.
35. Korman B, Krsek P, Duchowny M, Maton B, Pacheco-Jacome E, Rey G. Early seizure onset and dysplastic lesion extent independently disrupt cognitive networks. Neurology. 2013;81:745–51.
36. Ma Y, Chen G, Wang Y, Xu K. Language dysfunction is associated with age of onset of benign epilepsy with centrotemporal spikes in children. Eur Neurol. 2015;73:179–83.
37. Hermann B, Seidenberg M, Bell B, Rutecki P, Sheth R, Ruggles K, et al. The neurodevelopmental impact of childhood-onset temporal lobe epilepsy on brain structure and function. Epilepsia. 2002;43:1062–71.
38. Rutter M, Bailey A, Lord C. The Social Communcation Questionnaire. 1st ed. Western Psychological Services: Los Angeles, CA; 2003.
39. Richards C, Powis L, Moss J, Stinton C, Nelson L, Oliver C. Prospective study of autism phenomenology and the behavioural phenotype of Phelan-McDermid syndrome: comparison to fragile X syndrome, Down syndrome and idiopathic autism spectrum disorder. J Neurodev Disord. 2017;9:37.
40. Charman T, Baird G, Simonoff E, Loucas T, Chandler S, Meldrum D, Pickles A. Efficacy of three screening instruments in the identification of autistic-spectrum disorders. Br J Psychiatry. 2007;191:554–9.
41. Valente KD, Koiffmann CP, Fridman C, Varella M, Kok F, Andrade JQ. Epilepsy in patients with angelman syndrome caused by deletion of the chromosome 15q11-13. Arch Neurol. 2006;63:122–8.
42. Buoni S, Grosso S, Pucci L, Fois A. Diagnosis of Angelman syndrome: clinical and EEG criteria. Brain and Development. 1999;21:296–302.
43. Curatolo P, Moavero R, de Vries PJ. Neurological and neuropsychiatric aspects of tuberous sclerosis complex. Lancet Neurol. 2015;4:733–45.

44. Chonchaiya W, Au J, Schneider A, Hessl D, Harris SW, Laird M, et al. Increased prevalence of seizures in boys who were probands with the FMR1 premutation and co-morbid autism spectrum disorder. Hum Genet. 2012;131:581–9.
45. Bolton PF, Carcani-Rathwell I, Hutton J, Goode S, Howlin P, Rutter M. Epilepsy in autism: features and correlates. Br J Psychiatry. 2011;198:289–94.
46. Danielsson S, Gillberg IC, Billstedt E, Gillberg C, Olsson I. Epilepsy in young adults with autism: a prospective population-based follow-up study of 120 individuals diagnosed in childhood. Epilepsia. 2005;46:918–23.
47. Klein B, Levin BE, Duchowny MS, Llabre MM. Cognitive outcome of children with epilepsy and malformations of cortical development. Neurology. 2000; 55:230–5.
48. Bourgeois BF, Prensky AL, Palkes HS, Talent BK, Busch SG. Intelligence in epilepsy: a prospective study in children. Ann Neurol. 1983;14:438–44.

5

Facial expression recognition as a candidate marker for autism spectrum disorder: how frequent and severe are deficits?

E. Loth[1,2*], L. Garrido[3], J. Ahmad[2], E. Watson[2], A. Duff[2] and B. Duchaine[4]

Abstract

Background: Impairments in social communication are a core feature of Autism Spectrum Disorder (ASD). Because the ability to infer other people's emotions from their facial expressions is critical for many aspects of social communication, deficits in expression recognition are a plausible candidate marker for ASD. However, previous studies on facial expression recognition produced mixed results, which may be due to differences in the sensitivity of the many tests used and/or the heterogeneity among individuals with ASD. To ascertain whether expression recognition may serve as a *diagnostic marker* (which distinguishes people with ASD from a comparison group) or a *stratification marker* (which helps to divide ASD into more homogeneous subgroups), a crucial first step is to move beyond identification of mean group differences and to better understand the frequency and severity of impairments.

Methods: This study tested 46 individuals with ASD and 52 age- and IQ-matched typically developing (TD) participants on the Films Expression Task, which combines three key features of real-life expression recognition: naturalistic facial expressions, a broad range of simple and complex emotions, and short presentation time. Test-retest reliability was assessed in 28 individuals who did not participate in the main study and revealed acceptable reliability (ICC $r = .74$).

Results: Case-control comparisons showed highly significant mean group differences for accuracy ($p = 1.1 \times 10^{-10}$), with an effect size (Cohen's $d = 1.6$), more than twice as large as the mean effect size reported in a previous meta-analysis (Uljarevic and Hamilton, 2012, *J Autism Dev Disord*). The ASD group also had significantly increased mean reaction times overall ($p = .00015$, $d = .83$) and on correct trials ($p = .0002$, $d = .78$). However, whereas 63% of people with ASD showed severe deficits (they performed below two standard deviations of the TD mean, a small subgroup (15.3%) performed normally (within one standard deviation of the mean).

Conclusion: These findings indicate that the majority of people with ASD have severe expression recognition deficits and that the Films Expression Test is a sensitive task for biomarker research in ASD. Future work is needed to establish whether ASD subgroups with and without expression recognition deficits differ from one another in terms of their symptom profile or neurobiological underpinnings.

Keywords: Autism Spectrum disorder, Facial expression recognition, Biomarker

* Correspondence: Eva.loth@kcl.ac.uk
[1]Sackler Institute for Translational Neurodevelopment, Institute of Psychiatry, Psychology and Neuroscience, King's College London, De Crespigny Park, Denmark Hill, London SE5 8AF, UK
[2]Department of Forensic and Neurodevelopmental Sciences, Institute of Psychiatry, Psychology and Neuroscience, King's College London, London, UK
Full list of author information is available at the end of the article

Background

Autism spectrum disorder (ASD) is a life-long neurodevelopmental disorder, behaviourally defined by impairments in social communication and the presence of repetitive and restricted behaviours and interests [1]. The considerable variability in the quality and severity of symptoms between individuals with ASD is widely recognized [2]. For example, social communicative impairments can be manifested in a range of difficulties in social-emotional reciprocity, in non-verbal communicative behaviours, and in developing and maintaining social relationships [1]. Recognition of this heterogeneity has begun to cast doubt as to whether a truly diagnostic biological or behavioural marker for ASD exists (which differentiates all or the majority of people with ASD from typically developing individuals or those with other neurodevelopmental/psychiatric conditions) and prompted an increasing interest in the identification of *stratification markers* to parse ASD into more homogeneous subgroups [3]. Biomarkers have been defined as "a characteristic that is objectively measured and evaluated as an indication of normal biological processes, pathogenic processes, or pharmacologic responses to a therapeutic intervention" [4]. Here we use the term "biomarker" in a broad sense to refer to measures of any modality, including cognitive/behavioural tests [4]. *Stratification biomarkers* are then characteristics that vary between ASD subgroups and that map onto differences in their symptom presentation, etiology, need for particular treatments, and/or treatment response.

Because the ability to infer other people's emotions from their facial expressions is critical for many aspects of social communication, deficits in expression recognition have long been suggested to represent a core impairment in ASD [5]. However, over the past three decades, behavioural studies of facial expression recognition in ASD have produced mixed findings, ranging from reports of profound deficits to apparently intact expression recognition skills (see e.g., [6, 7] for recent reviews). A review of this literature suggests that in ASD, the presence and severity of expression recognition deficits on experimental tests is influenced by both participant characteristics—age and ability level—and task requirements [7]. On the whole, deficits in recognizing *basic* emotion expressions appear to be predominantly found in children and low-functioning individuals (i.e., people with ASD who also have intellectual disabilities) [5, 8]. By contrast, high-functioning individuals with ASD (with IQ in the normal range) usually perform well on tests that depict facial expressions in a prototypical manner and that used relatively long presentation times [9–11]. However, some studies reported group-level deficits in recognizing expressions of *complex* emotions (e.g., guilt, defiance) [9, 12], expressions that were presented only briefly [13] or subtle expressions displayed with low intensities [14] using morphs [15, 16]. Furthermore, speed-accuracy trade-offs [17], abnormal gaze fixation patterns [18], and differences in underlying neural processes as measured by EEG [19] and fMRI have also been reported [20, 21]. However, some inconsistencies remain even within the different methodologies and sample types. For example, some studies have found mean group deficits in adult ASD samples with IQ in the normal range on tasks that required labeling basic emotions with unlimited presentation times [20, 22, 23], while others reported no deficits in the recognition of complex emotions [24].

Recently, a formal meta-analysis of 48 papers concluded that there is an emotion recognition difficulty in "autism", with a mean effect size of Cohen's $D = 0.80$, yet this was estimated to decrease to around 0.40 after adjusting for publication biases [6]. Hence, it remains unclear whether differences in study findings reflect variability in the nature or sensitivity of the many behavioural tests used to assess expression recognition in ASD and/or differences in the severity of deficits among people with ASD.

To ascertain the value of expression recognition deficits as a candidate diagnostic or stratification biomarker we need, first, sensitive tests that incorporate several real-life characteristics. For example, in daily life, facial expressions are usually more subtly displayed than those depicted in most standard stimuli of "prototypical" facial emotion expressions. People also often reveal their emotions for only a very brief time. The observer is then required to identify the facial emotion expression quickly to react appropriately to the person's feelings. Second, the field needs to move away from a sole focus on mean between-group differences to better understand the frequency and severity of expression recognition deficits among individuals with ASD. For example, in case-control studies, a significant p value (especially in combination with small or medium effect sizes) could either reflect (small) deficits in most cases (say, around 1 SD below the typically developing (TD) mean) or may be driven by a subgroup of individuals with severe deficits. Obviously these two scenarios have profoundly different implications for the potential utility of the test in clinical practice.

Hence, the aim of this study was to investigate the frequency and severity of deficits in the recognition of facial expressions of emotion using a task that is more sensitive and naturalistic than previous tests. The Films Expression Task [25] uses still images captured from movie scenes and combines three elements that appear to be challenging for people with ASD: depiction of naturalistic facial expressions, inclusion of a range of both basic and complex emotions, and brief presentation times.

Methods

The Films Expression Task

The Films Expression Task [25] consists of 58 trials. In each trial, participants were first presented with an adjective describing an emotional state (e.g., confident, pleased). They were then briefly shown three images one after the other (500 ms each, with a 500 ms blank screen between images). The images were taken from films made in non-English-speaking countries to decrease the probability that participants had seen them or were familiar with the actors.

Within each trial, images present the same actor or actress, but with different emotional expressions. Participants were asked to indicate, by key press, which of the images best matched the target word. In 14 trials, the target emotion was a basic emotion (happy, angry, sad, afraid, surprised, disgusted). In the remaining 44 trials, the target emotion was complex (e.g., mocking, hurt, disappointed, resentful, see Additional file 1 for the list of target emotions). In trials with both basic and complex target emotions, the foils were selected to be similar to the targets in terms of perceptual features and intensity of the expression (see supplementary information [25]). Basic vs. complex emotion trials were presented interleaved, in a fixed-random order. Participants were instructed to respond as *quickly* and *accurately* as possible.

Immediately before the task, participants were presented with the definitions for each word describing a target emotion (e.g., guilty). They were encouraged to ask questions if they were unfamiliar with or did not understand any of the words. Participants were also allowed to review these definitions at the start of each trial, after presentation of the target word.

Task development and validation of the stimuli is described in [25] (supplementary information). Briefly, in pilot phase 1, three researchers suggested adjectives to describe 122 pictures of facial expressions taken from 18 films. In pilot phase 2, 32 native English speakers rated how well each adjective described the facial expression on a scale from 1 to 5 (1 = "it doesn't match at all", 5 = "it matches very well"). Adjectives were only carried forward if they had received at least a mean rating of 3.5 or a median rating of at least 4. Ten of these participants then also rated the intensity of the target expression from 1 to 5 (1 = "not intense" to 5 = "very intense") as well as the intensity of the expressions intended as foils. Targets and foils were then matched based on their expression intensity. In pilot phase 3, 30 different native English speakers were asked to choose one of two simultaneously presented expressions (the target and a foil) that best matched an adjective. Distractors were only included if participants had selected them less than 30% of the time. A fourth final pilot phase included ten new participants and employed the intended task procedure in which three pictures were presented sequentially, one target and two distractors. Only trials with equal or less than 30% errors were carried forward, which resulted in 58 trials with targets taken from 15 films.

IQ measures

Verbal, performance, and full-scale IQ were assessed using the Wechsler Abbreviated Scale of Intelligence-2nd edition (WASI-II; Wechsler, [26]) or a four-subtest short-form of the Wechsler Adult Intelligence Scale-Third Edition (WAIS-III; [27]). In both instances, the tests included two verbal subscales (vocabulary, similarities) and two non-verbal subscales (block design, matrix reasoning). Standardized scores from the WASI-II and WAIS are comparable.

Autism Spectrum Quotient

The Autism Spectrum Quotient (AQ) [28] is a self-report questionnaire to assess whether adults of average intelligence have symptoms associated with autism spectrum disorder. The test consists of 50 statements and participants indicate whether they "definitely agree", "slightly agree", "slightly disagree", or "definitely disagree" with each statement. Approximately half the items are worded to usually elicit an "agree" response from neurotypical individuals and half to usually elicit a "disagree" response. The questions cover five different domains associated with the autism spectrum: social skills, communication skills, imagination, attention to detail, and attention switching/ tolerance of change.

Test-retest reliability of the films expression test

Thirty-one participants took part in a test-retest study to assess the reliability of the Films Expression Test. We aimed to recruit participants with a range of expression recognition abilities to ensure that test-retest reliability on this task was stable at both high and low performance scores. Because we hypothesized that individuals with ASD would have lower accuracy scores than typically developing individuals, four participants were recruited from an autism support group. Hence, 27 participants were typically developing, three had a formal diagnosis of autism, and one was suspected of having autism.

Two participants exceeded the intended maximum retest interval of 6 weeks and did not complete the retest, one participant's retest data was not available after a technical error. This left 28 participants (20 females and 8 males, mean age = 33.48 years; range = 20–57 years, four from the autism support group). Out of the 28 participants, English was a second language for six but all participants described themselves as fluent English speakers. The retest interval ranged from 14 to 34 days, with an average interval of 18.11 days.

All test-retest participants also completed a two-subtest (vocabulary and matrix reasoning) short-form of the Wechsler Abbreviated Scale of Intelligence (WASI-II; [26]). The mean two-scale IQ was 113.07 (range 87–146).

Test-retest analysis revealed an intra-class correlation coefficient of ICC = .74, indicating acceptable reliability. The mean accuracy score at time 1 was 86.64% (SD = 7.49, range 62.07–98.28%) and at time 2 was also 86.64% (SD = 7.93, range 62.07–94.83%). Individual difference scores, calculated between time 1 and time 2 performance, showed that 17 (60.71%) participants had a difference score less than .5 SDs, 6 (21.43%) were between .5 and 1 SD, and 5 were (17.86%) greater than 1 SD.

Participants

In the main study, participants consisted of 46 adolescents or adults with ASD (34 male, 12 female) and 53 typically developing (TD) individuals (33 male, 20 female). Eighteen TD participants were tested as part of a previous study [25]. Although the ASD group included a higher proportion of males than the TD group, the difference in the sex ratio between the groups was not statistically significant (χ^2 = 1.5, p = .21). Mean age of the ASD group was 30.2 years (SD 9.4, 15–50 years) and of the TD group was 27.5 years (SD 7.8, range 14–55 years). Two participants in the ASD group (15 and 17 years) and two participants in the TD group (15 and 14 years) were younger than 18 years. IQ data was available for 42 out of 46 participants with ASD and all participants in the TD group. Mean verbal and full-scale IQ in the ASD group were 113.9 (range 85–140) and 116.0 (range 87–135), respectively, and in the TD group were 114.0 (range 74–146) and 115.5 (range 85–143). The groups did not significantly differ from each other in terms of age (t(86) = 2.3, p = .12), full-scale IQ (t(86) = .02, p = .87), verbal IQ (t(86) = .0004, p = .98), or performance IQ (t(86) = .002, p = .96). The four individuals with ASD for whom no IQ data were available had attended mainstream schools, which suggests that their IQ was within the normal range.

All participants with ASD except one were native English speakers. In the TD group, 37 of 53 participants were native English speakers. All TD participants for whom English was not their first language described their current English language level as "fluent". Fourteen individuals performed within 1 SD of the TD mean or above, one individual below 1 SD, and two individual below 2 SDs of the TD mean. Of these two TD participants, one had an above-average verbal IQ (VIQ) (124), indicative of adequate language comprehension and was therefore not excluded. The other TD participant had an accuracy score of more than 4 SDs below the TD mean (male, 32 years, VIQ = 92, first language Uzbek) and was excluded from the analyses reported below. This left 46 people with ASD and 52 people with TD. The study was approved by the South London and Maudsley NHS Trust ethics committee and the UCL Research Ethics Committee. All participants or a parent in the case of participants who were minors gave informed written consent before study participation.

Results

Case-control comparisons

Descriptive statistics are provided in Additional file 2. The ASD group accurately identified an average of 70.8% (SD = 13.5) of the briefly presented emotion expressions, compared to 87.5% (SD = 5.5) in the control group (see Fig. 1a). The Welch test, which does not assume equal variances, showed that this mean group difference was highly significant (t(58.1) = – 7.8, p = 1.1×10^{-10}). The effect size (Cohen's d) was 1.62. We used bootstrapping in Matlab version 8.3.0.532 (Mathworks, Natick, MA) to estimate the 95% confidence interval around this point estimate. We drew 10,000 resamples from the original sample using random sampling with replacement. We obtained a distribution of effect sizes for all the resamples, and using the percentile method (i.e. using the 2.5 and 97.5 percentiles as lower and upper bounds of the CI), the 95% CI was [1.30 2.05].

Analyses of *reaction times* (RT) revealed that the ASD group also responded significantly more slowly (M = 1459 ms, SD = 899) than the TD group (M = 878 ms, SD = 414) across all trials (t(61.5) = 4.02, p = .00015, Cohen's d = .83, 95% CI [0.49 1.19]) as well as on their correct trials (ASD: M = 1279 ms, SD = 812; TD: M = 767 ms, SD = 352) (t(df = 59.7) = 3.96, p = .0002, Cohen's d = 0.82, 95% CI [0.49 1.17]). These findings remain unchanged when adolescents below the age of 18 years were excluded (accuracy: ASD = 70.2%, TD = 87.7%; t(53.5) = 7.9, p = 1.4×10^{-10}) (see Fig. 1b).

Sex differences

Given previous reports of sex differences on several social-cognitive tasks in the typical population and in ASD [29], we performed 2 (group) × 2 (sex) ANOVAs to test whether accuracy, overall RT, or RT on correct trials differed between males and females overall or in either group. These tests confirmed the significant effects of group on accuracy (F(1,97) = 65.0, $p = 2.3 \times 10^{-12}$) and RTs (all ps < .00007) but there were no significant effects of sex (all ps > .5)) or group by sex interactions (all ps > .11). This finding indicates that the overall case-control difference cannot be attributed to differences in the slightly higher male:female ratio in the ASD than those in the control group.

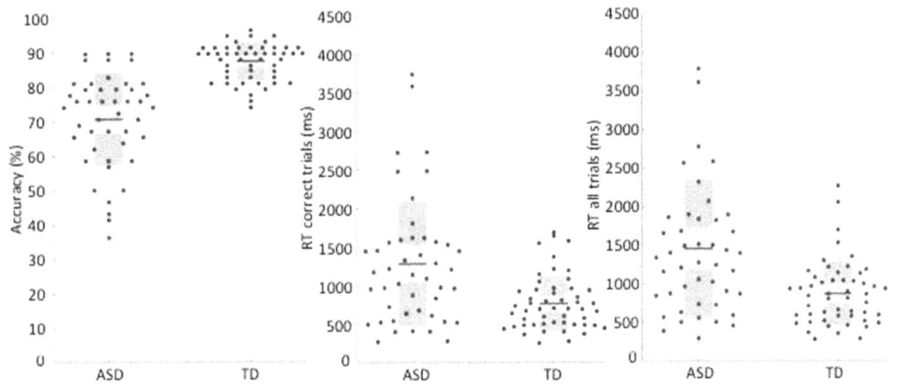

Fig. 1 a Accuracy: percentage of correct trials, by group. **b** Mean reaction time of correct trials and mean reaction time overall, by group

Basic vs. complex emotions

Next, we explored whether in the ASD group, the expression recognition impairments reported above were driven by specific problems in identifying complex emotional expressions. To do so, we separately analysed trials with simple vs. complex target emotions (see Additional file 1).

A 2 (group) × 2 (emotion category) repeated-measures ANOVA revealed the above reported significant main effect of group ($F(1,96) = 70.7$, $p = 3.8 \times 10^{-13}$) and a significant effect of emotion category ($F(1,96) = 5.9$, $p = .016$) on response accuracy, such that on average, both groups were better at recognizing simple than complex emotions. The group x emotion category interaction was not significant $F(1,96) = .14$, $p = .7$) (see Fig. 2).

Correlations between accuracy and RT scores with age and IQ

Next, we tested whether age, verbal, performance, or full-scale IQ were related to accuracy or reaction time (RT overall or on correct trials) on the Films Expressions Test. In the ASD group, we found no significant relationships between expression recognition variables and age or IQ (all $p > .09$). In the TD group, there was a marginally significant relationship between accuracy scores and FIQ ($r(52) = .26$, $p = .057$), such that participants with higher intelligence also had higher expression recognition scores.

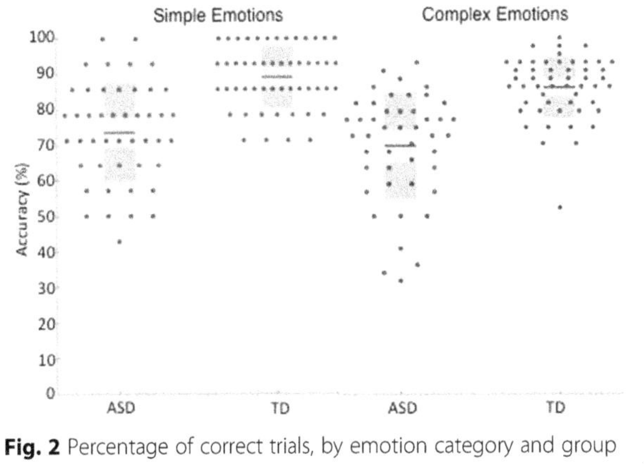

Fig. 2 Percentage of correct trials, by emotion category and group

Frequency and severity of expression recognition deficits in ASD

To establish the frequency and severity of expression recognition deficits in the ASD group, we calculated how far the accuracy score for each individual with ASD deviated from the TD group mean. Analyses of the scores showed that 63% of people with ASD performed more than 2 SDs below the TD mean. Of those, 23.9% performed between 2 and 3 SDs below the TD mean and 39.1% performed more than 3 SDs below the TD mean (see Fig. 3). 21.7% of people with ASD performed between 1 to 2 SDs below the TD mean while 15.3% had accuracy scores within the TD range. The 17-year-old with ASD performed within the 1 SD of the TD range, while the 15-year-old with ASD performed between 2 and 3 SDs below the TD range. As shown in Fig. 4, in the ASD group, accuracy and RT scores were negatively correlated such that individuals with ASD who had higher accuracy scores were also able to correctly recognize the emotion faster than those with low accuracy scores. Therefore, there was no evidence of speed-accuracy trade-off for most of the ASD participants who performed accurately on the task. These results suggest that the majority (63%) of individuals with ASD had severe deficits, while a small subgroup of around 15% of people with ASD showed intact expression recognition skills on this test.

Correlations between accuracy and RT scores and ASD symptoms

Finally, we investigated correlations with ASD symptoms in a subset of $N = 53$ participants (ASD = 25, TD = 28) for whom AQ data was available (see Fig. 5). When both groups were collapsed, we found a significant negative

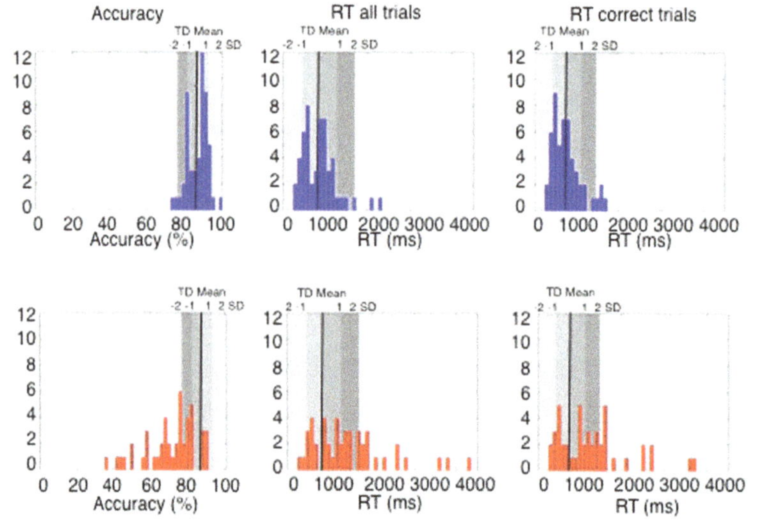

Fig. 3 Upper panel: Distribution of TD performance on percentage of accuracy. Lower panel: Distribution ofASD performance on percentage of accuracy. Grey bars denote − 2 to + 2 SDs of the TD means on percentage of correct expression recognition

correlation between the percentage of correct responses on the Films Expression Task and higher ASD symptoms $r(53) = -.48$, $p = .0002$. However, when the ASD and TD groups were considered separately, there were no significant relationships in either group (ASD $r(25) = .09$, $p = .66$, TD $r(28) = .03$, $p = .88$). This suggests that the negative correlation for the overall sample could be explained by the performance differences between the two groups.

A somewhat different picture emerged for RTs. We found that longer reaction times on correct trials were associated with more ASD symptoms. This was significant overall, i.e., when both groups were collapsed ($RT_{correct\ trials}$: overall $r(53) = .53$, $p = .00003$) and in the TD group (TD $r(28) = .48$, $p = .012$). Although a similar pattern was found in the ASD group, it did not reach statistical significance (ASD $r(25) = .29$, $p = .16$).

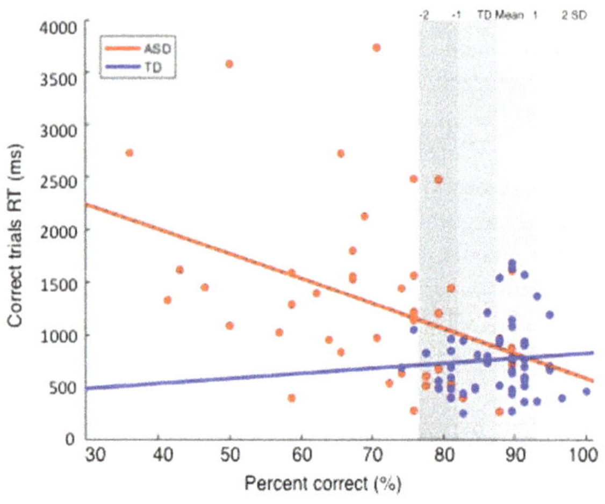

Fig. 4 Scatterplot showing percentage of accuracy and RT on correct trials, by group. Grey bars denote − 2to + 2 SDs of the TD means on percentage of correct expression recognition

Likewise, for overall RTs, we found a significant relationship with ASD symptoms when both groups were collapsed ($RT_{overall}$: overall: $r(53) = .54$, $p = .000026$). When the TD and ASD groups were analysed separately, similar but non-significant patterns were found (TD: $r(28) = .31$, $p = .10$, ASD: ($r(25) = .29$, $p = .16$).

Discussion

This study investigated the frequency and severity of impairments in facial expression recognition in ASD using a test that captured several features of expression recognition in daily life. A test-retest study showed reliability of .74, which is considered adequate for a test to be of use in clinical settings [30, 31]. At the group level, we found highly significant differences in accuracy and response times between a group of high-functioning adults and adolescents with ASD and an age- and IQ-matched TD control group. Effect sizes of the accuracy scores were more than twice as large as those estimated in a recent meta-analysis of studies on emotion recognition in ASD and more than four times larger than estimates that accounted for publication biases [6].

As a first step towards ascertaining whether deficits in expression recognition may serve as a diagnostic or stratification marker for ASD, we investigated the frequency and severity of these deficits. This revealed that 63% of people with ASD had severe deficits, which would be expected to create substantial social communicative difficulties. For example, participants who performed below 3 SDs of the TD mean failed to identify the briefly displayed target emotion expression in 3–7 out of 10 trials. Translated into real-life settings, it is

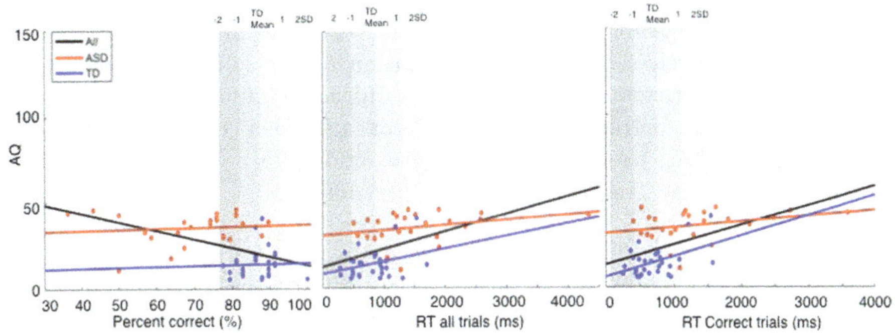

Fig. 5 Scatterplot showing the relationship between AQ scores and **a** accuracy scores, **b** overall RTs, and c RTs for correct responses. Regression lines are plotted overall, and for the ASD and TD groups separately. Grey bars denote − 2 to + 2 SDs of the TD means on percentage of correct expression recognition, RTs, and RTs on correct trials

easy to see how this may impact the ability to, for example, modulate a conversation or to respond empathically [32]. However, we also found considerable variability in that 21.7% performed between 1 to 2 SDs below the TD mean and 15.3% evidenced expression recognition skills indistinguishable from TD individuals (within 1 SD of the TD mean) as indexed by the combination of both accuracy and RT scores. This variability in expression recognition skills among individuals with ASD was unrelated to age or IQ (verbal or non-verbal). However, it should be borne in mind that the IQ range in the current sample was restricted to the normal range, so that this finding may not generalize to individuals with ASD and intellectual disabilities.

The present findings are broadly consistent with other recent efforts to parse heterogeneity in ASD. In particular, Lombardo and colleagues [33] used unsupervised hierarchical clustering approaches to identify ASD subgroups on the basis of item-level performance on the Reading the Mind in the Eyes Test (RMET).The RMET is a widely used mentalising task that also involves a strong emotion recognition component [34] as it requires participants to identify the mental or emotional state of a person from their eye region only. The study (which comprised a discovery and replication cohort) identified five ASD subgroups and four TD subgroups. For individuals with ASD, 45–62% showed what the authors termed "clear to immediate impairments", while two subgroups (19–36%) performed more than 2 and up to 11 SDs below the TD means - depending on the TD subgroup that was used as comparison. It would be valuable for future studies to directly compare performance on the RMET and Films Expression Tasks or combine information from both measures to derive a composite score.

A second requirement for a quantitative stratification marker is to demonstrate clinical relevance, for example, that people who fall within a certain range of deficits differ from those without abnormalities (normal range) in terms of symptom severity. To begin to address this, we conducted correlation analyses between severity of expression recognition deficits and ASD symptom severity, as measured by the AQ. When the ASD and TD groups were combined, we found both lower accuracy in expression recognition and higher RTs to be moderately related to greater severity of autism traits. However, whereas accuracy scores were not sensitive to the severity of ASD symptoms within the ASD and TD groups, respectively, longer reaction times on correct trials were significantly related to greater ASD symptoms in the TD group. A similar relationship was found in the ASD group with moderate correlation coefficients which, however, did not reach statistical significance. These correlation analyses should be viewed as preliminary, because AQ scores were only available in about half of the participants. As a consequence, the sample sizes were small when split by group, which reduced our power to detect a significant effect. In addition, the AQ is a composite measure of a range of autism-related traits, including features such as intolerance of changes that may not be expected to relate to expression recognition. This may have diluted potentially higher associations with more specific social communicative impairments.

In sum, our findings revealed that the majority of individuals with ASD had severe deficits in expression recognition deficits but also that a sub-sample of individuals with ASD had no behavioural impairments on this task. This indicates that expression recognition may more likely serve as a stratification as opposed to diagnostic marker, subject to further substantiation that subgroups with/without expression recognition deficits also differ in symptom severity or adaptive behavior. One implication of the current findings is that intervention programmes that specifically target expression recognition may be valuable for a substantial proportion of people with this disorder.

Study limitations and future directions

Several potential limitations of the current study as well as implications for future research should be considered. First, we deliberately chose a task that incorporated several factors crucial for expression recognition in real-life situations, including a wide range of simple and complex target emotions, and relatively short presentation times. As a consequence, could factors unrelated to expression recognition per se have contributed to the deficits observed in some of the ASD participants, for example, comprehension of the target words or other cognitive impairments/ anomalies?

If difficulties in comprehending some of the emotion words accounted for performance impairments, one would expect larger group differences in trials with complex target emotions than basic emotions. However, separate analyses, split by emotion target (simple vs complex), showed significant impairments in the ASD group on trials with basic as well as complex emotions. Basic emotion words are typically understood by the age of 6 years or earlier. Also most of the complex emotions used here are typically understood by age 8 (see Additional file 1), and the ASD participants had verbal IQs within (and mostly above) the population average. However, recognition of complex emotions also requires an understanding of the mental states they describe [34] and some high-functioning individuals with ASD may also have deficits in theory of mind [35]. Therefore, future studies should probe comprehension of the different emotion words and account for individual differences in understanding particular words and their emotional state—independent from recognition of their manifestation in facial expressions.

Previous studies reported that expression recognition deficits varied with the type of emotion, such that recognition of fear has been found to be more impaired than happiness (see [6] for a review). The naturalistic character of the task did not enable us to systematically analyse recognition of different types of emotion expressions (fear, anger, disappointment, etc.) as 34 different emotion adjectives were included, and many of the target emotions were only used once. However, descriptive trial-by-trial analyses, split by group (see Fig. 6) suggest that the mean percentages of correct response not only varied *between* target emotions but in some instances also *within* target emotions. For example, among the ASD group "angry" and "happy" trials had the highest percentages of correct responses whereas trials with the target emotions "disappointed", "tentative", and "disbelieving" had the

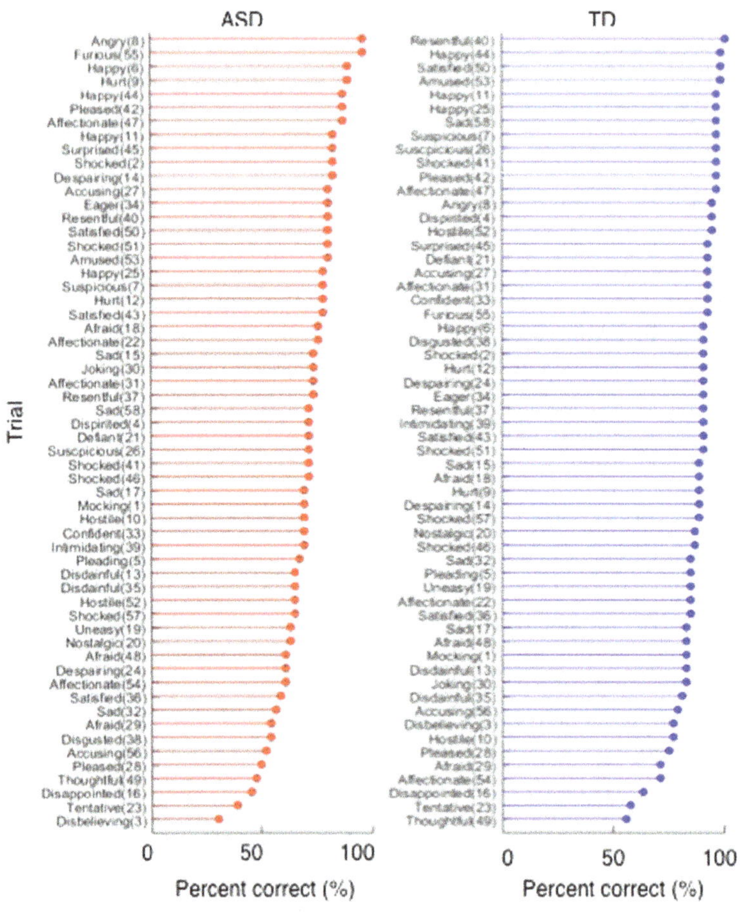

Fig. 6 Percentage of correct responses, by trial. **a** ASD group. **b** TD group

lowest percentages. For "sad" trials, correct recognition ranged from 56.5 to 73.9%. The latter finding may be due to the fact that the difficulty level of a trial is influenced by the nature of the target emotion and also by the expressions in the distractor stimuli used in a trial.

Could more general problems in rapid visual processing have contributed to deficits in recognizing relatively briefly presented (500 ms) facial expressions of emotions? This alternative explanation seems unlikely for two reasons. Several previous studies reported no deficits in rapid visual processing in ASD [13, 36]. For example, a study that tested recognition of micro-facial expressions, using much faster presentation times (15 and 30 ms) than those employed here reported specific deficits in identifying facial expressions, but not objects in an ASD group [37]. Moreover, as indicated above, our trial-by-trial analyses (see Fig. 6) showed quite variable performance scores between trials in the ASD group, with two trials being correctly identified by over 90% of the ASD participants. This pattern of largely intact expression recognition on some trials but impairments on others would be inconsistent with general problems in rapid visual processing. However, it remains a possibility that other cognitive abnormalities previously reported in (some people with) ASD, such as a detail-focused processing style [38] abnormalities in top-down processing [39] or difficulties with other aspects of face perception [40], may have contributed to behavioural impairments in expression recognition.

The present finding raises the question of what may account for the differences between people with ASD with/without expression recognition deficits. This question cannot be settled here but we discuss potential factors and outline some avenues for future research. A likely possibility is that (some) people with ASD have problems in the neurocognitive mechanisms that represent facial expression information and/or multi-modal expression information. One hypothesis that recently gained prominence is the notion that expression recognition deficits in ASD may be linked to the high frequency of comorbid alexithymia [41, 42], estimated to affect around 50% of people with ASD [43, 44]. Alexithymia is a sub-clinical trait characterized by difficulties in identifying and describing one's own emotional state [45]. Future work—ideally with larger samples—will be needed to ascertain whether some or all individuals with ASD who exhibit substantial expression recognition deficits also have higher rates of trait alexithymia. Other potential underlying mechanisms may include differences in attention (e.g., to the eye region [11, 46]), or brain structural/functional anomalies [20]. To identify the factors that underpin expression recognition impairments at an individual level will require multi-modal studies and/or designs that assess a range of cognitive functions within each individual. We have included an abridged version of the Films Expression Test and a companion child version in the follow-up assessment battery of the EU-AIMS Longitudinal European Autism Project [47, 48] to test whether the current findings can be replicated in an independent sample more diverse in age and ability level, to further determine the clinical usefulness of our findings, and to investigate potential underlying mechanisms.

Conclusion

Taken together, our findings show highly significant mean case-control differences in facial expression recognition, with one of the largest effect sizes ever reported in the expression recognition literature of ASD. This suggests that problems with expression recognition are more widespread than currently thought, likely owing to the more naturalistic character of the tasks used here. Nevertheless, we also highlight important variability in expression recognition skills among individuals with this condition and showed that a minority of people with ASD had no behavioural impairments. This finding indicates that the Films Expression Test may serve as a valuable tool to study expression recognition as a candidate stratification marker for ASD.

Abbreviations

AQ: Autism Spectrum Quotient; ASD: Autism Spectrum Disorder; IQ: Intelligence Quotient; RT: Reaction time; SD: Standard deviation; TD: Typically developing; WAIS: Wechsler Adult Intelligence Scales; WASI: Wechsler Abbreviated Scales of Intelligence

Acknowledgements

We thank all participants and their families for their help with this study, as well as Raka Tavashmi, Hannah Hayward, Daisy Crawley, Jessica Sabet, Jessica Faulkner, Claire Ellis, and Antonia San Jose Caceres for their help with volunteer recruitment and/or assessment.

Funding

This study was supported by an Economic and Social Research Council (ESRC) project grant (RES-000- 22-1123) and by EU-AIMS (European Autism Interventions), which receives support from the Innovative Medicines Initiative Joint Undertaking under grant agreement no. 115300, the resources of which are composed of financial contributions from the European Union's Seventh Framework Programme (grant FP7/2007-2013), from the European Federation of Pharmaceutical Industries and Associations companies' in-kind contributions, and from Autism Speaks.

Authors' contributions

EL designed the study and wrote the first and final draft. LG designed the study materials and contributed to the writing of the manuscript. JA carried out the test-retest reliability study, contributed to data collection, prepared all figures, and contributed to the writing of the manuscript. EW contributed to data collection and commented on the manuscript. ACD contributed to the data collection and commented on the manuscript. BD designed the study and contributed to the writing of the manuscript. All authors read and approved the final manuscript.

Competing interests

The authors declare that they have no competing interests.

Author details

[1]Sackler Institute for Translational Neurodevelopment, Institute of Psychiatry, Psychology and Neuroscience, King's College London, De Crespigny Park, Denmark Hill, London SE5 8AF, UK. [2]Department of Forensic and Neurodevelopmental Sciences, Institute of Psychiatry, Psychology and Neuroscience, King's College London, London, UK. [3]Division of Psychology, Department of Life Sciences, Brunel University, London, UK. [4]Department of Psychological and Brain Sciences, Dartmouth College, Hanover, USA.

References

1. American Psychiatric Association. Diagnostic and statistical manual of mental disorders. Fifth ed. Arlington: American Psychiatric Publishing; 2013.
2. Charman T. Variability in neurodevelopmental disorders: evidence from autism. In: Riby D, Van Herwegen J, editors. Applied research and key issues in neurodevelopmental disorders. Hove: Routledge Psychology Press; 2015. p. 177–40.
3. Loth E, Spooren W, Ham LM, Isaac MB, Auriche-Benichou C, Banaschewski T, Baron-Cohen S, Broich K, Bolte S, Bourgeron T, et al. Identification and validation of biomarkers for autism spectrum disorders. Nat Rev Drug Discov. 2016;15:70–3.
4. Biomarkers Definition Working Group. Biomarkers and surrogate endpoints: preferred definitions and conceptual framework. Clin Pharmacol Ther. 2001; 69:89–95.
5. Hobson RP. The autistic child's appraisal of expressions of emotion. J Child Psychol Psychiatry. 1986;27:321–42.
6. Uljarevic M, Hamilton A. Recognition of emotions in autism: a formal meta-analysis. J Autism Dev Disord. 2012;43(7):1517-26.
7. Harms MB, Martin A, Wallace GL. Facial emotion recognition in autism spectrum disorders: a review of behavioral and neuroimaging studies. Neuropsychol Rev. 2010;20:290–322.
8. Celani G, Battacchi MW, Arcidiacono L. The understanding of the emotional meaning of facial expressions in people with autism. J Autism Dev Disord. 1999;29:57–66.
9. Baron-Cohen S, Jolliffe T, Mortimore C, Robertson M. Another advanced test of theory of mind: evidence from very high functioning adults with autism or Asperger syndrome. J Child Psychol Psychiatry. 1997;38:813–22.
10. Castelli F. Understanding emotions from standardized facial expressions in autism and normal development. Autism. 2005;9:428–49.
11. Rutherford MD, Towns AM. Scan path differences and similarities during emotion perception in those with and without autism spectrum disorders. J Autism Dev Disord. 2008;38:1371–81.
12. Capps L, Yirmiya N, Sigman M. Understanding of simple and complex emotions in non-retarded children with autism. J Child Psychol Psychiatry. 1992;33:1169–82.
13. Clark TF, Winkielman P, McIntosh DN. Autism and the extraction of emotion from briefly presented facial expressions: stumbling at the first step of empathy. Emotion. 2008;8:803–9.
14. Wingenbach TSH, Ashwin C. Brosnan: diminished sensitivity and specificity at recognising facial emotion expressions of varying intensity underlie emotion-specific recognition deficits in autism spectrum disorders. Res Autism Spectr Disord. 2017;34:52–61.
15. Kennedy DP, Adolphs R. Perception of emotions from facial expressions in high-functioning adults with autism. Neuropsychologia. 2012;50:3313 9.
16. Wang S, Adolphs R. Reduced specificity in emotion judgment in people with autism spectrum disorder. Neuropsychologia. 2017;99:286–95.
17. Sucksmith E, Allison C, Baron-Cohen S, Chakrabarti B, Hoekstra RA. Empathy and emotion recognition in people with autism, first-degree relatives, and controls. Neuropsychologia. 2013;51:98–105.
18. Pelphrey KA, Sasson NJ, Reznick JS, Paul G, Goldman BD, Piven J. Visual scanning of faces in autism. J Autism Dev Disord. 2002;32:249–61.
19. Dawson G, Webb SJ, Carver L, Panagiotides H, McPartland J. Young children with autism show atypical brain responses to fearful versus neutral facial expressions of emotion. Dev Sci. 2004;7:340–59.
20. Ashwin C, Baron-Cohen S, Wheelwright S, O'Riordan M, Bullmore ET. Differential activation of the amygdala and the 'social brain' during fearful face-processing in Asperger syndrome. Neuropsychologia. 2007;45:2–14.
21. Wang AT, Dapretto M, Hariri AR, Sigman M, Bookheimer SY. Neural correlates of facial affect processing in children and adolescents with autism spectrum disorder. J Am Acad Child Adolesc Psychiatry. 2004;43:481–90.
22. Macdonald H, Rutter M, Howlin P, Rios P, Le Conteur A, Evered C, Folstein S. Recognition and expression of emotional cues by autistic and normal adults. J Child Psychol Psychiatry. 1989;30:865–77.
23. Boraston Z, Blakemore SJ, Chilvers R, Skuse D. Impaired sadness recognition is linked to social interaction deficit in autism. Neuropsychologia. 2007;45:1501–10.
24. Buitelaar JK, van der Wees M, Swaab-Barneveld H, van der Gaag RJ. Theory of mind and emotion-recognition functioning in autistic spectrum disorders and in psychiatric control and normal children. Dev Psychopathol. 1999;11:39–58.
25. Garrido L, Furl N, Draganski B, Weiskopf N, Stevens J, Tan GC, Driver J, Dolan RJ, Duchaine B. Voxel-based morphometry reveals reduced grey matter volume in the temporal cortex of developmental prosopagnosics. Brain. 2009;132:3443–55.
26. Wechsler D. Wechsler Abbreviated Scale of Intelligence - Second Edition (WASI-II). London: Pearson; 2011.
27. Wechsler D. Wechsler Adult Intelligence Scale. Third ed. London: Pearson; 1997.
28. Baron-Cohen S, Wheelwright S, Skinner R, Martin J, Clubley E. The autism-spectrum quotient (AQ): evidence from Asperger syndrome/high-functioning autism, males and females, scientists and mathematicians. J Autism Dev Disord. 2001;31:5–17.
29. Lai MC, Lombardo MV, Auyeung B, Chakrabarti B, Baron-Cohen S. Sex/gender differences and autism: setting the scene for future research. J Am Acad Child Adolesc Psychiatry. 2015;54:11–24.
30. George D, Mallery P. SPSS for Windows step by step: a simple guide and reference. Boston: Allyn & Bacon; 2003.
31. Kaplan R, Saccuzzo D. Psychological testing: principles, applications and issues (5th ed). Belmont: Wadsworth; 2001.
32. Baron-Cohen S. Autism: the empathizing-systemizing (E-S) theory. Ann N Y Acad Sci. 2009;1156:68–80.
33. Lombardo MV, Lai M-C, Auyeung B, Holt RJ, Allison C, Smith P, Chakrabarti B, Ruigrok ANV, Suckling J, Bullmore E, et al. Unsupervised data-driven stratification of mentalizing heterogeneity in autism. Sci Rep Oct. 2016;18:18.
34. Oakley BF, Brewer R, Bird G, Catmur C. Theory of mind is not theory of emotion: a cautionary note on the reading the mind in the eyes test. J Abnorm Psychol. 2016;125:818–23.
35. Castelli F, Frith C, Happe F, Frith U. Autism, Asperger syndrome and brain mechanisms for the attribution of mental states to animated shapes. Brain. 2002;125:1839–49.
36. Rinehart N, Tonge B, Brereton A, Bradshaw J. Attentional blink in young people with high-functioning autism and Asperger's disorder. Autism. 2010; 14:47–66.
37. Wright B, Clarke N, Jordan J, Young AW, Clarke P, Miles J, Nation K, Clarke L, Williams C. Emotion recognition in faces and the use of visual context in young people with high-functioning autism spectrum disorders. Autism. 2008;12:607–26.
38. Happe F, Frith U. The weak coherence account: detail-focused cognitive style in autism spectrum disorders. J Autism Dev Disord. 2006;36:5–25.
39. Loth E, Gómez JC, Happé F. When seeing depends on knowing: adults with autism spectrum conditions show diminished top-down processes in the visual perception of degraded faces but not degraded objects. Neuropsychologia. 2010;48:1227–36.
40. Verhallen RJ, Bosten JM, Goodbourn PT, Lawrance-Owen AJ, Bargary G, Mollon JD. General and specific factors in the processing of faces. Vis Res. 2017;141: 217-27.

41. Bird G, Cook R. Mixed emotions: the contribution of alexithymia to the emotional symptoms of autism. Transl Psychiatry. 2013;3:e285.
42. Cook R, Brewer R, Shah P, Bird G. Alexithymia, not autism, predicts poor recognition of emotional facial expressions. Psychol Sci. 2013;24:723–32.
43. Berthoz S, Haviland MG, Riggs ML, Perdereau F, Bungener C. Assessing alexithymia in French-speaking samples: psychometric properties of the Observer Alexithymia Scale-French translation. Eur Psychiatry. 2005;20:497–502.
44. Lombardo MV, Barnes JL, Wheelwright SJ, Baron-Cohen S. Self-referential cognition and empathy in autism. PLoS One. 2007;2:e883.
45. Nemiah JC, Freyberger H, Sifneos PE. Alexithymia: a view of the psychosomatic process. In: Hill OW, editor. Modern trends in psychosomatic medicine. London: Butterworths; 1976.
46. Klin A, Jones W, Schultz R, Volkmar F, Cohen D. Visual fixation patterns during viewing of naturalistic social situations as predictors of social competence in individuals with autism. Arch Gen Psychiatry. 2002;59:809–16.
47. Loth E, Charman T, Mason L, Tillmann J, Jones EJH, Wooldridge C, Ahmad J, Auyeung B, Brogna C, Ambrosino S, et al. The EU-AIMS Longitudinal European Autism Project (LEAP): design and methodologies to identify and validate stratification biomarkers for autism spectrum disorders. Mol Autism. 2017;8:24. https://doi.org/10.1186/s13229-017-0146-8.
48. Charman T, Loth E, Tillmann J, Crawley D, Wooldridge C, Goyard D, Ahmad J, Auyeung B, Ambrosino S, Banaschewski T, et al. The EU-AIMS Longitudinal European Autism Project (LEAP): clinical characterisation. Mol Autism. 2017; 8:27. https://doi.org/10.1186/s13229-017-0145-9.

6

Network-specific sex differentiation of intrinsic brain function in males with autism

Dorothea L. Floris[1], Meng-Chuan Lai[2,3], Tanmay Nath[1], Michael P. Milham[4,5] and Adriana Di Martino[1*]

Abstract

Background: The male predominance in the prevalence of autism spectrum disorder (ASD) has motivated research on sex differentiation in ASD. Multiple sources of evidence have suggested a neurophenotypic convergence of ASD-related characteristics and typical sex differences. Two existing, albeit competing, models provide predictions on such neurophenotypic convergence. These two models are testable with neuroimaging. Specifically, the Extreme Male Brain (EMB) model predicts that ASD is associated with enhanced brain maleness in both males and females with ASD (i.e., a shift-towards-maleness). In contrast, the Gender Incoherence (GI) model predicts a shift-towards-maleness in females, yet a shift-towards-femaleness in males with ASD.

Methods: To clarify whether either model applies to the intrinsic functional properties of the brain in males with ASD, we measured the statistical overlap between typical sex differences and ASD-related atypicalities in resting-state fMRI (R-fMRI) datasets largely available in males. Main analyses focused on two large-scale R-fMRI samples: 357 neurotypical (NT) males and 471 NT females from the 1000 Functional Connectome Project and 360 males with ASD and 403 NT males from the Autism Brain Imaging Data Exchange.

Results: Across all R-fMRI metrics, results revealed coexisting, but network-specific, shift-towards-maleness and shift-towards-femaleness in males with ASD. A shift-towards-maleness mostly involved the default network, while a shift-towards-femaleness mostly occurred in the somatomotor network. Explorations of the associated cognitive processes using available cognitive ontology maps indicated that higher-order social cognitive functions corresponded to the shift-towards-maleness, while lower-order sensory motor processes corresponded to the shift-towards-femaleness.

Conclusions: The present findings suggest that atypical intrinsic brain properties in males with ASD partly reflect mechanisms involved in sexual differentiation. A model based on network-dependent atypical sex mosaicism can synthesize prior competing theories on factors involved in sex differentiation in ASD.

Keywords: Autism spectrum disorder, Resting-state fMRI, Sex differentiation, Sex mosaicism, Extreme Male Brain, Gender Incoherence

* Correspondence: Adriana.dimartino@nyumc.org
[1]Hassenfeld Children's Hospital at NYU Langone Health, Department of Child and Adolescent Psychiatry, Child Study Center, 1 Park Avenue, New York City, NY 10016, USA
Full list of author information is available at the end of the article

Background

Substantial evidence supports models of autism spectrum disorder (ASD) as a condition characterized by altered brain connectivity [1, 2]. Yet, the striking heterogeneity of ASD has challenged efforts to profile the mechanisms underlying ASD-related dysconnections. One significant source of heterogeneity in ASD is biological sex [3, 4], as highlighted by the 3–4:1 male preponderance in prevalence [5, 6]. However, the impact of biological sex on ASD-related dysonnections remains poorly understood. In recent years, resting-state functional magnetic resonance imaging (R-fMRI) has demonstrated its feasibility in capturing typical sex differences in various aspects of the intrinsic connectome [7–9] and has emerged as a robust tool for substantiating the functional dysconnectivity hypothesis of ASD [1, 2]. This has motivated initial R-fMRI studies to characterize the contribution of biological sex to the neurobiology of ASD [10, 11]. Preliminary evidence suggests that both sex-dependent and sex-independent dysconnections coexist in ASD [12].

Here, in considering sex-dependent factors, we focused on investigating the neurophenotypic convergence of ASD-related characteristics and typical sex differences [13, 14]. Our focus was motivated by (1) genetic evidence emphasizing shared mechanisms between vulnerability to ASD and typical sexual differentiation [15] and (2) two current theoretical models whose predictions on neurophenotypic convergence can be assessed with neuroimaging. One model is the Extreme Male Brain (EMB) theory, which emerges from observations at the cognitive-behavioral level that individuals with ASD, regardless of sex, show “masculinized” or “hypermasculinized” profiles of empathizing and systemizing [16, 17]. Neurophenotypic prediction from the EMB model is that ASD brain characteristics will be associated with enhanced brain maleness (i.e., *shift-towards-maleness*) in both males and females with ASD. The other model is the Gender Incoherence (GI; [18]) theory. This is grounded on anthropometric and physiological findings that adult males and females with ASD are more androgynous than same-sex neurotypical peers [18]. The neurophenotypic prediction of the GI model is that a *shift-towards-maleness* is limited to females with ASD and that males with ASD instead show a *shift-towards-femaleness.*

While neuroimaging studies have begun to consider the mechanisms underlying sex differentiation in ASD in the context of these two models [14], only two studies have focused on intrinsic functional properties of the connectome. Both R-fMRI studies converged on a neural shift-towards-maleness in females with ASD, consistent with a prior volumetric study [3]. However, these earlier studies diverged in regard to males with ASD. Ypma et al. [11] reported a shift-towards-maleness within the default network (DN) in individuals with ASD regardless of their biological sex—a pattern consistent with EMB predictions. Results showed that both males and females with ASD exhibited hypo-connectivity within DN compared to typical males, who, in turn, showed lower intrinsic functional connectivity (iFC) than typical females. Alaerts et al. [10] found a similar pattern of a shift-towards-maleness in females with ASD in the voxel-wise iFC of the posterior superior temporal sulcus and posterior cingulate cortex (PCC). However, they also observed a shift-towards-femaleness in males with ASD—as predicted by GI. The disparities in these R-fMRI studies may reflect their moderate sample sizes. They employed a two-factorial design (i.e., testing sex-by-diagnosis interactions), with sample size generally including $n \sim 40$ individuals per cell. This is due to the scarcity of available ASD female datasets even in large repositories such as the Autism Brain Imaging Data Exchange (ABIDE).

Conjunction (spatial overlap) analyses can be a useful alternative and complementary approach in the identification of potential associations between ASD-related atypicalities and typical sex difference maps [3, 14]. This is particularly true in instances of limited availability of female datasets. Factorial designs can provide information about factors related to typical sex differentiation in regions that *differ* between males and females with ASD relative to NT males and females (i.e., by testing for regions showing significant sex-by-diagnosis interactions) and brain regions showing main effects of sex (ignoring diagnostic group) or ASD (ignoring sex). However, it is still possible that regions showing ASD-related atypicalities do not differ between males and females with ASD relative to NT males and females but are still related to typical sex differentiation. These nuances can be captured in the examination of specific spatial overlap scenarios of effects predicted by hypothetical links between ASD atypicalities (separately for ASD males and ASD females, whenever data is available) and typical sex differences.

We applied conjunction analyses to the large ABIDE I male R-fMRI dataset, thus allowing to address concerns on sample size as well as prior inconsistencies in sex-dependent intrinsic functional brain properties in males with ASD [10, 11]. We focused on five key whole-brain voxel-wise R-fMRI indices in regard to (a) typical sex differences in a neurotypical (NT) sample from the 1000 Functional Connectome Project (FCP) [19] and (b) ASD-related differences among males from ABIDE I [1]. We conducted an unbiased whole-brain exploration given reports of multiple networks involved in ASD including and beyond DN. To ensure that findings were not dependent on the specific NT sample employed, we examined replicability using the Brain Genomics Superstruct Project (GSP) [20] sample.

Methods

Analytical overview

Using conjunction analyses, we explored whether atypical intrinsic brain properties in males with ASD showed significant spatial overlap with those exhibiting typical sex differences. Primary analyses used group difference Z-statistics maps from two published large-scale R-fMRI studies [1, 19]. Applying a more stringent statistical voxel-level threshold of $Z \geq 2.58$ (cluster level $p < 0.05$) yielded highly similar findings as original results; see Additional file 1: Figure S1 for illustrative purposes. These studies were selected for their large sample sizes and for the representativeness of their findings in regard to typical sex differentiation (e.g., [7–9, 21, 22]) as well as ASD-related atypicalities [2, 23–25] (for complete reviews, see [26]). Five R-fMRI metrics were examined which have been reported to reflect typical sex differences [7–9, 19] and ASD-related intrinsic brain properties [1, 24, 27, 28]: (1) regional homogeneity (ReHo) [29], (2) voxel-mirrored homotopic connectivity (VMHC) [30], (3) network degree centrality (DC) [31], (4) PCC-iFC, and (5) fractional amplitude of low frequency fluctuations (fALFF) [32] (for details on each measure, see Additional file 2: Supplementary methods). Validation and replication analytical strategies were conducted to address the possible confounds related to samples and preprocessing differences (Table 1).

Conjunction analyses

For all analyses across primary as well as validation and replication analytical strategies, we applied a voxel-level thresholding consistent with prior work [3, 33, 34]. Z-maps were voxel-level-thresholded across 500 successive thresholds ranging from $p < 0.05$ to $p < 0.0001$ decrementing by 0.0001. This multi-threshold approach illustrates whether findings are stable and consistent across thresholds. No cluster-level thresholds were applied, as different statistical comparisons in independent cohorts (ABIDE I and FCP) can result in different spatial extent thresholds [3, 33, 34]. Spatial overlap was obtained by conjunction analyses of each voxel-level thresholded Z-maps with logical "AND" masking [35]. The extent of overlap for each conjunction contrast was quantified as the average of the proportion of the total number of suprathreshold voxels for each map (Additional file 2: Supplementary methods) [3, 33, 34].

We then verified that spatial overlaps were not random by contrasting them against a null distribution of random overlaps derived from Monte Carlo simulations with 5000 iterations, for all successive 500 voxel-level thresholds ($p = 0.05$ to $p = 0.0001$) [3, 34, 36]. For each iteration, two whole gray matter maps were created, with the same voxel resolutions as the observed maps filled with values randomly sampled from a Gaussian distribution. Their spatial smoothness was then adjusted based on the average smoothness across the two observed maps. This estimation was done using the AFNI command *3dFWHMx*, and resulting values were averaged across ABIDE I and FCP, and across ABIDE I and GSP. Simulated maps were also thresholded along 500 voxel-level thresholds as the observed maps, and their overlap percentage was calculated. For each R-fMRI metric, further inferences were based on the spatial overlaps consistently above the 99.5th percentile of the null distribution for at least 70% of the 500 tested thresholds (i.e., at least 350 out of 500 instances). All computations were run with MATLAB version 2013a (The MathWorks Inc., Natick, MA, USA).

Spatial overlap scenarios

Across all analytical strategies, spatial overlaps between ASD-related atypicality Z-maps and typical sex difference Z-maps may underlie distinct scenarios depending on the directionality of the contrasts utilized—i.e., ASD♂ > NT♂ and ASD♂ < NT♂ and NT♂ > NT♀ and NT♂ < NT♀. As illustrated in Fig. 1, four scenarios could emerge; two met the EMB predictions and two met the GI predictions, as detailed below.

1. Shift-towards-maleness (STM) ASD-related increases (*EMB 1*; ASD ♂ > NT ♂ and NT ♂ > NT ♀): Males with ASD have higher values on examined R-fMRI metrics (i.e., higher iFC in ReHo, PCC-iFC, DC, and VMHC and higher regional amplitude in fALFF) than typical males, and typical males have higher values than typical females;

Table 1 Overview of analysis strategies

Strategy	Description of overlapping maps	Addressed potential confounds	Samples
Strategy 1 *Originally published Z-maps*	Z-maps obtained from original ABIDE I and FCP samples	–	ABIDE I: $N = 763$ (ASD = 360; NT = 403) FCP: $N = 828$ (NT M = 357; NT F = 471)
Strategy 2 *Adjusting analytical pipelines*	Z-maps obtained after aligning processing with samples similar to strategy 1	Differences in MRI analytical methods (i.e., preprocessing and group model)	ABIDE I: $N = 759$ (ASD = 356; NT = 403) FCP: $N = 824$ (NT M = 356; NT F = 468)
Strategy 3 *Adjusting age*	Z-maps obtained in age-matched ABIDE I and FCP subsamples	Differences in sample age and MRI analytical methods	ABIDE I: $N = 199$ (ASD = 93; NT = 106) FCP: $N = 439$ (NT M = 183; NT F = 256)
Strategy 4 *Independent NT sample*	Z-maps of ABIDE I subsample as strategy 3 and an independent sex difference sample from Brain Genomics Superstruct Project (GSP)	Differences in sample age and MRI analytical methods	ABIDE I: $N = 199$ (ASD = 93; NT = 106) GSP: $N = 742$ (NT M = 320; NT F = 422)

ABIDE Autism Brain Imaging Data Exchange, *FCP* 1000 Functional Connectome Project, *GSP* Brain Genomics Superstruct Project, *ASD* autism spectrum disorder, *NT* neurotypicals, *M* males, *F* females

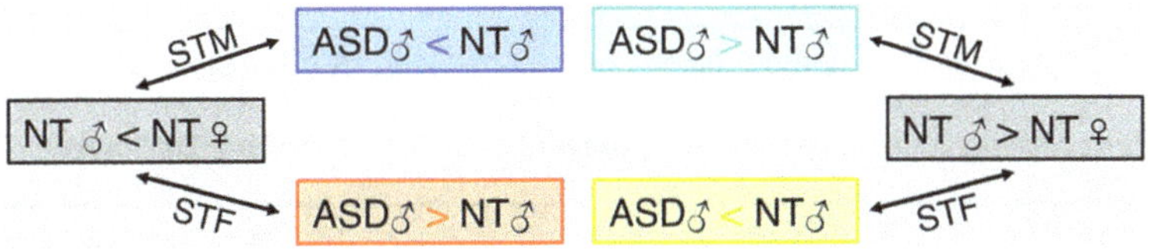

Fig. 1 Spatial overlap scenarios. Depending on the combination of statistical contrasts being overlapped, four different scenarios can emerge. Decreases or increases of R-fMRI metrics in males with autism spectrum disorder (ASD) relative to neurotypical males (NT M) lead to different scenarios depending on whether they overlap with increases or decreases in NT M relative to NT females (F) (gray boxes). Following the predictions of the Extreme Male Brain (EMB) theory and Gender Incoherence (GI) theory, two scenarios fit the EMB model predicting a shift-towards-maleness (STM) in males with ASD (see blue and turquois boxes) and two scenarios fit the GI model predicting a shift-towards-femaleness (STF) in males with ASD (see orange and yellow boxes)

2. Shift-towards-maleness (STM) ASD-related decreases (*EMB 2*; ASD ♂ < NT ♂ and NT ♂ < NT ♀): Males with ASD have lower values on examined R-fMRI metrics than typical males, and typical males have lower values than typical females;
3. Shift-towards-femaleness (STF) ASD-related increases (*GI 1*; ASD ♂ > NT ♂ and NT ♂ < NT ♀): Males with ASD have higher values on examined R-fMRI metrics than typical males, and typical males have lower values than typical females;
4. Shift-towards-femaleness (STF) ASD-related decreases (*GI 2*; ASD ♂ < NT ♂ and NT ♂ > NT ♀): Males with ASD have lower values on examined R-fMRI metrics than typical males, and typical males have higher values than typical females.

Primary analysis (strategy 1): originally published *Z*-maps

Statistical *Z*-maps were obtained from previously published analyses in Di Martino et al. [1] for the ASD-related difference male sample (ABIDE I) and Yan et al. [19] for the typical sex difference sample (FCP). The ABIDE I study included 763 males (360 ASD♂ and 403 NT♂; aged 6–58 years). The typical sex difference study (FCP), which included 828 NT selected from the 1000 Functional Connectome Project, comprised of 357 NT♂ and 471 NT♀ between 8 and 78 years of age (Table 2). Details of data acquisition can be found on the ABIDE I and FCP websites, http://fcon_1000.projects.nitrc.org/indi/abide and http://fcon_1000.projects.nitrc.org/fcpClassic/FcpTable.html, respectively, and a summary of the analyses and results can be found in Additional files 2 and 3: Supplementary methods and results.

Validation analysis (strategy 2): adjusting for differences in analytical pipelines

To account for possible confounds in the primary analyses (strategy 1) due to partially different preprocessing pipelines and statistical group models between ABIDE I and FCP studies, both original datasets were reanalyzed using version 0.3.9.1 of the Configurable Pipelines for the Analysis of Connectomes (C-PAC) [37]. Briefly, nuisance regression included white matter and cerebrospinal fluid signals, 24 motion parameters based on Friston 24-Parameter Model [38], and linear and quadratic trends. All derivatives were smoothed by a 6-mm FWHM Gaussian kernel. Statistical *Z*-maps were generated within study-specific functional volume masks including voxels (in MNI space) present across all subjects in a given study sample (ABIDE I and FCP). Group-level analyses were conducted for each sample separately using a general linear model including diagnosis (ABIDE I) or sex (FCP) as the regressor of interest and age, site, mean framewise displacement [39], and individual subject means of each R-fMRI derivative as the nuisance covariates (Additional file 2: Supplementary methods). We then used the resulting *Z*-maps for voxel-level conjunction analyses as detailed above.

Validation analysis (strategy 3): age-matched samples

To account for differences in age distribution between the ABIDE I and FCP samples, we applied the same analytical pipeline used for strategy 2 on subsamples matched for age (range 17.5–37 years). The age-matched ABIDE I sample comprised 199 individuals (93 ASD♂; 106 NT♂), whereas the age-matched FCP sample included 439 neurotypical individuals (183 NT♂; 256 NT♀) (Additional file 4: Figure S2 and Additional file 5: Table S1). Group analyses were conducted as described in strategy 2. We then used the resulting *Z*-maps for voxel-level conjunction analyses as detailed above.

Replication analysis (strategy 4): replication with an independent typical sex differences sample

Data were obtained from the GSP [20], matched for age based on the same criteria of strategy 3, resulting in a sample of 742 individuals comprising 320 NT♂ and 422 NT♀ ranging between 18 and 35 years of age (Additional file 5: Table S1). Analyses were conducted as in strategy 2. We then used the resulting *Z*-maps for voxel-level conjunction analyses as detailed above.

Results

Overview

Conjunction analyses revealed overlaps between intrinsic brain properties characterizing typical sex differences and

Table 2 Characterization of the original ABIDE I and FCP samples

ABIDE I	Sites[a] N	ASD (n=360) N/Mean (SD) [Range]	NT (n=403) N/Mean (SD) [Range]	Statistics
Sex	17	360 males	403 males	-
Age	17	16.4 (7.4) [7 – 58]	16.3 (6.53) [6.5 – 48]	t_{761}=0.1, p=.9
Full-Scale IQ[b]	17	106.4 (14.64) [78 – 139]	111 .1(11.44) [79 – 139]	t_{665}=-4.9, p<.001
Verbal IQ[c]	13	105.3 (15.57) [69 – 149]	111.6 (12.69) [67 – 147]	t_{582}=-5.6, p<.001
Performance IQ[d]	14	106.2 (15.37) [64 – 149]	107.8 (12.34) [67 – 137]	t_{581}=-1.5, p=.1
ADI-R				
Social[e]	13	20.0 (5.27) [7 – 30]	-	-
Communication[f]	13	15.9 (4.36) [4 – 26]	-	-
RRB[f]	13	6.3 (2.58) [0 – 13]	-	-
ADOS-G (Lord et al.)				
Communication[g]	11	3.8 (1.48) [0 – 8]	-	-
Social[h]	11	7.4 (3.45) [0 – 14]	-	-
RRB[i]	8	2.1 (1.59) [0 – 8]	-	-
Comorbidity	2	33 (NYU)[j]; 11 (KKI)[k]	-	-
FCP[l]	**Sites[m] N**	**Males (n=357) N/Mean (SD) [Range]**	**Females (n=471) N/Mean (SD) [Range]**	**Statistics**
Sex	18	357 males	471 females	-
Age	18	25.3 (9.77) [9 – 74]	24.5 (9.14) [8 – 78]	t_{826}=1.3, p=.2

[a]ABIDE I data collections (sites): KKI, Leuven 1, Leuven 2, MaxMun, NYU, OHSU, OLIN, PITT, SDSU, Stanford, Trinity, UCLA 1, UCLA 2, UM 1, UM 2, USM, and Yale
[b]FIQ was available for 354 individuals with ASD and 401 neurotypical (NT) controls
[c]VIQ was available for 302 individuals with ASD and 324 NT
[d]PIQ was available for 304 individuals with ASD and 337 NT
[e]ADI-R Social scale score was available for 245 individuals with ASD
[f]ADI-R Communication and ADI-R restricted repetitve bevhavior scale scores were available for 246 individuals with ASD
[g]ADOS-G Communication scores were available for 238 individuals with ASD
[h]ADOS-G Social scores were available for 261 individuals with ASD
[i]ADOS-G RRB scores were available for 202 individuals with ASD
[j]Attention deficit hyperactivity disorder (ADHD; N = 10), oppositional defiant disorder (ODD; N = 1), mood disorder (N = 10), anxiety disorders (N = 11)
[k]ADHD (N = 6), ODD (N = 2), mood disorder (N = 1), anxiety disorders (N = 2)
[l]There was no information available on IQ in the FCP sample
[m]FCP data collections: Baltimore, Bangor, Beijing, Berlin, Cambridge, Cleveland, ICBM, Leiden 1, Leiden 2, Leipzig, Munchen, Newark, New York 1, New York 2, Orangeburg, Oulu, Queensland, and Saint Louis

those characterizing ASD vs. NT differences in males (Fig. 2). Examining overlaps along successive voxel-level thresholds showed that they were significant above the 99.5th percentile of the null distribution across all R-fMRI measures. Depending on the R-fMRI metric, on average, 13 to 31% of those voxels characterized by ASD-related differences overlapped with those characterized by typical sex differences (inter-quartile range across all 500 voxel-level thresholds = 25–35% for ReHo; 21–31% for PCC-iFC; 17–30% for DC; 13–21% for VMHC; 8–16% for fALFF). As detailed below, based on the directionality of the Z-map contrasts involved in these non-random overlaps, findings were consistent with GI and EMB in *distinct* functional regions. To functionally characterize these spatial overlaps, we mapped them into the seven functional cortical networks as described by Yeo et al. [40] (Additional file 2: Supplementary methods). A double dissociation emerged. As illustrated in the maps

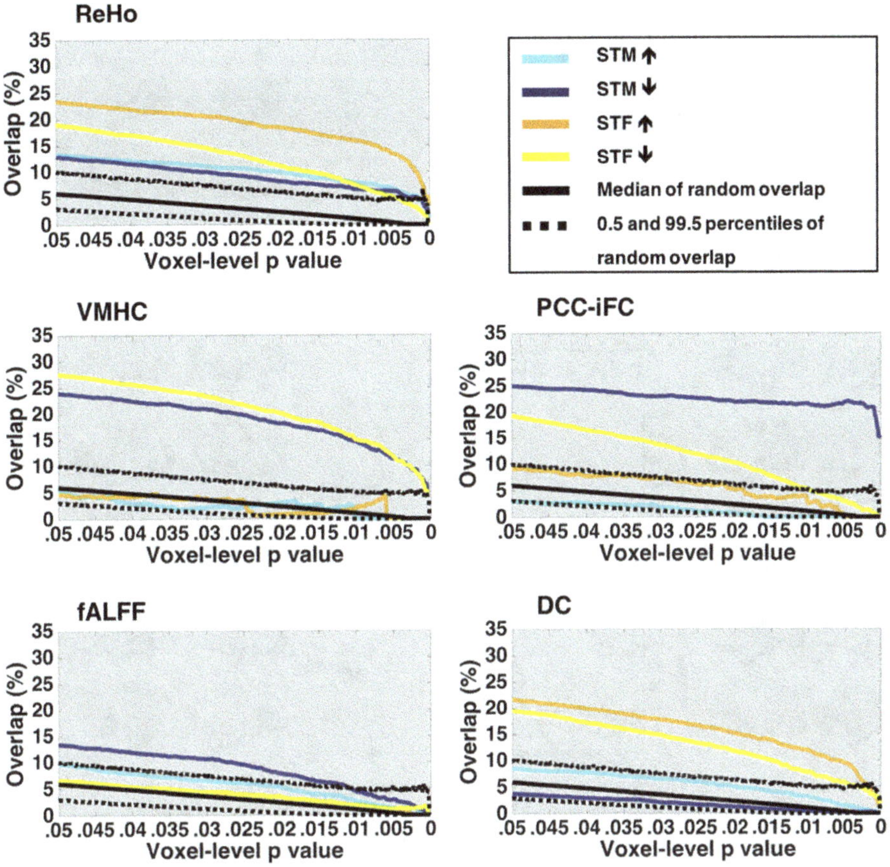

Fig. 2 Conjunction analyses. Plots (one per each resting-state fMRI metric [R-fMRI]) show the spatial overlap percentages across 500 successive statistical voxel-level thresholds for the four possible overlap scenarios (turquoise: shift-towards-maleness (STM) ASD-related increases (EMB 1; as indicated by the upward arrow) = ASD♂ > NT♂ and NT♂ > NT♀; blue: STM ASD-related decreases (EMB 2; as indicated by the downward arrow) = ASD♂ < NT♂ and NT♂ < NT♀; orange: shift-towards-femaleness (STF) ASD-related increases (GI 1; as indicated by the upward arrow) = ASD♂ > NT♂ and NT♂ < NT♀; yellow: STF ASD-related decreases (GI 2; as indicated by the downward arrow) = ASD♂ < NT♂ and NT♂ > NT♀). The black solid line represents the median of the null distribution of the random spatial overlap generated by 5000 Monte Carlo simulations for each threshold. The dotted lines mark the 0.5th and 99.5th percentiles of the null distribution of random spatial overlap. Only spatial overlaps consistently above the 99.5th percentile of the null distribution for at least 70% of the 500 tested thresholds were utilized for subsequent results' characterization. R-fMRI abbreviations: *DC* degree centrality, *fALFF* fractional amplitude of low frequency fluctuations, *ReHo* regional homogeneity, *VMHC* voxel-mirrored homotopic connectivity, *PCC-iFC* posterior cingulate cortex intrinsic functional connectivity

thresholded at $Z \geq 2.58$ in Fig. 3, regions matching EMB predictions mainly involved DN and related circuits involving higher-order socio-emotional and cognitive control processes. In contrast, regions matching GI predictions mainly centered around somatomotor (SM) circuits. This overall pattern of results was robust to permutation testing used as an alternative approach to Monte Carlo simulations (for generating the null distribution of random overlaps), as reported in supplementary post hoc analyses (Additional file 6: Table S2).

Shift-towards-maleness (EMB predictions)

A pattern of overlap consistent with a shift-towards-maleness (STM) characterized all R-fMRI metrics except DC (Fig. 2). Further, while only ASD-related increases in ReHo (EMB 1) significantly overlapped with typical sex differences, ASD-related decreases (EMB 2) did so for a wider range of R-fMRI metrics including ReHo, VMHC, PCC-iFC, and fALFF. These ASD-related decreases predominantly encompassed the DN—particularly the precuneus and PCC. The ASD-related hyper-connectivity in local iFC (i.e., ReHo) encompassed the fronto-parietal (FP) network and, to a lesser extent, the ventral attention (VA) network and DN including the frontal pole, middle frontal gyrus, and lateral occipital cortex (Fig. 3a and Additional file 7: Table S3).

Shift-towards-femaleness (GI predictions)

A pattern of overlap consistent with a shift-towards-femaleness (STF) characterized all R-fMRI metrics, except fALFF. Significant overlaps with typical sex differences involved ASD-related increases (GI 1) in ReHo and DC and

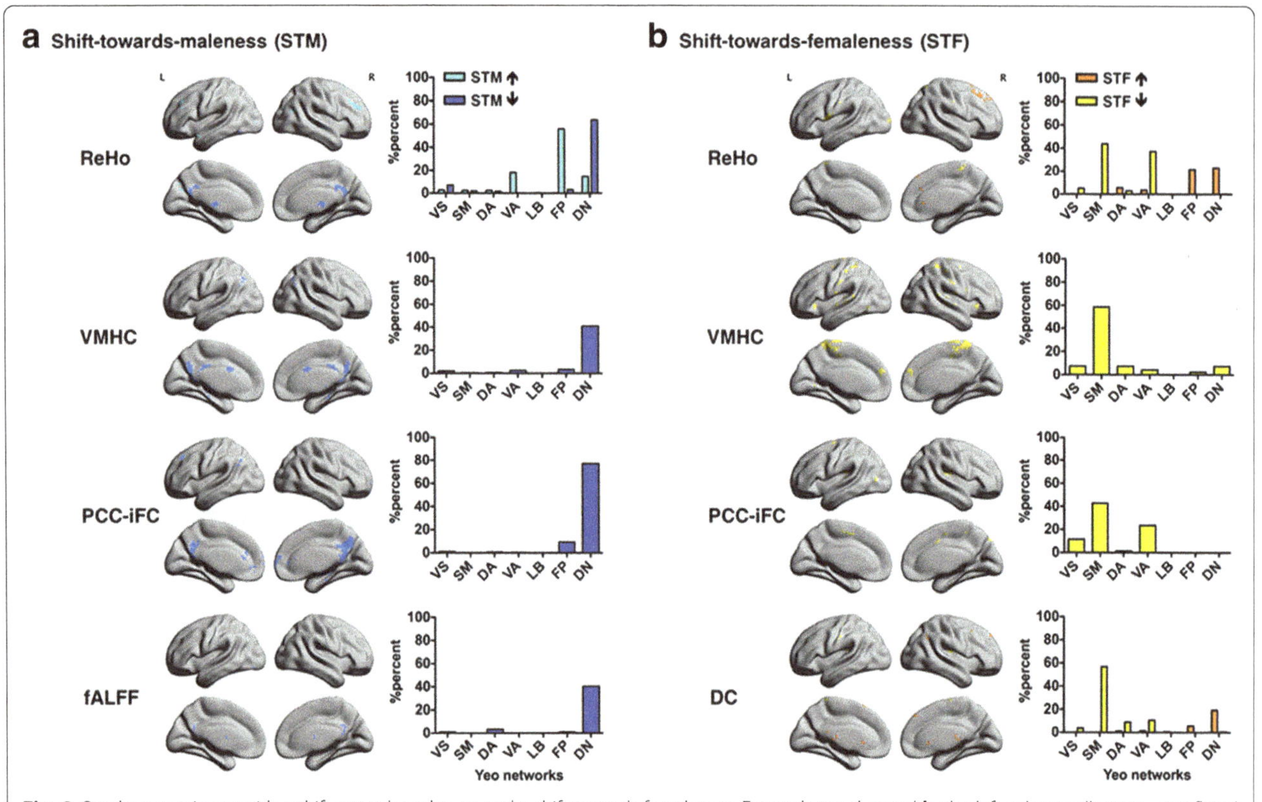

Fig. 3 Overlaps consistent with a shift-towards-maleness and a shift-towards-femaleness. For each panel, **a** and **b**, the left columns illustrate on inflated surface maps (BrainNet Viewer; https://www.nitrc.org/projects/bnv) the regions of significant spatial overlap based on the conjunction of statistical *Z*-maps resulting from the ABIDE I and FCP studies (voxel-level thresholded at $Z \geq 2.58$) for each resting-state fMRI (R-fMRI) metric. The histograms in the right column of each panel describe the percentage of voxels within the above clusters included in the seven functional cortical networks described by Yeo et al. [40]. R-fMRI abbreviations: *DC* degree centrality, *fALFF* fractional amplitude of low frequency fluctuations, *ReHo* regional homogeneity, *VMHC* voxel-mirrored homotopic connectivity, *PCC-iFC* posterior cingulate cortex intrinsic functional connectivity. Seven functional Yeo networks: *VS* visual network, *SM* somatomotor network, *DA* dorsal attention network, *VA* ventral attention network, *LB* limbic network, *FP* fronto-parietal network, *DN* default network. **a** Overlaps consistent with the Extreme Male Brain (EMB) theory: Hyper-connectivity consistent with a shift-towards-maleness (STM) was mainly present in the FP network for ReHo, whereas an STM hypo-connectivity for ReHo, VMHC, and PCC-iFC and decreased fALFF were mainly centered around the DN. Color codes: turquoise = STM ASD-related increases (EMB 1); blue = STM ASD-related decreases (EMB 2). **b** Overlaps consistent with the Gender Incoherence (GI) theory: Hyper-connectivity consistent with a shift-towards-femaleness (STF) was mainly in DN for DC and ReHo, whereas an STF hypo-connectivity across DC, ReHo, VMHC, and PCC-iFC was mainly centered around the SM network. Color codes: orange = STF ASD-related increases (GI 1); yellow = STF ASD-related decreases (GI 2)

decreases (GI 2) in ReHo, DC, VMHC, and PCC-iFC (Fig. 2). ASD-related R-fMRI decreases predominantly encompassed the SM network and to a lesser degree the ventral, visual, and dorsal attention networks, mainly centering around the postcentral gyrus, central and parietal operculum, and Heschl gyrus. ASD-related hyper-connectivity encompassed the DN and, to a lesser extent, the FP network, across DC and ReHo (Fig. 3b and Additional file 7: Table S3).

Cognitive ontology

To explore the cognitive domains implicated in the above regions, we quantified the percentage of their overlap with the 12 cognitive ontology maps by Yeo et al. [41] thresholded at $p = 1e{-}5$. We labeled each component based on the top five tasks it recruits. Consistent with the above functional network spatial distribution of our findings, a double dissociation was evident. In males with ASD, findings consistent with a shift-towards maleness involved higher-order social and cognitive processes, while those consistent with a shift-towards-femaleness mostly involved lower-order sensory and motor processes (Fig. 4 and Additional file 8: Table S4).

Validation and replication analyses

Results were highly similar across strategies, albeit greatest similarity was observed when analytical pipelines and age were aligned, i.e., strategies 3 and 4 (Additional files 9, 10, 11, and 12: Figures S3–S6 and Additional file 13: Table S5). A shift-towards-maleness in ASD-related decreases in PCC-iFC and VMHC was the most consistent findings across strategies, followed by those observed for ASD-related decreases in ReHo and, to a lesser extent, fALFF in

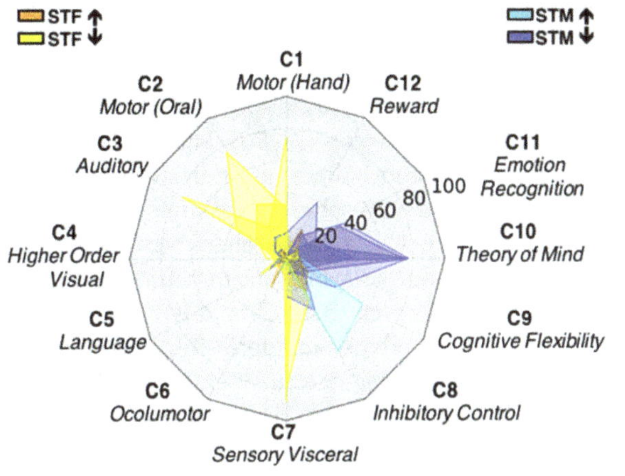

Fig. 4 Cognitive ontology maps. The polar plot shows the percentage (0–100%) of overlap between the significant conjunctions of statistical Z-maps (voxel-level thresholded at $Z \geq 2.58$) and the 12 Yeo cognitive ontology probability maps [41] (probability thresholded at $p = 1e{-5}$) for cognitive components C1–C12. We labeled each component based on the top five tasks reported to be most likely recruited by a given component. Results are summarized according to their consistency with the Extreme Male Brain (EMB) or Gender Incoherence (GI) models, regardless of the resting-state fMRI metric. Color codes: turquoise = shift-towards-maleness (STM) ASD-related increases (EMB 1); blue = STM ASD-related decreases (EMB 2); orange = shift-towards-femaleness (STF) ASD-related increases (GI 1); yellow = STF ASD-related decreases (GI 2)

DN (EMB 2) (Additional file 14: Table S6). For further details, see Additional file 3: Supplementary results.

Discussion

To characterize the neurophenotypic convergence of ASD-related intrinsic brain characteristics and typical sex differences, we examined the spatial overlap between neurotypical sex-related and ASD-related intrinsic brain properties in large independent samples [1, 19]. Results provided insights into two competing models of such convergence predicting either a shift-towards-maleness (EMB) [16] or a shift-towards-femaleness (GI) [18] in males with ASD. Across R-fMRI metrics, analyses revealed evidence consistent with both models, yet involving distinct functional neural networks. A shift-towards-maleness in males with ASD mostly involved DN and FP networks serving higher-order socio-emotional and cognitive control processes. In contrast, a shift-towards-femaleness in males with ASD predominantly centered around the SM network. These patterns remained stable across analytical strategies adjusting for differences in preprocessing pipelines and samples. The results suggest that previously reported R-fMRI abnormalities in males with ASD may partly result from atypical sexual differentiation in the brain, and these mechanisms act in a network-specific manner.

In typical individuals, a mosaic of brain region-specific masculinization and feminization exists across the sexes [42–45]. Our findings of coexisting shift-towards-maleness and shift-toward-femaleness of intrinsic brain properties in males with ASD suggest that biological mechanisms involved in sex mosaicism partly contribute to the neural characteristics of ASD. These may involve hormonal and non-hormonal factors [44, 46]. For example, estradiol can induce opposite effects in distinct brain regions by either initiating or preventing cell death and synaptogenesis, as well as by enhancing or dampening excitation [47]. Beyond hormonal factors, brain regional sexual differentiation is also driven by sex differential gene expression [46, 48]. Recent studies have shown that male differential expression of astrocyte and microglial genes are upregulated in ASD [13]. How these molecular phenomena affect the macro-scale intrinsic functional brain organization should be the focus of multilevel approaches that generate a unifying model of the relation between typical sex differentiation and ASD.

In regard to the macro-scale networks and functional processes involved, our most consistent finding was the shift-towards-maleness of DN, a network widely implicated in ASD [11, 23, 49–51]. In line with prior work [10, 11], we found that significant overlaps with typical sex differences encompassed PCC-iFC decreases along the DN midline. By extending our exploration to the whole brain, analyses revealed similar shift-towards-maleness exist for a range of intrinsic properties in the PCC. These included ASD-related decreases in local connectivity (ReHo) [52], homotopic inter-hemispheric interactions (VMHC) [30], and fractional amplitude of low frequency fluctuations (fALFF) [32]. These findings suggest that examinations of DN in ASD should consider sex-dependent biological factors.

Beyond DN ASD-related R-fMRI decreases, a shift-towards-maleness also involved other processes, especially ASD-related increases in FP local connectivity (ReHo). Notably, DN and FP networks subserve higher-order processes that are core to EMB theory's postulation that individuals with ASD are weaker "mentalizers" and stronger "systemizers" [16, 17, 53]. Consistent with the DN's role in social cognition and mentalizing, the shift-towards-maleness of atypical intrinsic properties in ASD mapped onto cognitive components associated with theory of mind and emotion recognition processes. Impairments in these domains are referred to as atypical mentalizing and characterize individuals with ASD [53]. On the other end, the FP network mapped onto inhibitory control and cognitive flexibility. Impairments in these domains have been attributed to weak central coherence, perseveration, and hyper-systemizing in ASD [54].

Our systematic examination of the intrinsic functional brain also revealed evidence of a shift-towards-femaleness in the male ASD brain in the SM network comprising motor and auditory cortices. Altered sensory-motor processing has often been observed in ASD [55, 56], and associated atypical intrinsic brain properties are emerging

[57–61]. Our findings suggest that a biological shift-towards-femaleness in the SM network may underlie these atypicalities [62, 63]. Alternatively, a SM shift-towards-femaleness might result from experience (e.g., being less engaged in motor activities). Longitudinal studies are required to clarify the impact of experiential factors [64], sex-specific biological factors, and their interactions. Finally, although in NT individuals motor and language processes are hemispherically specialized, NT females have greater bi-hemispheric integration compared to NT males [65]. Given prior reports of a reduction of typical asymmetries in males with ASD [58, 66, 67], our findings of a shift-towards-femaleness involving motor and auditory domains in males with ASD suggest that biological sex-related factors are likely involved in atypical inter-hemispheric interactions in this population.

With respect to specific R-fMRI features and atypical ASD-related differences, we note that shift-towards-femaleness or shift-towards-maleness in ASD did not affect any of the metrics differentially. Instead, echoing recent large-scale studies reconciling prior mixed findings of hypo- and hyper-connectivity in ASD [1, 24], results varied by the functional network involved. Our findings further suggest that sex-related biological factors contribute to the complex presentation of atypical iFC in ASD.

Results should be interpreted considering several limitations. First, a sufficiently large dataset was only available for males with ASD. While focusing on a large ASD male sample allowed us to address prior inconsistencies about a shift-towards-femaleness in males with ASD [10, 11], future large-scale characterizations of both females and males will provide insights into the role of typical sexual differentiation in ASD for both sexes [14, 68]. Second, while patterns of shift-towards-maleness and shift-towards-femaleness were similar across analytical strategies, aspects of the shift-towards-femaleness were more variable between the primary strategy and those adjusting for differences in age range. Speculatively, the shift-towards-maleness in ASD may therefore be related to *organizational* effects on neurodevelopment, as predicted by the EMB model that posits elevated prenatal steroidogenic processes [16, 69, 70]. An ASD-related shift-towards-femaleness in males could reflect later events even during and beyond puberty. This would be in line with the GI model which was mostly conceptualized based on postpubertal physiological measures [18]. As such, a shift-towards-femaleness may be more variable depending on the sample age. A cross-sectional examination of age effects would require a larger and more homogenous age distribution across data acquisition sites than the present one. Nevertheless, as we included age as a nuisance covariate in the statistical models used to generate the *Z*-maps overlapped, potential confounds on the present results are limited. Third, it was not possible to address the role of comorbid psychiatric conditions in our findings due to limited availability of this information across the ABIDE I datasets. Many comorbid conditions within ASD, such as attention deficit hyperactivity disorder, show a sex-biased prevalence ratio themselves [71, 72]. Further, recent studies considering comorbidities in individuals with ASD show brain connectivity patterns that are specific to ASD comorbidities [27]. This calls for characterization of both ASD core and comorbid symptoms in neuroimaging studies of ASD. Finally, given that FCP and ABIDE I aggregate data retrospectively across multiple sites, unknown confounds due to site differences may exist. We limited this concern by including sites as covariates at the group-level comparisons generating *Z*-maps used to assess spatial overlaps.

Conclusion

In conclusion, biological factors involved in typical sex differentiation are likely to affect the intrinsic functional properties of the male ASD connectome and manifest in both shift-towards-maleness and shift-towards-femaleness in different neural networks. The present findings suggest that a model based on network-dependent atypical sex mosaicism can synthesize seemingly competing EMB and GI theories. Given the heterogeneity of ASD, future studies combining multidimensional indices of shift-towards-maleness and shift-towards-femaleness and data-driven clustering methods can assess the extent to which sex mosaicism varies across individuals and may identify subgroups of ASD with different biological underpinnings.

Additional files

Additional file 1: ABIDE and FCP results.

Additional file 2: Supplementary methods.

Additional file 3: Supplementary results.

Additional file 4: Age Matching.

Additional file 5: Characterization of age-matched ABIDE I, FCP and GSP samples.

Additional file 6: Comparison of percentage of overlaps at $Z \geq 2.58$ for the real overlap, random overlap generated by 5000 Monte Carlo simulation, and random overlap generated by 1000 permutations, across R-fMRI metrics by model.

Additional file 7: Percentages of voxels within the conjunction maps (thresholded at $Z \geq 2.58$) overlapping with the seven functional cortical networks per Yeo et al. [40].

Additional file 8: Percentage of voxels within the conjunction maps (thresholded at $Z \geq 2.58$) and the 12 cognitive ontology maps defined Yeo et al. [41] (probability thresholded at $p = 1e\text{-}5$).

Additional file 9: Conjunction Analyses Across Strategies 2-4.

Additional file 10: Overlaps Consistent with a Shift-Towards-Maleness (EMB) across Strategies 2–4.

Additional file 11: Overlaps Consistent with a Shift-Towards-Femaleness (GI) across Strategies 2–4.

Additional file 12: Cognitive Ontology Maps for Strategies 2-4.

Additional file 13: Similarity across analytical strategies.

Additional file 14: Similarity across R-fMRI metrics by model across all analytical strategies.

Abbreviations

ABIDE: Autism Brain Imaging Data Exchange; ASD: Autism spectrum disorder; DC: Degree centrality; DN: Default network; EMB: Extreme Male Brain theory; fALFF: Fractional Amplitude of Low Frequency Fluctuations; FCP: 1000 Functional Connectome Project; FP: Fronto-parietal; GI: Gender Incoherence theory; GSP: Brain Genomics Superstruct Project; NT F: Neurotypical females; NT M: Neurotypical males; PCC-iFC: Posterior cingulate cortex intrinsic functional connectivity; ReHo: Regional homogeneity; SM: Somatomotor; STF: Shift-towards-femaleness; STM: Shift-towards-maleness; VMHC: Voxel-mirrored homotopic connectivity

Acknowledgements

We acknowledge the data donors and organizers of the 1000 Functional Connectome Project (http://fcon_1000.projects.nitrc.org/fcpClassic/FcpTable.html), Autism Brain Imaging Data Exchange I (http://fcon_1000.projects.nitrc.org/indi/abide), and Brain Genomics Superstruct Project (http://neuroinformatics.harvard.edu/gsp/) data repositories. We are grateful to Chao-Gan Yan for suggestions in earlier versions of this manuscript, Michael V. Lombardo for providing and assisting with the Monte Carlo simulation scripts, F. Xavier Castellanos for the helpful comments, Ting Xu for the helpful advice on permutation testing, and R. Cameron Craddock, John Pellman, and Steve Giavasis for the technical support with C-PAC.

Funding

Work for this study has been partly supported by NIMH (5R21MH107045 to ADM), by gifts to the Child Mind Institute from Phyllis Green, Randolph Cowen, and Joseph Healey, and by UO1 MH099059 (to MPM), the O'Brien Scholars Program within the Child and Youth Mental Health Collaborative at the Centre for Addiction and Mental Health and The Hospital for Sick Children, Toronto (to M-CL), and a Postdoctoral Training Award from the Autism Science Foundation (to DLF).

Authors' contributions

DLF, M-CL, ADM, and MPM designed the study and interpreted the results. DLF conducted the analyses. DLF and ADM drafted the manuscript. M-CL contributed the codes and assisted in the interpretation of the results. TN ran the pre-processing for the Brain Genomic Superstruct Dataset and helped with the permutation testing. All authors revised and approved the final manuscript.

Competing interests

The authors declare that they have no competing interests.

Author details

[1]Hassenfeld Children's Hospital at NYU Langone Health, Department of Child and Adolescent Psychiatry, Child Study Center, 1 Park Avenue, New York City, NY 10016, USA. [2]Child and Youth Mental Health Collaborative at the Centre for Addiction and Mental Health and The Hospital for Sick Children, Department of Psychiatry, University of Toronto, Toronto, ON M6J 1H4, Canada. [3]Autism Research Centre, Department of Psychiatry, University of Cambridge, Cambridge CB2 8AH, UK. [4]Center for the Developing Brain, Child Mind Institute, New York, NY 10022, USA. [5]Nathan S Kline Institute for Psychiatric Research, Orangeburg, NY 10962, USA.

References

1. Di Martino A, Yan CG, Li Q, Denio E, Castellanos FX, Alaerts K, Anderson JS, Assaf M, Bookheimer SY, Dapretto M, et al. The autism brain imaging data exchange: towards a large-scale evaluation of the intrinsic brain architecture in autism. Mol Psychiatry. 2014;19:659–67.
2. Picci G, Gotts SJ, Scherf KS. A theoretical rut: revisiting and critically evaluating the generalized under/over-connectivity hypothesis of autism. Dev Sci. 2016;19:524–49.
3. Lai MC, Lombardo MV, Suckling J, Ruigrok AN, Chakrabarti B, Ecker C, Deoni SC, Craig MC, Murphy DG, Bullmore ET, et al. Biological sex affects the neurobiology of autism. Brain. 2013;136:2799–815.
4. Lai MC, Lombardo MV, Ruigrok AN, Chakrabarti B, Wheelwright SJ, Auyeung B, Allison C, Baron-Cohen S, Consortium MA. Cognition in males and females with autism: similarities and differences. PLoS One. 2012;7:e47198.
5. Christensen DL, Baio J, Van Naarden BK, Bilder D, Charles J, Constantino JN, Daniels J, Durkin MS, Fitzgerald RT, Kurzius-Spencer M, et al. Prevalence and characteristics of autism spectrum disorder among children aged 8 years—autism and developmental disabilities monitoring network, 11 sites, United States, 2012. MMWR Surveill Summ. 2016;65:1–23.
6. Loomes R, Hull L, Mandy WPL. What is the male-to-female ratio in autism spectrum disorder? A systematic review and meta-analysis. J Am Acad Child Adolesc Psychiatry. 2017;56:466–74.
7. Biswal BB, Mennes M, Zuo XN, Gohel S, Kelly C, Smith SM, Beckmann CF, Adelstein JS, Buckner RL, Colcombe S, et al. Toward discovery science of human brain function. Proc Natl Acad Sci U S A. 2010;107:4734–9.
8. Tomasi D, Volkow ND. Gender differences in brain functional connectivity density. Hum Brain Mapp. 2012;33:849–60.
9. Satterthwaite TD, Wolf DH, Roalf DR, Ruparel K, Erus G, Vandekar S, Gennatas ED, Elliott MA, Smith A, Hakonarson H, et al. Linked sex differences in cognition and functional connectivity in youth. Cereb Cortex. 2015;25:2383–94.
10. Alaerts K, Swinnen SP, Wenderoth N. Sex differences in autism: a resting-state fMRI investigation of functional brain connectivity in males and females. Soc Cogn Affect Neurosci. 2016;11:1002–16.
11. Ypma RJ, Moseley RL, Holt RJ, Rughooputh N, Floris DL, Chura LR, Spencer MD, Baron-Cohen S, Suckling J, Bullmore ET, Rubinov M. Default mode hypoconnectivity underlies a sex-related autism spectrum. Biol Psychiatry Cogn Neurosci Neuroimaging. 2016;1:364–71.
12. Di X, Biswal BB. Sex-dependent and sex-independent brain resting-state functional connectivity in children with autism spectrum disorder. bioRxiv. 2016:038026. doi: https://doi.org/10.1101/038026 .
13. Werling DM, Parikshak NN, Geschwind DH. Gene expression in human brain implicates sexually dimorphic pathways in autism spectrum disorders. Nat Commun. 2016;7:10717.
14. Lai MC, Lerch JP, Floris DL, Ruigrok AN, Pohl A, Lombardo MV, Baron-Cohen S. Imaging sex/gender and autism in the brain: etiological implications. J Neurosci Res. 2017;95:380–97.
15. Mitra I, Tsang K, Ladd-Acosta C, Croen LA, Aldinger KA, Hendren RL, Traglia M, Lavillaureix A, Zaitlen N, Oldham MC, et al. Pleiotropic mechanisms indicated for sex differences in autism. PLoS Genet. 2016;12:e1006425.
16. Baron-Cohen S. The extreme male brain theory of autism. Trends Cogn Sci. 2002;6:248–54.
17. Baron-Cohen S, Cassidy S, Auyeung B, Allison C, Achoukhi M, Robertson S, Pohl A, Lai MC. Attenuation of typical sex differences in 800 adults with autism vs. 3,900 controls. PLoS One. 2014;9:e102251.
18. Bejerot S, Eriksson JM, Bonde S, Carlström K, Humble MB, Eriksson E. The extreme male brain revisited: gender coherence in adults with autism spectrum disorder. Br J Psychiatry. 2012;201:116–23.
19. Yan CG, Craddock RC, Zuo XN, Zang YF, Milham MP. Standardizing the intrinsic brain: towards robust measurement of inter-individual variation in 1000 functional connectomes. NeuroImage. 2013;80:246–62.
20. Holmes AJ, Hollinshead MO, O'Keefe TM, Petrov VI, Fariello GR, Wald LL, Fischl B, Rosen BR, Mair RW, Roffman JL, et al. Brain Genomics Superstruct Project initial data release with structural, functional, and behavioral measures. Sci Data. 2015;2:150031.
21. Filippi M, Valsasina P, Misci P, Falini A, Comi G, Rocca MA. The organization of intrinsic brain activity differs between genders: a resting-state fMRI study in a large cohort of young healthy subjects. Hum Brain Mapp. 2013;34:1330–43.
22. Bluhm RL, Osuch EA, Lanius RA, Boksman K, Neufeld RW, Théberge J, Williamson P. Default mode network connectivity: effects of age, sex, and analytic approach. Neuroreport. 2008;19:887–91.
23. Assaf M, Jagannathan K, Calhoun VD, Miller L, Stevens MC, Sahl R, O'Boyle JG, Schultz RT, Pearlson GD. Abnormal functional connectivity of default

mode sub-networks in autism spectrum disorder patients. NeuroImage. 2010;53:247–56.
24. Chen CP, Keown CL, Jahedi A, Nair A, Pflieger ME, Bailey BA, Müller RA. Diagnostic classification of intrinsic functional connectivity highlights somatosensory, default mode, and visual regions in autism. Neuroimage Clin. 2015;8:238–45.
25. Anderson JS, Druzgal TJ, Froehlich A, MB DB, Lange N, Alexander AL, Abildskov T, Nielsen JA, Cariello AN, Cooperrider JR, et al. Decreased interhemispheric functional connectivity in autism. Cereb Cortex. 2011;21:1134–46.
26. Vissers ME, Cohen MX, Geurts HM. Brain connectivity and high functioning autism: a promising path of research that needs refined models, methodological convergence, and stronger behavioral links. Neurosci Biobehav Rev. 2012;36:604–25.
27. Di Martino A, Zuo XN, Kelly C, Grzadzinski R, Mennes M, Schvarcz A, Rodman J, Lord C, Castellanos FX, Milham MP. Shared and distinct intrinsic functional network centrality in autism and attention-deficit/hyperactivity disorder. Biol Psychiatry. 2013;74:623–32.
28. Paakki JJ, Rahko J, Long X, Moilanen I, Tervonen O, Nikkinen J, Starck T, Remes J, Hurtig T, Haapsamo H, et al. Alterations in regional homogeneity of resting-state brain activity in autism spectrum disorders. Brain Res. 2010;1321:169–79.
29. Kendall MG, Gibbons JD. Rank correlation methods. 5th ed.: Edward Arnold; 1990.
30. Zuo XN, Kelly C, Di Martino A, Mennes M, Margulies DS, Bangaru S, Grzadzinski R, Evans AC, Zang YF, Castellanos FX, Milham MP. Growing together and growing apart: regional and sex differences in the lifespan developmental trajectories of functional homotopy. J Neurosci. 2010;30:15034–43.
31. Zuo XN, Ehmke R, Mennes M, Imperati D, Castellanos FX, Sporns O, Milham MP. Network centrality in the human functional connectome. Cereb Cortex. 2012;22:1862–75.
32. Zou QH, Zhu CZ, Yang Y, Zuo XN, Long XY, Cao QJ, Wang YF, Zang YF. An improved approach to detection of amplitude of low-frequency fluctuation (ALFF) for resting-state fMRI: fractional ALFF. J Neurosci Methods. 2008;172:137–41.
33. Holt RJ, Chura LR, Lai MC, Suckling J, von dem Hagen E, Calder AJ, Bullmore ET, Baron-Cohen S, Spencer MD. 'Reading the mind in the eyes': an fMRI study of adolescents with autism and their siblings. Psychol Med. 2014;44:3215–27.
34. Lai MC, Lombardo MV, Ecker C, Chakrabarti B, Suckling J, Bullmore ET, Happé F, Murphy DG, Baron-Cohen S, Consortium MA. Neuroanatomy of individual differences in language in adult males with autism. Cereb Cortex. 2015;25(10):3613–28.
35. Nichols T, Brett M, Andersson J, Wager T, Poline JB. Valid conjunction inference with the minimum statistic. NeuroImage. 2005;25:653–60.
36. Lombardo MV, Ashwin E, Auyeung B, Chakrabarti B, Taylor K, Hackett G, Bullmore ET, Baron-Cohen S. Fetal testosterone influences sexually dimorphic gray matter in the human brain. J Neurosci. 2012;32:674–80.
37. Craddock RC, Sikka S, Cheung B, Khanuja R, Ghosh SS, Yan C, Li Q, Lurie D, Vogelstein J, Burns R, et al. Towards automated analysis of connectomes: the Configurable Pipeline for the Analysis of Connectomes (C-PAC). In: Neuroinformatics. Stockholm: Frontiers; 2013.
38. Friston KJ, Williams S, Howard R, Frackowiak RS, Turner R. Movement-related effects in fMRI time-series. Magn Reson Med. 1996;35:346–55.
39. Jenkinson M, Bannister P, Brady M, Smith S. Improved optimization for the robust and accurate linear registration and motion correction of brain images. NeuroImage. 2002;17:825–41.
40. Yeo BT, Krienen FM, Sepulcre J, Sabuncu MR, Lashkari D, Hollinshead M, Roffman JL, Smoller JW, Zöllei L, Polimeni JR, et al. The organization of the human cerebral cortex estimated by intrinsic functional connectivity. J Neurophysiol. 2011;106:1125–65.
41. Yeo BT, Krienen FM, Eickhoff SB, Yaakub SN, Fox PT, Buckner RL, Asplund CL, Chee MW. Functional specialization and flexibility in human association cortex. Cereb Cortex. 2015;25:3654–72.
42. Joel D, Berman Z, Tavor I, Wexler N, Gaber O, Stein Y, Shefi N, Pool J, Urchs S, Margulies DS, et al. Sex beyond the genitalia: the human brain mosaic. Proc Natl Acad Sci U S A. 2015;112:15468–73.
43. Joel D, McCarthy MM. Incorporating sex as a biological variable in neuropsychiatric research: where are we now and where should we be? Neuropsychopharmacology. 2016;42(2):379–85.
44. Bale TL, Epperson CN. Sex as a biological variable: who, what, when, why, and how. Neuropsychopharmacology. 2016;42(2):386–96.
45. Joel D, Fausto-Sterling A. Beyond sex differences: new approaches for thinking about variation in brain structure and function. Philos Trans R Soc Lond Ser B Biol Sci. 2016;371:20150451.
46. McEwen BS, Milner TA. Understanding the broad influence of sex hormones and sex differences in the brain. J Neurosci Res. 2017;95:24–39.
47. McCarthy MM. The two faces of estradiol: effects on the developing brain. Neuroscientist. 2009;15:599–610.
48. Ellegren H, Parsch J. The evolution of sex-biased genes and sex-biased gene expression. Nat Rev Genet. 2007;8:689–98.
49. Lynch CJ, Uddin LQ, Supekar K, Khouzam A, Phillips J, Menon V. Default mode network in childhood autism: posteromedial cortex heterogeneity and relationship with social deficits. Biol Psychiatry. 2013;74:212–9.
50. Moseley RL, Ypma RJ, Holt RJ, Floris D, Chura LR, Spencer MD, Baron-Cohen S, Suckling J, Bullmore E, Rubinov M. Whole-brain functional hypoconnectivity as an endophenotype of autism in adolescents. Neuroimage Clin. 2015;9:140–52.
51. Spencer MD, Chura LR, Holt RJ, Suckling J, Calder AJ, Bullmore ET, Baron-Cohen S. Failure to deactivate the default mode network indicates a possible endophenotype of autism. Mol Autism. 2012;3:15.
52. Zang Y, Jiang T, Lu Y, He Y, Tian L. Regional homogeneity approach to fMRI data analysis. NeuroImage. 2004;22:394–400.
53. Baron-Cohen S. Autism: the empathizing-systemizing (E-S) theory. Ann N Y Acad Sci. 2009;1156:68–80.
54. Baron-Cohen S, Belmonte MK. Autism: a window onto the development of the social and the analytic brain. Annu Rev Neurosci. 2005;28:109–26.
55. Fournier KA, Hass CJ, Naik SK, Lodha N, Cauraugh JH. Motor coordination in autism spectrum disorders: a synthesis and meta-analysis. J Autism Dev Disord. 2010;40:1227–40.
56. Baum SH, Stevenson RA, Wallace MT. Behavioral, perceptual, and neural alterations in sensory and multisensory function in autism spectrum disorder. Prog Neurobiol. 2015;134:140–60.
57. Mostofsky SH, Powell SK, Simmonds DJ, Goldberg MC, Caffo B, Pekar JJ. Decreased connectivity and cerebellar activity in autism during motor task performance. Brain. 2009;132:2413–25.
58. Floris DL, Barber AD, Nebel MB, Martinelli M, Lai MC, Crocetti D, Baron-Cohen S, Suckling J, Pekar JJ, Mostofsky SH. Atypical lateralization of motor circuit functional connectivity in children with autism is associated with motor deficits. Mol Autism. 2016;7:35.
59. Nebel MB, Joel SE, Muschelli J, Barber AD, Caffo BS, Pekar JJ, Mostofsky SH. Disruption of functional organization within the primary motor cortex in children with autism. Hum Brain Mapp. 2014;35:567–80.
60. Nebel MB, Eloyan A, Nettles CA, Sweeney KL, Ament K, Ward RE, Choe AS, Barber AD, Pekar JJ, Mostofsky SH. Intrinsic visual-motor synchrony correlates with social deficits in autism. Biol Psychiatry. 2016;79:633–41.
61. Green SA, Hernandez L, Tottenham N, Krasileva K, Bookheimer SY, Dapretto M. Neurobiology of sensory overresponsivity in youth with autism spectrum disorders. JAMA Psychiat. 2015;72:778–86.
62. Hines M. Sex-related variation in human behavior and the brain. Trends Cogn Sci. 2010;14:448–56.
63. Yang CF, Shah NM. Representing sex in the brain, one module at a time. Neuron. 2014;82:261–78.
64. Thomas JR, French KE. Gender differences across age in motor performance a meta-analysis. Psychol Bull. 1985;98:260–82.
65. Hausmann M. Why sex hormones matter for neuroscience: a very short review on sex, sex hormones, and functional brain asymmetries. J Neurosci Res. 2017;95:40–9.
66. Kleinhans NM, Müller RA, Cohen DN, Courchesne E. Atypical functional lateralization of language in autism spectrum disorders. Brain Res. 2008;1221:115–25.
67. Floris DL, Lai MC, Auer T, Lombardo MV, Ecker C, Chakrabarti B, Wheelwright SJ, Bullmore ET, Murphy DG, Baron-Cohen S, Suckling J. Atypically rightward cerebral asymmetry in male adults with autism stratifies individuals with and without language delay. Hum Brain Mapp. 2016;37:230–53.
68. Lai M, Lombardo MV, Auyeung B, Chakrabarti B, Baron-Cohen S. Sex/gender differences and autism: setting the scene for future research. J Am Acad Child Adolesc Psychiatry. 2015;54:11–24.
69. Baron-Cohen S, Auyeung B, Nørgaard-Pedersen B, Hougaard DM, Abdallah MW, Melgaard L, Cohen AS, Chakrabarti B, Ruta L, Lombardo MV. Elevated fetal steroidogenic activity in autism. Mol Psychiatry. 2015;20:369–76.

70. Baron-Cohen S, Lombardo MV, Auyeung B, Ashwin E, Chakrabarti B, Knickmeyer R. Why are autism spectrum conditions more prevalent in males? PLoS Biol. 2011;9:e1001081.
71. Sassi RB. Attention-deficit hyperactivity disorder and gender. Arch Womens Ment Health. 2010;13:29–31.
72. Ramtekkar UP, Reiersen AM, Todorov AA, Todd RD. Sex and age differences in attention-deficit/hyperactivity disorder symptoms and diagnoses: implications for DSM-V and ICD-11. J Am Acad Child Adolesc Psychiatry. 2010;49:217–28. e211-213.

7

EHMT1 mosaicism in apparently unaffected parents is associated with autism spectrum disorder and neurocognitive dysfunction

Anneke de Boer[1,3†], Karlijn Vermeulen[1,2,3†], Jos I. M. Egger[4,5,6], Joost G. E. Janzing[3], Nicole de Leeuw[7], Hermine E. Veenstra-Knol[8], Nicolette S. den Hollander[9], Hans van Bokhoven[2,7], Wouter Staal[1,2,3,10,11] and Tjitske Kleefstra[2,7*]

Abstract

Background: Genetic mosaicism is only detected occasionally when there are no obvious health or developmental issues. Most cases concern healthy parents in whom mosaicism is identified upon targeted testing of a genetic defect that was initially detected in their children. A germline genetic defect affecting the euchromatin histone methyltransferase 1 (*EHMT1*) gene causes Kleefstra syndrome, which is associated with the typical triad of distinct facial appearance, (childhood) hypotonia, and intellectual disability. A high degree of psychopathology is associated with this syndrome. A few parents with a mosaic *EHMT1* mutation have been detected upon testing after a child was diagnosed with a germline *EHMT1* defect. At first glance, carriers of a mosaic *EHMT1* mutation appeared to function normally. However, recent studies have shown that de novo, postzygotic mutations in important developmental genes significantly contribute to autism spectrum disorder (ASD). Therefore, we hypothesized that *EHMT1* mosaicism could cause neuropsychiatric defects. To investigate this, we performed a detailed investigation of cognitive neuropsychiatric parameters in parents identified with *EHMT1* mosaicism.

Methods: Three adults (two males, one female) with a genetically confirmed diagnosis of *EHMT1* mosaicism were examined by means of a battery of tests and observational instruments covering both neurocognitive and psychiatric features. The battery included the following instruments: the Autism Diagnostic Observation Schedule (ADOS), the mini Psychiatric Assessment Schedules for Adults with Developmental Disabilities (mini PAS-ADD), the Vineland Adaptive Behavior Scales (VABS), and the Cambridge Neuropsychological Test Automated Battery (CANTAB). These measures were compared with our previously reported data from Kleefstra syndrome patients with confirmed (germline) *EHMT1* defects.

Results: All three subjects achieved maximum total scores on the VABS, indicative of adequate (adaptive) functioning. In all, scores above cutoff were found on the ADOS for ASD and on the mini PAS-ADD for major depressive disorder (lifetime). Finally, results on the CANTAB showed impaired cognitive flexibility in all subjects.

Conclusion: Individuals with *EHMT1* mosaicism seem to have increased vulnerability for developing severe psychopathology, especially ASD and mood disorders. Although at first glance they appear to be well-adapted in their daily functioning, they may experience significant psychiatric symptoms and show reduced cognitive flexibility in comparison to the general population.

Keywords: Kleefstra syndrome, *EHTM1*, Mosaicism, Cognition, Autism spectrum disorder, Major depressive disorder

* Correspondence: tjitske.kleefstra@radboudumc.nl
†Equal contributors
[2]Donders Institute for Brain, Cognition and Behavior, Centre for Neuroscience, Radboud University, Nijmegen, the Netherlands
[7]Department of Human Genetics, Radboud University Medical Center, P.O. Box 9101, 6500, HB, Nijmegen, the Netherlands
Full list of author information is available at the end of the article

Background

Kleefstra syndrome (KS; OMIM #610253) is caused by haploinsufficiency of the *euchromatin histone methyltransferase* 1 (*EHMT1*) gene located at chromosome 9q34.3. Almost all cases of KS are due to de novo microdeletions or intragenic loss-of-function mutations in this gene [1, 2]. So far, no inherited cases have been reported, except for a few cases on the basis of parental mosaicism. Mosaicism for *EHMT1* defects appears to be rare. At present, only four cases have been reported: three with a 9q34.3 microdeletion [3, 4] and one with a splice-site mutation in *EHMT1* [5]. These carriers of a genetic *EHMT1* mosaicism were reported to function normally in daily life. However, the focus of these reports was on the genetic and somatic features of the subjects. No data was presented on the possible psychopathology, which is the most pronounced comorbidity in patients with KS caused by a germline *EHMT1* defect [6–9].

The full KS phenotype is characterized by the core triad of intellectual disability (ID), (childhood) hypotonia, and distinct facial features. Additional clinical features include specific behavioral characteristics, heart and urogenital defects, epilepsy, and overweight [1, 2, 10]. Recently, we studied the specific profile of behavioral characteristics in KS, which led us to conclude that KS patients are extremely vulnerable to developing severe psychiatric disorders. In our cohort, the prevalence of autism spectrum disorder (ASD) is nearly 100% [6]. In addition, we found high prevalence of mood disorders and psychotic disorders. Moreover, patients above the age of 18 years in our cohort showed severe regression with a loss of at least 30–50% of their initial functioning [6, 8, 11]. Interestingly, recent studies have shown that de novo postzygotic mutations (PZM) in important developmental genes contribute to ASD [12, 13]. Based on this evidence, we set out to investigate the presence of psychopathology in the parents with an *EHMT1* mosaicism.

In this study, we examined three subjects with *EHMT1* mosaicism for the presence of psychopathology. All three subjects are seemingly unaffected parents of children diagnosed with KS caused by a germline *EHMT1* defect. We hypothesized that individuals with *EHMT1* mosaicism are vulnerable to psychopathology which may have significant clinical consequences.

Methods

Participants

Subjects with *EHMT1* mosaicism were invited by the Department of Human Genetics, Radboud University Medical Center, Nijmegen, the Netherlands, to participate in this study. Informed consent was obtained. The regional medical ethical committee (medical research ethics committee CMO/METC Arnhem-Nijmegen, the Netherlands) approved the study (NL43187.091.13), which was performed in full accordance with the Declaration of Helsinki.

Subject characteristics are summarized in Table 1.

Mosaic pattern detection

In all three subjects, the presence of mosaicism was detected upon carrier testing after the initial finding of a deletion in 9q34 by genome-wide arrays in their respective children. Subsequent confirmation by fluorescent in situ hybridization (FISH) and/or multiplex ligation-dependent probe amplification (MLPA) in blood or in additional tissue was performed in all three subjects.

Instruments

The instruments that were used in this case study are briefly described below. More extensive details can be found in the study of Vermeulen et al. [6] where the instruments have been applied previously in a large cohort of patients with the full KS phenotype.

The Autism Diagnostic Observation Schedule (ADOS) is a semi-structured observational method to assess autism features [14, 15]. It is performed by a certified psychologist or psychiatrist (in this cohort, the first author, KV) and consists of four modules, based on the (developmental) age and language capacity of the participant. Module 4 is designed for normal functioning adults and was used in the current study. A total cutoff score of 7 and above is suspect for an ASD.

The Dutch version of the mini Psychiatric Assessment Schedules for Adults with Developmental Disabilities (mini PAS-ADD) is a psychometrically adequate interview for the detection of psychiatric symptoms and disease in persons with developmental disabilities [16, 17]. It consists of 86 items on a 4-point scale: 0 (symptom not present) to 3 (symptom is severe). The interview is divided into seven subscales: major depressive disorder (MDD), anxiety, obsessive-compulsive disorder, hypomania/mania, psychosis, unspecified disorder, and autism. All criteria are based on the International Classification of Diseases (ICD-10). In this study, subjects were interviewed about themselves.

The Dutch adaptation of the Vineland Adaptive Behavior Scales (VABS) [18] is a widely used clinical interview, which determines the level of adaptive functioning. The age-equivalent scores aid in classifying intellectual and developmental disabilities. The VABS consists of three domains: communication skills, daily living skills, and social skills. This instrument has good reliability and validity [19]. In this study, the subjects were interviewed about themselves.

The Cambridge Neuropsychological Test Automated Battery (CANTAB) is a tablet-based neuropsychological test set comprising all major cognitive domains. Four subtests of the CANTAB were performed in the following sequence:

Table 1 Genetic, psychopathological, and neurocognitive subject characteristics of the subjects

	Subject 1	Subject 2	Subject 3
Sex/age (years)	Male/44	Female/43	Male/39
Genetic defect [*EHMT1* mosaicism]	~60 kb deletion exons 5–17 *EHMT1* 40% mosaicism in blood lymphocytes and buccal swab	~200 kb deletion exons 1–5 *EHMT1* 80% mosaicism buccal swab	~200 kb deletion exon 1 *EHMT1* 60% mosaicism blood lymphocytes
VABS (maximum score)			
Communication (134)	134	121	132
Daily living skills (184)	184	176	177
Socialization (132)	132	118	132
Raw score (450)	450	415	441
Mean developmental age in years	> 12	> 12	> 12
ADOS module 4 (cutoff score)			
Communication (2)	4	2	2
Social interaction (4)	7	10	9
Total score (7)	11	12	11
Classification	Autism spectrum disorder	Autism spectrum disorder	Autism spectrum disorder
Mini PAS-ADD			
Major depressive disorder	Past	Present and past	Present and past
Anxiety disorder	–	Present and past	–
(Hypo)mania	–	–	–
Obsessive compulsive disorder	–	Present and past	–
Psychosis	–	Present and past	–
Unspecified disorder	–	–	–
Autism spectrum disorder	–	–	–
CANTAB *			
MOT mean latency	85–90%	40–45%	80–85%
MOT error	70–75%	95–100%	40–45%
PRM	20–25%	0–5%	70–75%
IED error	30–35%	10–15%	10–15%
IED completed stages	15–20%	5–10%	10–15%
PAL	55–60%	0–5%	75–80%

VABS Vineland Adaptive Behavior Scales, *mini PAS-ADD* Psychiatric Assessment Schedules for Adults with Developmental Disabilities, *CANTAB* Cambridge Neuropsychological Test Automated Battery, *MOT* Motor Screening Test, *PRM* Pattern Recognition Memory, *IED* Intra-Extra Dimensional, *PAL* Paired Associate Learning

*The percentages represent the subjects' performance compared to the normative group. For example, a subject score of 10% means that 90% of the normative group has better scores on this item

1. The Motor Screening Test (MOT) is a training procedure designed to introduce the subject to the tablet touchscreen. In our cohort, it is also an estimate to reactivity, which could not be tested with an official reaction time test because of the complexity of the latter (pushing a button instead of the touch screen during the task).
2. The Pattern Recognition Memory (PRM) is a test of visual pattern recognition memory in a two-alternative forced choice discrimination paradigm. These patterns are designed in such a way so that they cannot easily be given verbal labels. This study presents the number of correct responses.
3. The Intra-Extra Dimensional Test Shift (IED) is a test of rule acquisition and reversal. Visual discrimination, cognitive flexibility, and sustained attention are tested. This study presents (1) total errors, a measure of the subject's efficiency in attempting the test, and (2) the number of completed stages.
4. Paired Associate Learning (PAL) assesses visual memory and new learning. It consists of eight stages.

Each stage is composed of several trials, consisting of the first presentation of the shape(s) and followed by representation when the subject makes an error. The clinical mode terminates after ten repeat presentations. This study presents the total number of errors.

Procedure

Subjects were visited at home. After obtaining informed consent, the study procedure consisted of two clinical interviews with the subjects (VABS and mini PAS-ADD), followed by a semi-structured observation (ADOS) and the tablet-based neurocognitive tests (CANTAB). These procedures were performed by a certified psychiatrist (KV).

Clinical reports

Subject 1 is a 44-year-old married male. He is a father of two children; the youngest son was diagnosed with KS. After finishing a higher professional education, he started working as a data engineer. He does not report social or communicative problems himself; meaningful social contacts are limited, even with family members and colleagues. He had a normal development. His medical history includes an inguinal hernia and hydrocele in childhood, both of which were surgically corrected. The family history does not mention any medical or developmental problems. At physical examination, no typical facial characteristics were observed.

Subject 2 is a 43-year-old female, mother of two children, and her youngest daughter was diagnosed with KS. The somatic characteristics of subject 2 and her youngest daughter have been previously described, represented as family 2 [3]. At the age of 13 years, the subject emigrated from Morocco to the Netherlands. She experienced learning difficulties and did not finish high school. Besides running the household, she started working as a care assistant for elderly people. She was not able to take care of her own financial administration, because of learning difficulties. Her psychiatric history reported a MDD during pregnancy for which fluoxetin was prescribed. Further medical history mentioned three spontaneous abortions, psoriasis, and nephritis. Additionally, she experiences sleep disturbances comprising apneas and frequent awakenings during the night.

Her social network was limited to her family. She had no friends and experienced problems in initiating and maintaining contacts and conversations. Small talk was difficult for her. At the time of examination, she was divorced and not able to work due to mental health problems, consisting of problems in social reciprocity, reactive depressive complaints, and overstimulation and burnout.

At the time of our investigations, she experienced a second major depressive episode with psychotic features (imperative hallucinations and delusions). The imperative hallucinations had led to a suicide attempt. Her general practitioner was informed after our examination, and intensive outreaching care was suggested based on our observation. Physical examination of this subject at the age of 43 years showed obesity and minor dysmorphic features as previously described, including a hypoplastic midface, small upslanting palpebral fissures, depressed nasal root, and anteverted nares.

Subject 3 is a 39-year-old male with three children; the second child was diagnosed with KS. There is no further family history of somatic or neuropsychiatric disorders. After finishing primary school, he struggled to finish high school (practical education level) because of learning disabilities. He went through different jobs, but at the time of the current evaluation, he was not able to work due to his impaired somatic and mental health. He lives an isolated life, together with his wife and children. Despite his social isolation, the patient did not experience any problems in social behavior.

His birth was complicated by a forceps delivery. The remaining medical history revealed atrial fibrillation, knee surgery, tonsillectomy, tympanostomy, and mild auditory and visual impairment. Pharmacotherapy started after the atrial fibrillation was diagnosed and comprised the following: metoprolol, acenocoumarol, simvastatin, and perindopril. Physical examination at the age of 39 years showed obesity, an occipito-frontal circumference of 59 cm (nearly + 1 SD), and minor dysmorphic features including a hypoplastic midface and synophrys.

Genetic analysis

Subject 1: After the detection of an intragenic *EHMT1* deletion in the son by routine array analysis, we performed an MLPA (kit P340-A1, MRC-Holland, Amsterdam, The Netherlands) analysis to confirm the deletion in subject 1. We detected an intragenic deletion of exons 5–17 of *EHMT1* in DNA from both blood lymphocytes and a buccal swab sample, with a mosaicism of 40%. In cultured fibroblasts, the level of mosaicism was 15–20% of cells carrying the deletion.

Subject 2: Results were presented in more detail in a previous study [3]. In summary, genome-wide array analysis on DNA from the daughter revealed an interstitial deletion of ~ 200 kb in 9q34.3 encompassing at least the first five exons of the *EHMT1* gene. Carrier testing by array in both parents showed that this deletion was inherited from subject 2 (the mother), but her array results showed a less pronounced loss, suggestive of mosaicism.

Interphase FISH analysis with two different FISH probes on a buccal swab sample from subject 2 showed the deletion in 80% of her cells (50–55 cells analyzed), indicating that she is a mosaic carrier of the 9q34.3 deletion: .nuc ish del(9)(q34.3q34.3)(RP11_417A4-)[37/55],(RP13_467E5-)[45/50].

Subject 3: After the detection of a 9q34.3 deletion in the son (arr [hg 19] 9q34.3(140350924 140551108)× 1), the array analysis on DNA from subject 3 suggested the presence of a mosaic deletion in 9q34.3. Subsequent FISH analyses on blood lymphocytes showed an abnormal signal pattern in 29 of 50 cells analyzed, suggesting 60% mosaicism: ish del(9)(q34.3q34.3)(RP11-48C7-)[29/50].

Results

The genetic, psychopathological, and neurocognitive characteristics are presented in Table 1.

Psychopathological and neurocognitive studies

The developmental age of all three mosaic carriers was 12 years or older. This maximum score on the clinical interview VABS is in line with the developmental age of the general population. Additionally, all subjects fulfilled the diagnostic criteria for ASD and MDD either currently and/or in the past. In contrast to the ADOS, the mini PAS-ADD did not formally determine ASD as the total subscale scores were just below the cutoff score. Notwithstanding, ASD items scored in the mini PAS-ADD were similar to the clinical observations of the ADOS. During the clinical observation, all participants scored on limited eye contact and minimum use of emotional gestures, when testing was focused on the communication. For social interaction, all three showed impaired social reciprocity, a limited range of facial expressed emotions, and an inadequate description of their role in social relations.

In addition to estimating the degree of psychopathology, we used the CANTAB to measure several cognitive functions of our subjects. The percentages represent the subjects' performance compared to the normative group with the same sex and age. Subject 1 had low scores on the PRM and IED. Subject 2 had overall low scores on the tests. Subject 3 experienced problems with the IED. Detailed results are presented in Table 1; all IED scores were lower than 35% of the peer group, indicating an impaired mental flexibility in all three subjects.

Discussion

In this report, we describe the consequences of *EHMT1* mosaicism on psychopathology in three adult subjects. The three seemingly unaffected parents included in this study had been referred to the clinical genetics department only because of the diagnostic trajectory of each parent's respective child. The discovery of *EHMT1* mosaicism in these subjects was unexpected [3–5]. The degree of mosaicism that was measured in different tissues varied from 15 to 40% (subject 1) to 80% (subject 2). It is difficult to predict the clinical consequences of mosaicism, as the patterns and distribution of abnormal cells can vary widely between different tissues, depending on the timing of the mutation events [20]. Despite this predicted variation, all three subjects had an ASD, a (prior) MDD, and other associated neurocognitive dysfunctions. Some features that can be seen in patients with a germline *EHMT1* mutation had a variable occurrence in the mosaic individuals. The results are indicative of a vulnerability to develop severe psychiatric disorders that carriers of an *EHMT1* mosaic mutation possess. This correlates with the high prevalence of psychopathology, which has been reported for individuals with the full KS phenotype due to a germline *EHMT1* mutation [6, 8, 21]. Based on the ADOS test, all mosaic subjects met the criteria for ASD and all had a (prior) MDD. This is further corroborated by our findings on the CANTAB. All subjects showed weaknesses in performance on the IED, which is suggestive of cognitive inflexibility. This might be related to the set-shifting problems often seen in subjects with ASD, although findings on executive function deficits in adults with ASD were inconsistent [22]. These deficiencies on the IED are on the continuum compared with a significant high dropout on the IED in our previous research on subjects with the full KS phenotype (unpublished data). Subject 3 had no other deviating scores compared to his norm group. Subject 1 showed performance problems on the PRM, but we could not clearly link this to his clinical profile. Subject 2 had low scores on all tasks, most likely due to (a combination of) her learning and mood problems.

Psychopathology has a direct impact on adaptive functioning. The adaptive behavior measured with the VABS implies a developmental age above 12 years, consistent with adult functioning, for all of our subjects. Nevertheless, all three of them struggle to fulfill their role in society, most likely as a direct consequence of their neurodevelopmental problems. They became socially isolated and experienced difficulties in finding the right type of education and employment that would suit their strengths and weaknesses. Therefore, the clinical relevance for diagnosing these subjects with *EHMT1* mosaicism and consequent neuropsychiatric assessment is significant. Optimal treatment of the psychopathology may improve daily functioning and positively influence the well-being of the individuals treated and their families, including the child with KS, as well as their participation in society. Based on our findings, personalized psychiatric evaluation and treatment should be considered for subjects diagnosed with *EHMT1* mosaicism. The diagnostic procedure should include a special attention to ASD and mood disorders. Furthermore, these cases illustrate that presence of mosaic deletions could potentially be missed, since the genetic defects were only discovered during the diagnostic phase of the children with the full KS phenotype. None of the subjects had been referred to a medical specialist for their own psychiatric problems prior to our studies. These subjects tend to have a more subtle presentation, but this can nevertheless cause impaired (social) functioning. Therefore, our study also demonstrates that genetic analysis should be considered in patients with a psychiatric disorder and other characteristics of KS without the classic appearance.

Despite the similarities in psychopathology between our subjects, the consequences of mosaicism in general are widespread and unique for each individual [23]. The phenotypic expression of somatic mosaicism has been investigated and reported in several studies including mosaic trisomy 21 (Down syndrome) and mosaic fragile X syndrome [24, 25]. These studies show severe phenotypic expression, as well as somatic mosaicism without clinical consequences. The expression of the behavioral phenotype is also variable. In mosaic trisomy 21, for example, the social adaptive skills were significantly better in the subjects with a mosaicism compared to non-mosaic subjects with Down syndrome. However, the intellectual performance did not relate to the level of mosaicism [24]. This necessitates interpretative caution, especially since we assessed the psychopathology of only three subjects with an *EHMT1* mosaicism and each had different levels of mosaic expression. Interestingly, in recent studies, it was shown that rare postzygotic mutations in important developmental genes contribute significantly to ASD [12, 13]. Our present results obtained for three ASD subjects with such a rare mosaic defect in *EHMT1* are in line with these reports. *EHMT1* is an important developmental gene that is extremely intolerant to loss-of-function mutations (http://exac.broadinstitute.org) [26]. Further clinical studies are warranted to provide more insight into the wide spectrum of the *EHMT1* mosaicism, although the extremely low prevalence of such mosaic defects hampers the careful collection of symptoms in larger cohorts. For future research, we recommend to include more specific measures on IQ, ASD, and mood disorders in subjects with an *EHMT1* mosaicism. These measures should be in addition to a (semi)structured clinical observation as people with neurodevelopmental disorders, like ASD, are more likely to have deviating scores on questionnaires [27, 28]. Thus, clinical interviews and observations should always be performed to gain a more comprehensive and objective insight into the psychopathology.

Conclusion

Subjects with *EHMT1* mosaicism seem vulnerable to developing psychiatric disorders, especially ASD and mood disorders. However, since the behavioral outcome of mosaicism is unpredictable, these results should be interpreted with caution. Based on our findings in this small but unique cohort, we recommend screening subjects with an *EHMT1* mosaicism for psychopathology. In our experience, multidisciplinary care, combining expertise in psychiatry, clinical genetics, and clinical neuropsychology, is of additional value in these complex cases where a broad perspective is required. Ideally, a careful diagnostic assessment of psychopathology, cognition, and physical health should be performed to provide an integrative diagnosis. Deficits in daily functioning and behavioral problems may well be a result of an underlying genetic or otherwise somatic cause, which is often not clearly present. Clinical considerations should therefore include the possibility of a genetic mosaicism in parents who have one or more children with a neurodevelopmental disorder of genetic origin and a typical combination of complaints, as illustrated in this study.

Abbreviations

ADOS: Autism Diagnostic Observation Schedule; ASD: Autism spectrum disorder; CANTAB: Cambridge Neuropsychological Test Automated Battery; EHMT1: Euchromatin histone methyltransferase 1; ICD-10: International Classification of Diseases-10; ID: Intellectual disability; IED: Intra-Extra Dimensional Test Shift; KS: Kleefstra syndrome; MDD: Major depressive disorder; MOT: Motor Screening Test; PAL: Paired Associate Learning; PAS-ADD: Psychiatric Assessment Schedules for Adults with Developmental Disabilities; PRM: Pattern Recognition Memory; PZM: Postzygotic mutations; VABS: Vineland Adaptive Behavior Scales

Acknowledgements

We are thankful for the participation of our patients. Furthermore, we are grateful to the local caregivers, who provided treatment for the diagnosed disorders. Thanks are extended to the Vincent van Gogh Institute and Cambridge Cognition for the kind provision of the simplified versions of the subtests. This study arose from collaboration among the departments of Human Genetics and Psychiatry of the Radboud University Medical Center, Karakter Child and Adolescent Psychiatry, all located in Nijmegen, and the Vincent van Gogh Centre of Excellence for Neuropsychiatry, Venray, the Netherlands. The study was funded by the Donders Institute for Brain, Cognition and Behavior, Radboud University Nijmegen, the Netherlands.

Funding

The study was funded by a grant of the Donders Institute for Brain, Cognition and Behaviour.

Authors' contributions

The study was designed and directed by TK, KV, and JGEJ. Patient referral and recruitment were carried out by KV, TK, HVK, and NSdH. The home visits were performed by KV and AdB. The data and results were interpreted by AdB, KV, TK, WS, JIME, JGEJ, and HvB. Microarray analyses, DNA sequencing, validation, and genotyping were carried out and interpreted by TK, HVK, NSdH, and NdL. The manuscript was written by AdB, KV, TK, WS, JIME, JGEJ, and HvB, with all authors refining and approving the final version of it.

Competing interests

The authors declare that they have no competing interests.

Author details

[1]Karakter Child and Adolescent Psychiatry University Centre, Nijmegen, the Netherlands. [2]Donders Institute for Brain, Cognition and Behavior, Centre for Neuroscience, Radboud University, Nijmegen, the Netherlands. [3]Department of Psychiatry, Radboud University Medical Center, Nijmegen, the Netherlands. [4]Centre of Excellence for Neuropsychiatry, Vincent van Gogh Institute for Psychiatry, Venray, the Netherlands. [5]Behavioural Science Institute, Radboud

University, Nijmegen, the Netherlands. [6]Donders Institute for Brain, Cognition and Behaviour, Centre for Cognition, Radboud University, Nijmegen, the Netherlands. [7]Department of Human Genetics, Radboud University Medical Center, P.O. Box 9101, 6500, HB, Nijmegen, the Netherlands. [8]Department of Genetics, University Medical Centre Groningen, University of Groningen, Groningen, the Netherlands. [9]Department of Clinical Genetics, Leiden University Medical Center, Leiden, the Netherlands. [10]Faculty of Social Sciences, Leiden University, Leiden, the Netherlands. [11]Leiden Institute for Brain and Cognition, Leiden University, Leiden, the Netherlands.

References

1. Willemsen MH, Vulto-van Silfhout AT, Nillesen WM, Wissink-Lindhout WM, van Bokhoven H, Philip N, Berry-Kravis EM, Kini U, van Ravenswaaij-Arts CM, Delle Chiaie B, et al. Update on Kleefstra syndrome. Mol Syndromol. 2012;2:202–12.
2. Kleefstra T, Brunner HG, Amiel J, Oudakker AR, Nillesen WM, Magee A, Genevieve D, Cormier-Daire V, van Esch H, Fryns JP, et al. Loss-of-function mutations in euchromatin histone methyl transferase 1 (EHMT1) cause the 9q34 subtelomeric deletion syndrome. Am J Hum Genet. 2006;79:370–7.
3. Willemsen MH, Beunders G, Callaghan M, de Leeuw N, Nillesen WM, Yntema HG, van Hagen JM, Nieuwint AW, Morrison N, Keijzers-Vloet ST, et al. Familial Kleefstra syndrome due to maternal somatic mosaicism for interstitial 9q34.3 microdeletions. Clin Genet. 2011;80:31–8.
4. Herve B, Roume J, Cognard S, Fauvert D, Molina-Gomes D, Vialard F. Low-level mosaicism of a de novo derivative chromosome 9 from a t(5;9)(q35.1; q34.3) has a major phenotypic impact. Eur J Med Genet. 2015;58:346–50.
5. Rump A, Hildebrand L, Tzschach A, Ullmann R, Schrock E, Mitter D. A mosaic maternal splice donor mutation in the EHMT1 gene leads to aberrant transcripts and to Kleefstra syndrome in the offspring. Eur J Hum Genet. 2013;21:887–90.
6. Vermeulen K, de Boer A, Janzing JGE, Koolen DA, Ockeloen CW, Willemsen MH, Verhoef FM, van Deurzen PAM, van Dongen L, van Bokhoven H, et al. Adaptive and maladaptive functioning in Kleefstra syndrome compared to other rare genetic disorders with intellectual disabilities. Am J Med Genet A. 2017. https://doi.org/10.1002/ajmg.a.38280. Epub ahead of print.
7. Vermeulen K, Staal W, Janzing J, Buitelaar J, van Bokhoven H, Egger J, Kleefstra T. From a single gene defect towards a cross species neurocognitive phenotype: the *EHMT1* disruption example (Kleefstra syndrome). Austin J Autism Relat Disabil. 2015;1(2):1009.
8. Verhoeven WM, Egger JI, Vermeulen K, van de Warrenburg BP, Kleefstra T. Kleefstra syndrome in three adult patients: further delineation of the behavioral and neurological phenotype shows aspects of a neurodegenerative course. Am J Med Genet A. 2011;155a:2409–15.
9. Schmidt S, Nag HE, Hunn BS, Houge G, Hoxmark LB. A structured assessment of motor function and behavior in patients with Kleefstra syndrome. Eur J Med Genet. 2016;59(4):240–8.
10. Kleefstra T, van Zelst-Stams WA, Nillesen WM, Cormier-Daire V, Houge G, Foulds N, van Dooren M, Willemsen MH, Pfundt R, Turner A, et al. Further clinical and molecular delineation of the 9q subtelomeric deletion syndrome supports a major contribution of EHMT1 haploinsufficiency to the core phenotype. J Med Genet. 2009;46:598–606.
11. Kleefstra T, Nillesen WM, Yntema HG. Kleefstra Syndrome. In: Pagon RA, Adam MP, Ardinger HH, Wallace SE, Amemiya A, Bean LJH, Bird TD, Ledbetter N, Mefford HC, Smith RJH, Stephens K, editors. GeneReviews(R). Seattle: University of Washington; 1993.
12. Lim ET, Uddin M, De Rubeis S, Chan Y, Kamumbu AS, Zhang X, D'Gama AM, Kim SN, Hill RS, Goldberg AP, et al. Rates, distribution and implications of postzygotic mosaic mutations in autism spectrum disorder. Nat Neurosci. 2017;20:1217–24.
13. Krupp DR, Barnard RA, Duffourd Y, Evans SA, Mulqueen RM, Bernier R, Riviere JB, Fombonne E, O'Roak BJ. Exonic mosaic mutations contribute risk for autism spectrum disorder. Am J Hum Genet. 2017;101:369–90.
14. Lord C, Rutter M, Goode S, Heemsbergen J, Jordan H, Mawhood L, Schopler E. Autism diagnostic observation schedule: a standardized observation of communicative and social behavior. J Autism Dev Disord. 1989;19:185–212.
15. Lord C, Rutter M, PC DL, Risi S. Autism diagnostic observation schedule. Manual. Los Angeles: WPS; 1999.
16. Janssen R, Maes B. Psychometric evaluation of a Dutch version of the mini PAS-ADD for assessing psychiatric disorders in adults with different levels of intellectual disability. J Intellect Disabil Res. 2013;57:689–702.
17. Prosser H, Moss S, Costello H, Simpson N, Patel P, Rowe S. Reliability and validity of the mini PAS-ADD for assessing psychiatric disorders in adults with intellectual disability. J Intellect Disabil Res. 1998;42(Pt 4):264–72.
18. Sparrow SS, Balla DA, Cicchetti DV. Vineland Adaptive Behavior Scales. Minneapolis: American Guidance Services; 1984.
19. de Bildt A, Kraijer D, Sytema S, Minderaa R. The psychometric properties of the Vineland Adaptive Behavior Scales in children and adolescents with mental retardation. J Autism Dev Disord. 2005;35:53–62.
20. De S. Somatic mosaicism in healthy human tissues. Trends Genet. 2011; 27:217–23.
21. Mitra AK, Dodge J, Van Ness J, Sokeye I, Van Ness B. A de novo splice site mutation in EHMT1 resulting in Kleefstra syndrome with pharmacogenomics screening and behavior therapy for regressive behaviors. Mol Genet Genomic Med. 2017;5:130–40.
22. Chen SF, Chien YL, Wu CT, Shang CY, Wu YY, Gau SS. Deficits in executive functions among youths with autism spectrum disorders: an age-stratified analysis. Psychol Med. 2016;46:1625–38.
23. Cohen AS, Wilson SL, Trinh J, Ye XC. Detecting somatic mosaicism: considerations and clinical implications. Clin Genet. 2015;87:554–62.
24. Papavassiliou P, Charalsawadi C, Rafferty K, Jackson-Cook C. Mosaicism for trisomy 21: a review. Am J Med Genet A. 2015;167a:26–39.
25. Pretto D, Yrigollen CM, Tang HT, Williamson J, Espinal G, Iwahashi CK, Durbin-Johnson B, Hagerman RJ, Hagerman PJ, Tassone F. Clinical and molecular implications of mosaicism in FMR1 full mutations. Front Genet. 2014;5:318.
26. Tachibana M, Ueda J, Fukuda M, Takeda N, Ohta T, Iwanari H, Sakihama T, Kodama T, Hamakubo T, Shinkai Y. Histone methyltransferases G9a and GLP form heteromeric complexes and are both crucial for methylation of euchromatin at H3-K9. Genes Dev. 2005;19:815–26.
27. Havdahl KA, Hus Bal V, Huerta M, Pickles A, Øyen AS, Stoltenberg C, Lord C, Bishop SL. Multidimensional influences on autism symptom measures: implications for use in etiological research. J Am Acad Child Adolesc Psychiatry. 2016;55:1054–63. e3
28. Vermeulen K, JIM E, JGE J, van Dongen L, van Bokhoven H, Kleefstra T, Staal WG. The context of symptom measures: interpretation and clinical diagnosis of autism spectrum disorders in intellectual disabilities. J Am Acad Child Adolesc Psychiatry. 2017;56:618–9.

8

Association between maternal antidepressant use during pregnancy and autism spectrum disorder

Xi-Hong Zhou[1], Yong-Jiang Li[2,3], Jian-Jun Ou[4] and Ya-Min Li[1*]

Abstract

Studies have investigated the risk of autism spectrum disorder (ASD) in children exposed in utero to antidepressant, with inconsistent results. Given the substantial public health implications on this topic, here, we presented an updated meta-analysis of the association between maternal antidepressant use during pregnancy and ASD. Cochrane Library, EMBASE, PsycINFO, and PubMed databases were systematically searched. A random effects model was used to pool the adjusted relative risk (RR) for cohort studies and the adjusted odds ratio (OR) for case-control studies as well as their corresponding 95% confidence intervals (CIs). Meta-analysis restricted to sibling studies was also conducted. Publication bias was systematically assessed. Fourteen studies were identified (eight cohort studies and six case-control studies). Pooled adjusted RR for cohort studies ($n = 2{,}839{,}980$) was 1.13 (0.93–1.39) showed a non-significant association; while two studies were potentially missing from the test of publication bias, filled estimates also showed a non-significant association (filled RR 0.97, 95% CI 0.79–1.19). Pooled OR was 1.51 (1.15–1.99) for case-control studies ($n = 117{,}737$) showed a significant association; two studies were potentially missing; however, the filled estimates suggested a non-significant association (filled OR 1.26, 95% CI 0.98–1.62). Analyses restricted to sibling studies also showed a non-significant association (RR 0.99, 95% CI 0.81–1.22). In summary, we did not evidence a significant association between maternal antidepressant use during pregnancy and ASD.

Keywords: Antidepressant exposure, Autism spectrum disorder, Offspring, Meta-analysis

Introduction

Nearly 15% of pregnant women have depression [1]. Untreated depression during pregnancy may lead to significant obstetrical and developmental issues, including gestational diabetes, hypertension, preeclampsia, postnatal complications and suicidal ideation on mothers, hyperactivity and irregular heart rate on developing fetus, increased rates of premature deaths on newborns as well as internalizing and externalizing problems on children [2]. Therefore, treatment of depression during pregnancy is of great significance for both mothers and children.

Antidepressants are widely used medications for the treatment of prenatal depression, and selective serotonin reuptake inhibitors (SSRIs) were the most commonly prescribed. With the considerably increased prevalence of antidepressant use during pregnancy, confusion continued regarding the appropriate use of antidepressants during this critical period in consideration of maternal and fetal outcomes.

Previous meta-analyses have evaluated the association between antidepressant use during pregnancy and the risk of autism spectrum disorders (ASDs) in children [3–9], all reported a significant association. However, those meta-analyses concluded a positive association did not cover several important eligible studies, including the cohort study by Malm et al. [10] and other four newly published large-scale cohort studies [11–14].

* Correspondence: aminny@csu.edu.cn
[1]Clinical Nursing Teaching and Research Section, The Second Xiangya Hospital, Central South University, Changsha 410011, Hunan, China
Full list of author information is available at the end of the article

Further, publication bias has not been comprehensively examined in previous meta-analyses.

In recent two large-scale cohort studies that aimed to further disentangled the associations of maternal depression, antidepressant exposure during pregnancy, and ASD risk in offspring [11, 12], researchers reported that their data analysis of large, population-based sample with adequate statistical power showed that maternal antidepressant exposure was not associated with ASD. Also, they emphasized the fact that regardless of antidepressant treatment, maternal depression without treatment remains at increased risk for developmental disorders in children.

As the use of antidepressants is likely to be remained widely for the treatment of depression during pregnancy, the precise estimation of the potential risk has substantial public health implications. Hence, we presented an updated meta-analysis based on current evidence to first evaluate whether maternal antidepressant use during pregnancy is a risk factor for ASD and to second comprehensively assess the publication bias.

Method

Search strategies and eligibility criteria

A systematic literature search of Cochrane Library, EMBASE, PsycINFO, and PubMed databases was conducted in July 2017, using the combination of Medical Subject Headings and relevant keywords as follows: autism/autistic/asperger/autism spectrum disorder/ASD and antidepressant/antidepressive agents/selective serotonin uptake inhibitor/SSRI/ and maternal/pregnancy/fetal/children/offspring. Reference lists from articles as well as meta-analyses identified by the search were also screened to identify additional studies. Two reviewers performed the searches, screened title/abstracts, and reviewed full text independently. Articles were included if they reported original case-control or cohort studies that investigated the risk of ASD in children exposed in utero to antidepressant; articles were excluded if they reported cases or case series.

Data extraction

The baseline characteristics of included studies, including the first author's name, publication year, study design, data source, sample size, adjusted covariates, and main findings (adjusted estimates and their corresponding 95% CIs), were reviewed and extracted.

Quality assessment

The improved Newcastle-Ottawa Scale [15] was used for quality assessment of included studies. Three domains were evaluated, including selection, comparability, and exposure. Each satisfactory answer was assigned one "star," and studies with six or more stars were considered of high quality. Two authors independently assessed study quality. Consensus was reached by discussion with the primary author.

Data analysis

We first analyzed the overall impact of any antidepressant exposure and second analyzed the specific impact of SSRIs to investigate whether the association between SSRI exposure and ASD would be influenced by other antidepressants. After careful review of the reported data from the original publications, the exposure period of prepregnancy, first trimester, second and/or third trimester, and the whole pregnancy were investigated in cohort studies. While for case-control studies, the exposure period of prepregnancy, first trimester, second trimester, third trimester, and the whole pregnancy were investigated. Therefore, in consideration of methodological heterogeneity between cohort studies and case-control studies, data from cohort studies and case-control studies were separately pooled.

A random effects model was used for meta-analyses. Heterogeneity was evaluated with the I^2 statistic, P value, and tau value. Funnel plots were produced to evaluate publication bias. If potential publication bias was observed by visually examining the asymmetry of the funnel plots, then the "trim and fill" method would be applied to adjust the funnel plot and further to recalculate the pooled estimates. In addition, to test the robustness of the pooled estimates, sensitivity analyses were performed for studies with overlapping data sources by deleting each study and rerunning meta-analysis. Confounding by indication was first addressed by excluding studies that did not include maternal psychiatric conditions as covariates, and second addressed by performing meta-analysis on cohort studies employing more rigorous controls such as sibling controls or controls of children exposed to maternal psychiatric disorder but no antidepressant use during pregnancy. All data analyses were performed using Stata statistical software (version 12.0; Stata Corporation, College Station, TX, USA).

Results

Study selection and baseline characteristics

Flow diagram of the study selection process was presented in Additional file 1: Figure S1. Briefly, 213 records were retrieved from our systematic literature search. After removing duplicates and irrelevant titles, 23 articles remained for full-text screening. Eight studies that did not report original investigations and one study did not address the outcome of interest were excluded. Finally, 14 studies met the eligibility criteria were included [10–14, 16–24]. Baseline characteristics of the included studies were presented in Additional file 2: Table S1. Three out of six case-control studies, two out of eight cohort studies reported a positive association.

Two case-control studies did not include maternal psychiatric disorders as covariates in their multivariate analysis [16, 21]. In quality assessment, NOS scores for all included studies were high and all were rated as high quality (Additional file 3: Table S2).

Meta-analysis

Pooled adjusted RR for cohort studies ($n = 2{,}839{,}980$) was 1.13 (95% CI 0.93–1.39) with moderate between-study heterogeneity ($I^2 = 61.4\%$, $P = 0.016$) showed a non-significant association between prenatal antidepressants exposure and ASD (Fig. 1). Pooled adjusted OR for case-control studies ($n = 117{,}737$) was 1.51 (95% CI 1. 15–1.99) with moderate between-study heterogeneity ($I^2 = 44.6\%$, $P = 0.108$) showed a statistically significant association (Fig. 2).

Results of meta-analyses stratified by pregnancy period and medication were summarized in Table 1. A non-significant association was found for pooled RR for cohort studies, while the pooled ORs for case-control studies showed a significant association. As for different trimesters, the pooled results did not alter for both cohort studies and case-control studies. The effect of SSRI was slightly larger than the combined effect of any antidepressant. Although there were two cohort studies with overlapping data sources [17, 19], the sample was not duplicated as data were not pooled in any subgroup in our analysis. As for confounding by indication, the pooled OR was changed to 1.41 (95% CI 1.00–1.99) after excluding the two case-control studies that did not include maternal psychiatric disorders as covariates in their multivariate analysis (Additional file 4: Figure S2). The pooled RR for cohort studies with sibling controls or controls of children exposed to maternal psychiatric disorder, but no antidepressant use during pregnancy was 0.99 (95% CI 0.81–1.22), with substantially decreased heterogeneity between studies ($I^2 = 9.0\%$, $P = 0.355$) (Additional file 5: Figure S3).

Publication bias

Although the number of included studies was limited, funnel plots for cohort studies and case-control studies were produced separately for assessment of publication bias, and all were obviously asymmetry, suggesting potential publication bias (Additional file 6: Figure S4; Additional file 7: Figure S5). Therefore, "trim and fill" analysis was performed to estimate the number of missing studies. As a result, for both cohort studies and case-control studies, two potential missing studies were detected by adjusting the funnel plot (Figs. 3 and 4). However, both filled estimates demonstrated a non-significant association (filled RR for cohort studies 0.97, 95% CI 0.79–1.19; filled OR for case-control studies 1. 26, 95% CI 0.98–1.62).

Discussion

Our meta-analysis is based on published observational studies pertaining to ASD risk of in utero exposure to antidepressant. Data from cohort studies and case-control studies were synthesized separately due to inconsistent study design, which is a significant source of heterogeneity. Results from our meta-analysis showed that no association was found for cohort studies; while the pooled OR for case-control studies showed a

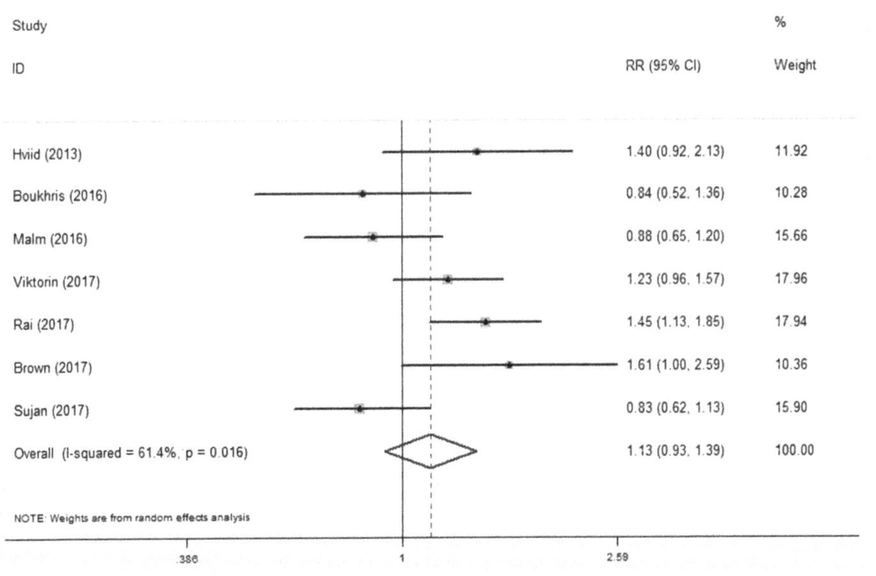

Fig. 1 Forest plot of the meta-analysis of cohort studies on the effects of prenatal antidepressant exposure and autism spectrum disorder

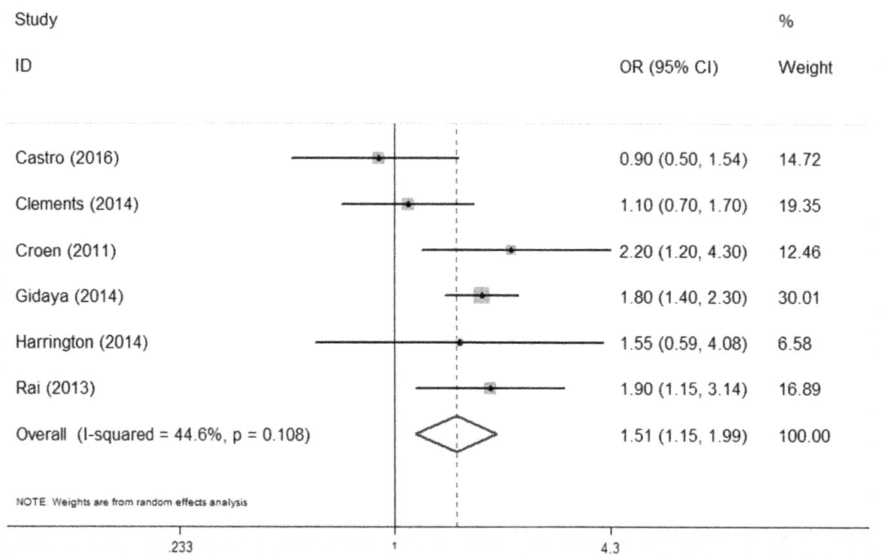

Fig. 2 Forest plot of the meta-analysis of case-control studies on the effects of prenatal antidepressant exposure and autism spectrum disorder

Table 1 Summary of the meta-analyses performed on fetal antidepressant exposure during pregnancy and autism spectrum disorders

	Medication	No. of studies	Overall effect			Heterogeneity		
			OR/HR (95% CI)	*Z*	*P* value	I^2 (%)	*P*	Tau
Cohort studies								
Pregnancy	Any antidepressant	7	1.13 (0.93–1.39)	1.22	0.224	61.4	0.016	0.0437
	Any SSRI	3	1.22 (0.83–1.79)	0.99	0.320	64.7	0.059	0.0749
First trimester	Any antidepressant	5	1.01 (0.82–1.24)	0.06	0.953	31.9	0.209	0.0174
	Any SSRI	3	1.04 (0.81–1.34)	0.32	0.747	42.7	0.155	0.027
Second and/or third trimester	Any antidepressant	4	1.35 (0.96–1.90)	1.75	0.080	46.4	0.133	0.0552
	Any SSRI	3	1.43 (0.84–2.42)	1.32	0.187	71.6	0.030	0.1549
Prepregnancy	Any antidepressant	2	1.26 (0.91–1.74)	1.40	0.160	67.1	0.081	0.0365
	Any SSRI	1	1.46 (1.17–1.81)					
Case-control studies								
Pregnancy	Any antidepressant	6	1.51 (1.15–1.99)	3.00	0.003	44.6	0.108	0.0478
	Any SSRI	4	1.81 (1.46–2.23)	5.50	< 0.001	0.0	0.908	< 0.0001
First trimester	Any antidepressant	5	1.69 (1.17–2.44)	2.81	0.005	46.3	0.114	0.0756
	Any SSRI	2	2.08 (1.54–2.81)	4.78	< 0.001	7.2	0.340	0.0098
Second trimester	Any antidepressant	5	1.62 (1.22–2.16)	3.31	0.001	8.6	0.358	0.0107
	Any SSRI	3	1.94 (1.41–2.68)	4.04	< 0.001	0.0	0.413	< 0.0001
Third trimester	Any antidepressant	5	1.47 (0.88–2.44)	1.48	0.140	60.0	0.040	0.1843
	Any SSRI	3	2.32 (1.63–3.30)	4.68	< 0.001	0.0	0.515	< 0.0001
Prepregnancy	Any antidepressant	4	1.70 (1.43–2.02)	6.04	< 0.001	0.0	0.897	< 0.0001
	Any SSRI	2	1.81 (1.43–2.29)	4.92	< 0.001	0.0	0.896	< 0.0001

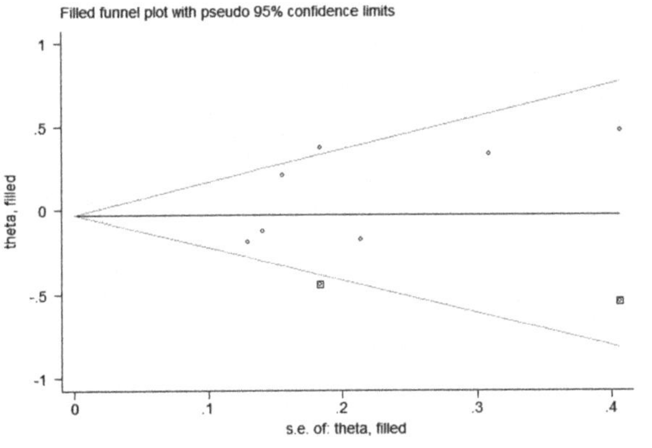

Fig. 3 Filled funnel plot of included cohort studies showing number of potential missing studies

significant association, the filled OR was dramatically changed and the association was changed accordingly to be non-significant.

Our systematic literature search identified seven published meta-analyses on this topic [3–9], all reported a significant association from their data analysis. However, those meta-analyses did not include all eligible original investigations, especially for several newly published large scale cohort studies [10–14], and thus concluded a positive association. Besides, publication bias was not systematically evaluated in previous meta-analyses due to insufficient number of eligible studies. Hence, the weight of case-control studies was very high and may thus lead to a false-positive result and a misleading conclusion. Most cohort studies did not replicate such a significant association reported in most case-control studies. Compared with cohort studies, case-control studies were generally retrospective and unable to control for important confounding factors (i.e., indication) thus less likely to evidence a causal association. In addition, the pooled sample size of case-control studies

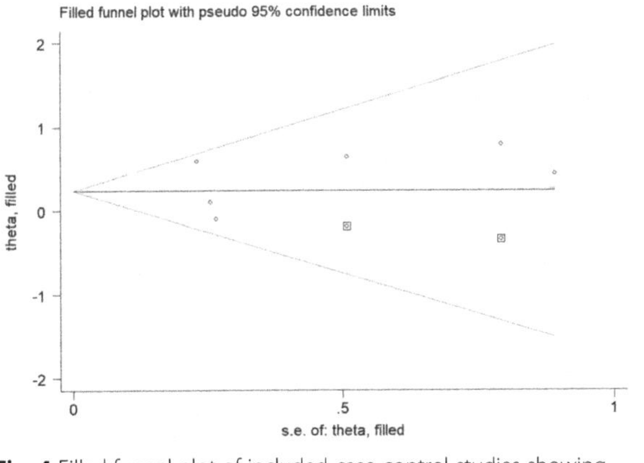

Fig. 4 Filled funnel plot of included case-control studies showing number of potential missing studies

(n = 117,737) was much smaller than that of cohort studies (n = 2,839,980).

The combined effect of confounding by indication and publication bias may explain the difference between cohort studies and case-control studies. After excluding the two case-control studies that did not include maternal psychiatric disorders as covariates [16, 21], the pooled estimate was significantly changed (OR 1.41, 95% CI 1.00–1.99). Results of meta-analysis on cohort studies with sibling controls or controls of children exposed to maternal psychiatric disorder but no antidepressant use during pregnancy showed a non-significant association (RR 0.99, 95% CI 0.81–1.22) with less heterogeneity (I^2 = 9.0%, P = 0. 355) suggested that the residual confounding of maternal psychiatric disorders might be an important source of heterogeneity. More importantly, in our test of publication bias, two potential missing studies were detected by "trim and fill" method for both cohort studies and case-control studies, and the filled estimates for cohort studies still suggested a non-significant association between maternal antidepressant use and ASD, but the filled estimates for case-control studies dramatically changed and demonstrated a non-significant association.

Findings from studies should be treated with caution in consideration of study limitations and in case of false-positive results. Indeed, medication use during pregnancy has been concern of clinicians and mother-to-be. Nevertheless, the devastating effects of untreated depression during pregnancy on the mothers as well as on the developing children have been widely studied and reported [2]. More seriously, prenatal depression is characterized by a relatively high frequency of somatic symptoms and suicide ideation that may lead to grave consequences [25].

The limitation for this meta-analysis is the unexplored validity of the test of publication bias as it contributed significantly to our conclusions. The "trim and fill" method for testing and adjusting publication bias is funnel-plot-based. The number of missing studies and their effect sizes were estimated and calculated rather than retrieved. Therefore, the filled studies may not match reality in any close way and the filled estimates may not reflect the precision.

In conclusion, this meta-analysis based on current best evidence and conducted with an appropriate approach quantitatively concluded that maternal antidepressant exposure may not be associated with ASD. In this case, we do not suggest pregnant women diagnosed with severe depression discontinuing their antidepressant use for fear of an uncertain risk. Nevertheless, despite the non-significant association we currently concluded, information about doses of antidepressant exposure and severity of ASD symptoms is less, and the absence of population-level, individual-specific data on depression, and ASD warranted further investigations.

Additional files

Additional file 1: Figure S1. PRISMA diagram for the study selection process.

Additional file 2: Table S1. Baseline characteristics and main findings of included studies in the meta-analysis.

Additional file 3: Table S2. Quality assessment of the included studies by the improved Newcastle–Ottawa Scale.

Additional file 4: Figure S2. Forest plot for case-control studies adjusted for maternal psychiatric disorders in their multivariate analysis.

Additional file 5: Figure S3. Forest plot for cohort studies with sibling controls or controls of children exposed to maternal psychiatric disorder but no antidepressant use during pregnancy.

Additional file 6: Figure S4. Funnel plot of included cohort studies.

Additional file 7: Figure S5. Funnel plot of included case-control studies.

Abbreviations
ASD: Autism spectrum disorder; CI: Confidence interval; OR: Odds ratio; RR: Relative risk

Funding
None.

Authors' contributions
LYM conceived of the study; ZXH, LYJ, and OJJ conducted the literature search; ZXH, LYJ, and OJJ extracted the data; LYJ analyzed the data; and ZXH and LYJ drafted and reviewed the manuscript. All authors read and approved the final manuscript.

Competing interests
The authors declare that they have no competing interests.

Author details
[1]Clinical Nursing Teaching and Research Section, The Second Xiangya Hospital, Central South University, Changsha 410011, Hunan, China. [2]Department of Pharmacy, The Second Xiangya Hospital, Central South University, Changsha 410011, Hunan, China. [3]Institute of Clinical Pharmacy, Central South University, Changsha 410011, Hunan, China. [4]Mental Health Institute, The Second Xiangya Hospital, Central South University, Changsha 410011, Hunan, China.

References
1. Yonkers KA, Wisner KL, Stewart DE, Oberlander TF, Dell DL, Stotland N, Ramin S, Chaudron L, Lockwood C. The management of depression during pregnancy: a report from the American Psychiatric Association and the American College of Obstetricians and Gynecologists. Gen Hosp Psychiatry. 2009;31:403–13.
2. Gentile S. Untreated depression during pregnancy: short- and long-term effects in offspring. A systematic review. Neuroscience. 2017;342:154–66.
3. Man KK, Tong HH, Wong LY, Chan EW, Simonoff E, Wong IC. Exposure to selective serotonin reuptake inhibitors during pregnancy and risk of autism spectrum disorder in children: a systematic review and meta-analysis of observational studies. Neurosci Biobehav Rev. 2015;49:82–9.
4. Kaplan YC, Keskin-Arslan E, Acar S, Sozmen K. Prenatal selective serotonin reuptake inhibitor use and the risk of autism spectrum disorder in children: a systematic review and meta-analysis. Reprod Toxicol. 2016;66:31–43.
5. Kobayashi T, Matsuyama T, Takeuchi M, Ito S. Autism spectrum disorder and prenatal exposure to selective serotonin reuptake inhibitors: a systematic review and meta-analysis. Reprod Toxicol. 2016;65:170–8.
6. Brown HK, Hussain-Shamsy N, Lunsky Y, Dennis C, Vigod SN. The association between antenatal exposure to selective serotonin reuptake inhibitors and autism: a systematic review and meta-analysis. J Clin Psychiatry. 2017;78:e48.
7. Mezzacappa A, Lasica P-A, Gianfagna F, Cazas O, Hardy P, Falissard B, Sutter-Dallay A-L, Gressier F. Risk for autism spectrum disorders according to period of prenatal antidepressant exposure: a systematic review and meta-analysis. JAMA Pediatr. 2017;171(6):555–63.
8. Andalib S, Emamhadi M, Yousefzadeh-Chabok S, Shakouri S, Høilund-Carlsen P, Vafaee M, Michel T, Maternal SSRI. Exposure increases the risk of autistic offspring: a meta-analysis and systematic review. Eur Psychiatry. 2017;45:161–6.
9. Rais TB, Rais A. Association between antidepressants use during pregnancy and autistic spectrum disorders: a meta-analysis. Innov Clin Neurosci. 2014;11:18.
10. Malm H, Brown AS, Gissler M, Gyllenberg D, Hinkka-Yli-Salomäki S, McKeague IW, Weissman M, Wickramaratne P, Artama M, Gingrich JA. Gestational exposure to selective serotonin reuptake inhibitors and offspring psychiatric disorders: a national register-based study. J Am Acad Child Adolesc Psychiatry. 2016;55:359–66.
11. Brown HK, Ray JG, Wilton AS, Lunsky Y, Gomes T, Vigod SN. Association between serotonergic antidepressant use during pregnancy and autism spectrum disorder in children. JAMA. 2017;317:1544–52.
12. Sujan AC, Rickert ME, Öberg AS, Quinn PD, Hernández-Díaz S, Almqvist C, Lichtenstein P, Larsson H, D'Onofrio BM. Associations of maternal antidepressant use during the first trimester of pregnancy with preterm birth, small for gestational age, autism spectrum disorder, and attention-deficit/hyperactivity disorder in offspring. JAMA. 2017;317:1553–62.
13. Viktorin A, Uher R, Reichenberg A, Levine S, Sandin S. Autism risk following antidepressant medication during pregnancy. Psychol Med. 2017;47(16): 2787–96.
14. Rai D, Lee BK, Dalman C, Newschaffer C, Lewis G, Magnusson C. Antidepressants during pregnancy and autism in offspring: population based cohort study. BMJ. 2017;358:j2811.
15. Wells G, Shea B, O'connell D, Peterson J, Welch V, Losos M, Tugwell P: The Newcastle-Ottawa Scale (NOS) for assessing the quality of nonrandomised studies in meta-analyses. Ottawa Hospital Research Institute, 2014. oxford. ASp; 2015.
16. Croen LA, Grether JK, Yoshida CK, Odouli R, Hendrick V. Antidepressant use during pregnancy and childhood autism spectrum disorders. Arch Gen Psychiatry. 2011;68:1104–12.
17. Hviid A, Melbye M, Pasternak B. Use of selective serotonin reuptake inhibitors during pregnancy and risk of autism. N Engl J Med. 2013;369:2406–15.
18. Rai D, Lee BK, Dalman C, Golding J, Lewis G, Magnusson C. Parental depression, maternal antidepressant use during pregnancy, and risk of autism spectrum disorders: population based case-control study. BMJ. 2013;346:f2059.
19. Sørensen MJ, Grønborg TK, Christensen J, Parner ET, Vestergaard M, Schendel D, Pedersen LH. Antidepressant exposure in pregnancy and risk of autism spectrum disorders. Clin Epidemiol. 2013;5:449.
20. Gidaya NB, Lee BK, Burstyn I, Yudell M, Mortensen EL, Newschaffer CJ. In utero exposure to selective serotonin reuptake inhibitors and risk for autism spectrum disorder. J Autism Dev Disord. 2014;44:2558–67.
21. Harrington RA, Lee L-C, Crum RM, Zimmerman AW, Hertz-Picciotto I, Prenatal SSRI. Use and offspring with autism spectrum disorder or developmental delay. Pediatrics. 2014;133:e1241–8.
22. Clements CC, Castro VM, Blumenthal SR, Rosenfield HR, Murphy SN, Fava M, Erb JL, Churchill SE, Kaimal AJ, Doyle AE. Prenatal antidepressant exposure is associated with risk for attention deficit-hyperactivity disorder but not autism spectrum disorder in a large health system. Mol Psychiatry. 2015;20:727.
23. Boukhris T, Sheehy O, Mottron L, Bérard A. Antidepressant use during pregnancy and the risk of autism spectrum disorder in children. JAMA Pediatr. 2016;170:117–24.
24. Castro V, Kong S, Clements C, Brady R, Kaimal A, Doyle A, Robinson E, Churchill S, Kohane I, Perlis R. Absence of evidence for increase in risk for autism or attention-deficit hyperactivity disorder following antidepressant exposure during pregnancy: a replication study. Transl Psychiatry. 2016;6:e708.
25. Gavin AR, Tabb KM, Melville JL, et al. Prevalence and correlates of suicidal ideation during pregnancy. Arch Womens Ment Health. 2011;14:239–46.

9

Subcellular organization of UBE3A in human cerebral cortex

Alain C. Burette[1*], Matthew C. Judson[2], Alissa N. Li[3,4], Edward F. Chang[5], William W. Seeley[3,4], Benjamin D. Philpot[2,6] and Richard J. Weinberg[2]

Abstract

Background: Loss of UBE3A causes Angelman syndrome, whereas excess UBE3A activity appears to increase the risk for autism. Despite this powerful association with neurodevelopmental disorders, there is still much to be learned about UBE3A, including its cellular and subcellular organization in the human brain. The issue is important, since UBE3A's localization is integral to its function.

Methods: We used light and electron microscopic immunohistochemistry to study the cellular and subcellular distribution of UBE3A in the adult human cerebral cortex. Experiments were performed on multiple tissue sources, but our results focused on optimally preserved material, using surgically resected human temporal cortex of high ultrastructural quality from nine individuals.

Results: We demonstrate that UBE3A is expressed in both glutamatergic and GABAergic neurons, and to a lesser extent in glial cells. We find that UBE3A in neurons has a non-uniform subcellular distribution. In somata, UBE3A preferentially concentrates in euchromatin-rich domains within the nucleus. Electron microscopy reveals that labeling concentrates in the head and neck of dendritic spines and is excluded from the PSD. Strongest labeling within the neuropil was found in axon terminals.

Conclusions: By highlighting the subcellular compartments in which UBE3A is likely to function in the human neocortex, our data provide insight into the diverse functional capacities of this E3 ligase. These anatomical data may help to elucidate the role of UBE3A in Angelman syndrome and autism spectrum disorder.

Keywords: Angelman syndrome, E6-AP, Axon terminal, Mitochondria, Euchromatin

Background

Protein degradation through the ubiquitin-proteasome pathway (UPP) is important for a wide range of functions in the nervous system [1, 2]. In UPP processing, the protein substrate is marked by covalent attachment of the small protein ubiquitin for subsequent degradation by the proteasome, a specialized proteolytic complex. The process starts with the activation of ubiquitin by E1 ubiquitin ligase enzymes [3, 4]. E2 enzymes then transfer the activated ubiquitin to E3 ubiquitin ligases, which attach the ubiquitin to the substrate. The E3 ligases determine the substrate specificity of ubiquitination.

Two major classes of E3s have been defined: HECT (homologous to E6-AP carboxyl-terminus) domain E3s and RING finger E3s. UBE3A, the first E3 discovered in the HECT class [5], is of special interest, because failure to maintain appropriate levels of UBE3A in the brain is directly linked to severe clinical disorders. The loss of UBE3A function causes Angelman syndrome (AS) [6, 7], characterized by profound intellectual and developmental disabilities [8]. On the other hand, increased UBE3A activity (via gene duplication or gain-of-function mutation) is implicated in several forms of autism [9–15], implying that UBE3A must be expressed at precise levels to allow proper neuronal function.

Despite its clinical importance, our current understanding of UBE3A's function in the brain remains limited. UBE3A has been implicated in regulation of Golgi acidification [16] and mitochondrial function [17–19], as

* Correspondence: alain.burette@gmail.com
[1]Department of Cell Biology and Physiology, University of North Carolina at Chapel Hill, 314 Taylor Hall, Campus, Box 7545, Chapel Hill, NC 27599-7545, USA
Full list of author information is available at the end of the article

well as synaptic transmission and plasticity [20–26]. Several potential interactors and substrates for its ubiquitin ligase activity have been identified, including the RhoA guanine nucleotide exchange factors Pbl/ECT2 and Ephexin5 [24, 27, 28], RAD23A, (an enzyme involved in excision repair of damaged DNA [29]), and the estrogen receptor [30]. UBE3A has also been shown to regulate the levels of Cbln1 in excitatory neurons, which in turn can influence sociability [26]. Finally, UBE3A can interact directly with the proteasome to influence its degradative activity [15, 31–35], suggesting potentially wide-ranging roles for UBE3A in cellular functions that remain to be fully defined.

Crucial for the elucidation of UBE3A's functions is to determine where the protein actually lies within the cell. Previous immunohistochemical studies in rodents found a broad distribution of UBE3A, but emphasized its nuclear expression in mature neurons, consistent with a proposed role for UBE3A in the regulation of transcription [26, 36–38]. However, patterns of UBE3A expression in humans may not be fully conserved, considering the 100 million years of divergent evolution between rodents and primates. Unique patterns of UBE3A expression within the cerebral cortex could have important functional implications, especially given the cognitive manifestations of both AS and autism. Here, we explore this intriguing possibility by investigating the subcellular distribution of UBE3A in the human temporal cortex.

Methods

Human brain tissue

All procedures regarding human tissue were performed with the approval of the UCSF Committee on Human Research and the University of Maryland Institutional Review Board. Nine small blocks from postmortem temporal cortex were obtained from the UCSF Neurodegenerative Disease Brain Bank (NDBB) and the NIH NeuroBioBank, including autopsy materials from all three adults with AS currently available for study. Details are listed in Table 1. Interpretability of immunohistochemical results depends on the quality of the tissue. To assess structural preservation, we used transmission electron microscopy of fixed samples embedded in epoxy plastic.

The ultrastructural integrity of all postmortem tissue was seriously compromised. In the best preserved samples, most subcellular structures were identifiable, but the tissue contained abnormal holes, neurons were vesiculated, cytoplasm was disrupted, nucleoplasm appeared abnormally condensed, membranes were distorted, and mitochondria were swollen (Fig. 1a, b). The overall impression was of substantial deterioration of the material surrounding a "skeleton" of residual organization. Notwithstanding the suboptimal integrity of this material, it was far superior to that of the available postmortem samples from persons with AS (Fig. 1c, d). This material was markedly degraded, with severe disruption and a global lack of ultrastructural integrity. A few elements remained identifiable, including many synapses, but these resembled biochemically isolated preparations; synaptic membranes and synaptic vesicles were typically lost or distorted. We concluded that despite their inherent clinical importance, the available AS samples were unsuitable for micro-anatomical study, while autopsy material from neurotypical controls was acceptable for specific purposes if results were interpreted with caution. Unexpectedly, the structural preservation and RIN score (RNA integrity number) were not always correlated (Table 1), further emphasizing the value of ultrastructural assessment.

Choosing to focus on well preserved material, we obtained 9 surgical biopsies. Because of limited tissue availability, all nine were from patients undergoing surgery to remove epileptic foci in the hippocampus (Table 2). The temporal cortex from these patients was intact, displaying normal activity in intraoperative electrocorticography, and removed only to gain access to the pathological hippocampal tissue beneath it. Small pieces of the neocortex overlying the epileptic focus were immersion-fixed for 24 h at 4 °C in 1–4% paraformaldehyde (PFA)/1% glutaraldehyde in phosphate buffer (PB), 2% PFA/2–4% glutaraldehyde in 0.1 M sodium cacodylate + 0.1% $CaCl_2$ and

Table 1 Autopsy cases included in this study

Repository	Case ID	Sex	Age (years)	Clinical diagnosis	Time to fixation (hours)	RIN
UCSF NDBB	P2321.10	M	77	MCI	4.9	3–3.6
UCSF NDBB	P2394.12	M	76	Control	8.2	5.2–6.1
UCSF NDBB	P2698	M	81	MCI	10	–
Maryland	5363	F	28	Control	11	–
Maryland	5659	M	17	Control	10	6.8
Maryland	5758	F	43	Control	18–23	–
Maryland	1494	F	43	AS	21	–
Maryland	5743	M	19	AS	18–23	–
Maryland	3854	F	21	AS	21	–

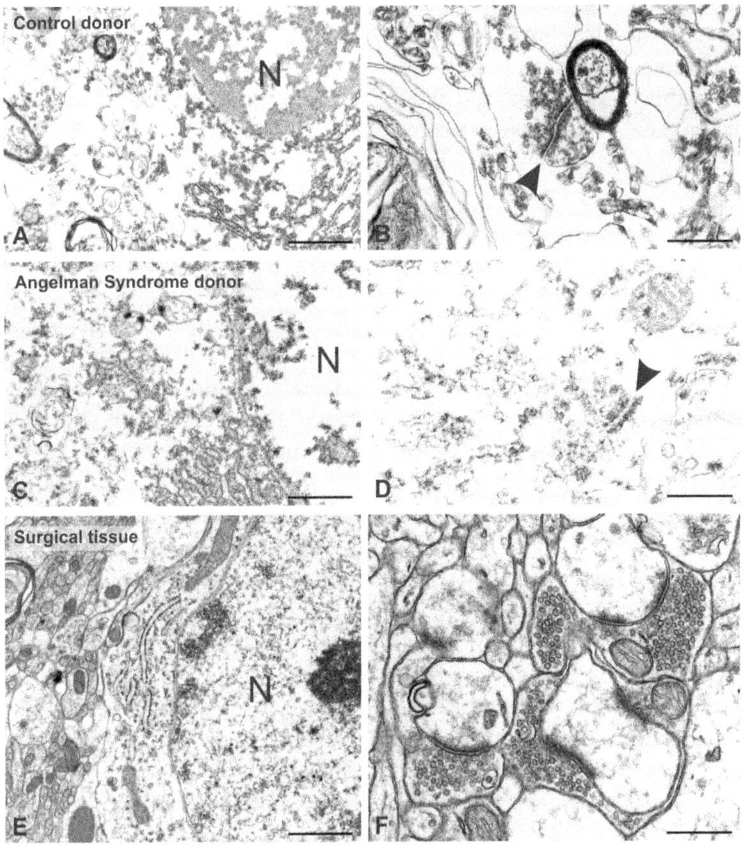

Fig. 1 Ultrastructural integrity of human tissue samples from different sources. Ultrastructural integrity is low in postmortem material from a control donor, though major organelles such as nuclei (N) remain identifiable (low-magnification view, **a**). At high magnification, synapses (arrowhead) are damaged but clearly defined (**b**). Material from an Angelman syndrome donor is virtually uninterpretable (reflecting the practical difficulty of obtaining and curating such material), though damaged mitochondria and traces of nuclear structure remain (N in panel **c**); hints of synaptic specializations may be identified even in this material (arrowhead, **d**). In contrast, tissue from biopsy specimens obtained during surgeries for epilepsy shows very good preservation, as documented by features including intact mitochondria, well-aligned rough endoplasmic reticulum, and intact chromatin (**e**). The well-preserved neuropil (**f**) contrasts with that of the autopsy specimens above. Tissue from case no. 5758 for **a** and **b**, 1494 for **c** and **d**, and Q1012 for **e** and **f**. Scale bar = 1 μm in **a**, **c**, and **e** and 500 nm in **b**, **d**, and **f**

2.5% DMSO, or 4% PFA in 0.1 M sodium cacodylate + 0.1% $CaCl_2$ and 2.5% DMSO. Following fixation, the samples were stored in PO_4-buffered saline (PBS) at 4 °C. Sections were cut at 50 μm on a Vibratome and collected in cold PB.

In contrast to the postmortem tissue, the ultrastructural integrity of the biopsy samples was generally good, and in many cases, comparable to that obtained from perfusion-fixed mice (Fig. 1e, f). Since the biopsies were from patients undergoing surgery to remove epileptic

Table 2 Biopsy cases included in this study

Case no.	Sex	Age (years)	Clinical diagnosis	Time to fixation (minutes)
Q1010	M	30	Epilepsy	15
Q1011	M	44	Epilepsy	6
Q1012	M	58	Epilepsy	10
Q1013	F	38	Epilepsy	6
Q1014	F	48	Epilepsy	10
Q1015	F	66	Epilepsy	7
Q1017	M	46	Epilepsy	7
Q1018	F	20	Epilepsy	5
Q1019	F	51	Epilepsy	4

foci, we took the added precaution of staining each sample for parvalbumin, GABA, and glial fibrillary acidic protein (GFAP), three markers which may undergo pathological changes in epileptic tissues; we restricted our analysis to regions from each biopsy that appeared normal, as assessed by comparison with immunostaining in perfusion-fixed rodents.

Animals

All procedures related to the care and treatment of animals were in accordance with institutional and NIH guidelines, and all animal use protocols were reviewed and approved by the UNC Institutional Animal Care and Use Committee. AS model mice (*Ube3a*$^{m-/p+}$), which maternally inherit the *Ube3a* knock-out allele, were generated by mating wild-type (*Ube3a*$^{m+/p+}$) male mice to female mice with paternal inheritance of the *Ube3a* knock-out allele (*Ube3a*$^{m+/p-}$), which themselves are phenotypically normal [39, 40]. After inducing deep anesthesia with sodium pentobarbital (80 mg/kg, i.p.), adult (P60–P100) male mice were intracardially perfused with 50 ml of 4% freshly depolymerized paraformaldehyde in phosphate buffer (PB, 0.1 M, pH 7.4), then post-fixed overnight at 4 °C in the same buffer. To mimic the biopsy procedure in human patients, we anesthetized mice with pentobarbital (80 mg/kg) and quickly removed the brain. One hemisphere was immediately submerged in fixative, while the other half was exposed to room air for 15 min prior to immersion in fixative. After 24 h in the fixative, the brains were rinsed in PB, sectioned at 50 or 100 µm on a Vibratome, and collected in cold PB.

Antibodies

To identify UBE3A, we used a mouse monoclonal antibody (3E5, Sigma-Aldrich, cat. no. SAB1404508, RRID:AB_10740376) raised against a peptide corresponding to mouse UBE3A isoforms 1 and 3 (a.a. 315–415) and isoform 2 (a.a. 336–436). Importantly, this immunogen shares 100% sequence identity with human UBE3A isoforms 1 (a.a. 318–417), 2 (a.a. 341–441), and 3 (a.a. 338–437). We used this antibody because we had previously verified its specificity against AS model and UBE3A KO mice [41].

To identify GABA, we used a rabbit polyclonal antibody (Sigma, St. Louis, MO; A2052, lot 052K4827) developed using GABA-BSA as the immunogen. The antibody was affinity-purified using the immunogen. It showed positive binding with GABA and GABA-KLH in a dot blot assay and negative binding with bovine serum albumin (BSA) (manufacturer's technical information).

To identify GFAP, we used a rabbit polyclonal anti-GFAP (Chemicon, AB5804) developed against purified bovine GFAP. This antibody recognizes a 51 kDa band on immunoblot of rat spinal cord.

To identify Oligodendrocyte Transcription Factor 2 (Olig2), we used a rabbit polyclonal anti-Olig2 (Millipore, AB9610) developed using a recombinant mouse Olig-2. This antibody specifically labels cells of oligodendrocyte lineage [42], consistent with our own observations [43].

Light microscopy

Free-floating sections were treated for 30 min in 1% sodium borohydride, followed by 30 min with 3% H_2O_2 in phosphate-buffered saline (PBS, 0.1 M, pH 7.4). After preincubation in 10% normal donkey serum (to block secondary antibody binding sites), sections were incubated in UBE3A (1:500 to 1:5000) overnight on a shaker at room temperature.

For immunoperoxidase microscopy, sections were then incubated overnight on a shaker at room temperature in biotinylated secondary antibody (1:200; Jackson ImmunoResearch, West Grove, PA) and for 4 h in ExtrAvidin-peroxidase complex (1:5000; Sigma, St. Louis, MO); peroxidase was histochemically visualized with diaminobenzidine. Processed sections were mounted on gelatin-coated slides, air dried, and cleared with xylene before being coverslipped with D.P.X. Mountant (BDH Chemicals, Poole, England).

For immunofluorescence, antigenic sites were visualized with donkey IgG conjugated to DyLight 549 (1:200, Jackson ImmunoResearch; West Grove, PA). For double labeling, the second primary antibody (1:10,000 GABA, 1:1000 Olig2, or 1:2000 GFAP) was applied overnight and visualized by a secondary antibody conjugated to Alexa 488 (1:200, Invitrogen). Some sections were then counterstained with DAPI (1:10,000, Sigma-Aldrich, cat. no. D9542) to visualize nuclei, and with NeuroTrace 640–660 (1:1000, Invitrogen, Thermo Fisher Scientific, Rockford, IL; cat. no. N21483) to visualize neuronal somata. Sections were examined with a Zeiss LSM 880 confocal microscope with Airyscan.

Electron microscopy

To assess structural preservation, sections were processed for reduced osmium according to the Knott protocol [44, 45]. Briefly, sections were washed in cacodylate buffer (0.1 M, pH 7.4) and post-fixed for 40 min in 1.5% potassium ferrocyanide and 1% osmium tetroxide, followed by 1 h in 1% osmium tetroxide alone, rinsed in water, then incubated 40 min in 1% uranyl acetate in water, rinsed in water, dehydrated in an ethanol series, and infiltrated and embedded in resin (Spurr's low viscosity epoxy with ERL-4221, Electron Microscopy Sciences, Hatfield, PA; cat. no. 14300).

For immunohistochemistry, sections were treated with 1% sodium borohydride/PBS, followed by 3% H_2O_2/PBS, then 0.025% Triton X-100/PBS, then blocked with 10%

normal goat serum (NGS), and incubated overnight in primary antibody (UBE3A, 1:200 to 1:1000). Sections were rinsed, and blocked again in 2% NGS, then incubated overnight with biotinylated goat-anti mouse IgG (1:2000, Vector Laboratories, Burlingame, CA; cat. no. BA-9200), rinsed, and incubated for 2 h in 1.4 nm gold particles conjugated to streptavidin (1:100; Nanoprobes, Yaphank, NY; cat. no. 2016). After rinsing, binding was stabilized by treating 30 min in 2% glutaraldehyde/PBS; sections were washed again and transitioned into 0.05 M sodium acetate (to remove phosphate and chloride ions), followed by silver enhancement with HQ Silver (Nanoprobes, Yaphank, NY; cat. no. 2012). After rinsing in sodium acetate and transitioning to PB, sections were post-fixed in 0.5% osmium tetroxide in 0.1 M PB for 45 min, rinsed and transitioned to 0.1 M maleate buffer, pH 6, and then incubated for 45 min with 1% uranyl acetate in maleate buffer (0.1 M, pH 6.0).

After processing, sections were dehydrated in a graded ethanol series and infiltrated with a low viscosity epoxy resin (Spurr's with ERL-4221, Electron Microscopy Sciences, Hatfield, PA) and flat-mounted between sheets of ACLAR® fluoropolymer (Electron Microscopy Sciences, Hatfield, PA; cat. no. 50425) within glass slides. Sixty-nanometer sections were cut and mounted on 200 mesh copper grids. For double labeling with GABA, nickel grids were pretreated 15 min at 60 °C in 0.01 M citrate buffer, pH 6, rinsed in water, blocked in 1% BSA in Tris-buffered saline, pH 7.6, with 0.005% Tergitol NP-10, and incubated overnight at 21–24 °C room temperature with the primary antibody (GABA, 1:10,000 to 1:50,000). Grids were rinsed, blocked in 1% normal goat serum in TBS, pH 8.2, with Tergitol NP-10, and incubated in secondary antibodies for 2 h (goat antibody to rabbit IgG conjugated to 20 nm gold particles, BBI, UK, cat. no. EM.GAR20). Grids were then rinsed in buffer, then water, and counterstained with 1% uranyl acetate in water, followed by Sato's lead. Electron microscopy was performed with a Philips Tecnai transmission electron microscope.

Controls

Biopsy specimens are subject to an unavoidable delay (for our material, 5–15 min, Table 2) prior to immersion in the fixative. Delayed fixation could in principle lead to misleading artifacts in immunolocalization, particularly for a protein involved in proteasomal degradation like UBE3A. Accordingly, we verified that similarly delayed immersion fixation in mice does not significantly affect UBE3A distribution or cause other unforeseen issues. We compared the overall distribution of UBE3A in mouse brains fixed by perfusion, immediate immersion fixation, and immersion fixation after a delay of 15 min (Fig. 2). We found that UBE3A staining was similar in all three cases: it was expressed throughout all layers of the neocortex, with strong nuclear staining and weaker staining in somata and dendrites. Vascular artifacts and subtle indications of cytoplasmic condensation after delayed fixation did not significantly affect the pattern of immunostaining.

To verify antibody specificity, we performed the same procedures on AS model mice (maternal UBE3A knock-out); only a very weak background staining could be detected in these mice (Fig. 2e, f). We conclude that a 15-min delay in fixation does not significantly alter the distribution of UBE3A.

Image analysis

To compare the level of nuclear UBE3A between excitatory neurons and GABAergic neurons, we acquired 58 random fields of human cortical layers II/III (100 μm × 100 μm, from Q1010, Q1011, and Q1012) from material quadruple-stained for UBE3A, GABA, NeuroTrace, and DAPI. To minimize artifacts arising from limited penetration, confocal images were acquired just below the section surface. For each neuron, the intensity of UBE3A staining in the nucleus (defined by DAPI) was computed using FIJI [46]. To control for possible local variations of immunostaining intensity arising from immersion fixation, we computed the ratio of staining in GABA-positive and GABA-negative neurons from each field individually, reasoning that NeuroTrace-positive neurons that were immunonegative for GABA were very likely to be excitatory.

To examine the quantitative relationship between staining for UBE3A and DAPI, we performed intensity correlation analysis as described by Li et al. [47], using FIJI. The analysis was performed on 92 random nuclei from human cortical layers II/III (from Q1010, Q1011, and Q1012, which yielded particularly robust immunostaining for UBE3A). The imaging was done with the Airyscan mode.

Results

The overall pattern of staining was consistent across biopsy samples from all 9 subjects. UBE3A was found in neurons throughout the depth of cerebral cortex (Fig. 3a–c). Staining within neurons concentrated in the nucleus, but could also be seen in somata and proximal dendrites, and punctate staining was observed in neuropil (Fig. 3d, e). The apparent lack of nuclear staining in some neurons was interpreted as an artifact arising from limited antibody penetration, since it was not seen in neurons whose nucleus lay at the section edge. Examination of thin (< 300 nm) sections showed that much of the nuclear staining was organized into discrete tiny aggregates of DAB reaction product distributed through the nucleus (Fig. 3f).

GABAergic deficits have been implicated in the pathogenesis of neocortical hyperexcitability and epilepsy in AS model mice [25, 48], and GABA transporter-1 has

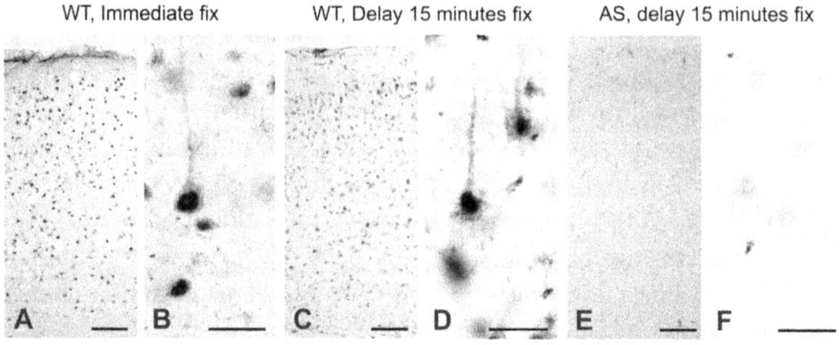

Fig. 2 Immunohistochemistry for UBE3A in mouse cerebral cortex following different methods of fixation. UBE3A staining in tissue fixed by perfusion (**a**, **b**). **c**, **d** Immersion fixation of mouse cortex after a delay of 15 min (similar to the fixation for our surgical material) shows only modest differences, including a subtle condensation of immunopositive cytoplasm. In both cases, UBE3A is expressed through all layers of the neocortex, with strong nuclear staining and weaker staining in somata and dendrites. UBE3A staining is nearly absent in the brain of an AS model mouse fixed by immersion after a delay of 15 min (**e**, **f**), further confirming specificity of the UBE3A antibody in brain tissue harvested under conditions similar to surgical biopsy. Scale bar = 100 μm in **a**, **c**, and **e** and 25 μm in **b**, **d**, and **f**

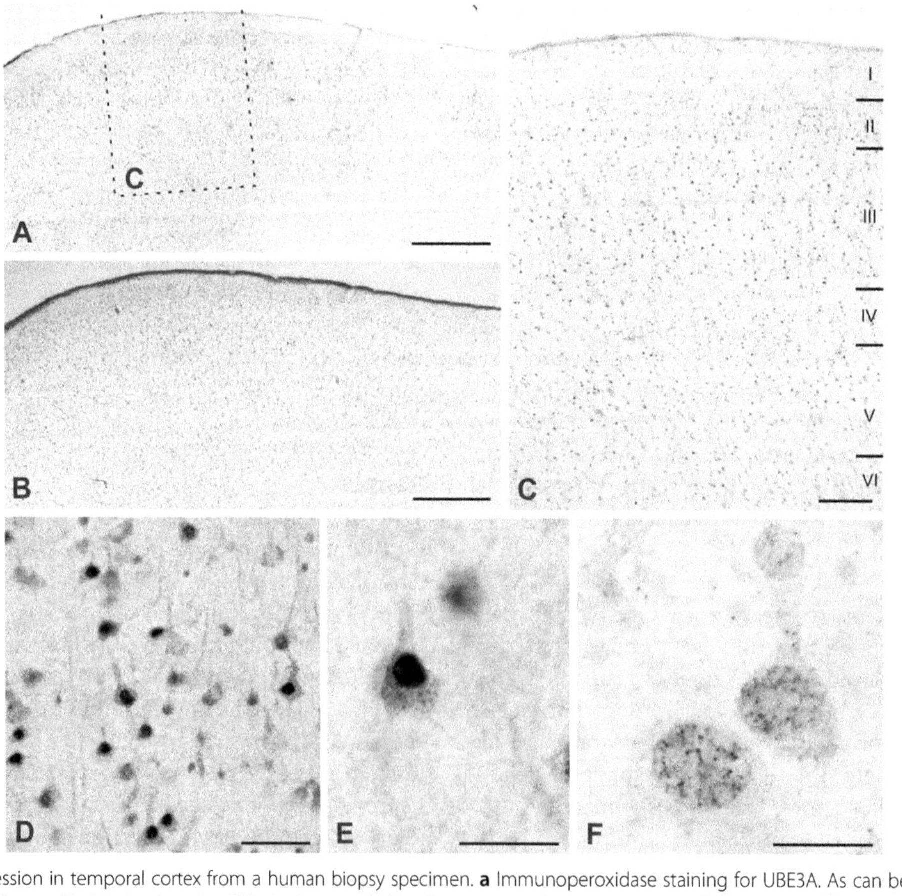

Fig. 3 UBE3A expression in temporal cortex from a human biopsy specimen. **a** Immunoperoxidase staining for UBE3A. As can be seen by comparison with adjacent Nissl-stained section (**b**), the large majority of neurons are immunopositive. **c** Enlargement of boxed area from **a**; UBE3A is expressed throughout all layers of temporal cortex. **d**, **e** Higher magnification micrographs show UBE3A concentrating in nuclei. Antigen is also visible in somata and neuropil, but at lower levels. **f** High magnification micrograph of a 250-nm plastic section shows discrete grains of immunoperoxidase reaction product scattered through most of the nucleus, but seemingly excluded from certain regions. Tissue from case no. Q1019. Scale bar = 1 mm in **a** and **b**, 250 μm in **c**, 50 μm in **d**, 25 μm in **e**, and 10 μm in **f**

been proposed as a potential UBE3A substrate [49]. To determine whether UBE3A is expressed in inhibitory neurons of the human neocortex, as it is in mice, we performed double labeling with GABA (Fig. 4). We found that GABAergic neurons, like pyramidal neurons, express higher levels of UBE3A in their nuclei than in their somata. However, quantitative analysis of biopsy material from three subjects revealed that the concentration of nuclear UBE3A is ~ 40% (38 ± 6.4%, $n = 51$) higher in pyramidal neurons than in GABAegic neurons. In addition, colocalization was observed in fine processes and puncta distributed through the neuropil (Fig. 4c, d).

In mice, UBE3A is expressed not only in neurons but also neuroglia. To evaluate its distribution in non-neuronal cells in the human temporal cortex, we performed double staining with Olig2, to identify oligodendrocytes (Fig. 5a, b). Indeed Olig2-positive somata were consistently immunopositive for UBE3A, though to a lesser degree than seen in neurons. We also performed double staining with GFAP to identify astrocytes, finding that astrocytes also expressed UBE3A, though generally at lower levels than either neurons or oligodendrocytes (Fig. 5c, d). These patterns were reminiscent of UBE3A staining of neuroglia in the mouse brain [43].

To get a better understanding of the subcellular organization of UBE3A, we performed high-resolution immunofluorescence microscopy. In images prepared using an Airyscan confocal microscope (Fig. 6), UBE3A staining appeared as discrete puncta whose density was high in the nucleus and also present (though at lower densities) in somata and proximal dendrites; scattered puncta of immunolabel were seen in neuropil (Fig. 6a). In the nucleus, UBE3A puncta were interspersed with DAPI "hotspots," but did not overlap with them (Fig. 6b, c). Likewise, UBE3A staining seemed to be excluded from nucleoli (*Nu*, Fig. 6b). To more directly test the relationship between UBE3A and DNA condensation, we computed the intensity correlation quotient [47] (ICQ, computed such that − 0.5 represents perfect negative covariance and 0.5 represents perfect positive covariance between two antigens) for 92 nuclei from 3 humans Q1010, Q1011, and Q1012 (Fig. 7). We found an average ICQ of − 0.04 ± 0.005, showing that UBE3A and DAPI staining negatively co-vary, confirming our qualitative impression that UBE3A is excluded from regions of condensed DNA.

We used electron microscopy to examine the subcellular organization of UBE3A with higher precision, using pre-embedding immunogold labeling followed by silver

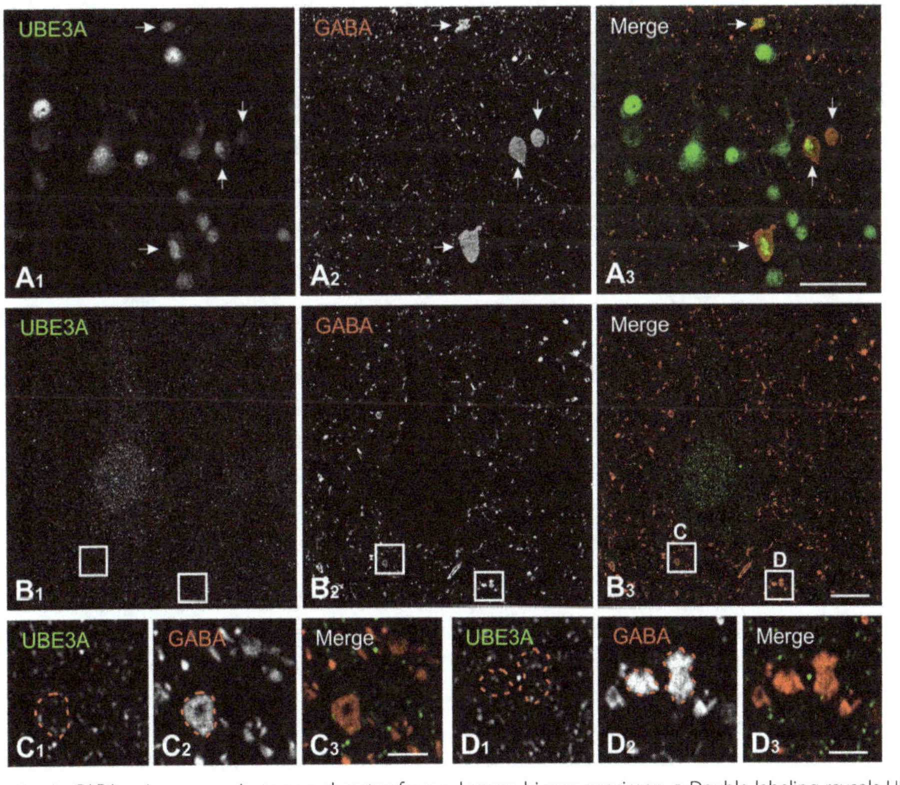

Fig. 4 UBE3A expression in GABAergic neurons in temporal cortex from a human biopsy specimen. **a** Double labeling reveals UBE3A in the nuclei and somata of GABAergic neurons (arrows). **b** A pyramidal neuron immunopositive for UBE3A is surrounded by numerous GABA-positive structures likely to represent cross sections of dendrites and axon terminals. Enlargements in **c** and **d** show the presence of UBE3A in some of these small GABA-positive structures. Tissue from case no. Q1010. Scale bar = 50 μm in **a**, 10 μm in **b**, and 2 μm in **c** and **d**

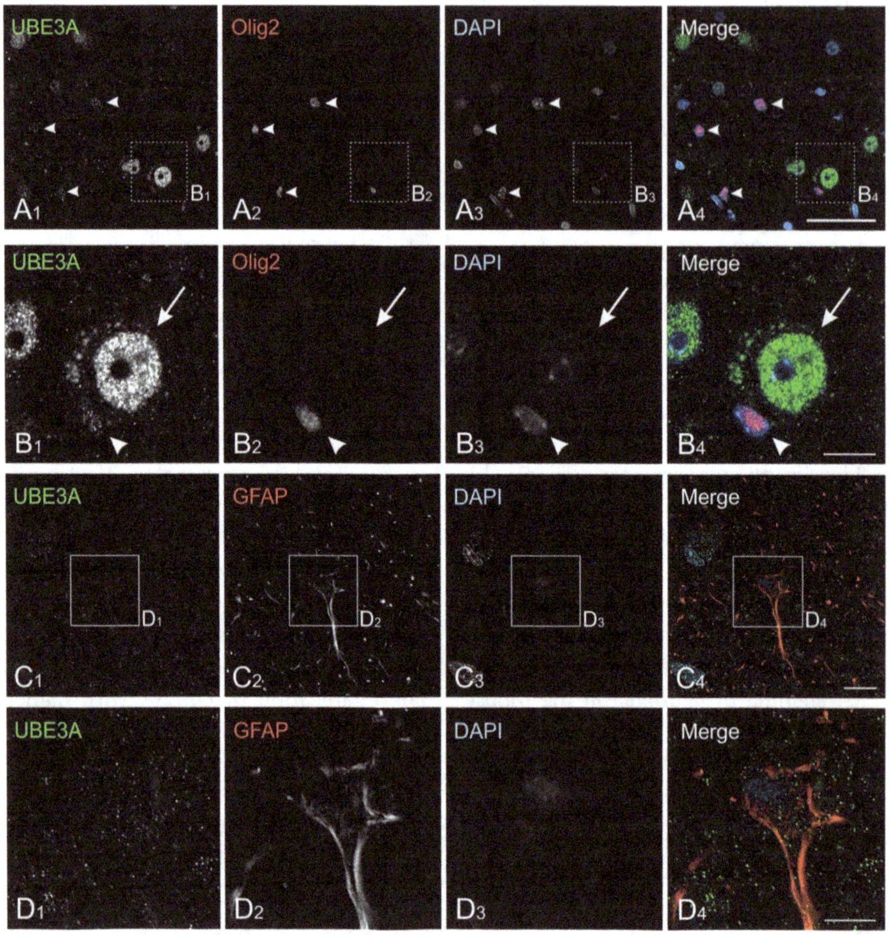

Fig. 5 UBE3A expression in neuroglia in temporal cortex from human biopsy specimen. **a, b** Double labeling reveals UBE3A in the nuclei and somata of Olig2-positive glia (oligodendrocytes, arrowheads). However, UBE3A staining in Olig2-positive glia (**b**, arrowhead) is appears weaker than in neurons (**b**, arrow). **c** Double labeling reveals UBE3A in the nuclei and somata in GFAP-positive cells (astrocytes). UBE3A in GFAP-positive cells is at lower levels than in neurons and Olig2-positive glia. Tissue from case no. Q1010. Scale bar = 50 μm in **a**, 10 μm in **b** and **c**, and 5 μm in **d**

intensification (Fig. 8). We focused our attention on layers II–III as we had done previously for mouse [41]. Labeling was prominent in nuclei but was also present in somatic cytoplasm and neuropil, echoing the results from light microscopy (Fig. 6). In the nucleus, UBE3A labeling was largely restricted to euchromatin domains; very little labeling was found over electron-dense heterochromatin zones (Fig. 8a, b), as was predicted by our ICQ analysis of UBE3A/DAPI colocalization (Fig. 7). UBE3A was also excluded from nuclear organelles such as nucleoli. Occasional gold/silver particles were associated with the nuclear membrane. In neuronal cytoplasm, UBE3A was seen decorating the Golgi apparatus and was associated with the outer mitochondrial membrane (Fig. 8c, d). In dendrites, labeling was often associated with the plasma membrane and with poorly defined tubulo-vesicular endomembranous structures. In dendritic spines, labeling was within the spine head and neck, including the spine apparatus, but was not found at the PSD (Fig. 8e). The majority of labeling within the neuropil was found in axon terminals making axospinous, axodendritic, and axosomatic synapses (Fig. 8e, f). In axon terminals, UBE3A associated with the plasma membrane and over clusters of presynaptic vesicles, but did not show a special affinity for the active zone. Double labeling experiments showed that UBE3A is expressed in GABAergic terminals (Fig. 8g).

Discussion

While previous studies have examined human UBE3A expression using Western blot analysis [50, 51] and in human-induced pluripotent stem cells [52, 53], the present work provides the first high-resolution description of the subcellular distribution of UBE3A in the human brain. Though reporting only the presence of a molecule, not its functional level of activity, immunohistochemistry can shed light on important aspects of human neurophysiology and neuropathology inaccessible

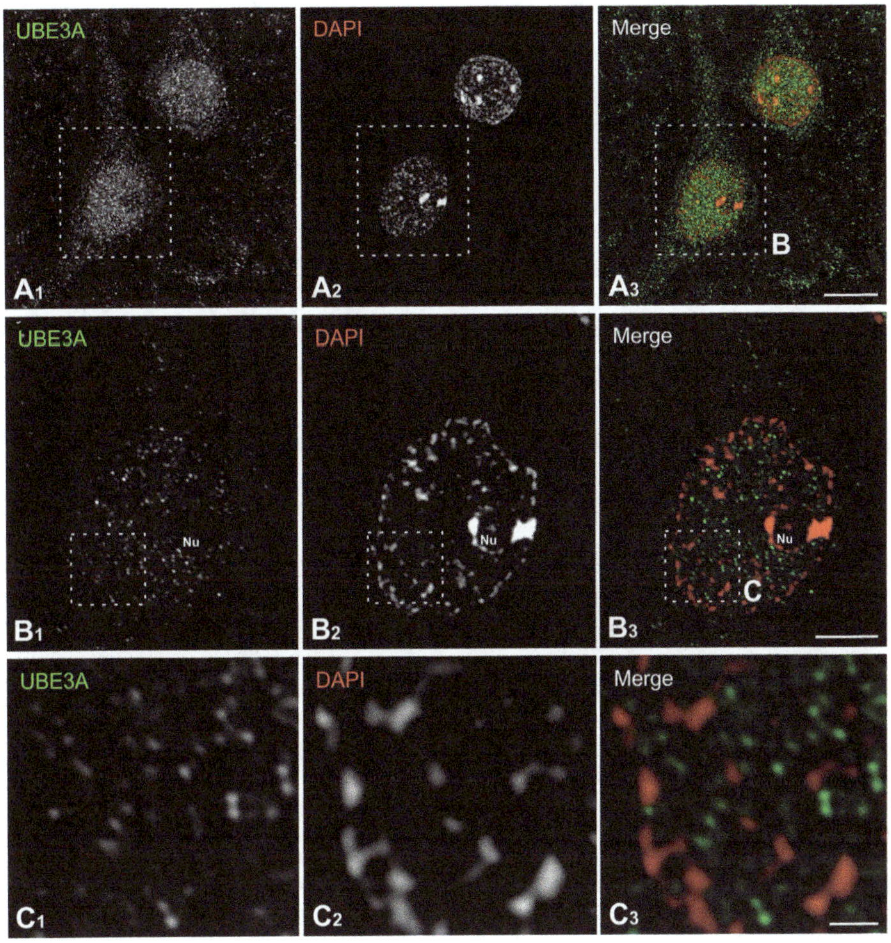

Fig. 6 High magnification immunofluorescence, showing UBE3A (green) in two pyramidal neurons in layer V in temporal cortex from human biopsy specimen (**a**). Sections were counterstained with DAPI (red) to visualize nuclei. UBE3A staining is organized into small puncta that concentrate in neuronal nuclei. Small UBE3A-positive puncta are visible in somata and proximal dendrites, and throughout the neuropil. Successive enlargements (**b**, **c**) show that UBE3A puncta are excluded from the nucleolus (Nu) and from DAPI "hotspots." Scale bar = 10 μm in **a**, 5 μm in **b**, and 1 μm in **c**. Tissue from case no. Q1019

by even the most sensitive contemporary methods of live brain imaging. However, immunohistochemistry may be misleading unless tissue of excellent quality is studied. The potential for error is particularly troublesome when tissue of poor quality is examined using super-resolution methods. Several indirect methods are customarily used to assess the quality of human histological material including tissue pH and specific markers of RNA quality [54]. We used electron microscopy to assess tissue quality directly, finding that histological and immunocytochemical staining at the light microscopic level can appear to be satisfactory even in material that has been severely degraded, potentially resulting in misleading results.

Based on examination of surgically resected tissue of high ultrastructural quality, we conclude that UBE3A is broadly expressed by both excitatory (pyramidal) and inhibitory (GABAergic) neurons of the human cerebral cortex. Epilepsy, a common comorbidity in AS, is thought to reflect a disrupted balance between excitatory and inhibitory neurotransmission. We recently demonstrated in an animal model that selective deletion of *Ube3a* in GABAergic neurons causes both circuit hyperexcitability and seizures; the presence of UBE3A in inhibitory neurons of the human neocortex further supports the hypothesis that GABAergic neurons play a key role in precipitating the electroencephalographic abnormalities and epilepsy seen in AS.

UBE3A may also serve important functions in glia. For example, flies with glia-specific overexpression of Dube3a (the fly UBE3A homolog) display a robust seizure phenotype, suggesting a possible role for glial UBE3A in Dup15q pathophysiology [55]. Our finding

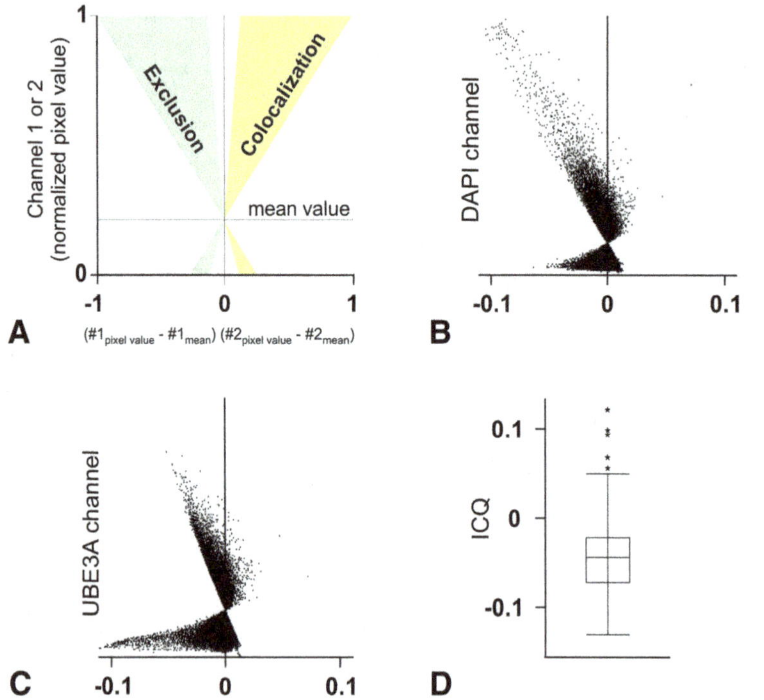

Fig. 7 Quantification of the reciprocal localization of UBE3A and DAPI in human neuronal nuclei. To analyze the relationship between UBE3A and DAPI in neuronal nuclei, we used the intensity correlation analysis approach of Li et al. [47]. Analyses are presented as intensity correlation plots: the x value, (channel 1 pixel value–channel 1 mean value) × (channel 2 value–channel 2 mean value), reflect the covariance of both channels, and the y value reflects the intensity of channels 1 or 2. Pixels with values situated left of the $x = 0$ line do not colocalize or have inversely correlated intensities, whereas pixels situated on the right side colocalize (see diagram in **a**). Scatterplot in **b** and **c** corresponds to the nuclear region of the sections used for illustration in Fig. 6b (Scatterplots are from raw confocal images, while contrast and brightness were adjusted in the micrographs). Panel **c** shows DAPI with respect to UBE3A, and **d** shows UBE3A with respect to DAPI. Both plots are skewed toward negative values, implying that UBE3A and DAPI pixel intensity co-varies in opposite directions. **d** Box and whiskers plot of intensity correlation quotient (ICQ, [47]) from 92 nuclei from layers II–III. ICQ values ~ 0 imply random staining, $0 > ICQ \geq -0.5$ indicate segregated (negatively correlated) staining, and $0 < ICQ \leq +0.5$ indicate dependent (positively correlated) staining. We found an average ICQ of -0.04 ± 0.005, showing that UBE3A and DAPI staining negatively co-vary

that UBE3A is also expressed in glia in the human brain (though at a lower level than in neurons) is consistent with this possibility.

We found that UBE3A is expressed in multiple subcellular compartments. In neurons, it concentrates in euchromatin-rich domains within the nucleus, where it is positioned to regulate the expression of active genes, possibly exerting cell-wide global effects. A recent study shows that increasing UBE3A in the nucleus downregulates the glutamatergic synapse organizer Cbln1 [26], leading to weakened glutamatergic transmission; the same study found impaired sociability in these mutant mice, providing a possible explanation for how UBE3A overexpression might lead to autism spectrum disorder. Nuclear UBE3A may also perform additional roles. Like other ubiquitin E3 ligases, UBE3A may modulate the abundance and activity of transcriptional activators via its ubiquitin-protein ligase activity, thus modulating the formation of transcriptional complexes at genes and regulating chromatin structure [56]. UBE3A might also act more directly within the nucleus as a transcriptional co-regulator [36, 57–59].

UBE3A labeling was also associated with mitochondria. Loss of UBE3A has been linked to key enzymatic deficits in the mitochondrial respiratory chain [17, 18]. A role for mitochondrial abnormalities in the pathogenesis of autism spectrum disorders has also been suggested [60], and mitochondrial dysfunction has been shown in autistic patients with 15q inverted duplication [61].

The enrichment of UBE3A that we observed in both excitatory and GABAergic axon terminals and (to a lesser extent) in dendritic spines is of special interest since both Dup15q and AS mouse models show synaptic deficits [13, 25, 62]. Postsynaptically, abnormal function of excitatory synapses in UBE3A mutant mice has been linked to decreased UBE3A-mediated proteasomal degradation of the RhoA guanine exchange factor Ephexin5 and to pathways modulated by the synaptic protein Arc [23, 24, 58, 63]. UBE3A has also been shown to target the small-conductance potassium channel SK2 for

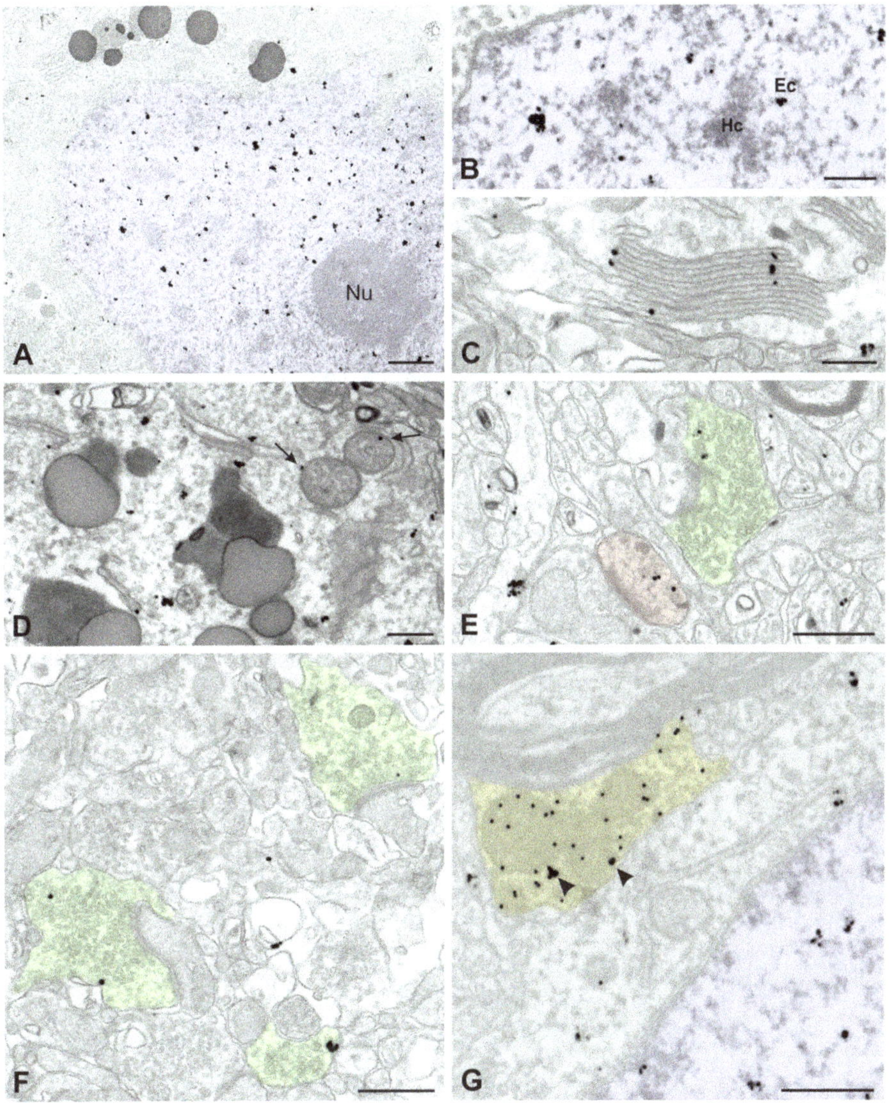

Fig. 8 Pre-embedding immunogold labeling for UBE3A in layer II/III lateral temporal cortex from human biopsy specimen. **a**, **b** UBE3A labeling in nucleus (colorized in blue); labeling is over euchromatin (Ec) domains, but is not associated with heterochromatin (Hc) or nucleoli (Nu). **c** UBE3A labeling associated with endomembranes of the Golgi apparatus. **d** UBE3A labeling in cytoplasm; arrows point to label associated with mitochondria. **e**, **f** UBE3A labeling in presynaptic terminals (colorized in green) and a dendritic spine (colorized in red). **g** A GABAegic terminal (colorized in yellow) labeled for UBE3A (pre-embedding, irregular 30–50 nm particles of silver-intensified immunogold, arrowheads) and GABA (post-embedding, 20 nm gold). Tissue from case no. Q1010 in **a**, **c**, **d**, **e**, and **f** and Q1019 in **b** and **g**. Scale bar = 1 μm in **a** and **b**, 250 nm in **c** and **g**, and 500 nm in **d**–**f**

degradation. Decreased NMDA receptor activation due to an elevated SK2 protein level may underlie the impaired LTP seen in AS model mice [62]. Presynaptically, the localization of UBE3A over vesicle clusters is surprising, since no integral synaptic vesicle proteins have yet been identified as targets for UBE3A [64]. However, UBE3A does appear to modulate the degradation of α-synuclein, a protein closely associated with synaptic vesicles [65–68], and loss of UBE3A can alter rates of synaptic depression [25, 48]. Although the mechanistic basis of UBE3A-associated synaptic disruption remains unclear, our data support a role for UBE3A in regulating synapses in the human neocortex.

The overall pattern of UBE3A immunoreactivity we found in human temporal cortex is generally consistent with that seen in previous studies of rodent cortex, reinforcing the idea that mice offer a valuable model in which to study the role of UBE3A in the brain. Mouse models of AS display many Angelman-like phenotypes, including learning and memory deficits, motor dysfunction, and seizures, while transgenic mice expressing UBE3A at increased dosages manifest several core autistic behavioral traits [26]. Nevertheless, some divergence between mouse and human UBE3A expression is likely. In particular, regulatory elements may have evolved in humans to sculpt UBE3A expression (which is spatiotemporally ubiquitous in the mouse) into unique and discrete patterns across the neocortex and throughout the cerebrum during development [69]. This remains to be tested in diverse samples of the developing and adult human brain.

Conclusions

That UBE3A is expressed at high levels in both excitatory and inhibitory neurons in the human cerebral cortex points to the many ways that its dysregulation might disrupt circuit function, while its concentration at synapses and in nuclei offers intriguing functional clues. UBE3A in axon terminals presumably regulates the function of individual synapses; in contrast, its concentration in euchromatin-rich nuclear domains suggests that UBE3A may also mediate global effects on neuronal physiology, by regulating gene transcription. This information identifies axon terminals and nuclei as two distinct potential targets for future clinical intervention.

Abbreviations

DMSO: Dimethyl sulfoxide; E6-AP: E6AP ubiquitin-protein ligase; GABA: γ-Aminobutyric acid; GFAP: Glial fibrillary acidic protein; HECT: Homologous to E6-AP carboxyl-terminus; NDBB: Neurodegenerative disease brain bank; Olig2: Oligodendrocyte transcription factor 2; PB: Phosphate buffer; PBS: Phosphate-buffered saline; PFA: Paraformaldehyde; RAD23A: Rad23 homolog A, nucleotide excision repair protein; RIN: RNA integrity number; UBE3A: Ubiquitin-protein ligase E3A; UPP: Ubiquitin-proteasome pathway

Acknowledgements

We thank the subjects who donated brain tissue for their invaluable contribution to neuroscientific research. Imaging was supported by the Hooker Imaging Core at UNC.

Funding

This work was supported by the National Institutes of Health (NS039444 and NS092474 to R.J.W. and R56-NS097831 and R01HD093771 to B.D.P.) and the Angelman Syndrome Foundation (to B.D.P.). The UCSF NDBB receives funding support from NIH grants P01AG019724 and P50AG023501, the Consortium for Frontotemporal Dementia Research, and the Tau Consortium.

Authors' contributions

ANL, EFC, and WWS provided human samples. ACB and MCJ performed the experiments. ACB analyzed the data and drafted the manuscript. ACB, BDP, MCJ, and RJW wrote the manuscript. All authors reviewed the manuscript. All authors read and approved the final manuscript.

Competing interests

The authors declare that they have no competing interests.

Author details

[1]Department of Cell Biology and Physiology, University of North Carolina at Chapel Hill, 314 Taylor Hall, Campus, Box 7545, Chapel Hill, NC 27599-7545, USA. [2]Department of Cell Biology and Physiology and Neuroscience Center, University of North Carolina, Chapel Hill, NC 27599, USA. [3]Department of Neurology, University of California, San Francisco, CA, USA. [4]Department of Pathology, UCSF Weill Institute for Neurosciences, University of California, San Francisco, CA, USA. [5]Department of Neurological Surgery, University of California, 505 Parnassus Avenue, Box 0112, San Francisco, CA 94143-0112, USA. [6]Neuroscience Curriculum, Carolina Institute for Developmental Disabilities, University of North Carolina at Chapel Hill, Chapel Hill, NC 27599, USA.

References

1. Hegde AN, Haynes KA, Bach SV, Beckelman BC. Local ubiquitin-proteasome-mediated proteolysis and long-term synaptic plasticity. Front Mol Neurosci. 2014;7:96.
2. Hegde AN. The ubiquitin-proteasome pathway and synaptic plasticity. Learn Mem. 2010;17:314–27.
3. Pelzer C, Kassner I, Matentzoglu K, Singh RK, Wollscheid HP, Scheffner M, Schmidtke G, Groettrup M. UBE1L2, a novel E1 enzyme specific for ubiquitin. J Biol Chem. 2007;282:23010–4.
4. Shang F, Deng G, Obin M, Wu CC, Gong X, Smith D, Laursen RA, Andley UP, Reddan JR, Taylor A. Ubiquitin-activating enzyme (E1) isoforms in lens epithelial cells: origin of translation, E2 specificity and cellular localization determined with novel site-specific antibodies. Exp Eye Res. 2001;73:827–36.
5. Beer-Romero P, Glass S, Rolfe M. Antisense targeting of E6AP elevates p53 in HPV-infected cells but not in normal cells. Oncogene. 1997;14:595–602.
6. Matsuura T, Sutcliffe JS, Fang P, Galjaard RJ, Jiang YH, Benton CS, Rommens JM, Beaudet AL. De novo truncating mutations in E6-AP ubiquitin-protein ligase gene (UBE3A) in Angelman syndrome. Nat Genet. 1997;15:74–7.
7. Kishino T, Lalande M, Wagstaff J. UBE3A/E6-AP mutations cause Angelman syndrome. Nat Genet. 1997;15:70–3.
8. Bird LM. Angelman syndrome: review of clinical and molecular aspects. Appl Clin Genet. 2014;7:93–104.
9. Glessner JT, Wang K, Cai G, Korvatska O, Kim CE, Wood S, Zhang H, Estes A, Brune CW, Bradfield JP, et al. Autism genome-wide copy number variation reveals ubiquitin and neuronal genes. Nature. 2009;459:569–73.
10. Hogart A, Wu D, LaSalle JM, Schanen NC. The comorbidity of autism with the genomic disorders of chromosome 15q11.2-q13. Neurobiol Dis. 2010;38: 181–91.
11. Nurmi EL, Bradford Y, Chen Y, Hall J, Arnone B, Gardiner MB, Hutcheson HB, Gilbert JR, Pericak-Vance MA, Copeland-Yates SA, et al. Linkage disequilibrium at the Angelman syndrome gene UBE3A in autism families. Genomics. 2001;77:105–13.
12. Baron CA, Tepper CG, Liu SY, Davis RR, Wang NJ, Schanen NC, Gregg JP. Genomic and functional profiling of duplicated chromosome 15 cell lines reveal regulatory alterations in UBE3A-associated ubiquitin-proteasome pathway processes. Hum Mol Genet. 2006;15:853–69.
13. Smith SE, Zhou YD, Zhang G, Jin Z, Stoppel DC, Anderson MP. Increased gene dosage of Ube3a results in autism traits and decreased glutamate synaptic transmission in mice. Sci Transl Med. 2011;3:103ra197.
14. Noor A, Dupuis L, Mittal K, Lionel AC, Marshall CR, Scherer SW, Stockley T, Vincent JB, Mendoza-Londono R, Stavropoulos DJ. 15q11.2 duplication encompassing only the UBE3A gene is associated with developmental delay and neuropsychiatric phenotypes. Hum Mutat. 2015;36:689–93.
15. Yi JJ, Berrios J, Newbern JM, Snider WD, Philpot BD, Hahn KM, Zylka MJ. An autism-linked mutation disables phosphorylation control of UBE3A. Cell. 2015;162:795–807.
16. Condon KH, Ho J, Robinson CG, Hanus C, Ehlers MD. The Angelman syndrome protein Ube3a/E6AP is required for Golgi acidification and surface protein sialylation. J Neurosci. 2013;33:3799–814.
17. Su H, Fan W, Coskun PE, Vesa J, Gold JA, Jiang YH, Potluri P, Procaccio V, Acab A, Weiss JH, et al. Mitochondrial dysfunction in CA1 hippocampal neurons of the UBE3A deficient mouse model for Angelman syndrome. Neurosci Lett. 2011;487:129–33.
18. Llewellyn KJ, Nalbandian A, Gomez A, Wei D, Walker N, Kimonis VE. Administration of CoQ10 analogue ameliorates dysfunction of the mitochondrial respiratory chain in a mouse model of Angelman syndrome. Neurobiol Dis. 2015;76:77–86.
19. Santini E, Turner KL, Ramaraj AB, Murphy MP, Klann E, Kaphzan H.

Mitochondrial superoxide contributes to hippocampal synaptic dysfunction and memory deficits in Angelman syndrome model mice. J Neurosci. 2015; 35:16213–20.

20. Weeber EJ, Jiang YH, Elgersma Y, Varga AW, Carrasquillo Y, Brown SE, Christian JM, Mirnikjoo B, Silva A, Beaudet AL, Sweatt JD. Derangements of hippocampal calcium/calmodulin-dependent protein kinase II in a mouse model for Angelman mental retardation syndrome. J Neurosci. 2003;23:2634–44.
21. van Woerden GM, Harris KD, Hojjati MR, Gustin RM, Qiu S, de Avila Freire R, Jiang YH, Elgersma Y, Weeber EJ. Rescue of neurological deficits in a mouse model for Angelman syndrome by reduction of alphaCaMKII inhibitory phosphorylation. Nat Neurosci. 2007;10:280–2.
22. Yashiro K, Riday TT, Condon KH, Roberts AC, Bernardo DR, Prakash R, Weinberg RJ, Ehlers MD, Philpot BD. Ube3a is required for experience-dependent maturation of the neocortex. Nat Neurosci. 2009;12:777–83.
23. Greer PL, Hanayama R, Bloodgood BL, Mardinly AR, Lipton DM, Flavell SW, Kim TK, Griffith EC, Waldon Z, Maehr R, et al. The Angelman syndrome protein Ube3A regulates synapse development by ubiquitinating arc. Cell. 2010;140:704–16.
24. Margolis SS, Salogiannis J, Lipton DM, Mandel-Brehm C, Wills ZP, Mardinly AR, Hu L, Greer PL, Bikoff JB, Ho HY, et al. EphB-mediated degradation of the RhoA GEF Ephexin5 relieves a developmental brake on excitatory synapse formation. Cell. 2010;143:442–55.
25. Wallace ML, Burette AC, Weinberg RJ, Philpot BD. Maternal loss of Ube3a produces an excitatory/inhibitory imbalance through neuron type-specific synaptic defects. Neuron. 2012;74:793–800.
26. Krishnan V, Stoppel DC, Nong Y, Johnson MA, Nadler MJ, Ozkaynak E, Teng BL, Nagakura I, Mohammad F, Silva MA, et al. Autism gene Ube3a and seizures impair sociability by repressing VTA Cbln1. Nature. 2017;543:507–12.
27. Reiter LT, Seagroves TN, Bowers M, Bier E. Expression of the Rho-GEF Pbl/ECT2 is regulated by the UBE3A E3 ubiquitin ligase. Hum Mol Genet. 2006; 15:2825–35.
28. Sell GL, Margolis SS. From UBE3A to Angelman syndrome: a substrate perspective. Front Neurosci. 2015;9:322.
29. Kumar S, Talis AL, Howley PM. Identification of HHR23A as a substrate for E6-associated protein-mediated ubiquitination. J Biol Chem. 1999;274: 18785–92.
30. Ramamoorthy S, Nawaz Z. E6-associated protein (E6-AP) is a dual function coactivator of steroid hormone receptors. Nucl Recept Signal. 2008;6:e006.
31. Martinez-Noel G, Galligan JT, Sowa ME, Arndt V, Overton TM, Harper JW, Howley PM. Identification and proteomic analysis of distinct UBE3A/E6AP protein complexes. Mol Cell Biol. 2012;32:3095–106.
32. Tomaic V, Banks L. Angelman syndrome-associated ubiquitin ligase UBE3A/E6AP mutants interfere with the proteolytic activity of the proteasome. Cell Death Dis. 2015;6:e1625.
33. Jacobson AD, MacFadden A, Wu Z, Peng J, Liu CW. Autoregulation of the 26S proteasome by in situ ubiquitination. Mol Biol Cell. 2014;25:1824–35.
34. Lee SY, Ramirez J, Franco M, Lectez B, Gonzalez M, Barrio R, Mayor U. Ube3a, the E3 ubiquitin ligase causing Angelman syndrome and linked to autism, regulates protein homeostasis through the proteasomal shuttle Rpn10. Cell Mol Life Sci. 2014;71:2747–58.
35. Martinez A, Ramirez J, Osinalde N, Arizmendi JM, Mayor U. Neuronal proteomic analysis of the ubiquitinated substrates of the disease-linked E3 ligases Parkin and Ube3a. Biomed Res Int. 2018;2018:3180413.
36. Nawaz Z, Lonard DM, Smith CL, Lev-Lehman E, Tsai SY, Tsai MJ, O'Malley BW. The Angelman syndrome-associated protein, E6-AP, is a coactivator for the nuclear hormone receptor superfamily. Mol Cell Biol. 1999;19:1182–9.
37. Bernassola F, Karin M, Ciechanover A, Melino G. The HECT family of E3 ubiquitin ligases: multiple players in cancer development. Cancer Cell. 2008;14:10 21.
38. Pal P, Lochab S, Kanaujiya JK, Kapoor I, Sanyal S, Behre G, Trivedi AK. E6AP, an E3 ubiquitin ligase negatively regulates granulopoiesis by targeting transcription factor C/EBPalpha for ubiquitin-mediated proteasome degradation. Cell Death Dis. 2013;4:e590.
39. Jiang YH, Armstrong D, Albrecht U, Atkins CM, Noebels JL, Eichele G, Sweatt JD, Beaudet AL. Mutation of the Angelman ubiquitin ligase in mice causes increased cytoplasmic p53 and deficits of contextual learning and long-term potentiation. Neuron. 1998;21:799–811.
40. Mulherkar SA, Jana NR. Loss of dopaminergic neurons and resulting behavioural deficits in mouse model of Angelman syndrome. Neurobiol Dis. 2010;40:586 92.
41. Burette AC, Judson MC, Burette S, Phend KD, Philpot BD, Weinberg RJ. Subcellular organization of UBE3A in neurons. J Comp Neurol. 2017;525: 233–51.
42. McTigue DM, Tripathi RB. The life, death, and replacement of oligodendrocytes in the adult CNS. J Neurochem. 2008;107:1–19.
43. Judson MC, Sosa-Pagan JO, Del Cid WA, Han JE, Philpot BD. Allelic specificity of Ube3a expression in the mouse brain during postnatal development. J Comp Neurol. 2014;522:1874–96.
44. Knott G, Rosset S, Cantoni M. Focussed ion beam milling and scanning electron microscopy of brain tissue. J Vis Exp. 2011;53:e2588.
45. Knott G, Marchman H, Wall D, Lich B. Serial section scanning electron microscopy of adult brain tissue using focused ion beam milling. J Neurosci. 2008;28:2959–64.
46. Schindelin J, Arganda-Carreras I, Frise E, Kaynig V, Longair M, Pietzsch T, Preibisch S, Rueden C, Saalfeld S, Schmid B, et al. Fiji: an open-source platform for biological-image analysis. Nat Methods. 2012;9:676–82.
47. Li Q, Lau A, Morris TJ, Guo L, Fordyce CB, Stanley EF. A syntaxin 1, Galpha(o), and N-type calcium channel complex at a presynaptic nerve terminal: analysis by quantitative immunocolocalization. J Neurosci. 2004;24:4070–81.
48. Judson MC, Wallace ML, Sidorov MS, Burette AC, Gu B, van Woerden GM, King IF, Han JE, Zylka MJ, Elgersma Y, et al. GABAergic neuron-specific loss of Ube3a causes Angelman syndrome-like EEG abnormalities and enhances seizure susceptibility. Neuron. 2016;90:56–69.
49. Egawa K, Kitagawa K, Inoue K, Takayama M, Takayama C, Saitoh S, Kishino T, Kitagawa M, Fukuda A. Decreased tonic inhibition in cerebellar granule cells causes motor dysfunction in a mouse model of Angelman syndrome. Sci Transl Med. 2012;4:163ra157.
50. Williams K, Irwin DA, Jones DG, Murphy KM. Dramatic loss of Ube3A expression during aging of the mammalian cortex. Front Aging Neurosci. 2010;2:18.
51. Daily J, Smith AG, Weeber EJ. Spatial and temporal silencing of the human maternal UBE3A gene. Eur J Paediatr Neurol. 2012;16:587–91.
52. Chamberlain SJ, Chen PF, Ng KY, Bourgois-Rocha F, Lemtiri-Chlieh F, Levine ES, Lalande M. Induced pluripotent stem cell models of the genomic imprinting disorders Angelman and Prader-Willi syndromes. Proc Natl Acad Sci U S A. 2010;107:17668–73.
53. Stanurova J, Neureiter A, Hiber M, de Oliveira Kessler H, Stolp K, Goetzke R, Klein D, Bankfalvi A, Klump H, Steenpass L. Angelman syndrome-derived neurons display late onset of paternal UBE3A silencing. Sci Rep. 2016;6: 30792.
54. Stan AD, Ghose S, Gao XM, Roberts RC, Lewis-Amezcua K, Hatanpaa KJ, Tamminga CA. Human postmortem tissue: what quality markers matter? Brain Res. 2006;1123:1–11.
55. Hope KA, LeDoux MS, Reiter LT. Glial overexpression of Dube3a causes seizures and synaptic impairments in Drosophila concomitant with down regulation of the Na(+)/K(+) pump ATPalpha. Neurobiol Dis. 2017;108:238–48.
56. Geng F, Wenzel S, Tansey WP. Ubiquitin and proteasomes in transcription. Annu Rev Biochem. 2012;81:177–201.
57. Khan OY, Fu G, Ismail A, Srinivasan S, Cao X, Tu Y, Lu S, Nawaz Z. Multifunction steroid receptor coactivator, E6-associated protein, is involved in development of the prostate gland. Mol Endocrinol. 2006;20:544–59.
58. Kuhnle S, Mothes B, Matentzoglu K, Scheffner M. Role of the ubiquitin ligase E6AP/UBE3A in controlling levels of the synaptic protein Arc. Proc Natl Acad Sci U S A. 2013;110:8888–93.
59. El Hokayem J, Weeber E, Nawaz Z. Loss of Angelman syndrome protein E6AP disrupts a novel antagonistic estrogen-retinoic acid transcriptional crosstalk in neurons. Mol Neurobiol. 2018;55:7187–200.
60. Hollis F, Kanellopoulos AK, Bagni C. Mitochondrial dysfunction in autism Spectrum disorder: clinical features and perspectives. Curr Opin Neurobiol. 2017;45:178–87.
61. Filipek PA, Juranek J, Smith M, Mays LZ, Ramos ER, Bocian M, Masser-Frye D, Laulhere TM, Modahl C, Spence MA, Gargus JJ. Mitochondrial dysfunction in autistic patients with 15q inverted duplication. Ann Neurol. 2003;53:801–4.
62. Sun J, Zhu G, Liu Y, Standley S, Ji A, Tunuguntla R, Wang Y, Claus C, Luo Y, Baudry M, Bi X. UBE3A regulates synaptic plasticity and learning and memory by controlling SK2 channel endocytosis. Cell Rep. 2015;12:449–61.
63. Mandel-Brehm C, Salogiannis J, Dhamne SC, Rotenberg A, Greenberg ME. Seizure-like activity in a juvenile Angelman syndrome mouse model is attenuated by reducing Arc expression. Proc Natl Acad Sci U S A. 2015;112: 5129–34.

64. Takamori S, Holt M, Stenius K, Lemke EA, Gronborg M, Riedel D, Urlaub H, Schenck S, Brugger B, Ringler P, et al. Molecular anatomy of a trafficking organelle. Cell. 2006;127:831–46.
65. Maroteaux L, Campanelli JT, Scheller RH. Synuclein: a neuron-specific protein localized to the nucleus and presynaptic nerve terminal. J Neurosci. 1988;8:2804–15.
66. Jensen PH, Nielsen MS, Jakes R, Dotti CG, Goedert M. Binding of alpha-synuclein to brain vesicles is abolished by familial Parkinson's disease mutation. J Biol Chem. 1998;273:26292–4.
67. Mulherkar SA, Sharma J, Jana NR. The ubiquitin ligase E6-AP promotes degradation of alpha-synuclein. J Neurochem. 2009;110:1955–64.
68. Ham A, Kim DW, Kim KH, Lee SJ, Oh KB, Shin J, Mar W. Reynosin protects against neuronal toxicity in dopamine-induced SH-SY5Y cells and 6-hydroxydopamine-lesioned rats as models of Parkinson's disease: reciprocal up-regulation of E6-AP and down-regulation of alpha-synuclein. Brain Res. 2013;1524:54–61.
69. King MC, Wilson AC. Evolution at two levels in humans and chimpanzees. Science. 1975;188:107–16.

10

Assessing subtypes of restricted and repetitive behaviour using the Adult Repetitive Behaviour Questionnaire-2 in autistic adults

Sarah L. Barrett[1*], Mirko Uljarević[2], Catherine R. G. Jones[1] and Susan R. Leekam[1]

Abstract

Background: The majority of previous research into restricted and repetitive behaviours (RRBs) has focussed on children, partly due to a lack of suitable measures for RRBs in adults. This study aimed to explore the psychometric properties of the Adult Repetitive Behaviour Questionnaire-2 (RBQ-2A) in a large sample of autistic adults using a self-report questionnaire method.

Methods: The RBQ-2A and Autism-Spectrum Quotient (AQ) were administered online. Data from 275 autistic adults aged 18–66 ($M = 36.56$, SD = 12.24; 100 men and 171 women) were analysed using polychoric principal components analysis (PCA). Reliability and validity were assessed using Cronbach's alpha and correlation analyses.

Results: PCA resulted in two components of the RBQ-2A, interpretable as repetitive sensory and motor behaviours (RSMB) and insistence on sameness (IS). Both components showed acceptable internal consistency ($\alpha = .70$ and .81 respectively) and were significantly moderately correlated with scores on the AQ ($r_s = .25$ and .42). Participants' scores on IS were higher than their scores on RSMB. RSMB, but not IS, was negatively associated with age, particularly in older adults (≥ 50 years). There were no gender differences.

Conclusions: The RBQ-2A is a reliable and valid self-report measure of RRBs in the present sample of autistic adults. As one of the few measures of RRBs aimed at adults, it is suitable for adults with the ability to read and complete a self-report questionnaire. Results build on previous work with children using the Repetitive Behaviour Questionnaire-2 (RBQ-2).

Keywords: Repetitive behaviours, Insistence on sameness, Repetitive sensory and motor behaviours, Adults, Principal components analysis, Questionnaire

Introduction

Restricted and repetitive behaviours (RRB) are an essential diagnostic criterion for autism spectrum disorder (ASD; [1]). RRBs encompass a wide variety of behaviours from motor stereotypes to maintaining order and sameness, and are seen across different situations and settings. This heterogeneous group of behaviours has been found to divide into two subtypes: Repetitive Sensory and Motor Behaviours (RSMB) and Insistence on Sameness (IS). This structure has been identified in factor-analytic studies of autistic populations [2–5] and typically developing (TD) and community populations [6–8]. However, some studies find between three and six subtypes [9–12], which may be a result of the use of different measures of RRBs, and the inclusion of children at different developmental stages in each study [13].

Previous research has focussed on RRBs in younger children, although they can be measured in adults [14, 15], including neurotypical (NT) adults [6, 16]. However, there are only two currently published measures of RRBs that have been developed with the aim of assessing RRBs in an adult population; the Adult Repetitive Behaviour

* Correspondence: BarrettSL2@cardiff.ac.uk
[1]Wales Autism Research Centre, School of Psychology, Cardiff University, Cardiff, UK
Full list of author information is available at the end of the article

Questionnaire-2 (RBQ-2A; [16]), and the Adult Routines Inventory (ARI; [6]). This paper aims to build on previous findings using the RBQ-2A by establishing the RBQ-2A's reliability and validity in a larger sample of autistic adults, as well as exploring the presentation of RRBs in adulthood in relation to age and gender. It should be noted that the cognitive demands of completing a self-report questionnaire necessarily limits the representative nature of our sample to adults with competent levels of reading fluency and comprehension.

As previous research into RRBs has generally focussed on children, little is known about the expression and trends of RRBs across autistic adulthood, as well as how RRBs differ according to age and gender in autistic adults; therefore, we will consider some of the relevant findings in children as well as in adults. Although some previous factor analysis studies included adults, the age ranges of some of these studies are narrow and often limited to adults in their twenties (e.g. [17, 18]). Furthermore, there were no separate factor analyses of the adults alone. Only two studies have assessed the structure of RRBs in exclusively adult samples [6, 16], both of which found a two-dimensional structure corresponding to RSMB and IS. However, Barrett et al.'s [16] principal components analysis (PCA) was carried out on typical adults only, and Evans et al.'s [6] analysis was conducted on a large community sample that included adults with a range of neurodevelopmental and neuropsychiatric disorders as well as NT adults, with a low number of ASD individuals.

It is unclear the extent to which RRBs change with age in adulthood, although autistic traits in general are known to vary over time (e.g. [19]) and RRBs decrease in TD children after the age of 7 years (e.g. [8, 20]). There is evidence both for [15, 21] and against [22] the decrease of RRBs over time in autistic individuals. Esbensen et al. [14] reported a specific decrease in RSMBs with age compared to IS that was particularly pronounced in individuals with a learning disability (LD). Conversely, Georgiades et al. [2] found no difference in RSMBs between children and adults with ASD, but found that adults scored higher on IS. One study that exclusively assessed adults found no difference between older and younger adults with ASD [23], while another found that all RRBs decrease with age, particularly RSMBs [24]. Barrett et al. [16] did not find a significant association between age and RRBs in autistic or NT adults, although Evans et al. [6] found that all RRBs decreased with age in their cross-sectional sample of adults. Therefore, the precise relationship between age and RRBs is not clear in adulthood, although there is some evidence for IS behaviours being more common than RSMBs in adults.

In terms of gender, it has been shown that autistic women show significantly fewer RRBs than autistic men (e.g. [23, 25]). This has been supported in studies including children and adolescents [26]. There is some evidence that this varies according to RRB subtype and other factors such as concurrent mental health problems. For example, Evans et al. [6] found that while men scored higher on overall RRBs and RSMBs, there were no gender differences in terms of IS. Furthermore, in one study [27], girls and women scored higher in terms of IS as measured by the RBQ-2A compared to boys and men; this was potentially because the girls and women had higher self-reported anxiety, which is in turn positively associated with IS. However, our interpretation of this in relation to adults is limited by the inclusion of adolescents (14–18 years). In contrast, Barrett et al. [16] found no gender differences in RRBs, for either their NT or ASD group. The discrepancy in findings may be related to age, measurement and concurrent LDs. For example, all participants in Hattier et al.'s [23] study were diagnosed with LD, and they assessed RRBs using a caregiver-report measure, the Diagnostic Assessment for the Severely Handicapped [28], whereas Evans et al. [6] and Barrett et al. [16] used self-report measures and did not have exclusively LD samples. Moreover, the sample used by Uljarević et al. [27] focused on younger individuals with limited age range (15–25 years).

As the overview of the literature demonstrates, there is no clear consensus on the structure of RRBs in autistic adulthood and how it may differ according to age or gender. However, there are few dedicated measures to assess RRBs in adults to address these gaps. Although tools that have been employed to measure RRBs in autistic individuals, such as the Autism Diagnostic Interview-Revised (ADI-R [29]) and the Repetitive Behaviour Scale-Revised (RBS-R [30]) are reliable and valid, they are limited in other ways. For example, the ADI-R as a diagnostic instrument has been designed to be stable and reliable, but it samples a limited number of RRBs. Moreover, the ADI-R and RBS-R rely on caregiver-report which may be unreliable in the case of adults who have moved away from home, or unhelpful in the case of adults whose parents have passed away. Furthermore, observation measures, although reliable and valid in measuring RSMBs, are time-limited to the observational window and are limited in the measurement of IS behaviours [31].

The RBQ-2A was developed in response to the lack of suitable measures for assessing RRBs in adults and is based on the RBQ-2, a 20-item parent-report measure of the profile of RRBs in children. This measure was originally developed from the Diagnostic Interview for Social and Communication Disorders (DISCO [32, 33]) and the Repetitive Behaviours Interview (RBI [34]). The RBQ-2 demonstrates good reliability and validity, and a two-factor structure reflecting RSMB and IS. Strong psychometric properties and a stable factor structure have been reported in TD children at the ages of 15, 26, and 77 months (e.g. [8, 35]) and children and adolescents with ASD [36].

The adult version, the RBQ-2A, is similar to the child version with some questions reworded to be developmentally appropriate (see Barrett et al. [16] for details). The RBQ-2A was shown to be reliable and valid in a large sample of university students and a smaller sample comprising autistic and NT adults [16], as well as being reliable in adolescents and adults with ASD [27]. PCA of the university sample ([16] study 1) yielded a two-component solution; however, sensory items failed to load on either component. The two components were interpreted as IS and repetitive motor behaviours (RMB). This may be explained by the low endorsement of sensory items in the sample, reflecting that sensory symptoms are lower in NT compared to autistic individuals (e.g. [37, 38]). Conducting a PCA on a sample comprising only autistic adults will clarify the appropriate structure for the RBQ-2A.

The study presented here builds upon the findings of Barrett et al. [16] in two ways. Firstly, the study aimed to provide an additional assessment of the reliability and validity of the RBQ-2A by implementing PCA and assessing its correlational validity and internal consistency. It was expected that there would be two components corresponding to RSMB/RMB and IS as in previous research with the RBQ-2A. Secondly, we aimed to assess the profile of RRBs in autistic adults in terms of the different subtypes of RRBs and their differential association with gender and age, including differences between participants in early, middle and older adulthood.

Method

Participants

Participants were recruited through the Wales Autism Research Centre's webpages, and several United Kingdom (UK) ASD charities. Only those who self-reported a clinical diagnosis of ASD and living in or originally from the UK ($N = 352$) were included in the study. Participants were aged between 18 and 66 years ($M = 37.0$, $SD = 12.32$), and comprised 132 men, 215 women and 5 individuals with a non-binary gender identity. The majority reported a clinical diagnosis of Asperger's syndrome ($N = 198$; 56.3%). Most were white (92.6%) and lived in England (74.4%). Two hundred and seventy two (77.3%) participants had studied beyond the age of compulsory education in the UK (16 years). One hundred and forty-seven participants (41.8%) reported studying to degree level, and 66 participants (18.8%) had studied to postgraduate degree level. Two hundred and one participants (57.1%) were employed. Of the participants who reported the age of diagnosis ($N = 341$), 73.6% were diagnosed as an adult and 26.4% were diagnosed as a child. Since data collection was online, it was not possible to confirm diagnoses of participants; however, given there was no incentive to take part other than personal interest, it is unlikely that participants would dishonestly report a diagnosis of ASD. Nevertheless, participants were retained in the study only if their Autism-Spectrum Quotient (AQ [39]) score was at 26 or above [40].[1] The lower cut-off of 26 was implemented in order to maximise the number of participants included in the study and to take into account autistic participants who may show lower levels of autistic traits. Removing participants scoring below 26 resulted in 309 individuals remaining in the sample. Online data collection procedures also prevented the opportunity to confirm IQ levels of participants; however, the level of education and employment and capacity for self-completion of the questionnaire were indirect indicators of a higher level of cognitive ability within the sample. Table 1 below summarises the demographic data for these participants.

Table 1 Summary of demographic information for participants from the UK meeting the Autism-Spectrum Quotient (AQ) cut-off of 26 ($N = 309$)

Age (years)	$M = 37.44$, SD = 12.44 Range: 18–66
Gender	116 (37.5%) male
	188 (60.8%) female
	5 (1.6%) non-binary
Reported diagnosis	179 (57.9%) Asperger's syndrome
	78 (25.2%) Autism spectrum disorder (including ASD level one)
	32 (10.4%) High functioning autism
	20 (6.47%) Other[a]
Age at diagnosis	231 (74.8%) adult (18–66; $M = 36.02$, SD = 11.15)
	69 (22.3%) child (3–17; $M = 11.62$, SD = 4.16)
AQ score	$M = 38.31$, SD = 5.86, range: 26–50
Ethnicity	286 (92.6%) White
	22 (7.1%) mixed race, Asian, Black, Chinese or other
Location	230 (74.4%) England
	32 (10.4%) Wales
	43 (13.9%) Scotland, Northern Ireland or other
Education	Post-16: 239 (77.3%)
	Undergraduate degree 128 (41.4%)
Employed	171 (55.3%) employed
	137 (44.3%) unemployed

[a]Other includes atypical autism; autistic disorder; childhood autism; high-functioning autism/Asperger's syndrome; pathological demand avoidance; Pervasive Developmental Disorder–Not Otherwise Specified

Materials and procedure

The RBQ-2A comprises 20 items, scored on either a 3- or 4-point Likert scale. The fourth option is collapsed into option three while scoring [16]. A mean score across items is then calculated for each participant, with a maximum of 3. As with previous research, item 20 (*activities*) was not included in the PCA as it is qualitatively different from the other items [7, 36]. Although items 7 (*fascination*) and 12 (*collect*) are not included in studies with children due to failure to load in factor analysis studies, they were included here in order to test whether or not they load for autistic adults. The exact wordings of the 20 items comprising the RBQ-2A have previously been published [16].

The AQ is a 50-item self-report questionnaire that aims to assess traits and behaviours associated with ASD in the general population. Each participant receives a score out of 50, with higher scores indicating higher levels of autism traits. The AQ is not a diagnostic tool for ASD; however, it reliably distinguishes between autistic and NT individuals and shows good sensitivity and specificity [39, 40]. Demographic questions included age, gender, diagnostic information (specific diagnosis and age of diagnosis), educational level, employment, ethnicity, and country/region.

Participants completed the study online (via Google Documents), and received and completed the questionnaires in the fixed order of RBQ-2A; AQ; demographic questions. The study was approved by the Cardiff University School of Psychology Research Ethics Committee.

Statistical analyses

As Likert scales produce ordinal rather than interval data, the recommended polychoric PCA (e.g. [41]) was carried out using the program FACTOR [42] to determine the structure of the RBQ-2A. Parallel analysis [43] was used to determine the number of components that should be retained. Direct oblimin rotation was employed to allow correlation between the two components. An item loading threshold of .4 was employed [44]. The remaining analyses were carried out using SPSS 20.0. Internal consistency was assessed by calculating Cronbach's alpha (α) values. The correlational validity between AQ and RBQ-2A scores was assessed, along with the correlation between the RBQ-2A sub-scales. Finally, the effects of age and gender were explored.

Results

Descriptive statistics and data screening

Table 2 shows the endorsement, mean total scores and SDs for all 20 RBQ-2A items ($N = 309$). For every item, at least 18.2% of the sample endorsed one of the two higher response options (e.g. mild or marked). There were 34 (11.0%) participants with missing data across the relevant 19 items. Little's Missing Completely at Random test was non-significant ($\chi^2[369] = 400.39$, $p = .13$) so it was appropriate to remove these participants from the analysis.

The final sample comprised 275 participants, aged from 18 to 66 years ($M = 36.56$, SD = 12.24; positively skewed [SW(275) = .96, $p < .001$] with no outliers), 100 of whom were men and 171 women. The total AQ score ranged from 26 to 50 ($M = 38.51$, SD = 5.88) and was positively skewed (SW[275] = .98, $p < .001$) with no outliers. There were 20 participants who had missing data on the AQ (ranging from 1 [2%] to 4 items [8%]). Little's Missing Completely at Random test was non-significant ($\chi^2[681] = 716.01$, $p = .17$), so these participants were removed for analyses that included the total AQ score. The mean total RBQ-2A score ranged from 1.15 to 2.95 ($M = 2.11$, SD = .36), which was positively skewed (SW[275] = .98, $p = .002$) with no outliers. The internal consistency of all 20 RBQ-2A items was good ($\alpha = .84$). The mean total RBQ-2A score significantly correlated with AQ ($r_s = .43$, $p < .001$), but not with age ($r_s = -.01$, $p = .84$).

Principal components analysis

Initial screening indicated that the assumptions of sampling adequacy (KMO = .87), multicollinearity and factorability ($\chi^2[171] = 1437.8$, $p < .001$) were all met. The initial PCA solution resulted in four components with eigenvalues greater than 1, explaining 62.9% of the variance. Parallel analysis indicated that two components should be retained and the PCA was re-run with Direct Oblimin rotation. The correlation between components was .35, suggesting that oblique rotation was appropriate [45].

The final rotated solution explained 49.09% of the variance. Table 3 shows the pattern matrix of item loadings following Direct Oblimin rotation, along with the percentage of variance explained, Cronbach's alpha value and mean inter-item correlation for each component. The analysis was re-run removing participants who did not score 32 or above on the AQ, in line with the original cut-off for this questionnaire [39]). The results of the analysis were broadly similar, with the exception that items 1 (*arrange*) and 11 (*carry*) loaded onto RSMB rather than IS. Given the lack of differences between the two solutions in terms of percentage of variance explained and reliability, the original analysis was retained in order to preserve sample size and to take into account autistic adults who may score lower on measures of autistic traits; this is particularly important given the large proportion of women and individuals diagnosed as adults who took part in the study.

Table 4 shows the means and SDs, and the medians and IQRs for each component. The first component corresponds to IS, and the second component corresponds to RSMB. The internal consistency (Cronbach's alpha) of IS was good (.81) and acceptable for

Table 2 Frequencies, percentages, means and standard deviations (SD) of participants' responses to all twenty RBQ-2A items (N = 309)

	Never or rarely	Mild or occasional/one or more times daily	Marked or notable/15 or more times daily	Mean (SD)
1. Arrange	69 (22.3%)	182 (58.9%)	58 (18.8%)	1.96 (.64)
2. Fiddle[b]	38 (12.4%)	73 (23.8%)	196 (63.8%)	2.51 (.71)
3. Spin[a]	236 (76.6%)	56 (18.2%)	16 (5.2%)	1.29 (.56)
4. Rock[a]	125 (40.6%)	98 (31.8%)	85 (27.6%)	1.87 (.82)
5. Pace[a]	96 (31.2%)	121 (39.3%)	91 (29.5%)	1.98 (.78)
6. Hand/finger[b]	95 (30.9%)	83 (27.0%)	129 (42.0%)	2.11 (.85)
7. Fascination[b]	45 (14.7%)	117 (38.1%)	145 (47.2)	2.33 (.72)
8. Angles[d]	75 (24.6%)	144 (47.2%)	86 (28.2%)	2.04 (.73)
9. Smell[c]	132 (43.1%)	106 (34.6%)	68 (22.2%)	1.79 (.78)
10. Feel[d]	94 (30.8%)	105 (34.4%)	106 (34.8%)	2.04 (.81)
11. Carry[d]	124 (40.8%)	97 (31.9%)	83 (27.3%)	1.87 (.82)
12. Collect[b]	51 (16.6%)	93 (30.3%)	163 (53.1%)	2.36 (.75)
13. Home[b]	18 (5.9%)	65 (21.2%)	224 (73.0%)	2.67 (.58)
14. Change[c]	34 (11.1%)	88 (28.8%)	184 (60.1%)	2.49 (.69)
15. Routine[b]	20 (6.5%)	92 (30.0%)	195 (63.5%)	2.57 (.61)
16. Redoing[a]	16 (5.2%)	66 (21.4%)	226 (73.4%)	2.68 (.57)
17. TV/Music[b]	30 (9.8%)	83 (27.0%)	194 (63.2%)	2.53 (.67)
18. Clothes[d]	74 (24.3%)	106 (34.8%)	125 (41.0%)	2.17 (.79)
19. Food[b]	67 (21.8)	89 (29.0%)	151 (49.2%)	2.27 (.80)
20. Activities	11 (3.6%)	117 (37.9%)	181 (58.6%)	2.55 (.57)

Percentages given as valid percentages
[a]Missing = 1
[b]Missing = 2
[c]Missing = 3
[d]Missing ≥ 4

RSMB (.70). The mean inter-item correlation for both components was .29.

Subscale analyses

Both components were positively skewed. There was one outlier who scored more than three SDs below the mean on IS; however, removing this participant from the analyses did not affect the pattern of findings. A Wilcoxon signed-rank test demonstrated a significant difference between IS and RSMB ($Z = -11.0$, $p < .001$, $r = -.66$) with a large effect size.

Table 5 shows the correlations between the two components of the RBQ-2A, the AQ and age. Spearman's correlation analyses indicated significant associations between RSMB and IS ($r_s = .47$, $p < .001$), and both components were significantly correlated with total AQ score. Only RSMB significantly correlated with age, and this association was negative ($r_s = -.21$, $p < .001$).

Table 6 shows the means, SDs, medians and IQRs for the sample when divided into three age groups (18–34; 35–49; 50–66) based on an approximate tertile split. Kruskall-Wallis tests indicated that there was a significant difference between age groups in terms of RSMB ($\chi^2(2) = 12.34$, $p = .002$) but not IS ($\chi^2(2) = 1.67$, $p = .43$). Follow-up Mann-Whitney tests indicated significant differences between 18 and 34 and 50–66-year-olds ($Z = -3.64$, $p < .001$, $r = -.27$) and between 35 and 49 and 50–66-year-olds ($Z = -2.46$, $p = .014$, $r = .20$), but not between 18 and 34 and 35–49-year-olds ($Z = -.86$, $p = .39$).

Finally, there were no significant gender differences in terms of the RBQ-2A subscales (Table 7). However, in terms of the AQ, women ($M = 39.22$, SD = 5.77) scored significantly higher than men ($M = 37.48$, SD = 6.12) with a small effect size ($Z = -2.23$, $p = .026$, $r = -.14$). The two groups did not differ by age (men: $M = 37.27$ years, SD = 13.66; women: $M = 36.11$ years, SD = 11.23; $Z = -.61$, $p = .54$).

Discussion

This is the first PCA of self-reported RRB data from a sample of autistic adults aged 18 to 66 years. We examined the factor structure of the RBQ-2A and also the differential effects of age and gender on RRBs. A two-dimensional structure was identified using polychoric PCA, corresponding to IS and RSMB. This is in line with most RRB research, including findings from a

Table 3 Pattern matrix for polychoric PCA after Direct Oblimin rotation ($N = 275$)

Rotated item loadings:	Component 1	Component 2
	Insistence on Sameness (IS)	Repetitive sensory and motor behaviours (RSMB)
1. Arrange	*.402*	.377
2. Fiddle	.038	*.783*
3. Spin	−.156	*.800*
4. Rock	−.052	*.815*
5. Pace	.036	*.609*
6. Hand/finger	.051	*.709*
7. Fascination	*.537*	.247
8. Angles	.368	.361
9. Smell	.298	.254
10. Feel	.258	*.490*
11. Carry	*.441*	.389
12. Collect	*.670*	.128
13. Home	*.885*	−.140
14. Change	*.844*	−.115
15. Routine	*.722*	.025
16. Redoing	*.801*	−.042
17. TV/music	*.496*	.341
18. Clothes	*.493*	.311
19. Food	*.523*	.052
Percentage of variance explained:	37.6%	11.5%
Cronbach's alpha (α):	.81	.70
Mean inter-item correlation:	.29	.29

Items in italics met the item threshold (>.4) for that component

community sample of adults that included autistic adults [6]. Both components showed good reliability as well as being significantly associated with AQ, supporting the construct validity of the RBQ-2A. Age was found to be significantly associated with RSMB, but not IS, with RSMBs decreasing with age. In contrast to previous research, there were no significant gender differences in RRBs. Given the lack of research into RRBs in autistic adulthood, the discussion will focus on the comparison between the present study and the previous research using the RBQ-2A [16].

Overall, the PCA structure supports previous findings using a university student sample [16], but with some minor differences. In terms of the IS component, the present solution is the same as Barrett et al.'s analysis with two exceptions. Two additional items loaded on to IS: items 7 (*fascination*) and 1 (*arrange*), which may reflect the samples used. Neither fascination nor arrange were highly endorsed in Barrett et al.'s university student sample, whereas there were relatively common in the present ASD sample. Although ASD individuals show more marked RRBs compared to the general population (e.g. [46, 47]), the difference may be particularly pronounced for certain RRBs such as fascination with specific objects and arranging objects.

Table 4 The ranges, means and SDs, and medians and IQRs for RSMB and IS ($N = 275$)

	Range	Mean (SD)	Median (IQR)
RSMB	1.0–3.0	1.97 (.48)	2.0 (.67)
IS	1.0–3.0	2.36 (.41)	2.45 (.55)

Table 5 Correlations between the subscales of the RBQA, the AQ and age ($N = 275$)

	RSMB	AQ ($N = 255$)	Age
RSMB	–	.30[a]	−.21[a]
IS	.47[a]	.44[a]	.06

[a]Significant at the .01 level

The current RSMB component resembles the component RMB [16] with the exception of the exclusion of arrange and inclusion of item 10 (*feel*). The loading of a sensory item (*feel*) led to the decision to name the component RSMB rather than RMB. Again, endorsement of feel was much higher in the current sample compared to that in Barrett et al.'s participants. As well as differing in diagnosis, Barrett et al.'s participants were generally younger than in the present study (although spanned a similar age range from 18 to 50) and drawn only from university students, while the present sample was more evenly distributed in age and drawn from the general population.

Notably, two of the items that load differently across studies (*fascination* and *arrange*) were identified as sensory items in a study using an autistic child sample [36]. A relevant similarity between the two solutions is that sensory items 8 (*angles*) and 9 (*smell*) failed to load in either study. The unstable loading of four of the RBQ-2A's sensory items across the two studies may indicate an inherent weakness in the sensory items. Alternatively, this instability may reflect genuine structural differences in RRB between autistic and NT individuals. The RBQ-2A may not capture a wide enough range of sensory responses to detect variation in a typical sample. For example, the RBQ-2A's sensory items mainly focus on sensory-seeking rather than sensory-avoidant behaviours. There are also some modalities not included in the RBQ-2A that are included in other measures such as the Glasgow Sensory Profile [48], which includes auditory, vestibular and proprioceptive modalities. Indeed, studies using other measures find a relatively wide range of sensory behaviours in NT samples (e.g. [48, 49]). Further research directly comparing the performance of the RBQ-2A's sensory items in a large sample of autistic and NT individuals would be useful, as well as comparing

Table 6 Means, SDs, medians and IQRs for RSMB and IS by age group ($N = 275$)

	18–34 years ($N = 129$)		35–49 years ($N = 98$)		50–66 years ($N = 48$)	
	Mean (SD)	Median (IQR)	Mean (SD)	Median (IQR)	Mean (SD)	Median (IQR)
RSMB	2.05 (.47)	2.0 (.67)	1.98 (.51)	2.08 (.83)	1.76 (.40)	1.83 (.63)
IS	2.33 (.43)	2.45 (.55)	2.41 (.40)	2.5 (.64)	2.37 (.38)	2.45 (.45)

the RBQ-2A to more specific measures of sensory processing.

Apart from noted caveats that warrant further research, the results indicate that the RBQ-2A is a stable and reliable measure of RRBs in adults. The PCA findings presented here also generally reflect factor analytic findings by previous researchers using the child parent-report RBQ-2 [7, 8, 36], particularly in terms of IS. Again, there are some minor differences. First, *arrange* usually loads on to RSMB rather than IS. Second, in previous studies, *angles* has always loaded onto RSMB, whereas *smell* has loaded onto both RSMB [7, 8] and IS [36]. These differences may reflect the fluid nature of some RRBs, which can reflect either RSMB or IS depending on the intent and experience of the individual. This may also explain why two items in the present study (*arrange* and *carry*) load differently depending on whether the AQ cut-off of 26 or 32 is used. The desire to arrange items could be seen as an interest in patterns (RSMB) or a desire to impose order on the world (IS); similarly, an individual could be motivated to carry an object around because of a sensory property (RSMB), or because of a compulsion (IS). Overall, these minor differences between solutions do not undermine the conclusion that both the RBQ-2 and RBQ-2A can be conceptualised as a two-dimensional measure of RRB, comprising two subtypes of RSMB and IS. The two-dimensional solution supports the majority of findings using both interviews such as ADI-R as well as questionnaire measures (e.g. [3, 5, 50]).

Given the lack of data on the presentation of RRBs throughout autistic adulthood, the effect of age and gender on RBQ-2A scores was also examined. RSMB, but not IS, was significantly negatively correlated with age, and the sample scored significantly lower on the RSMB overall. When broken down into subgroups, older adults (50–66 years) scored significantly lower on RSMBs compared to the younger groups (18–34 years and 35–49 years), which did not differ from each other. Previous research has shown that while RRBs reduce across the lifetime, they remain more stable than social and communication traits [14, 15, 22]. Evans et al. [6] found significant negative associations between age, overall RRBs and both subtypes of RRBs in a community sample that included adults with ASD, as well as other neurodevelopmental and psychiatric conditions. However, there is also some evidence that RSMBs are particularly associated with younger individuals (e.g. [14, 51, 52]). The present results support and extend these findings, showing that RSMBs do not only occur less often in autistic adults compared to IS behaviours, but this difference is particularly pronounced in older adults.

Table 7 Means, SDs, medians and IQRs for the RBQ-2A and its subscales by gender

	Men ($N = 100$)		Women ($N = 171$)		
	Mean (SD)	Median (IQR)	Mean (SD)	Median (IQR)	
RSMB	1.95 (.49)	2.0 (.83)	1.98 (.47)	2.0 (.67)	$Z = -.47$ $p = .64$
IS	2.35 (.41)	2.45 (.52)	2.37 (.41)	2.45 (.55)	$Z = -.36$ $p = .72$

There were no significant gender differences on the RBQ-2A, which supports previous findings using the RBQ-2A in both autistic and NT participants [16]. However, one study [27] found that female participants scored higher than male participants on the IS subscale of the RBQ-2A; although as mentioned, this particular sample included adolescents and the girls and women in the group showed high levels of anxiety. In contrast, research with other measures of RRBs tends to find that autistic men score higher than autistic women (e.g. [23, 53]). This discrepancy could be interpreted in one of two ways; firstly, it may be that the RBQ-2A is more sensitive to RRBs in women and therefore women score higher in line with men. Secondly, it could be that unlike other measures the RBQ2-A is not biased towards men. This could be explored by assessing RRBs using more than one measure in men and women.

Strengths and limitations

The present study is the first to analyse the component structure of a sample that only comprises autistic adults, using polychoric PCA. Polychoric PCA is recommended for ordinal data, which is the form most questionnaire data takes, and yet the majority of factor analyses in this area are based on Pearson's correlation matrix, which assumes continuous data. However, future research using the RBQ-2A should employ confirmatory factor analysis, which would provide a stringent test of the structure of the RBQ-2A. An important future direction is to explore the performance of the RBQ-2A as a measure of RRBs in other neurodevelopmental and neuropsychiatric disorders in order to establish sensitivity and specificity for ASD. Another important direction for future research is to assess the developmental trajectory of the RBQ-2 and RBQ-2A from childhood to adulthood.

An important limitation of this study is the fact that the present sample is not representative of the adult autistic population. Given the online design of the study, it was not possible to ascertain IQ or cognitive ability. However, it is important to highlight the fact that it would have been difficult for an individual to access and complete this self-report questionnaire if they had a significant LD or a specific difficulty with reading fluency or comprehension, and many reported high education and employment. This indirectly indicates that the majority had high ability, and further research is needed to establish a more representative sample. Furthermore, the majority of the current participants were diagnosed as adults, whereas individuals with ASD are usually diagnosed as children [54]. Similarly, the majority of participants were female, whereas ASD is diagnosed much more commonly in boys and men (e.g. [55, 56]); although the gender ratio in ASD may be a result of gender bias in diagnostic tools, misdiagnosis of girls and women, or masking of symptoms [57]. However, this also represents a strength of the research as it allowed us to explore gender differences in adequate group sizes. Finally, the majority of the sample identified as white (93%), and the findings may not be representative of other ethnicities. The characteristics of this sample therefore prevent us from generalising the present findings to the wider autistic adult population. However, this should be addressed in future research, by developing the RBQ-2A to make it more accessible for use with a more diverse and representative sample.

All of the measures used in this study were self-report. Although it has been suggested that autistic individuals may struggle with insights into their own feelings and behaviours [58, 59], previous research demonstrates that autistic individuals complete self-report questionnaires in a reliable and valid manner [60, 61]. While comparisons between parent and self-completed questionnaires (RBQ-2 and a modified version of the RBQ-2A) have been conducted with autistic adolescents [62], future studies should collect RBQ-2A data from autistic adults and their relatives in order to check their correlational validity; although as noted earlier, parent-report may be less useful for reporting on adults compared to children.

Finally, despite the advantage of the online nature of the study allowing us to reach a large number of participants, there are some inherent limitations to online research. Notably, it was not possible to independently confirm diagnoses of ASD; participants were asked whether or not they had a clinical diagnosis of ASD, but they did not provide further details or evidence. Care was taken to only include participants who reported a clinical diagnosis of ASD and scored at 26 or above on the AQ, which has been shown to be a cut-off with good sensitivity and specificity for ASD [40]. Although the psychometric properties of the RBQ-2A have been assessed in a small number of autistic adults with confirmed diagnoses [16], these should be assessed in a larger sample.

Conclusion

The study presented here was the first to explore the factor structure of RRBs in a sample solely comprising autistic adults. Results suggest RBQ-2A to be a two-dimensional measure comprising RSMB and IS. This study also found that RSMBs, but not IS, decrease with age in autistic adults. In contrast to previous research, we did not find evidence of gender differences in terms of RRBs. One issue that remains for future research is whether or not to use the structure determined here in autistic adults or the structure identified by Barrett et al. [16] in university students. Given the use of the target ASD population, polychoric PCA, and a larger sample size in this study, we would recommend using the structure identified here. However, it would be important to carry out confirmatory factor analysis in an independent sample to test the best solution, especially given the instability of the sensory and carry items. Furthermore, future research should address the demographic limitations of the sample here as a priority before generalising the findings to the wider ASD population. Finally, an important step for future research is to consider the trajectory of RRBs from childhood to adulthood, and how the content of RSMB and IS may change over time. Our results show that RRBs reduce over adulthood, but the subtypes remain similar to those seen in children. Overall, the results reported here highlight preliminary evidence of the usefulness of the RBQ-2A as a reliable and valid measure of RRBs in self-reporting autistic adults.

Endnotes

[1]One participant had a score of 24 but missing data on two items, so may have reached the cut-off of 26. However, as it was not possible to know what their scores would have been, they were not included in the analysis.

Abbreviations

ADI-R: Autism Diagnostic Interview-Revised; AQ: Autism-Spectrum Quotient; ASD: Autism spectrum disorder; DISCO: Diagnostic Interview for Social and Communication Disorders; IQR: Inter-quartile range; IS: Insistence on Sameness; LD: Learning difficulty; NT: Neurotypical; PCA: Principal component analysis; RBQ-2: Repetitive Behaviour Questionnaire-2; RBQ-2A: Adult Repetitive Behaviour Questionnaire-2; RBS-R: Repetitive Behavior Scale-Revised; RMB: Repetitive motor behaviour; RRB: Restricted and repetitive behaviour; RSMB: Repetitive sensory and motor behaviour; SD: Standard deviation; TD: Typically developing; UK: United Kingdom

Acknowledgements
The authors would like to thank all of the autistic adults who participated in this research.

Funding
The research reported in this paper was supported by a PhD studentship jointly awarded by the Economic and Social Research Council and Cardiff University to the first author.

Authors' contributions
SB designed the study, collected and analysed the data, and wrote the manuscript. CJ and SL were major contributors to the design of the study, analytic plan for the data and writing of the manuscript. MU was a major contributor to the analytic plan for the data and writing of the manuscript. All authors read and approved the final manuscript.

Authors' information
Not applicable.

Competing interests
The authors declare that they have no competing interests.

Author details
[1]Wales Autism Research Centre, School of Psychology, Cardiff University, Cardiff, UK. [2]Department of Psychiatry and Behavioral Sciences, Stanford University School of Medicine, Stanford, California, USA.

References

1. American Psychiatric Association. Diagnostic and statistical manual of mental disorders (DSM-5®). Washington: American Psychiatric Pub; 2013.
2. Georgiades S, Papageorgiou V, Anagnostou E. Brief report: repetitive Behaviours in Greek individuals with autism spectrum disorder. J Autism Dev Disord. 2010;40:903–6.
3. Mooney EL, Gray KM, Tonge BJ, Sweeney DJ, Taffe JR. Factor analytic study of repetitive Behaviours in young children with pervasive developmental disorders. J Autism Dev Disord. 2009;39:765–74.
4. Richler J, Huerta M, Bishop SL, Lord C. Developmental trajectories of restricted and repetitive behaviors and interests in children with autism spectrum disorders. Dev Psychopathol. 2010;22:55–69.
5. Tao Y, Gao H, Ackerman B, Guo W, Saffen D, Shugart YY. Evidence for contribution of common genetic variants within chromosome 8p21.2-8p21. 1 to restricted and repetitive behaviors in autism spectrum disorders. BMC Genomics. 2016;17:163.
6. Evans DW, Uljarević M, Lusk LG, Loth E, Frazier T. Development of two dimensional measures of restricted and repetitive behavior in parents and children. J Am Acad Child Adolesc Psychiatry. 2017;56:51–8.
7. Leekam S, Tandos J, McConachie H, Meins E, Parkinson K, Wright C, Turner M, Arnott B, Vittorini L, Couteur AL. Repetitive behaviours in typically developing 2-year-olds. J Child Psychol Psychiatry. 2007;48:1131–8.
8. Uljarević M, Arnott B, Carrington SJ, Meins E, Fernyhough C, McConachie H, Le Couteur A, Leekam SR. Development of restricted and repetitive behaviors from 15 to 77 months: stability of two distinct subtypes? Dev Psychol. 2017;53:1859–68.
9. Honey E, McConachie H, Randle V, Shearer H, Couteur ASL. One-year change in repetitive behaviours in young children with communication disorders including autism. J Autism Dev Disord. 2008;38:1439–50.
10. Lam KSL, Bodfish JW, Piven J. Evidence for three subtypes of repetitive behavior in autism that differ in familiality and association with other symptoms. J Child Psychol Psychiatry. 2008;49:1193–200.
11. Lam KSL, Aman MG. The repetitive behavior scale-revised: independent validation in individuals with autism spectrum disorders. J Autism Dev Disord. 2007;37:855–66.
12. Scahill L, Dimitropoulos A, McDougle CJ, Aman MG, Feurer ID, McCracken JT, Tierney E, Pu J, White S, Lecavalier L, et al. Children's Yale–Brown obsessive compulsive scale in autism Spectrum disorder: component structure and correlates of symptom checklist. J Am Acad Child Adolesc Psychiatry. 2014;53:97 107.e101.
13. Leekam SR, Prior MR, Uljarevic M. Restricted and repetitive behaviors in autism spectrum disorders: a review of research in the last decade. Psychol Bull. 2011;137:562–93.
14. Esbensen AJ, Seltzer MM, Lam KSL, Bodfish JW. Age-related differences in restricted repetitive behaviors in autism spectrum disorders. J Autism Dev Disord. 2009;39:57–66.
15. Fecteau S, Mottron L, Berthiaume C, Burack JA. Developmental changes of autistic symptoms. Autism. 2003;7:255–68.
16. Barrett SL, Uljarević M, Baker EK, Richdale AL, Jones CR, Leekam SR. The Adult Repetitive Behaviours Questionnaire-2 (RBQ-2A): a self-report measure of restricted and repetitive behaviours. J Autism Dev Disord. 2015;45:3680–92.
17. Cuccaro ML, Shao Y, Grubber J, Slifer M, Wolpert CM, Donnelly SL, Abramson RK, Ravan SA, Wright HH, DeLong GR, Pericak-Vance MA. Factor analysis of restricted and repetitive behaviors in autism using the Autism Diagnostic Interview-R. Child Psychiatry Hum Dev. 2003;34:3–17.
18. Papageorgiou V, Georgiades S, Mavreas V. Brief report: cross-cultural evidence for the heterogeneity of the restricted, repetitive Behaviours and interests domain of autism: a Greek study. J Autism Dev Disord. 2008;38: 558–61.
19. Seltzer MM, Shattuck P, Abbeduto L, Greenberg JS. Trajectory of development in adolescents and adults with autism. Ment Retard Dev Disabil Res Rev. 2004;10:234–47.
20. Evans DW, Leckman JF, Carter A, Reznick JS, Henshaw D, King RA, Pauls D. Ritual, habit, and perfectionism: the prevalence and development of compulsive-like behavior in Normal young children. Child Dev. 1997;68:58–68.
21. Seltzer MM, Krauss MW, Shattuck PT, Orsmond G, Swe A, Lord C. The symptoms of autism spectrum disorders in adolescence and adulthood. J Autism Dev Disord. 2003;33:565–81.
22. Piven J, Harper J, Palmer PAT, Arndt S. Course of behavioral change in autism: a retrospective study of high-IQ adolescents and adults. J Am Acad Child Adolesc Psychiatry. 1996;35:523–9.
23. Hattier MA, Matson JL, Tureck K, Horovitz M. The effects of gender and age on repetitive and/or restricted behaviors and interests in adults with autism spectrum disorders and intellectual disability. Res Dev Disabil. 2011;32:2346–51.
24. Chowdhury M, Benson BA, Hillier A. Changes in restricted repetitive behaviors with age: a study of high-functioning adults with autism Spectrum disorders. Res Autism Spectr Disord. 2010;4:210–6.
25. Lai M-C, Lombardo MV, Pasco G, Ruigrok ANV, Wheelwright SJ, Sadek SA, Chakrabarti B, Consortium MA, Baron-Cohen S. A behavioral comparison of male and female adults with high functioning autism spectrum conditions. PLoS One. 2011;6:e20835.
26. Van Wijngaarden-Cremers PJM, van Eeten E, Groen WB, Van Deurzen PA, Oosterling IJ, Van der Gaag RJ. Gender and age differences in the core triad of impairments in autism spectrum disorders: a systematic review and meta-analysis. J Autism Dev Disord. 2014;44:627–35.
27. Uljarević M, Richdale AL, Evans DW, Cai RY, Leekam SR. Interrelationship between insistence on sameness, effortful control and anxiety in adolescents and young adults with autism spectrum disorder (ASD). Molecular autism. 2017;8:36.
28. Matson JL. Diagnostic assessment for the severely handicapped II. Baton Rouge: Disability Consultants, LLC; 1998.
29. Lord C, Rutter M, Le Couteur A. Autism diagnostic interview-revised: a revised version of a diagnostic interview for caregivers of individuals with possible pervasive developmental disorders. J Autism Dev Disord. 1994;24: 659–85.
30. Bodfish JW, Symons FJ, Lewis MH. The Repetitive Behavior Scale - Revised. Morganton: Western Carolina Center Research Reports; 1999.
31. Honey E, Rodgers J, McConachie H. Measurement of restricted and repetitive behaviour in children with autism spectrum disorder: selecting a questionnaire or interview. Res Autism Spectr Disord. 2012;6:757–76.
32. Leekam SR, Libby SJ, Wing L, Gould J, Taylor C. The diagnostic interview for social and communication disorders: algorithms for ICD-10 childhood autism and wing and Gould autistic spectrum disorder. J Child Psychol Psychiatry. 2002;43:327–42.
33. Wing L, Leekam SR, Libby SJ, Gould J, Larcombe M. The diagnostic interview for social and communication disorders: background, inter-rater reliability and clinical use. J Child Psychol Psychiatry. 2002;43:307–25.
34. Turner M. Repetitive behavior and cognitive functioning in autism. Cambridge: University of Cambridge; 1995.

35. Arnott B, McConachie H, Meins E, Fernyhough C, Couteur AL, Turner M, Parkinson K, Vittorini L, Leekam S. The frequency of restricted and repetitive behaviors in a community sample of 15-month-old infants. J Dev Behav Pediat. 2010;31:223–9.
36. Lidstone J, Uljarević M, Sullivan J, Rodgers J, McConachie H, Freeston M, Le Couteur A, Prior M, Leekam S. Relations among restricted and repetitive behaviors, anxiety and sensory features in children with autism spectrum disorders. Res Autism Spectr Disord. 2014;8:82–92.
37. Baranek GT, David FJ, Poe MD, Stone WL, Watson LR. Sensory experiences questionnaire: discriminating sensory features in young children with autism, developmental delays, and typical development. J Child Psychol Psychiatry. 2006;47:591–601.
38. Ben-Sasson A, Hen L, Fluss R, Cermak SA, Engel-Yeger B, Gal E. A meta-analysis of sensory modulation symptoms in individuals with autism spectrum disorders. J Autism Dev Disord. 2009;39:1–11.
39. Baron-Cohen S, Wheelwright S, Skinner R, Martin J, Clubley E. The autism-Spectrum quotient (AQ): evidence from Asperger syndrome/high-functioning autism, Males and females, scientists and mathematicians. J Autism Dev Disord. 2001;31:5–17.
40. Woodbury-Smith MR, Robinson J, Wheelwright S, Baron-Cohen S. Screening adults for Asperger syndrome using the AQ: a preliminary study of its diagnostic validity in clinical practice. J Autism Dev Disord. 2005;35:331–5.
41. Baglin J. Improving your exploratory factor analysis for ordinal data: a demonstration using FACTOR. Pract Assess Res Eval. 2014;19:2.
42. Lorenzo-Seva U, Ferrando PJ. FACTOR: a computer program to fit the exploratory factor analysis model. Behav Res Methods. 2006;38:88–91.
43. Horn JL. A rationale and test for the number of factors in factor analysis. Psychometrika. 1965;30:179–85.
44. Guadagnoli E, Velicer WF. Relation to sample size to the stability of component patterns. Psychol Bull. 1988;103:265–75.
45. Tabachnick BG, Fidell LS. Using multivariate statistics. 6th ed. London: Pearson New International Edition; 2014.
46. Morgan L, Wetherby AM, Barber A. Repetitive and stereotyped movements in children with autism spectrum disorders late in the second year of life. J Child Psychol Psychiatry. 2008;49:826–37.
47. South M, Ozonoff S, McMahon WM. Repetitive behavior profiles in Asperger syndrome and high-functioning autism. J Autism Dev Disord. 2005;35:145–58.
48. Robertson AE, Simmons DR. The relationship between sensory sensitivity and autistic traits in the general population. J Autism Dev Disord. 2013;43: 775–84.
49. Kent RG. Measuring autism spectrum disorder: associated features and diagnostic criteria. Cardiff: Cardiff University; 2014.
50. Smith CJ, Lang CM, Kryzak L, Reichenberg A, Hollander E, Silverman JM. Familial associations of intense preoccupations, an empirical factor of the restricted, repetitive behaviors and interests domain of autism. J Child Psychol Psychiatry. 2009;50:982–90.
51. Militerni R, Bravaccio C, Falco C, Fico C, Palermo MT. Repetitive behaviors in autistic disorder. Eur Child Adolesc Psychiat. 2002;11:210–8.
52. Moore V, Goodson S. How well does early diagnosis of autism stand the test of time?: follow-up study of children assessed for autism at age 2 and development of an early diagnostic service. Autism. 2003;7:47–63.
53. Wilson CE, Murphy CM, McAlonan G, Robertson DM, Spain D, Hayward H, Woodhouse E, Deeley PQ, Gillan N, Ohlsen JC, et al. Does sex influence the diagnostic evaluation of autism spectrum disorder in adults? Autism. 2016; 20:808–19.
54. Howlin P, Asgharian A. The diagnosis of autism and Asperger syndrome: findings from a survey of 770 families. Dev Med Child Neurol. 1999;41:834–9.
55. Begeer S, Mandell D, Wijnker-Holmes B, Venderbosch S, Rem D, Stekelenburg F, Koot HM. Sex differences in the timing of identification among children and adults with autism Spectrum disorders. J Autism Dev Disord. 2013;43:1151–6.
56. Werling DM, Geschwind DH. Sex differences in autism spectrum disorders. Curr Opin Neurol. 2013;26:146–53.
57. Wing L, Gould J, Gillberg C. Autism spectrum disorders in the DSM-V: better or worse than the DSM-IV? Res Dev Disabil. 2011;32:768–73.
58. Jackson P, Skirrow P, Hare DJ. Asperger through the looking glass: an exploratory study of self-understanding in people with Asperger's syndrome. J Autism Dev Disord. 2012;42:697–706.
59. Williams D. Theory of own mind in autism:evidence of a specific deficit in self-awareness? Autism. 2010;14:474–94.
60. Berthoz S, Hill EL. The validity of using self-reports to assess emotion regulation abilities in adults with autism spectrum disorder. Eur Psychiat. 2005;20:291 8.
61. Hesselmark E, Eriksson JM, Westerlund J, Bejerot S. Autism spectrum disorders and self-reports: testing validity and reliability using the NEO-PI-R. J Autism Dev Disord. 2015;45:1156–66.
62. Joyce C, Honey E, Leekam SR, Barrett SL, Rodgers J. Anxiety, intolerance of uncertainty and restricted and repetitive behaviour: insights directly from young people with ASD. J Autism Dev Disord. 2017;47:3789–802.

11

Neuroglia in the autistic brain: evidence from a preclinical model

Maria Rosanna Bronzuoli[1†], Roberta Facchinetti[1†], Davide Ingrassia[1], Michela Sarvadio[2], Sara Schiavi[2], Luca Steardo[1], Alexei Verkhratsky[3,4,5], Viviana Trezza[2] and Caterina Scuderi[1*]

Abstract

Background: Neuroglial cells that provide homeostatic support and form defence of the nervous system contribute to all neurological disorders. We analyzed three major types of neuroglia, astrocytes, oligodendrocytes, and microglia in the brains of an animal model of autism spectrum disorder, in which rats were exposed prenatally to antiepileptic and mood stabilizer drug valproic acid; this model being of acknowledged clinical relevance.

Methods: We tested the autistic-like behaviors of valproic acid-prenatally exposed male rats by performing isolation-induced ultrasonic vocalizations, the three-chamber test, and the hole board test. To account for human infancy, adolescence, and adulthood, such tasks were performed at postnatal day 13, postnatal day 35, and postnatal day 90, respectively. After sacrifice, we examined gene and protein expression of specific markers of neuroglia in hippocampus, prefrontal cortex, and cerebellum, these brain regions being associated with autism spectrum disorder pathogenesis.

Results: Infant offspring of VPA-exposed dams emitted less ultrasonic vocalizations when isolated from their mothers and siblings and, in adolescence and adulthood, they showed altered sociability in the three chamber test and increased stereotypic behavior in the hole board test. Molecular analyses indicate that prenatal valproic acid exposure affects all types of neuroglia, mainly causing transcriptional modifications. The most prominent changes occur in prefrontal cortex and in the hippocampus of autistic-like animals; these changes are particularly evident during infancy and adolescence, while they appear to be mitigated in adulthood.

Conclusions: Neuroglial pathological phenotype in autism spectrum disorder rat model appears to be rather mild with little signs of widespread and chronic neuroinflammation.

Keywords: Autism spectrum disorder, Astrocyte, Microglia, Oligodendrocyte, Valproic acid

Background

Autism spectrum disorder (ASD) is a heterogeneous set of neurodevelopmental disorders characterized by deficits in social communication and social interaction, stereotypies, and reduced patterns of behaviors [1, 2]. Even though ASD can be diagnosed at any age, symptoms generally appear in the childhood and last throughout a person's life. Although about 1% of the world population suffers from ASD [3], little is known on ASD etiology and pathogenesis. Genetic predispositions, maternal stressors, environmental factors, infectious agents, and the intake of specific drugs during pregnancy all have some degree of association with ASD [4]. One of the common environmental factors involved in the pathogenesis of ASD is maternal exposure to the anti-epileptic and mood stabilizer drug valproic acid (VPA). When given during pregnancy, VPA was reported to induce various congenital malformations [5, 6] including autistic-like features in the exposed children, such as impaired communication, reduced sociability and stereotyped behaviors [7, 8]. Based on these clinical observations, prenatal VPA exposure in rodents has been developed and became a widely used environmental preclinical model of ASD with face and construct validity [9–11].

Recent findings highlight contribution of neuroglia to the ASD pathophysiology. Glial cells are non-excitable

* Correspondence: caterina.scuderi@uniroma1.it
†Maria Rosanna Bronzuoli and Roberta Facchinetti contributed equally to this work.
[1]Department of Physiology and Pharmacology, "Vittorio Erspamer" SAPIENZA University of Rome, 00185 Rome, Italy
Full list of author information is available at the end of the article

homeostatic cells of the central nervous system (CNS), sub-classified into astrocytes, oligodendrocytes and their precursors (also known as NG-2 glia) and microglia; all types of glia sustain vital brain functions [12]. Specifically, astroglial cells are key cellular contributors to the homeostasis of the nervous tissue and the brain as an organ [13–16]. Astrocytes regulate pH and ion homeostasis, regulate functional hyperaemia and provide trophic and metabolic support to neurones. Astrocytes are important elements of the cytoarchitecture of the brain. These cells are essential for synaptogenesis [17, 18] as well as synaptic remodeling and are likely to contribute to various aspects of memory formation, storage, and retention [19]. Oligodendrocytes form the myelin sheath, thus maintaining the functional connectome of the brain and contributing to the optimal information processing in complex neural networks [20]. Microglia provide the immune and cellular defence in the brain. Through several surveillance mechanisms, microglia detect diverse pathological extracellular signals, and respond to them to protect the brain. These cells also contribute to the development of the nervous tissue, shaping neuronal ensembles and synaptic plasticity [21–24].

Increasing appreciation of the multifaceted physiological roles of glia in the developing and mature CNS suggests that abnormalities in glial functions contribute to neuropathology. Several preclinical models of diseases revealed the role of glia in neurodevelopmental diseases, from ASD to neuropsychiatric disorders. Pathological changes in neuroglia are complex and can be classified into reactive response (astrogliosis, activation of microglia, and Wallerian remodeling of oligodendrocytes), degeneration with atrophy and loss of function (characteristic for astrocytes and microglia), and pathological remodeling [25–27]. The contribution of glial cells to pathological development of cognitive and neuropsychiatric disorders, such as Alzheimer's disease, Parkinson's disease, depression, schizophrenia, and others, has been demonstrated [28–36]. The role of glia in ASD however is not clear and often the data available are limited to their involvement in the inflammatory response.

In this study, we performed an in-depth analysis of gene and protein expression of specific markers of astrocytes, oligodendrocytes, and microglia in the rats prenatally exposed to VPA (ASD animal model). We studied brain areas critically involved in ASD, namely, hippocampus (HPC), prefrontal cortex (PfC), and cerebellum (Cb) [37–39]. To account for human infancy, adolescence, and adulthood, brain tissues were analyzed at three different ages, at postnatal day (PND) 13, PND 35, and PND 90. Our results indicate that prenatal VPA exposure affects all types of neuroglia, mainly causing transcriptional modifications. The most significant changes occur in PfC and in the HPC of autistic-like animals; these changes are particularly evident during infancy and adolescence, while they appear to be mitigated in adulthood.

Methods

All animal procedures were performed in agreement with the guidelines of the Italian Ministry of Health (D.L. 26/2014) and with the European Parliament directive 2010/63/EU.

Animals

The offspring born from VPA-exposed dams was obtained as described previously [40]. Adult female Wistar rats (Charles River, Arbresle, France) were housed and raised under controlled conditions (22 ± 2 °C temperature, 55–65% relative humidity, 12-h light/12-h dark cycle with lights on at 07:00 h) in an enriched environment, with food and water available ad libitum. Rats weighing 250 ± 15 g were mated overnight, and the morning when spermatozoa were found was assigned as gestational day 1 (GD 1). Pregnant rats, singly placed in Macrolon cages (40 × 26 × 20 cm), on GD 12.5, received an intraperitoneal injection of either VPA (500 mg/kg in saline) or saline (Veh). This dose of VPA, administered at this developmental time point, is known to induce autistic-like traits in the exposed rat offspring at infancy, adolescence, and adulthood [41]. The day after birth (PND 1), the litters were culled to six males and two females to reduce the litter size-induced variability in the growth and development of pups during the postnatal period. However, epidemiological studies report a higher incidence of ASD in boys than in girls, and it has been shown that the autistic-like-behaviors displayed by rats prenatally exposed to VPA are more pronounced in the male than in the female offspring [42, 43]. For these reasons, only the male offspring was used in this study. After weaning on PND 21, pups were weaned and housed in groups of three. In order to perform the molecular analysis of the brains in infancy, adolescence, and adulthood, the male offspring (one rat/litter/treatment) was sacrificed on PND 13, PND 35, and PND 90, respectively. After decapitation, PfC, HPC, and Cb were rapidly isolated to perform western blot and real time-quantitative PCR (RT-qPCR); whereas, whole brains for immunofluorescence were flash-frozen in 2-methylbutane and stored at − 80 °C. The experimental design is outlined in Fig. 1a.

Behavioral tests

Isolation-induced ultrasonic vocalizations (USVs)

On PND 13, the USVs emitted by each pup removed from the nest and placed into a Plexiglas arena were detected for 3 min by an ultrasound microphone (Avisoft Bioacoustics, Germany) sensitive to frequencies between

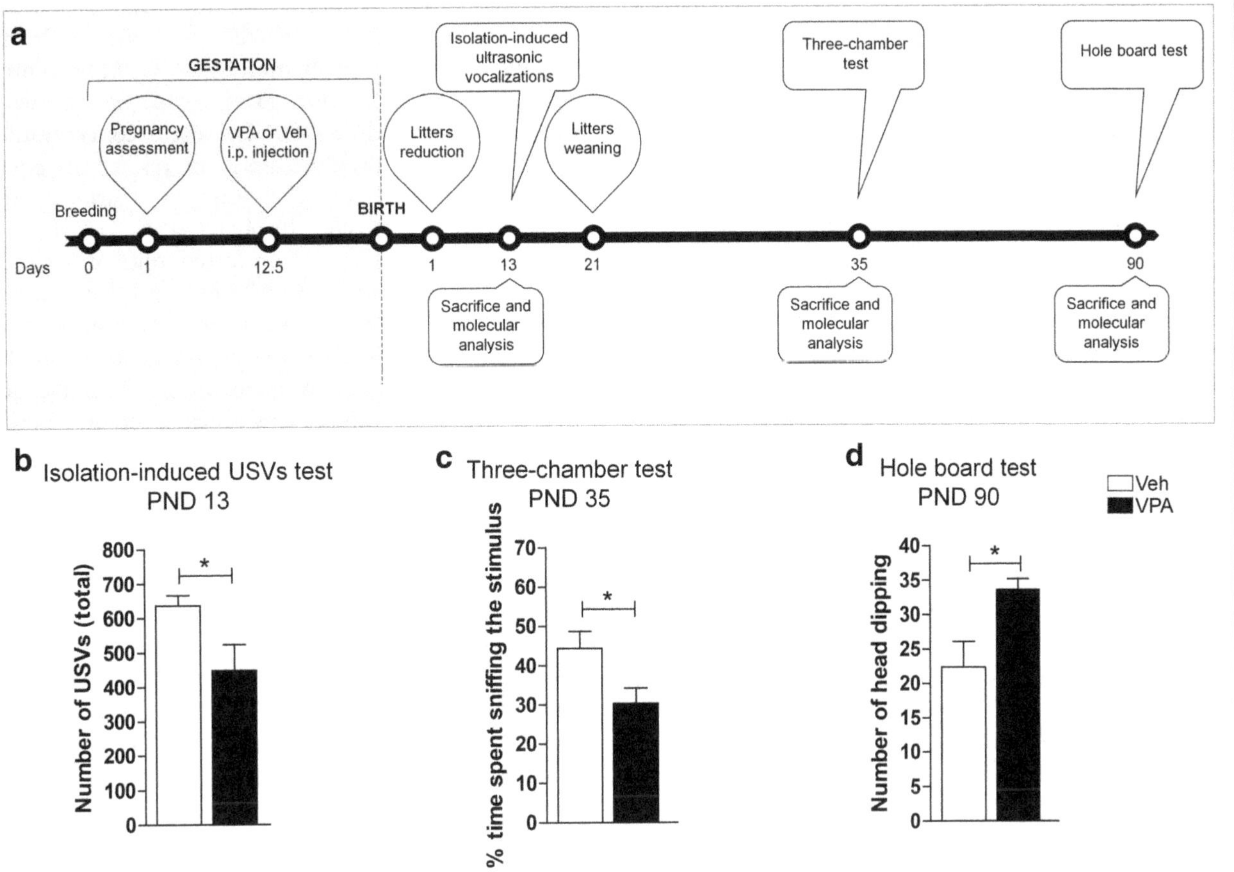

Fig. 1 Effect of prenatal VPA exposure on animals' behavior. Schematic representation of the experimental design (**a**). Assessment of the autistic-like phenotype in prenatally VPA-exposed rats through reduced isolation-induced USV emission at PND 13 (**b**), sociability in the three-chamber test at PND 35 (**c**), and induced stereotypic behavior in the hole-board test at PND 90 (**d**) (Veh $n = 5$, VPA $n = 5$). Data represent mean ± SEM. Statistical analysis was performed by t test ($^*p < 0.05$ vs Veh group)

10 and 200 kHz. The USVs were analyzed quantitatively using Avisoft Recorder software (Version 5.1).

Three-chamber test

The test was performed as previously described [40]. The apparatus was a rectangular three-chamber box, with two lateral chambers (30 l × 35 w × 35 h cm) connected to a central chamber (15 l × 35 w × 35 h cm). Each lateral chamber contained a small Plexiglas cylindrical cage. At PND 35, each experimental rat was individually allowed to explore the three-chamber apparatus for 10 min, and then confined in the central compartment. An unfamiliar stimulus animal was confined in a cage located in one chamber of the apparatus, while the cage in the other chamber was left empty. Both doors to the side chambers were then opened, allowing the experimental animal to explore the apparatus for 10 min. The percent of time spent in social approach (sniffing the stimulus animal) were scored using the Observer 3.0 software (Noldus, The Netherlands).

Hole board test

The apparatus was a gray square metal table (40 l × 40 w × 10 h cm) with 16 evenly spaced holes (4 cm in diameter), inserted in a Plexiglas arena (40 l × 40 w × 60 h cm). At PND 90, rats were individually placed in the apparatus and their behavior was observed for 5 min. Dipping behavior was scored by the number of times an animal inserted its head into a hole at least up to the eye level. Each session was recorded with a camera positioned above the apparatus for subsequent behavioral analysis performed using the Observer 3.0 software (Noldus Information Technology).

Real-time quantitative PCR (RT-qPCR)

Total mRNA of PfC, HPC, and Cb was isolated by TRI-Reagent (Sigma-Aldrich, Saint Louis, MO, USA) following the manufacturer's instructions. For each brain tissue, the total amount of the mRNA was quantified by D30 BioPhotometer spectrophotometer (Eppendorf AG, Hamburg, Germany). The first-strand cDNA synthesis kit, adding oligo (dT) 0.2 μM and random primers 0.05 μg/μl was used to perform revers transcription of 1 μg mRNA to obtain cDNA (Promega, Promega Corporation, WI, USA). Reverse transcription was carried out with the following thermal protocol: + 25 °C for 10 min and + 72 °C for 65 min. Samples were stored at + 4 °C and then processed for mRNA encoding for S100B, glial fibrillary acidic protein (GFAP), Olig2, Iba1 (Bio-Fab laboratories, Rome, Italy), and the cluster of differentiation 11b (CD11b) (Bio-Rad, Hercules, CA, USA).

To confirm pair's primers efficiency, the amplification products from each primer pair were tested with the melting curve analyses. The amounts of the amplicons were normalized against TATA-box binding protein (TBP) and hypoxanthine guanine phosphoribosyl transferase (HPRT) used as reference genes (all primers sequences are listed in Table 1). All amplifications were performed dissolving 500–800 nM primers and 75 ng cDNA in the iTaq Universal SYBR Green Supermix (Bio-Rad) using a CFX96 Touch thermocycler (Bio-Rad) according to the manufacturer's instructions. The detection of the fluorescent signals was assessed at the end of the + 60 °C extension period. For each sequence of interest, three independent experiments were performed in triplicate. Data are expressed as the fold difference in mRNA expression (ΔΔCq) calculated according to the Pflaffl method.

Western blot

Total protein amount of PfC, HPC, and Cb was isolated and processed as previously described [29, 30, 34]. Brain tissues were mechanically lysed in ice-cold hypotonic lysis buffer containing 50 mM Tris/HCl pH 7.5, 150 mM NaCl, 1 mM ethylenediamenetetraacetic acid (EDTA), 1% triton X-100, 1 mM phenylmethylsulfonyl fluoride (PMSF), 10 μg/ml aprotinin, and 0.1 mM leupeptin (all from Sigma-Aldrich), and then incubated for 40 min at + 4 °C. After centrifugation at 14000 rpm for 30 min, supernatants were collected and stored at − 80 °C. Protein concentration was calculated by Bradford assay to resolve an equal amount of proteins for each sample. Thirty micrograms were resolved through 12% acrylamide SDS-PAGE gel and then transferred onto nitrocellulose membranes with a trans-blot semi-dry transfer cell (Bio-Rad). From this step on, membranes were treated on an orbital shaker. Unspecific bound of the antibodies was avoided by incubating membranes for 1 h at room temperature in a blocking solution containing either 5% non-fat dry milk (Bio-Rad) or 5% bovine serum albumin (BSA, Sigma-Aldrich) in tris-buffered saline (TBS) (Corning, NY, USA) 0.1% tween 20 (TBS-T). Then, an overnight incubation with the proper primary antibodies against S100B, GFAP, Olig2, CD11b, or Iba1 was performed at + 4 °C (experimental conditions are reported in Table 2).

After removing the excess of antibody solution, the membranes were rinsed in TBS-T 0.05% and incubated for 1 h at room temperature with a specific secondary horseradish peroxidase (HRP)-conjugated antibody (Table 2) to detect immunocomplexes by an enhanced chemiluminescence (ECL) kit (GE Healthcare Life Sciences, Milan, Italy). Immunocomplexes were visualized using a Chemidoc XRS + and Image Lab software (Bio-Rad), and then quantified by ImageJ software. Values were normalized to those of β-actin.

For each protein of interest, three independent experiments were performed in triplicate. Data are expressed as percentage of control.

Table 1 Primer sequences and general conditions used to perform real-time qPCR

GENE	Primer (5′→3′)		Annealing (°C)	Efficiency (%)	R^2
S100B	Forward	TCAGGGAGAGAGGGTGACAA	60	94.6	.998
	Reverse	ACACTCCCCATCCCCATCTT			
GFAP	Forward	CGGCTCTGAGAGAGATTCGC	60	105.0	.989
	Reverse	GCAAACTTGGACCGATACCA			
Olig2	Forward	CCCGATGATCTTTTTCTGCC	60	98.8	.990
	Reverse	GCTTCTTATCTTTCTTGGTG			
CD11b	Forward	N/A (Cod. qRnoCID0002800, Bio-Rad)	60	94.0	.990
	Reverse				
Iba1	Forward	GTCCTTGAAGCGAATGCTGG	60	95.6	.994
	Reverse	CATTCTCAAGATGGCAGATC			
HPRT	Forward	TCCCAGCGTCGTGATTAGTGA	60	98.3	.992
	Reverse	CCTTCATGACATCTCGAGCAAG			
TBP	Forward	TGGGATTGTACCACAGCTCCA	60	99.7	.995
	Reverse	CTCATGATGACTGCAGCAAACC			

GFAP glial fibrillary acidic protein; *CD11b* cluster of differentiation 11b; *HPRT* hypoxanthine guanine phosphoribosyl transferase; *TBP* TATA-box binding protein

Table 2 Experimental conditions used to perform western blot experiments

Primary antibody	Brand/cat #	Dilution	Secondary antibody	Brand/cat #
Rabbit α-S100B	Genetex	1:1000	HRP conjugated goat anti-rabbit IgG 1:10000	Jackson ImmunoResearch
	GTX129573	5% BSA in TBS-T 0.1%	5% BSA in TBS-T 0.1%	111-035-045
Rabbit α-GFAP	Abcam	1:25000	HRP conjugated goat anti-rabbit IgG 1:10000	Jackson ImmunoResearch
	ab7260	5% milk in TBS-T 0.1%	5% milk in TBS-T 0.1%	111-035-045
Rabbit α-Olig2	Santa Cruz	1:500	HRP conjugated goat anti-rabbit IgG 1: 10000	Jackson ImmunoResearch
	sc-48817	5% milk in TBS-T 0.1%	5% milk in TBS-T 0.1%	111-035-045
Rabbit α-CD11b	Bioss	1:1000	HRP conjugated goat anti-rabbit IgG 1:10000	Jackson ImmunoResearch
	bs-1014R	5% BSA in TBS-T 0.1%	5% BSA in TBS-T 0.1%	111-035-045
Rabbit α-Iba1	Abcam	1:1000	HRP conjugated goat anti-rabbit IgG 1:10000	Jackson ImmunoResearch
	ab178846	5% milk in TBS-T 0.1%	5% milk in TBS-T 0.1%	111-035-045
Rabbit α-β-actin	Santa Cruz	1:1000	HRP conjugated goat anti-rabbit IgG 1:20000	Jackson ImmunoResearch
	sc-1616R	5% milk in TBS-T 0.1%	5% milk in TBS-T 0.1%	111-035-045

GFAP glial fibrillary acidic protein; *CD11b* cluster of differentiation 11b; *MAP2* microtubule associated protein; *BSA* bovine serum albumin; *TBS-T* tris buffered saline tween 20; *HRP* horseradish peroxidase

Immunofluorescence

Immunofluorescence was performed as previously described [30, 34, 44]. The assay was performed on 12-μm-thick coronal slices of PfC, HPC, and Cb. Tissues were rinsed in phosphate-buffered saline (PBS) and post-fixed with 4% paraformaldehyde (PFA). After the blocking step lasting 90 min at room temperature in 1% BSA dissolved in PBS/0.25% triton X-100, sections were incubated overnight with the primary antibody recognizing GFAP, Olig2, or Iba1 at +4 °C. Primary antibodies were diluted in 0.5% BSA in PBS/0.25% triton X-100. Tissues were rinsed in PBS and incubated for 2 h at room temperature with the proper secondary antibody. The staining of nuclei was performed with Hoechst (1:5000, Thermo Fisher Scientific, MA, USA). After rinses in PBS slices were mounted with Fluoromount aqueous mounting medium (Sigma-Aldrich). The experimental conditions are summarized in Table 3.

Cell count analysis

Cells labeled with the different markers were quantified in 4 serial coronal 12 μm sections, spaced 48 μm apart, in each brain region for each animal. We used three rats per experimental group ($N = 3$ vehicle and $N = 3$ VPA) for each age, for a total of 18 rats. The brain regions analyzed were the PfC, the molecular layer (ML) and the granular cell layer (GL) of the Cb, the stratum radiatum of the Ammon's horn 1 (CA1), CA2, CA3, and hilus of the dentate gyrus (DG) of the HPC. Nuclei were stained with Hoechst dye. Cells were identified as positive for a marker if they expressed immunoreactivity visually deemed to be above background. Images were captured using a ×20/0.50 magnification objective, and digitization was executed with a wide-field microscope (Eclipse E600; Nikon Instruments, Rome, Italy) connected to a QImaging camera with NIS-Elements BR 3.2 64-bit software. We used a 200 × 100 × 12 μm capture field of view to analyze the number of immunopositive cells within each field using the multi-point button of the Fiji Is Just ImageJ (FIJI) software. Cell count analyses, expressed as number of antibody positive cells in 2.4×10^5 μm^3 of tissue, were carried out by a blind observer.

Statistical analysis

GraphPad Prism 6 software (GraphPad Software, San Diego, CA, USA) was used for the statistical analyses. Student's t test was used to compare Veh and VPA

Table 3 Experimental conditions used to perform immunofluorescence

Primary antibody	Brand/cat #	Dilution	Secondary antibody	Brand/cat #
Rabbit α-GFAP	Abcam	1:200	FITC conjugated goat anti-rabbit IgG (H + L) 1:200, 5% BSA in PBS/0.25% triton X-100	Jackson ImmunoResearch
	ab7260	5% BSA in PBS/0.25% triton X-100		111-095-003
Rabbit α-Olig2	Santa Cruz	1:250	FITC conjugated goat anti-rabbit IgG (H + L) 1:200, 0.5% BSA in PBS/0.25% triton X-100	Jackson ImmunoResearch
	sc-48817	0.5% BSA in PBS/0.25% triton X-100		111-095-003
Rabbit α-Iba1	Wako	1:1000	FITC conjugated goat anti-rabbit IgG (H + L) 1:200, 0.5% BSA in PBS/0.25% triton X-100	Jackson ImmunoResearch
	019-19741	0.5% BSA in PBS/0.25% triton X-100		111-095-003

GFAP glial fibrillary acidic protein; *MAP2* microtubule associated protein; *BSA* bovine serum albumin; *FITC* fluorescein isothiocyanate; *PBS* phosphate buffered saline groups. Data are presented as mean ± SEM. Differences between means were considered as significant at $p < 0.05$.

Results

Behavioral tests

Animals prenatally exposed to VPA showed enduring impairments in the three core symptoms of autism. At infancy, VPA-exposed pups separated from the dam and siblings vocalized significantly less compared to Veh-exposed pups ($t = 2.334$; $p < 0.05$; df = 8, Fig. 1b). At adolescence, VPA-exposed rats showed decreased sociability in the three-chamber test, since they spent less time sniffing the stimulus animal compared to Veh-exposed animals ($t = -2.436$; $p < 0.05$; df = 8, Fig. 1c). At adulthood, VPA-exposed rats showed stereotypic behaviors in the hole board test, since they made more head dipping at PND 90 ($t = -2.781$; $p < 0.05$; df = 8, Fig. 1d).

In their entirety, these results confirm that prenatal exposure to VPA causes the manifestation of autistic-like behaviors that persist from infancy to early adulthood.

Astrocytes in ASD model rats

To investigate the effect of prenatal VPA exposure on astrocyte phenotype, we analyzed transcription and expression of the archetypal astroglial markers GFAP and the neurotrophin/Ca^{2+} binding protein S100B. At PND 13, we observed a significant reduction of S100B mRNA in the HPC of VPA-exposed rats compared to control animals, with no significant modification in its protein expression (Fig. 2a, b). At the same age, we detected a significant increase of GFAP mRNA in the HPC of VPA-exposed rats (Fig. 2c). No changes in GFAP protein were observed among all groups by western blot (Fig. 2d); however, immunofluorescence experiments revealed a significant increase of GFAP-positive cells in the PfC of VPA-exposed rats (Fig. 2e, f).

At PND 35 rats showed higher levels of S100B mRNA in both PfC and HPC of VPA-exposed rats, with a significant reduction in the Cb (Fig. 3a). A decreased level of GFAP mRNA was found in the PfC and in the Cb of VPA animals compared to controls (Fig. 3c). No modifications of S100B levels were found at protein level (Fig. 3b), whereas GFAP protein expression was higher in the PfC of VPA-exposed rats (Fig. 3d).The number of GFAP-positive cells was decreased in the GL of the Cb, and in the CA1 and DG hippocampal sub-regions, while a significant increase of GFAP-positive astrocytes was observed in the CA3 of VPA-exposed rats (Fig. 3e, f). Results obtained in adult rats demonstrate transcriptional modifications and some alterations in protein content. At PND 90, VPA-exposed animals showed higher levels of S100B mRNA in Cb and HPC (Fig. 4a). Conversely, GFAP mRNA was lower in the HPC and higher in the Cb of VPA-exposed rats compared to Veh animals (Fig. 4c). No changes in the protein expression of GFAP and S100B were detected (Fig. 4b, d). Finally, significantly higher number of GFAP-positive cells in the ML of the Cb and CA2 of the HPC of VPA-exposed rats was documented (Fig. 4e, f).

In summary, prenatal exposure to VPA differentially affects astrocytes in different brain regions, and causes transcriptional modifications of S100B and GFAP, which are particularly evident in adolescent and adult rats, where modified GFAP expression is also observed.

Oligodendrocytes in ASD model rats

We examined the effects of prenatal exposure to VPA on oligodendrocytes by testing Olig2, a transcriptional factor essential for oligodendrocyte development. Infant VPA-exposed rats showed higher levels of Olig2 mRNA in PfC and HPC, and a trend toward an increase of Olig2 protein expression (+ 76.77%) in PfC compared to age-matched control animals (Fig. 5a, b). No changes of Olig2-positive cells density were observed, except for the CA3 sub-region of the HPC where a significant decrease of their population was detected (Fig. 5c, d).

The RT-qPCR analysis revealed a significant increase of Olig2 in the PfC of VPA-exposed rats at PND 35, with a decrease of this transcription factor in the HPC of the same animals (Fig. 6a). These modifications were evident also at a protein level. In adolescent VPA-exposed rats, we observed a statistically significant increase of Olig2 protein expression in the PfC, a significant decrease in the Cb, and a trend toward a decrease in the HPC (–27.24%) (Fig. 6b). A more detailed analysis of the brain areas revealed subtler modifications in Olig2-positive cells distribution. In particular, in VPA-exposed rats we observed a significant increase in the number of Olig2-positive cells in the GL of the Cb and in the DG of the HPC, and a statistically significant reduction of Olig2-positive cells in the CA1 and CA2 of the same animals (Fig. 6c, d). In adult (PND 90) rats prenatally exposed to VPA, a significant decrease of Olig2 mRNA was observed solely in the HPC (Fig. 7a). On the contrary, the Olig2 protein was increased in the HPC of these animals (Fig. 7b). The VPA-exposed rats also showed more Olig2-positive cells in the ML of the Cb and in the CA1 (Fig. 7c, d).

Collectively, these results demonstrate that the prenatal exposure to VPA modifies oligodendrocytes at both the transcriptional and translational levels, and that these changes occur mainly in the PfC and in the HPC. Of note, these alterations are particularly evident during adolescence, but seem to be compensated in adulthood.

Microglia in ASD model rats

To characterize microglia in this rat model of ASD, we analyzed transcription and expression of CD11b, a

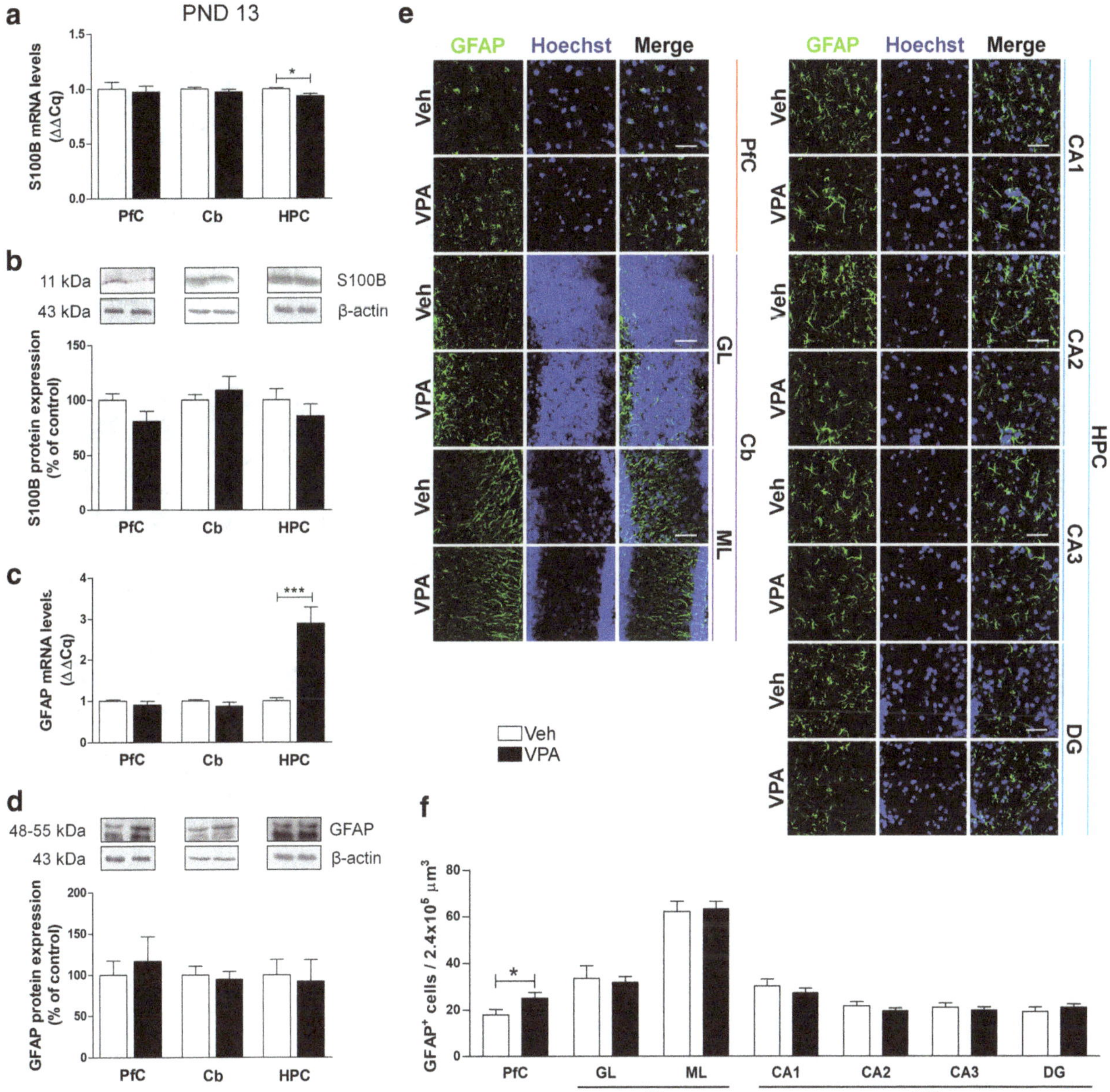

Fig. 2 Effect of prenatal VPA exposure on astrocytes in infancy. Analysis of the neurotrophin S100B and the GFAP in the PfC, Cb, and HPC of healthy- (open bars, Veh) and autistic-like (black bars, VPA) infant rats (PND 13). Representation of the relative concentration of S100B (**a**) and GFAP (**c**) in VPA animals compared to control (Veh), normalized to both TBP and HPRT (ΔΔCq; $N = 3$, in triplicate). Representative western blots for S100B (**b**) and GFAP (**d**) proteins, and densitometric analyses are normalized to β-actin used as loading control. Results are expressed as percentage of control (Veh) ($N = 3$, in triplicate). Representative fluorescence micrographs of GFAP (green) staining in the PfCGL and MLof Cb, and CA1, CA2, CA3, and the hilus of the DG of the HPC. Nuclei were stained with Hoechst (blue) (**e**). The images have been analyzed by counting the number of GFAP-positive cells in 2.4×10^5 μm^3 (scale bar 50 μm; $N = 3$, 4 times) (**f**). All data are presented as means ± SEM. Statistical analysis was performed by *t* test (**p* < 0.05; ****p* < 0.001 vs Veh group)

marker of microglia activation, and Iba1, a Ca^{2+}-binding protein constitutively expressed by both surveillant and activated microglia. In VPA-exposed rats at PND 13, we observed a significant increase of CD11b mRNA in PfC and HPC, and no substantial change in the protein expression except for a trend toward an increase of this marker in PfC (+ 54.36%) (Fig. 8a, b). At the same age, we detected a significant increase of Iba1 mRNA in the Cb of VPA-exposed rats (Fig. 8c). We also found a significant increase in the number of Iba-positive cells in the ML of the Cb of VPA-exposed rats with a significant decrease in the CA3 of the same animals (Fig. 8e, f).

Adolescent (PND 35) rats displayed more pronounced modifications. A significant increase of both transcription

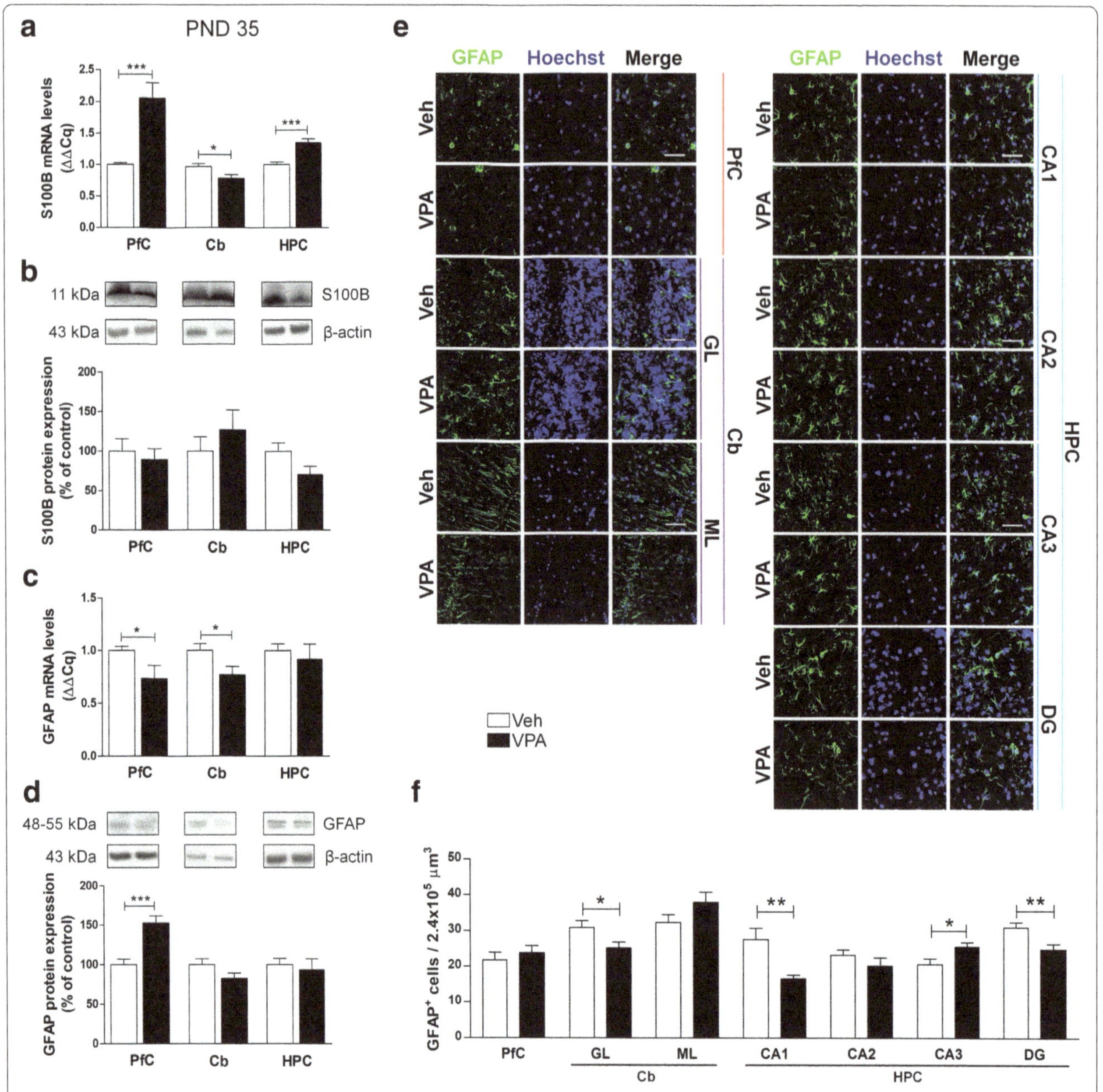

Fig. 3 Effect of the prenatal VPA exposure on astrocytes in adolescence. Evaluation of the neurotrophin S100B and the cytoskeletal GFAP in the PfC, Cb, and HPC of healthy- (open bars, Veh) and autistic-like (black bars, VPA) adolescent rats (PND 35). Representation of the relative concentration of S100B (**a**) and GFAP (**c**) in VPA animals compared to control (Veh), normalized to both TBP and HPRT (ΔΔCq; *N* = 3, in triplicate). Representative western blots for S100B (**b**) and GFAP (**d**) proteins, and densitometric analyses normalized to β-actin used as loading control. Results are expressed as percentage of control (Veh) (*N* = 3, in triplicate). Representative fluorescence micrographs of GFAP (green) staining in the PfC, GL and ML of Cb, and stratum radiatum of CA1, CA2, CA3, and the hilus of the DG of the HPC. Nuclei were stained with Hoechst (blue) (**e**). The images have been analyzed by counting the number of GFAP-positive cells in 2.4×10^5 μm^3 (scale bar 50 μm; *N* = 3, 4 times) (**f**). All data are presented as means ± SEM. Statistical analysis was performed by *t* test (**p* < 0.05; ***p* < 0.01; ****p* < 0.001 vs Veh group)

and expression of CD11b in the PfC of VPA-exposed animals compared to control rats was detected (Fig. 9a, b). Moreover, a significant increase of Iba1 mRNA was found in the PfC of VPA-exposed rats, whereas, in the same animals, we observed reduced transcription in the HPC (Fig. 9c). No changes of protein expression of Iba1 were observed (Fig. 9d). The number of Iba1-positive cells increased in the GL of the Cb and in the CA1 of adolescent (PND 35) VPA-exposed rats (Fig. 9e, f).

In adult rats (PND 90), no modifications of CD11b and Iba1 protein transcription and expression was observed, except for a trend toward an increase of CD11b expression in PfC (+ 47.04%) and Cb (+ 41.26%), and a significant decrease of Iba1 mRNA in the HPC of the

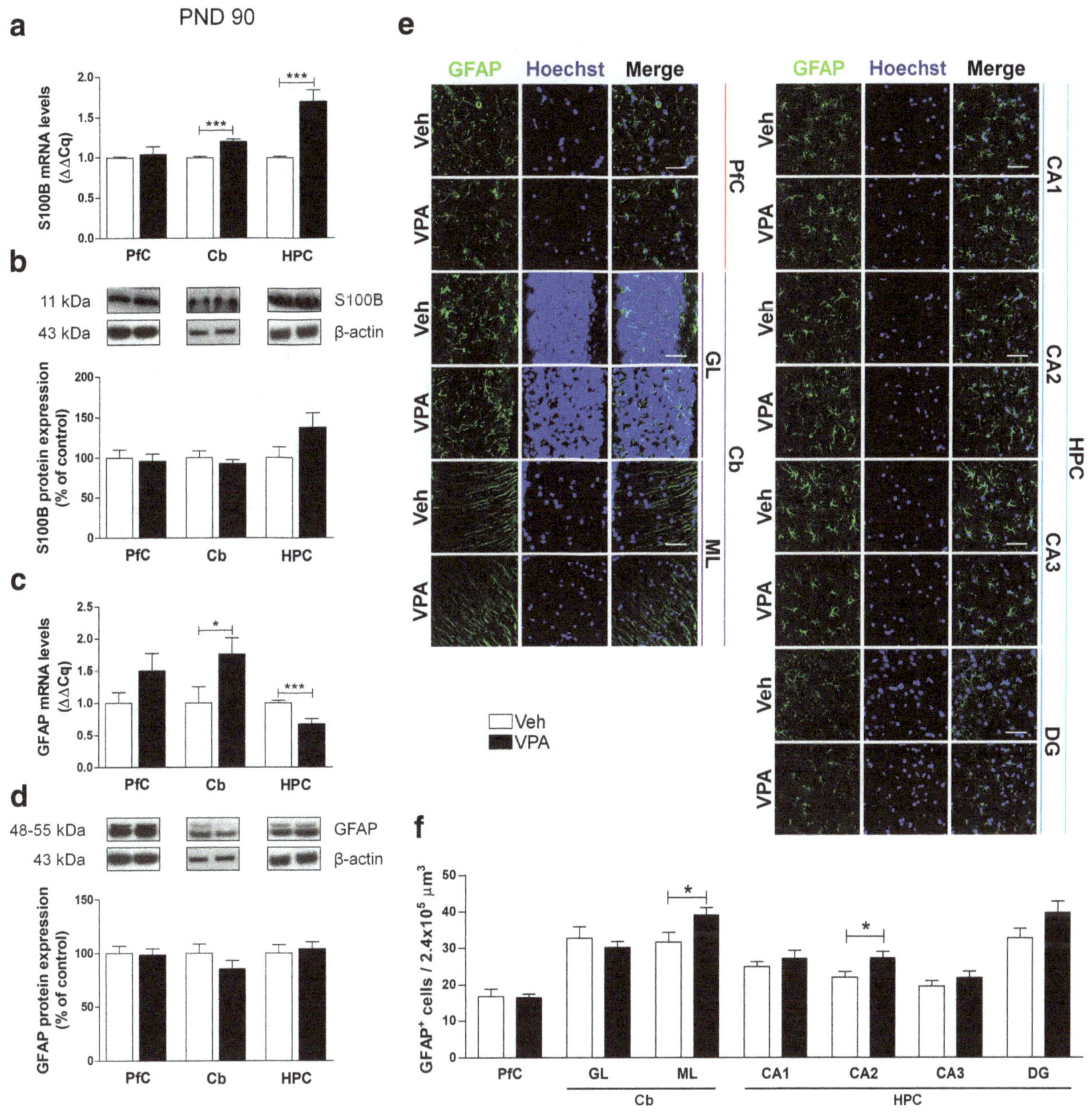

Fig. 4 Effect of the prenatal VPA exposure on astrocytes in adulthood. Evaluation of the neurotrophin S100B and the cytoskeletal GFAP in the PfC, Cb, and HPC of healthy- (open bars, Veh) and autistic-like (black bars, VPA) adult rats (PND 90). Representation of the relative concentration of S100B (**a**) and GFAP (**c**) in VPA animals compared to control (Veh), normalized to both TBP and HPRT (ΔΔCq; $N = 3$, in triplicate). Representative western blots for S100B (**b**) and GFAP (**d**) proteins, and densitometric analyses normalized to β-actin used as loading control. Results are expressed as percentage of control (Veh) ($N = 3$, in triplicate). Representative fluorescence micrographs of GFAP (green) staining in the PfC, GL and ML of Cb, and stratum radiatum of CA1, CA2, CA3, and the hilus of the DG of the HPC. Nuclei were stained with Hoechst (blue) (**e**). The images have been analyzed by counting the number of GFAP-positive cells in 2.4×10^5 μm^3 (scale bar 50 μm; $N = 3$, 4 times) (**f**). All data are presented as means ± SEM. Statistical analysis was performed by *t* test (*$p < 0.05$; ***$p < 0.001$ vs Veh group)

same animals (Fig. 10a–d). At PND 90, the number of Iba1-positive cells was significantly reduced in PfC, CA1, and CA2 of rats prenatally exposed to VPA, while more Iba1-positive cells were detected in the GL of the Cb of the same animals (Fig. 10e, f).

Taken together, these results indicate that the prenatal VPA exposure modifies microglia and that these changes occur mainly in the PfC and in the HPC. Moreover, we observed that the prenatal VPA exposure switches microglial phenotypes from resting to activated in infant

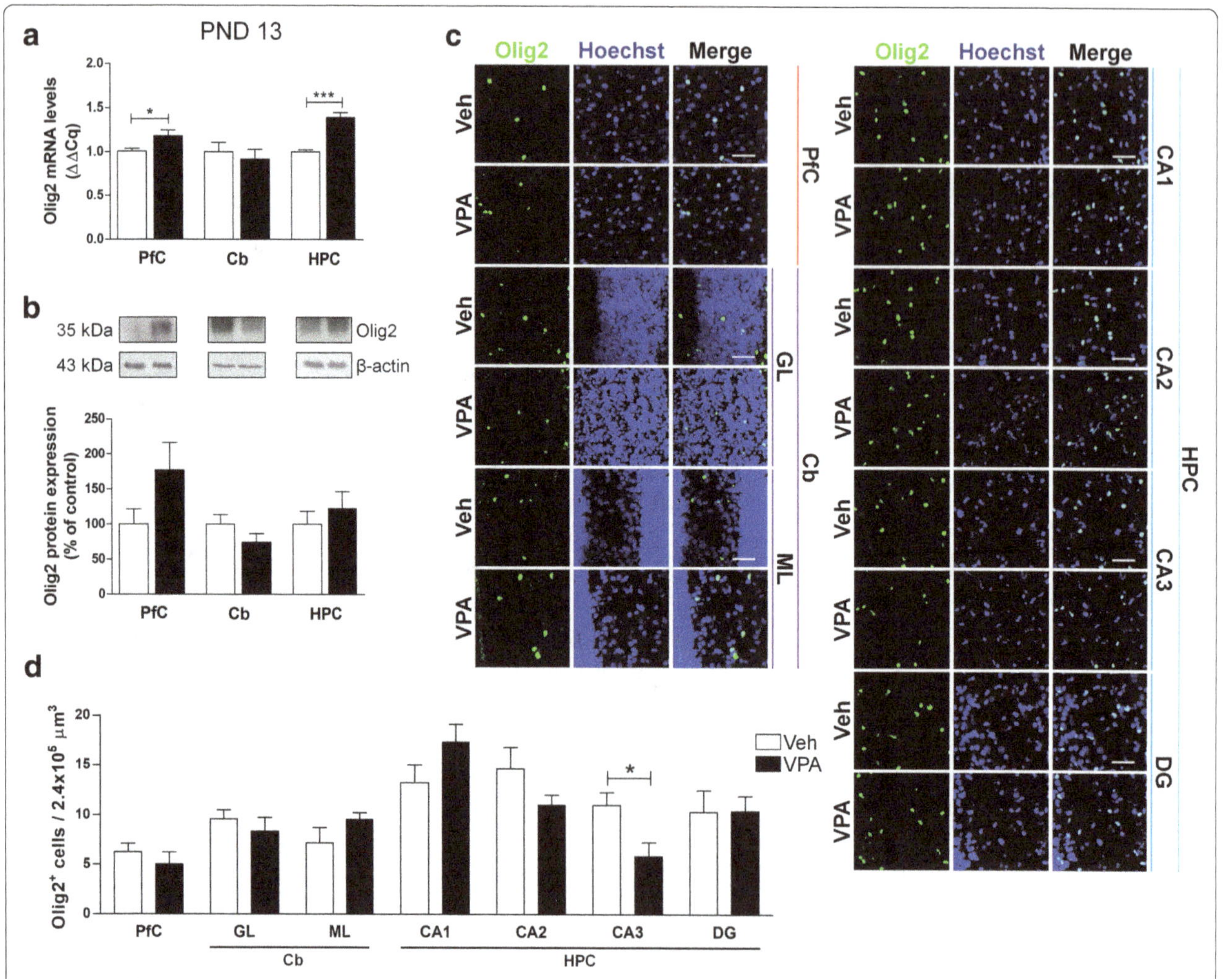

Fig. 5 Effect of the prenatal VPA exposure on oligodendrocytes in infancy. Evaluation of the transcription factor Olig2 in the PfC, Cb, and HPC of healthy- (open bars, Veh) and autistic-like (black bars, VPA) infant rats (PND 13). Representation of the relative concentration of Olig2 (**a**) in VPA animals compared to control (Veh), normalized to both TBP and HPRT (ΔΔCq; $N = 3$, in triplicate). Representative western blots for Olig2 protein and densitometric analyses normalized to β-actin used as loading control (**b**). Results are expressed as percentage of control (Veh) ($N = 3$, in triplicate). Representative fluorescence micrographs of Olig2 (green) staining in the PfC, GL and ML of Cb, and stratum radiatum of CA1, CA2, CA3, and the hilus of the DG of the HPC. Nuclei were stained with Hoechst (blue) (**c**). The images have been analyzed by counting the number of Olig2-positive cells in 2.4×10^5 μm^3 (scale bar 50 μm; $N = 3$, 4 times) (**d**). All data are presented as means ± SEM. Statistical analysis was performed by *t* test (*$p < 0.05$; ***$p < 0.001$ vs Veh group)

and adolescent rats while this phenomenon is somewhat mitigated in adulthood.

Discussion

All three types of neuroglia are critically important for normal development of the CNS and for formation of neuronal ensembles. Astrocytes assist synaptogenesis [17, 18], while astrocytes together with microglia shape neuronal networks through synaptic pruning and removal of redundant synaptic contacts [45–47]. Functional insufficiency of neuroglia leads to neurodevelopmental pathologies [48, 49]. The role of neuroglial components in ASD has received much attention recently, when several lines of evidence have demonstrated glia-specific alterations in animal models of ASD as well as in patients suffering from this disorder (for recent reviews see [48, 49]). The transcriptome analysis of the brains of ASD patients identified significant association of the pathology with genes linked to reactive gliosis and neuroinflammation [50]. Increased expression of astroglia-specific proteins aquaporin-4 and connexin43 has been found in the autistic human tissue [51]; increase in GFAP expression and astroglial hypertrophy was also observed with cerebellum demonstrating most prominent changes [52]. Microglial activation and increase in pro-inflammatory factors were other characteristic features of ASD brain tissue [52–54].

These findings support the notion of glia-related pathological developments that may exacerbate or even

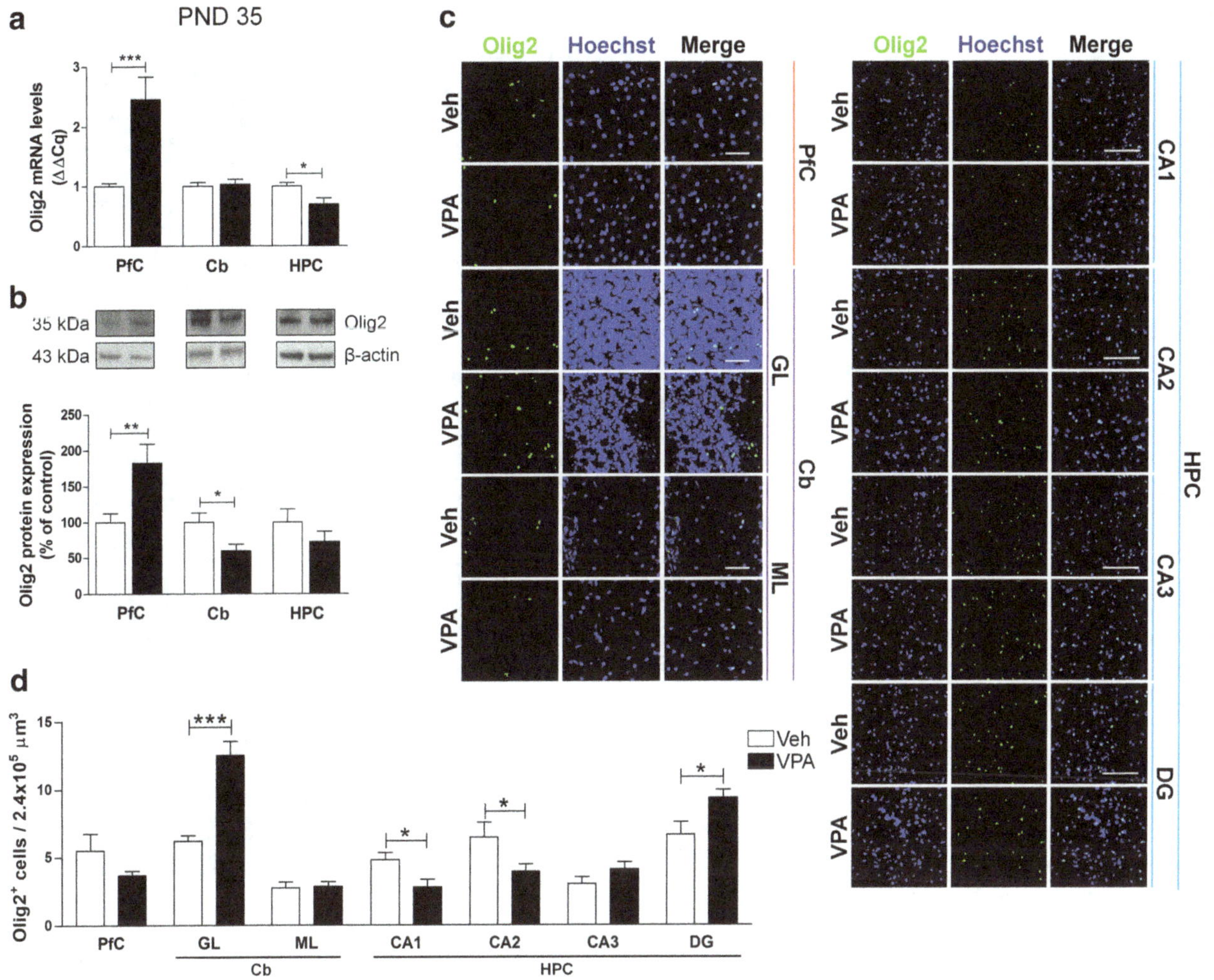

Fig. 6 Effect of the prenatal VPA exposure on oligodendrocytes in adolescence. Evaluation of the transcription factor Olig2 in the PfC, Cb, and HPC of healthy- (open bars, Veh) and autistic-like (black bars, VPA) adolescent rats (PND 35). Representation of the relative concentration of Olig2 (**a**) in VPA animals compared to control (Veh), normalized to both TBP and HPRT (ΔΔCq; $N = 3$, in triplicate). Representative western blots for Olig2 protein and densitometric analyses normalized to β-actin used as loading control (**b**). Results are expressed as percentage of control (Veh) ($N = 3$, in triplicate). Representative fluorescence micrographs of Olig2 (green) staining in the PfC, GL and ML of Cb, and stratum radiatum of CA1, CA2, CA3, and the hilus of the DG of the HPC. Nuclei were stained with Hoechst (blue) (**c**). The images have been analyzed by counting the number of Olig2-positive cells in 2.4×10^5 μm^3 (scale bar 50 μm; $N = 3$, 4 times) (**d**). All data are presented as means ± SEM. Statistical analysis was performed by *t* test (*$p < 0.05$; **$p < 0.01$; ***$p < 0.001$ vs Veh group)

drive ASD evolution. Indeed, the autistic brain is affected already at the early developmental stages, when loss of function of microglia and astrocytes can affect formation of synaptically connected neuronal networks. Equally important could be the contribution of oligodendrocytes, which shape the brain connectome. Expression of specific markers associated with cells of oligodendroglial lineage (including for example oligodendrocyte transcription factor 1/2 or myelin basic protein) is increased in the cerebella of autistic patients [55]. The single nucleotide polymorphisms of the central oligodendroglial differentiation regulator gene DUSP15 were identified in the brains of ASD patients [56], while many components of a molecular network associated with ASD are specifically enriched in oligodendroglia and white matter [57]. Changes in oligodendroglia and hence changes in white matter may be linked to a rather characteristic ASD-associated increase in the brain size (see for examples [58, 59]).

Astroglial as well as microglial abnormalities have been detected in animal models of several types of ASD associated with expression of pathologically modified genes; these include the Rett syndrome, fragile X syndrome, and tuberous sclerosis. In the Rett syndrome that arises from loss-of-function mutations in the X-linked MeCP2 encoding methyl-CpG-binding protein 2, the glial pathological phenotype has been clearly revealed. Microglial cells lacking MeCP2 triggered excitotoxicity

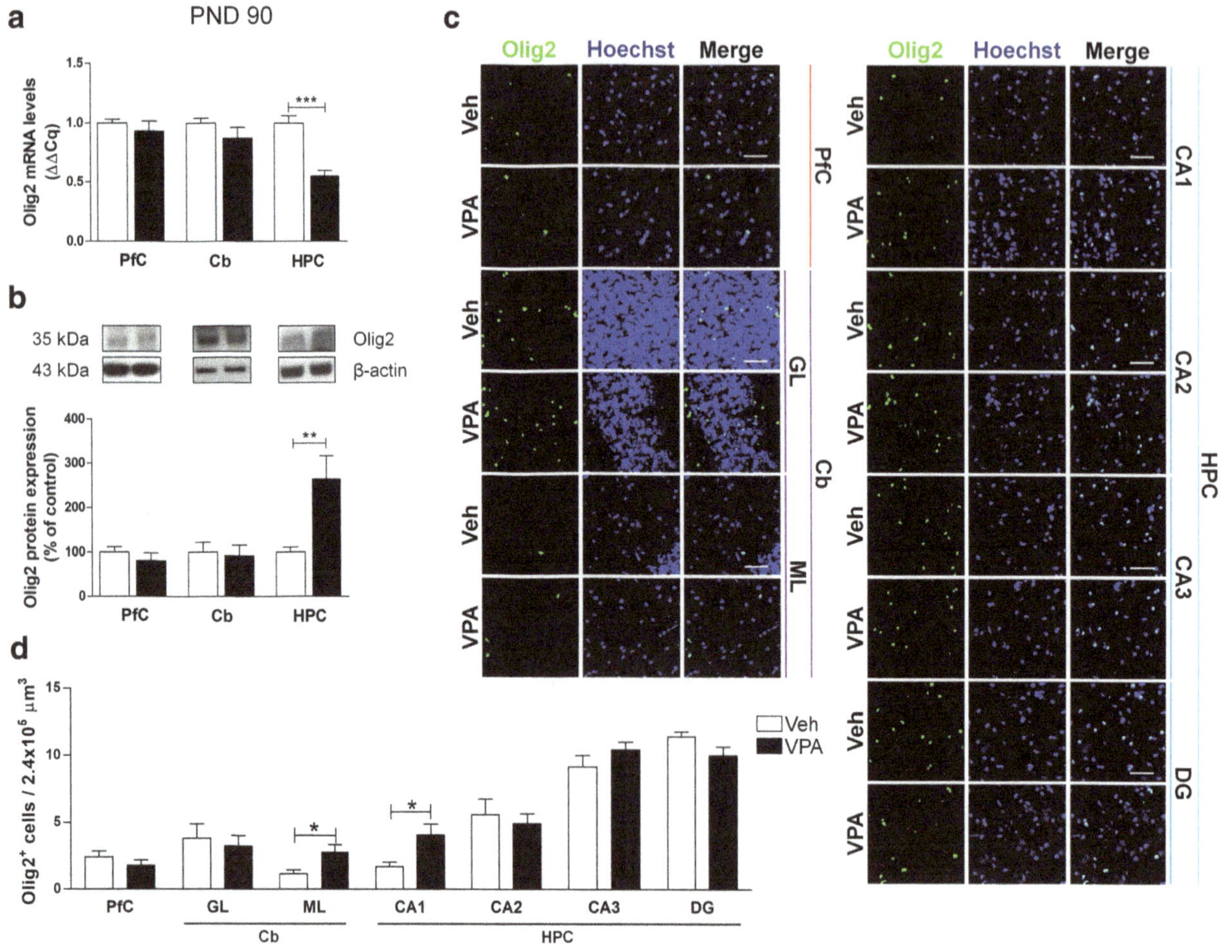

Fig. 7 Effect of the prenatal VPA exposure on oligodendrocytes in adulthood. Evaluation of the transcription factor Olig2 in the PfC, Cb, and HPC of healthy- (open bars, Veh) and autistic-like (black bars, VPA) adult rats (PND 90). Representation of the relative concentration of Olig2 (**a**) in VPA animals compared to control (Veh), normalized to both TBP and HPRT (ΔΔCq; $N = 3$, in triplicate). Representative western blots for Olig2 protein and densitometric analyses normalized to β-actin used as loading control (**b**). Results are expressed as percentage of control (Veh) ($N = 3$, in triplicate). Representative fluorescence micrographs of Olig2 (green) staining in the PfC, GL and ML of Cb, and stratum radiatum of CA1, CA2, CA3, and the hilus of the DG of the HPC. Nuclei were stained with Hoechst (blue) (**c**). The images have been analyzed by counting the number of Olig2-positive cells in 2.4×10^5 μm^3(scale bar 50 μm; $N = 3$, 4 times) (**d**). All data are presented as means ± SEM. Statistical analysis was performed by *t* test (*$p < 0.05$; **$p < 0.01$; ***$p < 0.001$ vs Veh group)

through excessive release of glutamate [60]; whereas MeCP2-deficient astrocytes lost their ability to support neuronal growth and dendritic ramifications in vitro [61]. In the fragile X syndrome (which results from the loss of Fmr1 gene function), increased astroglial reactivity has been observed (in mice with genetic deletion of Fmr1 gene) [62].

To summarize, the gliopathology in the ASD context is mainly represented by glial reactivity, which further highlights the contribution of neuroinflammation with both processes apparently having pathological significance. In this context, we asked ourselves whether the same reactive changes are pronounced in a rodent model of ASD resulting from in utero exposure to VPA, a widely used antiepileptic drug. The use of VPA has clinical significance as indeed VPA treatment during pregnancy has been related with a higher risk of ASD in the exposed children [7, 8]. Despite this evidence, recent epidemiological studies show that the public awareness of such an association is still limited [63].

Rodents prenatally exposed to VPA are widely used as a preclinical model of ASD [9, 11, 64]. The VPA-treated animals display several ASD-like symptoms in the course of development. These animals show impairment of the communicative capabilities, alteration of the social repertoire, stereotypical behavior, and anxiety [40, 65]. In particular, in line with previous studies [66, 67], we found that the infant male offspring born from VPA-treated rats exhibit reduced ability to interact with their mothers, since they emit less ultrasonic vocalizations when isolated

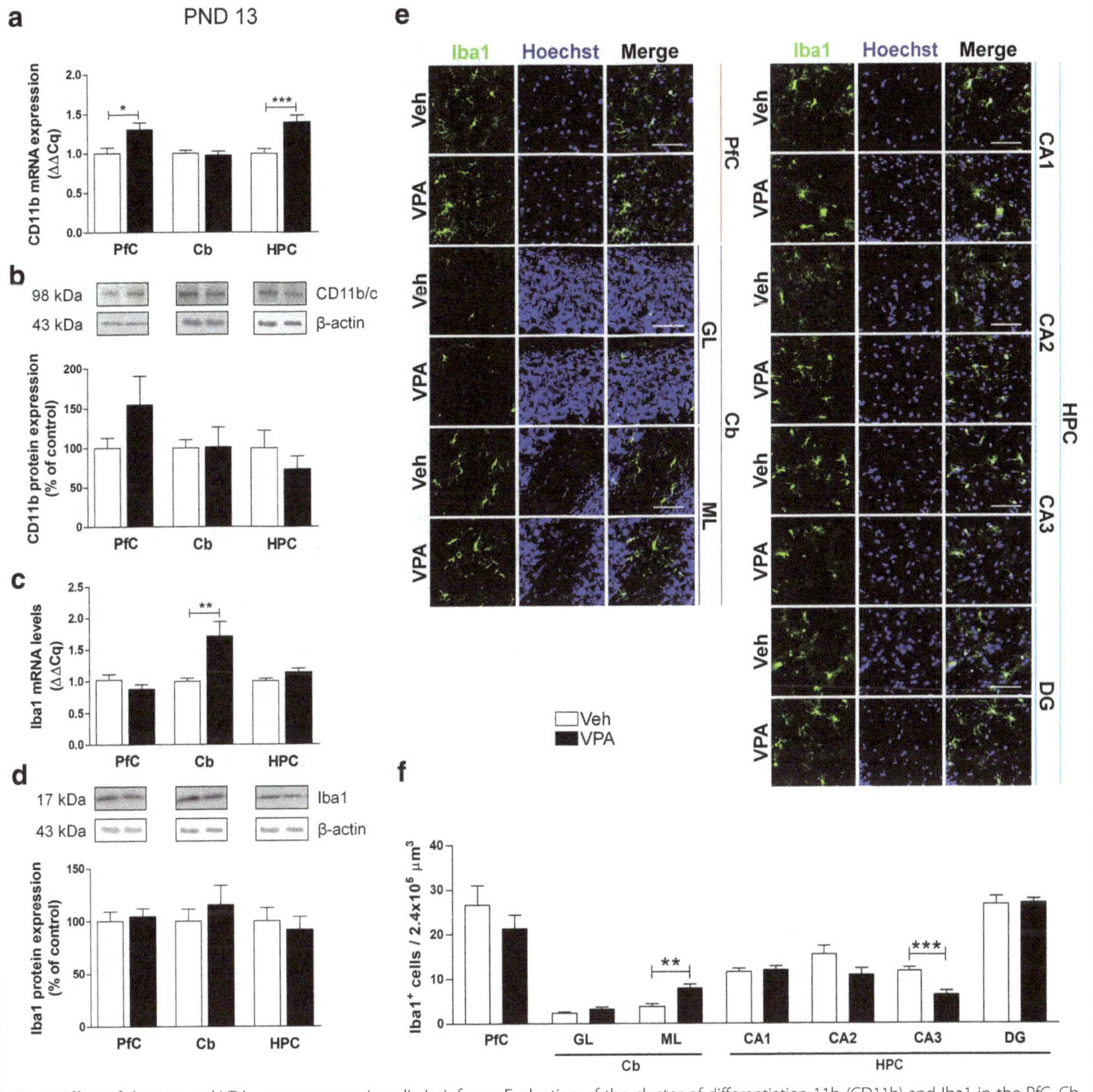

Fig. 8 Effect of the prenatal VPA exposure on microglia in infancy. Evaluation of the cluster of differentiation 11b (CD11b) and Iba1 in the PfC, Cb, and HPC of healthy- (open bars, Veh) and autistic-like (black bars, VPA) infant rats (PND 13). Representation of the relative concentration of CD11b (**a**) and Iba1 (**c**) in VPA animals compared to control (Veh), normalized to both TBP and HPRT (ΔΔCq; $N = 3$, in triplicate). Representative western blots for CD11b (**b**) and Iba1 (**d**) proteins, and densitometric analyses normalized to β-actin used as loading control. Results are expressed as percentage of control (Veh) ($N = 3$, in triplicate). Representative fluorescence micrographs of Iba1 (green) staining in the PfC, GL and ML of Cb, and stratum radiatum of CA1, CA2, CA3, and the hilus of the DG of the HPC. Nuclei were stained with Hoechst (blue) (**e**). The images have been analyzed by counting the number of Iba1-positive cells in 2.4×10^5 μm^3 (scale bar 50 μm; $N = 3$, 4 times) (**f**). All data are presented as means ± SEM. Statistical analysis was performed by *t* test (*$p < 0.05$; **$p < 0.01$; ***$p < 0.001$ vs Veh group)

from their mothers and siblings. This feature is accompanied by the inability of VPA-exposed pups to recognize familiar from unfamiliar odors, this being an early sign of the impairment in social recognition [66, 68, 69]. All these aspects negatively affect the social postnatal development of the VPA-exposed offspring and persist through adolescence and adulthood [40]. Indeed, VPA-exposed rats showed altered sociability in the three chamber test and increased stereotypic behavior in the hole board test. Our results are in agreement with those obtained by other researchers showing that a single injection of VPA to pregnant rats [65, 68, 70, 71] or mice [66, 72] on gestational day 12.5 yielded offspring with a behavioral pattern strikingly similar to that observed in autism. Beside behavioral

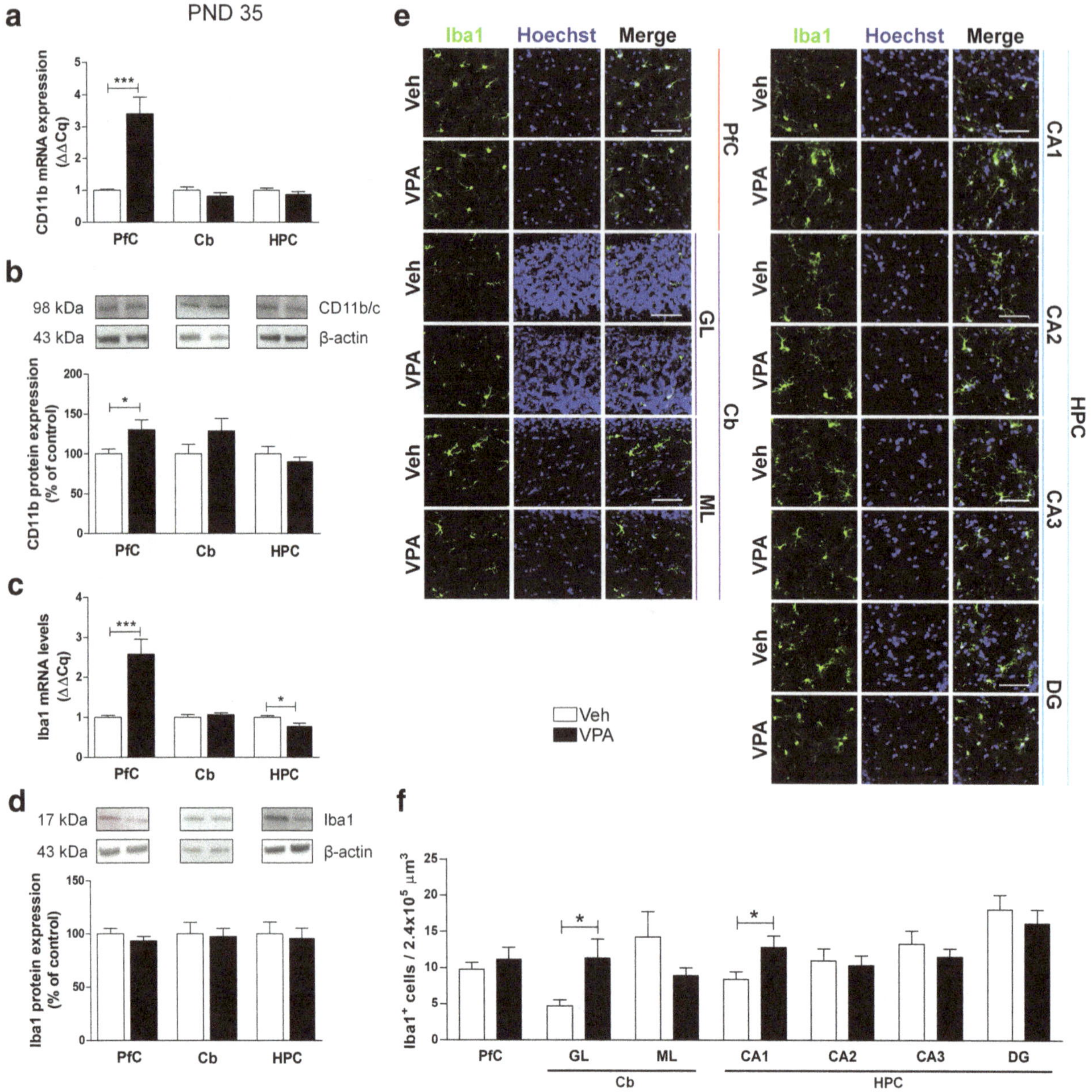

Fig. 9 Effect of the prenatal VPA exposure on microglia in adolescence. Evaluation of the cluster of differentiation 11b (CD11b) and Iba1 in the PfC, Cb, and HPC of healthy- (open bars, Veh) and autistic-like (black bars, VPA) adolescent rats (PND 35). Representation of the relative concentration of CD11b (**a**) and Iba1 (**c**) in VPA animals compared to control (Veh), normalized to both TBP and HPRT (ΔΔCq; $N = 3$, in triplicate). Representative western blots for CD11b (**b**) and Iba1 (**d**) proteins, and densitometric analyses normalized to β-actin used as loading control. Results are expressed as percentage of control (Veh) ($N = 3$, in triplicate). Representative fluorescence micrographs of Iba1 (green) staining in the PfC, GL and ML of Cb, and stratum radiatum of CA1, CA2, CA3, and the hilus of the DG of the HPC. Nuclei were stained with Hoechst (blue) (**e**). The images have been analyzed by counting the number of Iba1-positive cells in $2.4 \times 10^5\ \mu m^3$ (scale bar 50 µm; $N = 3$, 4 times) (**f**). All data are presented as means ± SEM. Statistical analysis was performed by *t* test (**p* < 0.05; ***p* < 0.01; ****p* < 0.001 vs Veh group)

alterations, rats exposed to VPA in utero demonstrate molecular and metabolic abnormalities. Very recent experiments demonstrated that VPA exposure impairs repair of DNA damage [41], modifies cholesterol/isoprenoid metabolism, and reduces the number of oligodendrocytes leading to lower myelin and cholesterol levels in the HPC of adolescent VPA-exposed rats [44].

Conclusions

Here, we extend this scenario by showing that prenatal VPA exposure induces autistic-like behaviors and does affect neuroglia. Modifications identified are brain region- and age-dependent. The changes in glia which we observed in VPA-exposed rats have been rather modest and occurred mostly at young ages; moreover, the

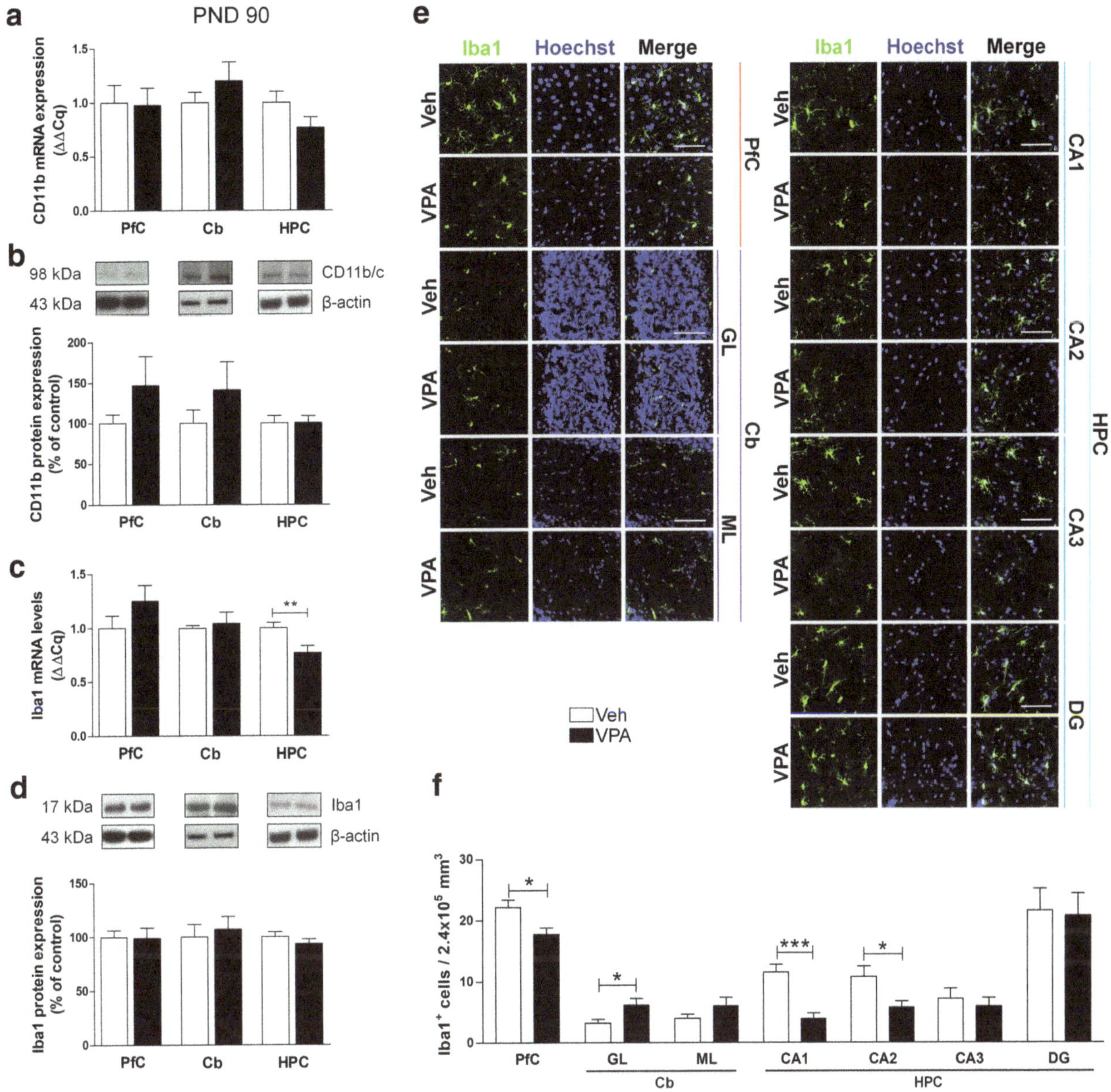

Fig. 10 Effect of the prenatal exposure to VPA on microglia in adulthood. Evaluation of the cluster of differentiation 11b (CD11b) and Iba1 in the PfC, Cb, and HPC of healthy- (open bars, Veh) and autistic-like (black bars, VPA) adult rats (PND 90). Representation of the relative concentration of CD11b (**a**) and Iba1 (**c**) in VPA animals compared to control (Veh), normalized to both TBP and HPRT (ΔΔCq; $N = 3$, in triplicate). Representative western blots for CD11b (**b**) and Iba1 (**d**) proteins, and densitometric analyses normalized to β-actin used as loading control. Results are expressed as percentage of control (Veh) ($N = 3$, in triplicate). Representative fluorescence micrographs of Iba1 (green) staining in the PfC, GL and ML of Cb, and stratum radiatum of CA1, CA2, CA3, and the hilus of the DG of the HPC. Nuclei were stained with Hoechst (blue) (**e**). The images have been analyzed by counting the number of Iba1-positive cells in 2.4×10^5 μm^3 (scale bar 50 μm; $N = 3$, 4 times) (**f**). All data are presented as means ± SEM. Statistical analysis was performed by *t* test (*$p < 0.05$; **$p < 0.01$; ***$p < 0.001$ vs Veh group)

changes were quite heterogeneous as they differ between brain regions, and often we have not seen obvious correlation between expression of mRNA and respective protein. In line with previous findings [24, 71], some hints for astrogliotic response were found in young animals, in which the density of GFAP-positive astrocytes has increased in the cortical regions. This increase went in parallel with elevated GFAP mRNA, without however changes in protein content. In adult rats, the number of GFAP-positive astrocytes was increased in CA3 but decreased in CA1 region and in cerebellum. Finally, in the mature rats, numbers of GFAP-positive cells were increased in Cb and CA2 hippocampal area, with no changes in expression of GFAP and S100B at a protein level. At the same time, the changes in expression of neuroglial markers seem to be rather mild, with neuroinflammatory phenotype being present mainly in young ages and being ameliorated in adulthood.

All in all, the results we obtained in VPA-exposed rats are heterogeneous and intricate and reflect the complexity of the molecular and cellular mechanisms underlying ASD. Indeed, autism is a complex disease, whose clinic features are multifaceted and intricate like equally complex and subtle should be the molecular changes causing these phenotypes.

Abbreviations

ASD: Autism spectrum disorder; BSA: Bovine serum albumin; Cb: Cerebellum; CD11b: Cluster of differentiation 11b; CNS: Central nervous system; DG: Dentate gyrus; ECL: Enhanced chemiluminescence; EDTA: Ethylenediaminetetraacetic acid; GD: Gestational day; GFAP: Glial fibrillary acidic protein; GL: Granular layer; HPC: Hippocampus; HPRT: Hypoxanthine guanine phosphoribosyl transferase; HRP: Secondary horseradish peroxidase; ML: Molecular layer; PBS: Phosphate-buffered saline; PFA: Paraformaldehyde; PfC: Prefrontal cortex; PMSF: Phenylmethylsulfonyl fluoride; PND: Postnatal day; RT-qPCR: Real-time quantitative PCR; TBP: TATA-box binding protein; TBS-T: Tris-buffered saline 0.1% tween 20; USVs: Isolation-induced ultrasonic vocalizations; Veh: Saline; VPA: Valproic acid

Funding

This work was supported by SAPIENZA University of Rome grant n.MA116154CD981DAE (CS), Marie Curie Career Reintegration Grant PCIG09-GA-2011-293589 (VT) and the Jerome Lejeune Foundation Research grant #1674 (VT).

Authors' contributions

MRB, RF, DI, and CS performed most of the molecular experiments and analyzed the data. MS, SS, and VT treated and housed the animals, and performed the behavioral tasks. VT, LS, AV, and CS supervised the experiments and discussed the results. MRB, RF, VT, AV, and CS wrote the manuscript. All authors contributed to and approved the final manuscript.

Competing interests

The authors declare that they have no competing interests.

Author details

[1]Department of Physiology and Pharmacology, "Vittorio Erspamer" SAPIENZA University of Rome, 00185 Rome, Italy. [2]Department of Science, Section of Biomedical Sciences and Technologies, University "Roma Tre", 00154 Rome, Italy. [3]Faculty of Biology, Medicine and Health, The University of Manchester, Manchester M13 9PT, UK. [4]Center for Basic and Translational Neuroscience, Faculty of Health and Medical Sciences, University of Copenhagen, 2200 Copenhagen, Denmark. [5]Achucarro Center for Neuroscience, IKERBASQUE, Basque Foundation for Science, 48011 Bilbao, Spain.

References

1. Gillott A, Standen PJ. Levels of anxiety and sources of stress in adults with autism. J Intellect Disabil. 2007;11(4):359–70.
2. Lai MC, Lombardo MV, Baron-Cohen S. Autism. Lancet. 2014;383(9920):896–910.
3. Christensen DL, Bilder DA, Zahorodny W, Pettygrove S, Durkin MS, Fitzgerald RT, et al. Prevalence and characteristics of autism spectrum disorder among 4-year-old children in the autism and developmental disabilities monitoring network. J Dev BehavPediatr. 2016;37(1):1–8.
4. Dietert RR, Dietert JM, Dewitt JC. Environmental risk factors for autism. Emerg Health Threats J. 2011;4:7111.
5. Kini U, Adab N, Vinten J, Fryer A, Clayton-Smith J. Liverpool and Manchester neurodevelopmental study group. Dysmorphic features: an important clue to the diagnosis and severity of fetal anticonvulsant syndromes. Arch Dis Child Fetal Neonatal. 2006;91:F90–5.
6. Kozma C. Valproic acid embryopathy: report of two siblings with further expansion of the phenotypic abnormalities and a review of the literature. Am J Med Genet. 2001;98(2):168–75.
7. Williams PG, Hersh JH. A male with fetal valproate syndrome and autism. Dev Med Child Neurol. 1997;39(9):632–4.
8. Williams G, King J, Cunningham M, Stephan M, Kerr B, Hersh JH. Fetal valproate syndrome and autism: additional evidence of an association. Dev Med Child Neurol. 2001;43(3):202–6.
9. Roullet FI, Lai JK, Foster JA. In utero exposure to valproic acid and autism--a current review of clinical and animal studies. Neurotoxicol Teratol. 2013;36:47–56.
10. Servadio M, Vanderschuren LJ, Trezza V. Modeling autism-relevant behavioral phenotypes in rats and mice: do 'autistic' rodents exist? Behav Pharmacol. 2015;26(6):522–40.
11. Nicolini C, Fahnestock M. The valproic acid-induced rodent model of autism. Exp Neurol. 2018;299:217–27.
12. Verkhratsky A, Butt AM. Glial physiology and pathophysiology. 1st ed: Wiley-Blackwell; 2013. Hoboken (NJ), USA
13. Wang DD, Bordey A. The astrocyte odyssey. Prog Neurobiol. 2008;86(4):342–67.
14. Parpura V, Heneka MT, Montana V, Oliet SH, Schousboe A, Haydon PG, et al. Glial cells in (patho)physiology. J Neurochem. 2012;121(1):4–27.
15. Verkhratsky A, Nedergaard M. The homeostatic astroglia emerges from evolutionary specialization of neural cells. Philos Trans R Soc Lond B Biol Sci. 2016;371(1700). https://doi.org/10.1098/rstb.2015.0428.
16. Verkhratsky A, Nedergaard M. Physiology of astroglia. Physiol Rev. 2018;98:239–389.
17. Eroglu C, Barres BA. Regulation of synaptic connectivity by glia. Nature. 2010;468:223–31.
18. Verkhratsky A, Nedergaard M. Astroglial cradle in the life of the synapse. Philos Trans R Soc Lond Ser B Biol Sci. 2014;369:20130595.
19. Zorec R, Horvat A, Vardjan N, Verkhratsky A. Memory formation shaped by astroglia. Front Integr Neurosci. 2015;9:56.
20. Nave KA. Myelination and support of axonal integrity by glia. Nature. 2010;468(7321):244–52.
21. Bessis A, Béchade C, Bernard D, Roumier A. Microglial control of neuronal death and synaptic properties. Glia. 2007;55(3):233–8.
22. Wake H, Moorhouse AJ, Jinno S, Kohsaka S, Nabekura J. Resting microglia directly monitor the functional state of synapses in vivo and determine the fate of ischemic terminals. J Neurosci. 2009;29(13):3974–80.
23. Kettenmann H, Hanisch UK, Noda M, Verkhratsky A. Physiology of microglia. Physiol Rev. 2011;91:461–553.
24. Salter MW, Stevens B. Microglia emerge as central players in brain disease. Nat Med. 2017;23(9):1018–27.
25. Pekny M, Pekna M, Messing A, Steinhauser C, Lee JM, Parpura V, et al. Astrocytes: a central element in neurological diseases. Acta Neuropathol. 2016;131:323–45.
26. Ferrer I. Diversity of astroglial responses across human neurodegenerative disorders and brain aging. Brain Pathol. 2017;27:645–74.
27. Verkhratsky A, Zorec R, Parpura V. Stratification of astrocytes in healthy and diseased brain. Brain Pathol. 2017;27:629–44.
28. Blank T, Prinz M. Microglia as modulators of cognition and neuropsychiatric disorders. Glia. 2013;61(1):62–70.
29. Scuderi C, Stecca C, Valenza M, Ratano P, Bronzuoli MR, Bartoli S, et al. Palmitoylethanolamide controls reactive gliosis and exerts neuroprotective functions in a rat model of Alzheimer's disease. Cell Death Dis. 2014;5:e1419.
30. Scuderi C, Bronzuoli MR, Facchinetti R, Pace L, Ferraro L, Broad KD, et al. Ultramicronized palmitoylethanolamide rescues learning and memory impairments in a triple transgenic mouse model of Alzheimer's disease by exerting anti-inflammatory and neuroprotective effects. Transl Psychiatry. 2018;8(1):32.
31. Verkhratsky A, Parpura V. Astrogliopathology in neurological, neurodevelopmental and psychiatric disorders. Neurobiol Dis. 2016;85:254–61.
32. Verkhratsky A, Zorec R, Rodriguez JJ, Parpura V. Astroglia dynamics in ageing and Alzheimer's disease. Curr Opin Pharmacol. 2016;26:74–9.

33. Zorec R, Parpura V, Vardjan N, Verkhratsky A. Astrocytic face of Alzheimer's disease. Behav Brain Res. 2017;322(Pt B):250–7.
34. Bronzuoli MR, Facchinetti R, Steardo L Jr, Romano A, Stecca C, Passarella S, et al. Palmitoylethanolamide dampens reactive astrogliosis and improves neuronal trophic support in a triple transgenic model of Alzheimer's disease: in vitro and in vivo evidence. Oxid Med Cell Longev. 2018;2018: 4720532.
35. Monzón M, Hernández RS, Garcés M, Sarasa R, Badiola JJ. Glial alterations in human prion diseases: a correlative study of astroglia, reactive microglia, protein deposition, and neuropathological lesions. Medicine (Baltimore). 2018;97(15):e0320.
36. Villadiego J, Labrador-Garrido A, Franco JM, Leal-Lasarte M, De Genst EJ, Dobson CM, et al. Immunization with α-synuclein/Grp94 reshapes peripheral immunity and suppresses microgliosis in a chronic Parkinsonism model. Glia. 2018;66(1):191–205.
37. Dichter GS, Felder JN, Green SR, Rittenberg AM, Sasson NJ, Bodfish JW. Reward circuitry function in autism spectrum disorders. Soc Cogn Affect Neurosci. 2012;7(2):160–72.
38. Donovan AP, Basson MA. The neuroanatomy of autism—a developmental perspective. J Anat. 2017;230(1):4–15.
39. Reim D, Distler U, Halbedl S, Verpelli C, Sala C, Bockmann J, et al. Proteomic analysis of post-synaptic density fractions from shank3 mutant mice reveals brain region specific changes relevant to autism spectrum disorder. Front Mol Neurosci. 2017;10:26.
40. Servadio M, Melancia F, Manduca A, di Masi A, Schiavi S, Cartocci V, et al. Targeting anandamide metabolism rescues core and associated autistic-like symptoms in rats prenatally exposed to valproic acid. Transl Psychiatry. 2016;6(9):e902.
41. Servadio M, Manduca A, Melancia F, Leboffe L, Schiavi S, Campolongo P, et al. Impaired repair of DNA damage is associated with autistic-like traits in rats prenatally exposed to valproic acid. Eur Neuropsychopharmacol. 2018; 28(1):85–96.
42. Kim KC, Kim P, Go HS, Choi CS, Park JH, Kim HJ, et al. Male-specific alteration in excitatory post-synaptic development and social interaction in pre-natal valproic acid exposure model of autism spectrum disorder. J Neurochem. 2013;124(6):832–43.
43. Melancia F, Schiavi S, Servadio M, Cartocci V, Campolongo P, Palmery M, et al. Sex-specific autistic endophenotypes induced by prenatal exposure to valproic acid involve anandamide signalling. Br J Pharmacol. 2018;175(18):3699–712.
44. Cartocci V, Catallo M, Tempestilli M, Segatto M, Pfrieger FW, Bronzuoli MR, et al. Altered brain cholesterol/isoprenoid metabolism in a rat model of autism spectrum disorders. Neuroscience. 2018;372:27–37.
45. Paolicelli RC, Bolasco G, Pagani F, Maggi L, Scianni M, Panzanelli P, et al. Synaptic pruning by microglia is necessary for normal brain development. Science. 2011;333:1456–8.
46. Tremblay ME, Stevens B, Sierra A, Wake H, Bessis A, Nimmerjahn A. The role of microglia in the healthy brain. J Neurosci. 2011;31:16064–9.
47. Kettenmann H, Kirchhoff F, Verkhratsky A. Microglia: new roles for the synaptic stripper. Neuron. 2013;77:10–8.
48. Zeidan-Chulia F, Salmina AB, Malinovskaya NA, Noda M, Verkhratsky A, Moreira JC. The glial perspective of autism spectrum disorders. Neurosci Biobehav Rev. 2014;38:160–72.
49. Petrelli F, Pucci L, Bezzi P. Astrocytes and microglia and their potential link with autism spectrum disorders. Front Cell Neurosci. 2016;10:21.
50. Voineagu I, Wang X, Johnston P, Lowe JK, Tian Y, Horvath S, et al. Transcriptomic analysis of autistic brain reveals convergent molecular pathology. Nature. 2011;474:380–4.
51. Fatemi SH, Folsom TD, Reutiman TJ, Lee S. Expression of astrocytic markers aquaporin 4 and connexin 43 is altered in brains of subjects with autism. Synapse. 2008;62:501–7.
52. Vargas DL, Nascimbene C, Krishnan C, Zimmerman AW, Pardo CA. Neuroglial activation and neuroinflammation in the brain of patients with autism. Ann Neurol. 2005;57:67–81.
53. Edmonson C, Ziats MN, Rennert OM. Altered glial marker expression in autistic post-mortem prefrontal cortex and cerebellum. Mol Autism. 2014;5:3.
54. Tetreault NA, Hakeem AY, Jiang S, Williams BA, Allman E, Wold BJ, et al. Microglia in the cerebralcortex in autism. J Autism Dev Disord. 2012;42: 2569–84.
55. Zeidan-Chulia F, de Oliveira BN, Casanova MF, Casanova EL, Noda M, Salmina AB, et al. Up-regulation of oligodendrocyte lineage markers in the cerebellum of autistic patients: evidence from network analysis of gene expression. Mol Neurobiol. 2016;53:4019–25.
56. Tian Y, Wang L, Jia M, Lu T, Ruan Y, Wu Z, et al. Association of oligodendrocytes differentiation regulator gene DUSP15 with autism. World J Biol Psychiatry. 2017;18:143–50.
57. Li J, Shi M, Ma Z, Zhao S, Euskirchen G, Ziskin J, et al. Integrated systems analysis reveals a molecular network underlying autism spectrum disorders. Mol Syst Biol. 2014;10:774.
58. Hardan AY, Libove RA, Keshavan MS, Melhem NM, Minshew NJ. A preliminary longitudinal magnetic resonance imaging study of brain volume and cortical thickness in autism. Biol Psychiatry. 2009;66:320–6.
59. Freitag CM, Luders E, Hulst HE, Narr KL, Thompson PM, Toga AW, et al. Total brain volume and corpus callosum size in medication-naive adolescents and young adults with autism spectrum disorder. Biol Psychiatry. 2009;66: 316–9.
60. Maezawa I, Jin LW. Rett syndrome microglia damage dendrites and synapses by the elevated release of glutamate. J Neurosci. 2010;30:5346–56.
61. Ballas N, Lioy DT, Grunseich C, Mandel G. Non-cell autonomous influence of MeCP2-deficient glia on neuronal dendritic morphology. Nat Neurosci. 2009; 12:311–7.
62. Yuskaitis CJ, Beurel E, Jope RS. Evidence of reactive astrocytes but not peripheral immune system activation in a mouse model of fragile X syndrome. Biochim Biophys Acta. 1802;2010:1006–12.
63. European Medicines Agency (EMA) New measures to avoid valproate exposure in pregnancy endorsed EMA/375438/2018. 2017. http://www.ema.europa.eu/docs/en_GB/document_library/Referrals_document/Valproate_2017_31/European_Commission_final_decision/WC500250216.pdf. Accessed 31 May 2018.
64. Ranger P, Ellenbroek BA. Perinatal influences of valproate on brain and behaviour: an animal model for autism. Curr Top BehavNeurosci. 2016;29: 363–86.
65. Markram K, Rinaldi T, La Mendola D, Sandi C, Markram H. Abnormal fear conditioning and amygdala processing in an animal model of autism. Neuropsychopharmacology. 2008;33:901–12.
66. Moldrich RX, Leanage G, She D, Dolan-Evans E, Nelson M, Reza N, et al. Inhibition of histone deacetylase in utero causes sociability deficits in postnatal mice. Behav Brain Res. 2013;257:253–64.
67. Wohr M, Schwarting RK. Affective communication in rodents: ultrasonic vocalizations as a tool for research on emotion and motivation. Cell Tissue Res. 2013;354:81–97.
68. Schneider T, Przewlocki R. Behavioral alterations in rats prenatally exposed to valproic acid: animal model of autism. Neuropsychopharmacology. 2005; 30:80–9.
69. Melo AI, Lovic V, Gonzalez A, Madden M, Sinopoli K, Fleming AS. Maternal and littermate deprivation disrupts maternal behavior and social-learning of food preference in adulthood: tactile stimulation, nest odor, and social rearing prevent these effects. Dev Psychobiol. 2006;48:209–19.
70. Schneider T, Turczak J, Przewlocki R. Environmental enrichment reverses behavioral alterations in rats prenatally exposed to valproic acid: issues for a therapeutic approach in autism. Neuropsychopharmacology. 2006;31:36–46.
71. Lucchina L, Depino AM. Altered peripheral and central inflammatory responses in a mouse model of autism. Autism Res. 2014;7(2):273–89.
72. Codagnone MG, Podestá MF, Uccelli NA, Reinés A. Differential local connectivity and neuroinflammation profiles in the medial prefrontal cortex and hippocampus in the valproic acid rat model of autism. Dev Neurosci. 2015;37(3):215–31.

12

Clinical phenotype of ASD-associated *DYRK1A* haploinsufficiency

Rachel K. Earl[1], Tychele N. Turner[2], Heather C. Mefford[3], Caitlin M. Hudac[1], Jennifer Gerdts[1], Evan E. Eichler[2,4] and Raphael A. Bernier[1,5*]

Abstract

Background: *DYRK1A* is a gene recurrently disrupted in 0.1–0.5% of the ASD population. A growing number of case reports with *DYRK1A* haploinsufficiency exhibit common phenotypic features including microcephaly, intellectual disability, speech delay, and facial dysmorphisms.

Methods: Phenotypic information from previously published *DYRK1A* cases (n = 51) and participants in an ongoing study at the University of Washington (UW, n = 10) were compiled. Frequencies of recurrent phenotypic features in this population were compared to features observed in a large sample with idiopathic ASD from the Simons Simplex Collection (n = 1981). UW *DYRK1A* cases were further characterized quantitatively and compared to a randomly subsampled set of idiopathic ASD cases matched on age and gender (n = 10) and to cases with an ASD-associated disruptive mutation to *CHD8* (n = 12). Contribution of familial genetic background to clinical heterogeneity was assessed by comparing head circumference, IQ, and ASD-related symptoms of UW *DYRK1A* cases to their unaffected parents.

Results: *DYRK1A* haploinsufficiency results in a common phenotypic profile including intellectual disability, speech and motor difficulties, microcephaly, feeding difficulties, and vision abnormalities. Eighty-nine percent of *DYRK1A* cases ascertained for ASD presented with a constellation of five or more of these symptoms. When compared quantitatively, *DYRK1A* cases presented with significantly lower IQ and adaptive functioning compared to idiopathic cases and significantly smaller head size compared to both idiopathic and *CHD8* cases. Phenotypic variability in parental head circumference, IQ, and ASD-related symptoms corresponded to observed variability in affected child phenotype.

Conclusions: Results confirm a core clinical phenotype for *DYRK1A* disruptions, with a combination of features that is distinct from idiopathic ASD. Cases with *DYRK1A* mutations are also distinguishable from disruptive mutations to *CHD8* by head size. Measurable, quantitative characterization of *DYRK1A* haploinsufficiency illuminates clinical variability, which may be, in part, due to familial genetic background.

Keywords: Autism, *DYRK1A*, Genetic syndrome, Genetically defined subtype, Disruptive mutation, Clinical phenotype

Background

Autism spectrum disorder (ASD) is characterized by tremendous clinical variability and causal heterogeneity. Historical efforts to behaviorally subtype ASD have been largely unsuccessful due to lack of meaningful treatment implications by subtype and inadequate consensus regarding clinical phenotype [1, 2]. Recent efforts have targeted the genetic causes of ASD to explore biologically defined subtypes [3, 4]. Advances in genetic sequencing technology have improved our ability to identify disease-causing mutations [5]. Chromosomal abnormalities, copy number variants (CNVs), and disruptive single nucleotide variants (SNVs), including nonsense, frameshift, and splice site mutations, have been associated with increased risk of ASD [6–9]. Most recently, work relating ASD risk to de novo disruptive SNVs suggests these single point mutations account for approximately 10% of ASD cases [6, 8]. These discoveries have prompted a shift in ASD research; instead of using extensive phenotyping prior to sequencing ASD populations, researchers have begun by identifying genes of

* Correspondence: rab2@u.washington.edu; rab2@uw.edu
[1]Department of Psychiatry and Behavioral Sciences, University of Washington, CHDD Box 357920, Seattle, WA 98195, USA
[5]Center on Human Development and Disability, University of Washington, Seattle, WA, USA
Full list of author information is available at the end of the article

interest in affected individuals and then exploring phenotype in specific gene cohorts [10].

The application of this genetics-first approach to subtyping ASD has successfully identified similar medical, behavioral, and dysmorphic features shared by individuals with disruptive variants in high-confidence ASD risk genes, such as *CHD8*, *ADNP*, *SCN2A*, and *DYRK1A* (e.g., [11–13]). Dual-specificity tyrosine phosphorylation-regulated kinase 1A, or *DYRK1A*, is a highly conserved gene in the Down syndrome critical region of chromosome 21 [6, 14], and appears to play a major role in brain development, specifically neurogenesis, neural plasticity, and cellular death [15]. *DYRK1A* haploinsufficiency was initially identified for its role in intellectual disability, which is clinically defined as childhood onset of significant cognitive and adaptive impairment [16]. Recurrent disruptions to *DYRK1A* have been found in as many as 0.5% of cases with ASD [14, 17]. In *Drosophila* models, truncating mutations to *DYRK1A* (*Drosophila* ortholog termed the Minibrain (*Mnb*) gene) result in microcephaly, including intact but smaller brain structures [18]. *Dyrk1A*-null mouse models (−/−) displayed growth deficiencies resulting in mid-gestational death [19]. Mice heterozygous for *Dyrk1A* (+/−) survived to adulthood but presented with reduced growth, developmental delays, motor and learning difficulties, and atypical behaviors, including anxiety [19, 20]. A consistent clinical phenotype appears in humans. Reported cases to date have exhibited microcephaly and intellectual disability; other features, including seizures, speech and motor delays, feeding difficulties, and distinct facial dysmorphology, have been noted as well [13, 15, 21–24].

Studies relying on medical record review have reported ASD diagnoses in up to 40% of cases with *DYRK1A* mutations, but many remaining cases have features consistent with ASD, such as stereotypies, reduced eye contact, and social anxiety [15, 21]. Few studies have conducted diagnostic evaluations of ASD and ASD-related symptoms as part of a clinical phenotyping battery. Diagnostic rates may be as high as 88% when ASD is directly evaluated as part of the study assessment process [13].

Literature on *DYRK1A* haploinsufficiency supports its association with ASD risk and suggests a complex phenotype that includes distinct dysmorphology as well as cognitive, neurological, and medical impairments. However, studies to date have only reported categorical descriptions of phenotype, which note the presence or absence of a common phenotype, such as ASD or no ASD. Quantitative assessments of ASD-related features in large cohorts and in relation to other ASD cohorts have not been examined. While previously published reports have noted an emerging phenotypic profile, variability in clinical presentation remains. Measurable data on medical, developmental, and behavioral characteristics are needed to better understand small variations in phenotype between individuals. Furthermore, varied clinical presentations of individuals with *DYRK1A* mutations have yet to be examined in the context of their familial phenotypic profile as a measure of remaining genetic background. This approach has been applied to other developmental disorders and to CNVs associated with ASD, but has yet to be applied to disruptive SNVs associated with ASD [25–28].

The aim of the proposed study was to examine a large cohort of cases with *DYRK1A* mutations, provide a summary of phenotype, and compare recurrent medical and behavioral features to (1) large idiopathic ASD samples and (2) a cohort with disruptive mutations to a different ASD-associated gene, *CHD8*. Alongside *DYRK1A*, *CHD8* is one of the most recurrent genes with disruptive SNVs implicated in ASD and provides a comparison group ascertained in the same way as the cases with *DYRK1A* mutations in this sample [6, 8]. Detection of phenotypic differences between these two groups could inform understanding of different biological profiles of ASD and illuminate key features unique to each disrupted gene. This study also explored the contribution of genetic background to phenotypic variability among individuals with disruptive *DYRK1A* mutations.

Methods

Participants

DYRK1A sample

Participants included 42 individuals with de novo, disruptive, pathogenic SNVs (nonsense, splice site, frameshift, and missense mutations) at the *DYRK1A* gene. (Fig. 1; see Additional files 1 and 2 for full variant information). The sample includes 10 individuals assessed as part of an ongoing study at the University of Washington (UW), including 7 new cases identified through clinical genetic testing and 3 previously published cases recruited from the Simons Simplex Collection (see below). In addition to the 3 previously published cases studied at UW, 32 other previously published cases with disruptive SNVs were included in the sample. All subjects were identified via clinical exome sequencing, or exome or targeted sequencing of research cohorts ascertained for a diagnosis of ASD or ID.

Those seen at UW (UW-SNV group; $n = 9$ de novo and $n = 1$ non-maternal; see Table 1 for variant information [29]) completed standardized behavioral measures and medical evaluations by clinicians naïve to gene group membership as part of a study evaluating individuals ages four and older with ASD-associated, disruptive mutations. Biological parents of the participants were also characterized.

Thirty-two previously published cases of *DYRK1A* disruptive SNVs (Pub-SNV group) included 31 de novo

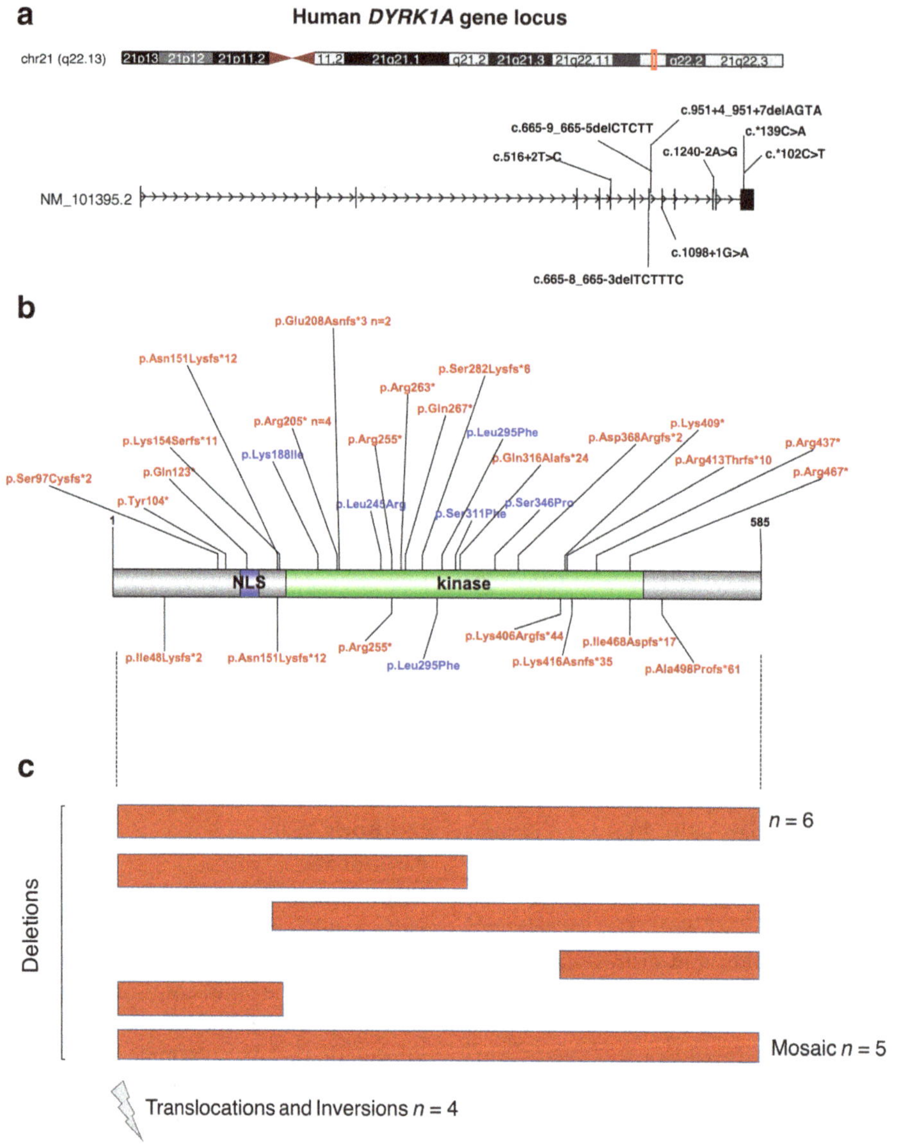

Fig. 1 Summary of *DYRK1A* gene variants. Schematic depicting the locations of disruptive variants (truncating, missense, and splice site mutations), copy number variations, and chromosomal rearrangements affecting *DYRK1A*. The ideogram of human chromosome 21 and isoform NM101395.2 coding sequence was obtained from the UCSC genome browser [54]. **a** NM101395.2 coding sequence with eight reported splice site mutations (presented in HGVS cDNA notation). Mutations below the sequence are UW-SNV participants, above are Pub-SNV mutation cases. **b** The *DYRK1A* protein (NP_567824.1) with truncating (red) and missense (blue) mutations (presented in HGVS notation). Mutations below the protein are UW-SNV cases, above are Pub-SNV mutation cases. **c** Copy number deletions and chromosomal rearrangements, including six deletions of entire gene, four partial deletions, five mosaic deletions, and four translocations/inversions (lightning bolt)

cases and 1 non-maternal case [13, 15, 21, 22, 30–32] with available medical history, physical features, and diagnoses.

Additionally, the phenotype of 19 previously published cases of de novo *DYRK1A* chromosomal rearrangements (Pub-CHR group), including microdeletions and translocations, was described and compared to those with disruptive SNVs [21, 24, 33–39]. See Table 2 for participant characteristics for the 61 total *DYRK1A* sample participants.

Comparison samples

Secondary data from an idiopathic subset of the Simons Simplex Collection (SSC), a large sample ascertained for ASD, were compared to the *DYRK1A* sample. The SSC was a cohort of 2446 simplex families including a single proband with ASD age 4–18, unaffected biological parents, and any unaffected siblings [40]. Probands were included in the idiopathic subset (n = 1981) if they had no known disruptive SNVs or deleterious CNVs, as determined by sequencing efforts by Sanders and colleagues

Table 1 *DYRK1A* variant information for UW-SNV mutation patients

Patient	Position	Type of mutation	cDNA	Protein	Inheritance
1	21:38865466	Splice site	c.1098+1G>A	–	De novo
2	21:38845116	Frameshift	c.143_144delTA	p.Ile48Lysfs*2	De novo
3	21:38877833	Frameshift	c.1491delC	p.Ala498Profs*61	De novo
4	21:38868533	Frameshift	c.1217_1220delAGAA	p.Lys406Argfs*44	De novo
5	21:38862575	Nonsense	c.763C>T	p.Arg255*	De novo
6	21:38877746	Frameshift	c.1401delAinsGG	p.Ile468Aspfs*17	De novo
7	21:38853064	Frameshift	c.452dupA	p.Asn151Lysfs*12	Not maternal
8	21:38862695	Missense	c.883C>T	p.Leu295Phe	De novo
9	21:38862463	Splice site	c.665-8_665-3delTCTTTC	–	De novo
10	21:38877590	Frameshift	c.1248delA	p.Lys416Asnfs*35	De novo

Variant information for UW-SNV patients using NCBI reference sequence for *DYRK1A* isoform NM_101395.2, GRCh37 (hg19) build version (Ensembl id: ENST00000338785). This isoform was selected because it was the highest expressing isoform in human tissues in the GTEx database [https://gtexportal.org/home/gene/DYRK1A]) [53]. Patients 1–3 were first identified through the Simons Simplex Collection, patients 4–10 underwent clinical genetic testing prior to research participation. cDNA and protein (NP_567824.1) annotation follows HGVS guidelines

in 2015, and not based on any phenotypic or behavioral profile [8]. In order to account for high rates of ID seen in the *DYRK1A* haploinsufficiency, a subset of the idiopathic group with full-scale IQ below 70 (n = 487) served as an additional comparison group. Also, a randomly selected age- and gender-matched subset (n = 10) of the full idiopathic sample was compared to the subset of *DYRK1A* cases assessed quantitatively at the UW. As part of the SSC, probands were assessed on measures of neurocognitive functioning, social communication behaviors, motor skills, physical features (e.g., head circumference), and medical history (measures described below).

Twelve individuals with disruptive SNVs at a different high-confidence ASD risk gene, *CHD8* (chromodomain helicase-DNA-binding protein 8), participating in the same UW characterization study and assessed by clinicians naïve to implicated gene disruption, served as a comparison cohort matched on ascertainment approach.

Measures

Categorical assessment of diagnostic history and developmental characteristics

Psychiatric and medical history, developmental milestones, and physiological characteristics were gathered from Pub-SNV and Pub-CHR cases. In addition to published data, supplemental case reports detailing medical history and developmental trajectory were reviewed when available.

For UW-SNV study participants, a structured caregiver interview, adapted from the SSC, was administered to gather information about developmental, psychiatric, and medical history. When caregiver-endorsed diagnoses required additional clarification, medical records were reviewed for confirmation. Using all available information, psychiatric diagnoses were either confirmed or newly diagnosed by a licensed clinical psychologist using the *Diagnostic and Statistical Manual of Mental Disorders, 5th Edition* (DSM-5) [16]. For research purposes, subjects were given an ASD diagnosis based on clinician observation and parent interview using standardized instruments (gold-standard assessment tools described below). A diagnosis of intellectual disability was given when a subject displayed childhood onset of deficits in both cognitive and adaptive functioning. When subjects were under the age of 5 and had failed to reach cognitive developmental milestones at the time of assessment, a diagnosis of Global Developmental Delay was given. A physical and dysmorphology exam was conducted by a licensed medical geneticist.

Table 2 Demographics

	DYRK1A sample			SSC idiopathic sample		*CHD8* sample
	Disruptive SNVs		*CHR*	No disruptive SNVs or deleterious CNVs		Disruptive SNVs
	Pub-SNV	UW-SNV	Pub-CHR	Total sample	IQ < 70	
Total *N* (male)	32 (22)	10 (4)	19 (9)	1981 (1705)	487 (407)	12(9)
Mean age in months (SD)	124.12 (128.85)	108.40 (69.12)	102.22 (88.06)	107.66 (42.34)	114.00 (44.00)	148.08 (64.56)

Participant demographics. *SNV* single nucleotide variant, *Pub-SNV* published disruptive SNV cases, *UW-SNV* UW study cases with disruptive SNVs, *Pub-CHR* published chromosomal rearrangement, *CNV* copy number variant. Note that there are three overlapping individuals in the Pub-SNV and UW-SNV groups ascertained from the Simons Simplex Collection. DYRK1A sample significantly differed from idiopathic ASD samples (total and IQ < 70) in gender ratio, χ^2 (1, n = 2042) = 66.88, $p < 0.001$ and χ^2 (1, n = 548) = 36.25, $p < 0.001$, respectively. Samples did not significantly differ in age, $p > 0.05$. No significant differences in age or gender for *DYRK1A* and *CHD8* samples

Quantitative assessment of *DYRK1A* UW-SNV (n = 10) and *CHD8* (n = 12)

Head circumference

Occipital frontal head circumference was measured and standardized values calculated using a normative population reference [41].

Cognitive functioning

Full-scale IQ was assessed in probands and unaffected parents. Probands ages 4 years, 0 months to 17 years, 11 months were administered the *Differential Abilities Scales, 2nd Edition* [42]. Probands 18 and older, as well as unaffected parents, were administered the Wechsler Abbreviated Scales of Intelligence [43]. For all assessments, IQ scores were generated using deviation (standard; mean = 100, SD = 15) or ratio scores (mental age equivalent/chronological age × 100). Ratio scores were derived using age equivalence values if standard scores were not possible to calculate due to subject's level of functioning.

Adaptive functioning

Caregivers were administered the *Vineland Adaptive Behavior Scales, 2nd edition* (VABS-2) to measure adaptive functioning across communication, daily living skills, and social domains [44].

ASD-specific assessment

Research-reliable clinicians administered the appropriate module of the *Autism Diagnostic Observation Schedule, 2nd Edition* (ADOS-2; [45, 46]) and *Autism Diagnostic Interview-Revised* (ADI-R; [47]). ADOS calibrated severity scores, and items regarding age of first words and age of first steps from the ADI-R were used in analyses. The total *T* score from the Social Responsiveness Scale (SRS-2; [48]) was used to quantify ASD-associated symptoms in all UW-SNV family members.

Analytic approach

Categorical variables

Fisher's exact tests were used to compare frequencies of features commonly found for *DYRK1A* mutations across disruptive SNV (Pub-SNV and UW-SNV) and chromosomal rearrangement (Pub-CHR) groups. These features included intellectual disability, speech delay (defined as first words after 24 months of age), motor deficits (e.g., delayed walking, poor coordination, abnormal gait), ASD-related deficits (e.g., ASD diagnosis, stereotypic behaviors, anxious behaviors), feeding difficulties, seizures, vision abnormalities, and microcephaly. The frequency of most common features (defined as present in 75% or more cases) was compared across *DYRK1A* and idiopathic ASD groups (total idiopathic sample and subset with IQ below 70). Only characteristics specifically noted in case reports were included in analyses; if a phenotypic characteristic was not reported, it was treated as missing for that individual. Total frequencies reflect cases with a reported presence or absence of a given characteristic.

Quantitative variables

UW-SNV *DYRK1A* participants were compared to (1) a randomly subsampled age and gender-matched subset of the SSC idiopathic sample and (2) a cohort with disruptive *CHD8* mutations on domains of functioning assessed quantitatively, including head circumference, IQ, adaptive functioning, ASD severity (ADOS calibrated severity score), age of first words (ADI-R), and age of first independent steps (ADI-R). Independent sample *t* tests were used to compare the *DYRK1A*, idiopathic, and *CHD8* groups, using the Bonferroni adjustment for multiple comparisons ($p < 0.002$).

Nonparametric Wilcoxon signed rank tests were used to compare parental and proband phenotype for UW-SNV participants in head circumference, IQ, and ASD symptoms (SRS). Gene "effect size," measured as the difference between parental and proband phenotype, was calculated as follows:

$$\text{Effect size} = \frac{\text{Proband mean} - \text{Unaffected biparental mean}}{\text{Unaffected biparental standard deviation}}$$

When both maternal and paternal data were available, biparental means were calculated as the average of maternal and paternal scores. If only one parent's data was available, that parent's score was used instead of a biparental mean.

Results

Clinical phenotype of *DYRK1A*

There were no significant differences between disruptive SNV (Pub-SNV and UW-SNV) and chromosomal rearrangement (Pub-CHR) groups on frequency of phenotypic characteristics (Table 3). Language delay was noted for 61/61 (100%); 21 individuals were nonverbal at the time of their evaluation. Intellectual disability and/or Global Developmental Delay (depending on age) were reported in 60/61 (98%) cases. The presence of motor difficulties, including delayed walking, abnormal gait, and poor coordination, was noted for 52/53 (98%). A common abnormal gait was observed across UW-SNV participants, specifically a lilting gait with a forward lean to the upper body, arms bent and held tight against the body, and hands splayed. Feeding difficulties in infancy, including poor suck, were observed in 51/54 (94%) of those with reports of feeding abilities in early development. Microcephaly, defined as head circumference two or more standard deviations below the mean for age, either primary (present throughout development) or

Table 3 Phenotypic characteristics of *DYRK1A*

	Pub-SNV and UW-SNV (n = 42)			Pub-CHR (n = 19)			Total (n = 61)			
Phenotypic characteristic	*N*	Total	%	*N*	Total	%	*N*	Total	%	Sig (Fisher's exact tests)
Intellectual disability or Global Developmental Delay	41	42	98	19	19	100	60	61	98	NS
Speech delay	42	42	100	19	19	100	61	61	100	NS
Motor difficulties	38	38	100	14	15	93	52	53	98	NS
Microcephaly	39	42	93	19	19	100	58	61	95	NS
Feeding difficulties	37	40	93	14	14	100	51	54	94	NS
Vision abnormalities	26	33	79	8	9	89	34	42	81	NS
Seizures	26	39	67	16	19	84	42	58	72	NS
ASD diagnosis	16	35	46	2	7	29	18	42	43	NS
Stereotyped behaviors	22	36	61	4	9	44	26	45	58	NS
Anxious behaviors	11	36	31	1	8	13	12	44	27	NS
Hyperactive behaviors	10	35	29	4	8	50	14	43	33	NS
Behavioral differences	35	42	83	7	19	37	42	61	69	NS
6+ symptoms including ASD	25	42	60	7	19	37	32	61	52	NS
6+ symptoms including broader behavioral difficulties	32	42	76	10	19	53	42	61	69	NS

Frequency of phenotypic features in cases with disruptive SNVs (Pub-SNV and UW-SNV) to *DYRK1A*, published chromosomal rearrangements (Pub-CHR) to *DYRK1A*, and total combined cases. Totals reflect those with complete data. Groups did not significantly differ in gender ratio (Fisher's exact test) or age (independent sample t test), $p > 0.05$. Fisher's exact tests used for group comparisons, *Sig* significance, *NS* not significant

acquired at a later age, was reported in 58/61 cases (95%). Vision abnormalities were identified in 34/42 (81%) cases, including impairments such as strabismus, astigmatism, optic nerve dysfunction, and corneal clouding. Febrile and non-febrile seizures were reported in 42/58 cases (72%).

Diagnoses of ASD were reported in 18/42 cases (43%), suggesting elevated risk well above the general population percentage of 1.5% [49]. The frequency increased to 42/61 cases (69%) when broadening the criteria to include ASD-related behaviors without a formal diagnosis, such as stereotypic behaviors (e.g., complex motor mannerisms, repetitive and self-stimulatory behaviors), limited eye contact (reported in those without known severe vision impairments), inappropriate laughter, and limited social engagement. Anxious behaviors were reported in 12/44 cases (27%), and hyperactivity was reported in 14/43 cases (33%). Seven of the ten UW-SNV cases were confirmed to have ASD; three who did not meet diagnostic criteria presented with notable stereotypies and socially anxious behaviors.

Co-occurrence of the seven most common phenotypic features (reported in 75% or more of cases) was evaluated: microcephaly, intellectual impairment, speech delay, motor difficulties, feeding difficulties, vision abnormalities, and ASD. Fifty-two percent of the total *DYRK1A* sample (32/61) possessed six or more features. Sixty-nine percent (42/61) presented with six or more features when the ASD category was broadened to include other behavioral difficulties, including stereotypic, anxious, and hyperactive behaviors.

Facial dysmorphisms were reported in 50/51 (98%) previously published cases (excluding UW-SNV cases who were previously published, n = 3). Similar dysmorphic facial features were observed in eight UW-SNV cases who participated in a standardized medical exam (five new cases, three previously published), including deep-set eyes with a hooded appearance, slightly upslanting palpebral fissures, bitemporal narrowing, prominent brow with high anterior hairline, tubular-shaped nose, prominent nasal bridge, retrognathic jaw, and small chin (Fig. 2a). Additionally, prominent, low-set, or malformed ears were also reported across cases; 4/8 UW-SNV cases presented with thick, overfolded ear helices (Fig. 2b). Foot anomalies were also noted across patients, including toe syndactyly (webbing of the toes), arachnodactyly, crooked toes, and proximal placement of the first toe (Fig. 2c). Observed commonalities in facial, ear, and foot characteristics in UW-SNV cases were consistent with reports of previously published cases. In the larger sample, spine or chest abnormalities, including pectus excavatum and scoliosis, were reported in 13/25 cases with documented skeletal observations.

Phenotypic comparisons of *DYRK1A* to idiopathic ASD

Rates of microcephaly, intellectual disability, speech delay, motor difficulties, vision impairments, and feeding difficulties were significantly higher in the total *DYRK1A* group (Pub-SNV, UW-SNV, and Pub-CHR combined) relative both to the full idiopathic SSC comparison cohort and the subset with IQ below 70 (Table 4; Fig. 3).

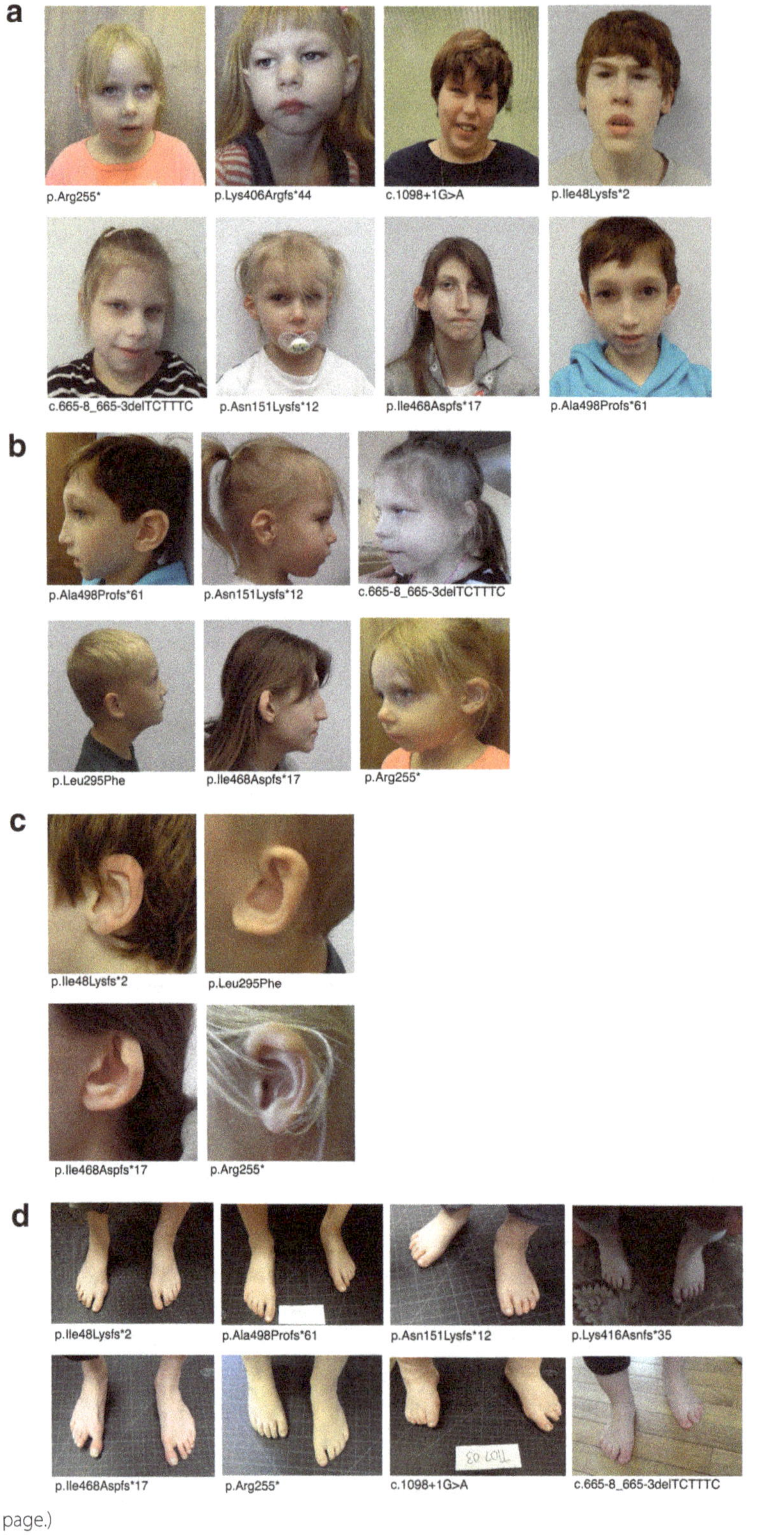

Fig. 2 (See legend on next page.)

(See figure on previous page.)
Fig. 2 Common dysmorphic features in UW-SNV patients with *DYRK1A* haploinsufficiency. **a** Facial features of eight UW-SNV patients with *DYRK1A* haploinsufficiency. Note common features across patients, including prominent brow with high anterior hairline, slightly upslanted palpebral fissures, retrognathic jaw, deep-set eyes with a hooded appearance, bitemporal narrowing, high nasal bridge with tubular-shaped, broad-tipped nose, and protruding ears. **b** Profiles of six UW-SNV patients. Note prominent brows with high anterior hairlines as well as low-set, posteriorly rotated ears in a subset of patients. **c** Ear abnormalities in four UW-SNV patients, including post-rotated and protruding ears with protruding thick and overfolded helices (i.e., outer fold of the ear). **d** Foot abnormalities in eight UW-SNV patients. Common features include proximal placement of the first toe, crooked toes, and syndactyly of the second and third toes. Frameshift, nonsense, and missense cases identified by HGVS protein notation; cases with splice site variants identified by HGVS cDNA notation

The majority of the *DYRK1A* group (79%) displayed five or more of these phenotypic features in combination. The percentages and group differences remain in the subset of individuals with *DYRK1A* mutations ascertained for an ASD diagnosis ($n = 18$, Fig. 3). Co-occurrence of five or more features increased to 89% in those with *DYRK1A* mutations ascertained for ASD.

Quantitative phenotype of *DYRK1A*

DYRK1A vs idiopathic ASD

Independent sample t tests revealed significant differences between UW-SNV and a matched idiopathic group on measures of head circumference, cognitive ability, and adaptive functioning (Table 5; Fig. 4). The UW-SNV group had significantly smaller head circumference ($p < 0.001$), significantly lower full-scale IQ ($p = 0.002$), and significantly lower adaptive abilities ($p = 0.001$) compared to the idiopathic group. There were no differences between groups on autism symptom severity (ADOS calibrated severity score), age of first words, or age of first independent steps. Outliers across the six phenotypic features of interest represented different UW-SNV individuals, highlighting the variability that is observed when exploring the phenotype quantitatively.

DYRK1A vs CHD8

No significant differences were found between *CHD8* and idiopathic groups. However, UW-SNV and *CHD8* groups differed significantly in head circumference ($p < 0.001$), such that *DYRK1A* cases had significantly smaller head size than *CHD8* cases. IQ, adaptive functioning, autism symptom severity, age of first words, and age of first steps were similar across groups (Table 5; Fig. 4).

Contribution of genetic background

When comparing parental and proband head circumference Z score, the presence of a *DYRK1A* mutation accounted for a 2.93 SD decrease in head size for probands. Wilcoxon signed rank tests showed that both mothers and fathers exhibited significantly larger head size, controlling for age and gender, compared to their affected child ($Z = -2.67$, $p = 0.008$ and $Z = -2.20$, $p = 0.028$, respectively (Fig. 5a)). When comparing ASD-related symptoms, *DYRK1A* accounted for a 5.51 SD increase in SRS total T score (more symptoms). Wilcoxon signed rank tests showed that both mothers and fathers display significantly lower SRS scores compared to their affected child ($Z = -3.62$, $p < 0.001$ and $Z = -3.41$, $p = 0.001$, respectively (Fig. 5b)). On measures of full-scale IQ, *DYRK1A* accounted for a 6.09 SD decrease in IQ for probands compared to biparental IQ. Wilcoxon signed rank tests showed that both mothers and fathers display significantly higher IQ compared to their affected child ($Z = -2.67$, $p = 0.008$ and $Z = -2.20$, $p = 0.028$, respectively (Fig. 5c)).

Discussion

This study of the *DYRK1A* haploinsufficiency phenotype, compiling previously published and newly identified cases, confirms a phenotype characterized by microcephaly, intellectual disability, speech delay, motor difficulties, feeding difficulties, and vision abnormalities. A common facial gestalt included deep-set eyes with a hooded appearance, slightly upslanted palpebral fissures, tubular-shaped nose with pronounced broad tip, high nasal bridge, prominent brow with high anterior hairline, retrognathic jaw, and small chin. Dysmorphic feet, including proximal placement of the first toe, syndactyly of the second and third toe, and unusually long and/or crooked toes, and protruding, post-rotated ears with overfolded, thick helices were also commonly observed. Those with de novo disruptive SNVs and chromosomal rearrangements did not differ in clinical features.

Of those case studies where ASD was mentioned and/or evaluated, 43% of probands received an ASD diagnosis. Among 15 cases who received gold-standard ASD assessment, rates increased to 73%. Additionally, features common to ASD, such as stereotypic and anxious behaviors, were noted in many cases where reference to an ASD diagnosis was absent. This suggests rates of ASD in *DYRK1A* cohorts may be higher in reality than reported in the total sample of *DYRK1A* cases published to date.

There are several reasons for the potential underestimated prevalence rate of ASD among published *DYRK1A* cases. First, most previously published cases relied on medical records, which varied greatly in the

Table 4 Phenotypic comparisons of *DYRK1A* to idiopathic ASD

Phenotypic characteristic	Total *DYRK1A* sample ($n = 61$)		*DYRK1A* ascertained for ASD ($n = 18$)		SSC idiopathic ascertained for ASD ($n = 1981$)		Sig (total DYRK1A vs idio total)	SSC idiopathic ASD with IQ < 70 ($n = 487$)		Sig (total DYRK1A vs idio IQ < 70)
	N/total	%	*N*/total	%	*N*/total	%		*N*	%	
Intellectual disability or Global Developmental Delay	60/61	98	18/18	100	487/1974	25	$p < 0.001$	487/487	100	–
Speech delay	61/61	100	18/18	100	1173/1981	59	$p < 0.001$	343/487	70	$p < 0.001$
Motor difficulties	52/53	98	18/18	100	963/1981	49	$p < 0.001$	253/487	52	$p < 0.001$
Microcephaly	58/61	95	16/18	89	31/1958	2	$p < 0.001$	10/485	2	$p < 0.001$
Feeding difficulties	51/54	94	16/18	89	386/1981	19	$p < 0.001$	112/487	15	$p < 0.001$
Vision abnormalities	34/42	81	16/18	67	355/1981	18	$p < 0.001$	60/487	12	$p < 0.001$
5+ symptoms	48/61	79	16/18	89	6/1981	0.30	–	5/487	1	–

Frequency of core phenotypic features (included if reported in 75% or more cases) observed in total *DYRK1A* sample (Pub-SNV, UW-SNV, and Pub-CHR) compared to frequency of same features in those with *DYRK1A* mutations ascertained for ASD, a large sample of cases with idiopathic ASD from the Simons Simplex Collection (ascertained for ASD), and a subset of idiopathic cases with IQ < 70. Totals reflect those with complete data. Fisher's exact tests used to compare total *DYRK1A* sample to both idiopathic samples on each phenotypic characteristic; all group differences significant, $p < 0.001$. *Sig* significance

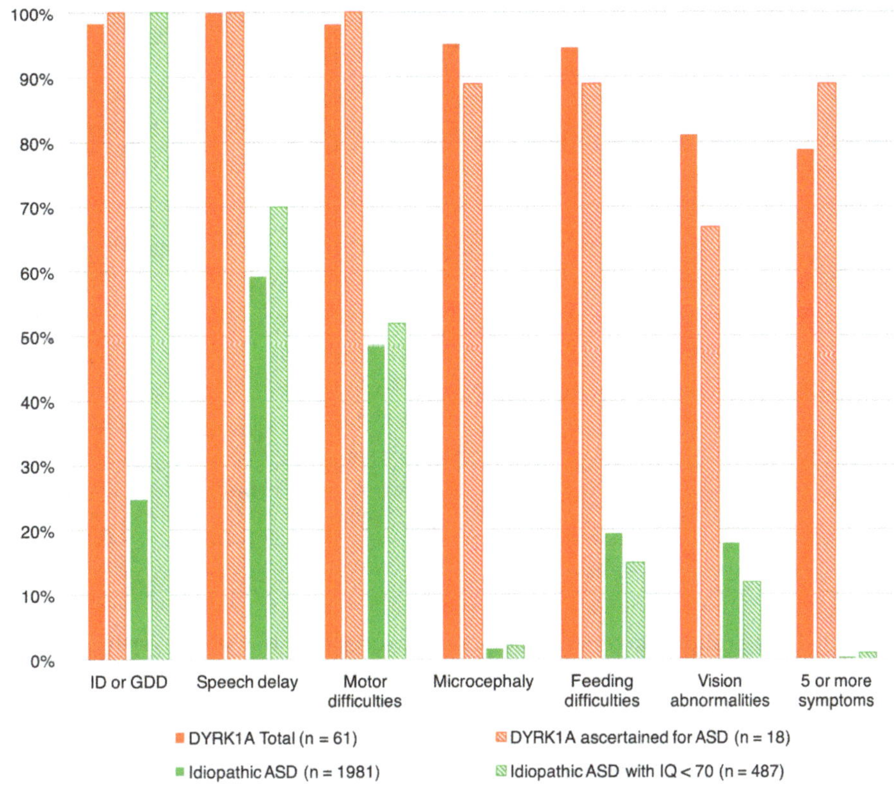

Fig. 3 Phenotypic features in total *DYRK1A* sample, *DYRK1A* sample ascertained for ASD, and idiopathic ASD samples. Bar graph presented frequencies of core phenotypic features observed in 75% or more of *DYRK1A* patients. Total *DYRK1A* sample (Pub-SNV, UW-SNV, Pub-CHR) and *DYRK1A* sample ascertained for ASD were compared to frequencies of features in idiopathic ASD samples (total and IQ < 70) using Fisher's exact tests ($p < 0.001$)

detail provided and discussion of comprehensiveness of prior evaluations; as such, it is unknown whether ASD was either evaluated and ruled out, or not evaluated at all. Second, it can be difficult to tease apart symptoms of ASD from those of intellectual disability and speech impairments without specialized training and experience with differential diagnosis within developmental disabilities, particularly in children with complex medical histories. Additionally, establishing an ASD diagnosis may not be the most pressing concern for families (and perhaps providers) given the array of impairments and medical conditions that often accompany children with a *DYRK1A* mutation. As *DYRK1A* haploinsufficiency continues to be explored within ASD risk, these factors need to be considered when determining rates in this population.

In an effort to situate the *DYRK1A* phenotype in the context of ASD, we found the *DYRK1A* group (Pub-

Table 5 Quantitative phenotype and group differences between *DYRK1A*, idiopathic, and *CHD8* groups

	DYRK1A (UW-SNV)			SSC idiopathic subset			*CHD8*			*t* statistics *DYRK1A* vs SSC		*t* statistics *DYRK1A* vs *CHD8*		*t* statistics *CHD8* vs SSC	
Phenotypic characteristic	Mean	SD	*N*	Mean	SD	*N*	Mean	SD	*N*	*t*	*d*	*t*	*d*	*t*	*d*
Head circumference *Z* score	– 3.62	2.17	10	1.21	0.39	10	1.76	2.9	11	6.94*	3.10	6.49**	2.84	NS	–
Full-scale IQ	45.30	18.14	10	81.20	26.12	10	60.91	27.39	11	3.57*	1.60	NS		NS	–
Overall adaptive functioning	54.80	9.04	10	70.50	9.40	10	65.00	18.49	12	3.81*	1.70	NS	–	NS	–
Autism severity (ADOS CSS)	6.50	2.80	10	7.70	1.25	10	8.18	1.78	11	NS	–	NS	–	NS	–
Age walked unaided	19.70	5.64	10	13.22	2.59	10	18.50	4.38	12	NS	–	NS	–	NS	–
Age of first single words	45.14	22.82	7	17.50	7.92	10	25.17	28.01	12	NS	–	NS	–	NS	–

Descriptives for phenotypic variables commonly impaired in *DYRK1A* haploinsufficiency for three groups: *DYRK1A* ($n = 10$), SSC idiopathic subset randomly samples and matched on age and gender ($n = 10$), and *CHD8* ($n = 12$). Group comparisons using independent sample *t* tests between (1) *DYRK1A* and SSC groups, (2) *DYRK1A* and *CHD8* groups, and (3) *CHD8* and SSC groups. *Significant differences between *DYRK1A* and idiopathic groups, $p < 0.002$; **Significant differences between *DYRK1A* and *CHD8* groups, $p < 0.001$. Independent sample *t* and Cohen's *d* values provided when significant, *p* value adjusted for multiple comparisons, *NS* not significant

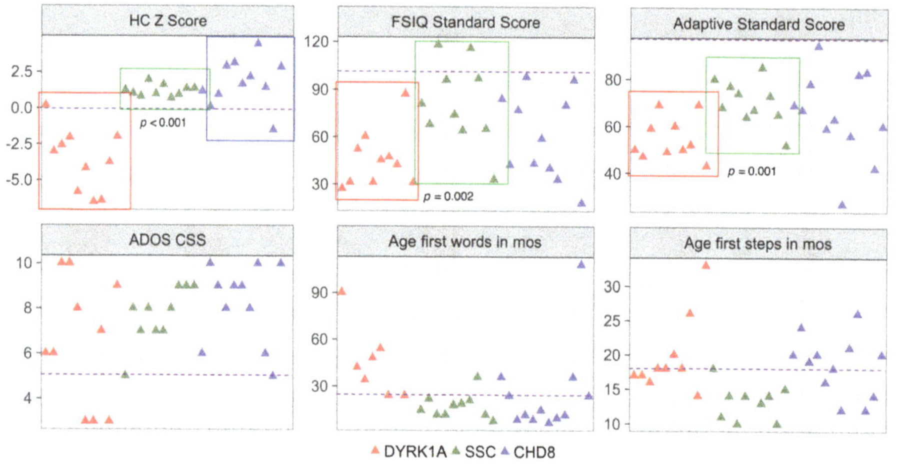

Fig. 4 Quantitative phenotype of *DYRK1A*, idiopathic, and *CHD8* samples. Scatterplots of core phenotypic features in UW-SNV *DYRK1A* sample, ($n = 10$), idiopathic subset matched for age and gender (randomly sample, $n = 10$), and *CHD8* sample ($n = 12$). Dotted lines designate conservative averages for typical population. *HC* head circumference, *FSIQ* full-scale IQ, *ADOS CSS* calibrated severity score. Independent sample *t* tests comparing *DYRK1A*, idiopathic, and *CHD8* groups, *p* value adjusted for multiple comparisons

SNV, UW-SNV, and Pub-CHR groups combined) exhibited significantly higher incidence of key features compared to those with idiopathic ASD: intellectual disability, speech delay, motor difficulties, vision abnormalities, feeding difficulties, and microcephaly. Frequency of these features also significantly differed between the *DYRK1A* group and the comparison group with idiopathic ASD and IQ below 70. This is consistent with prior evidence that disruptive SNVs and CNVs often result in significantly more impairing comorbidities than in idiopathic ASD [6, 8]. Notably, when those with *DYRK1A* mutations who were originally ascertained for an ASD diagnosis were compared to the idiopathic group (also ascertained for ASD), the profile remains the same. This provides further support that the phenotype commonly exhibited in individuals with *DYRK1A* disruptions and ASD is indeed distinct from idiopathic ASD. The co-occurrence of five or more of these phenotypic features in *DYRK1A* cases (79% of total sample, 89% of those ascertained for ASD) provides support for further exploration of *DYRK1A* haploinsufficiency in an individual presenting with concerns of ASD and this combination of phenotypic features.

Prior publications of *DYRK1A* mutation cases have relied on categorical data to describe clinical phenotype. Our exploration of a quantitative phenotype suggested that *DYRK1A* haploinsufficiency is differentiable from idiopathic ASD by measures of cognition, adaptive skills, and head size and distinguishable from a different ASD-associated gene mutation, *CHD8* by head size. It is possible that further phenotypic differences exist which have not been detected by current diagnostic tools given limits to the level of resolution inherent in clinical assessment. Markers relying on quantitative, brain-based measures may reveal gene-specific profiles. For instance, recent work highlights divergent information processing systems for children with 16p11.2 CNVs [50] and children with an early-emerging disruptive SNV [51]. Considering the intellectual disability associated with *DYRK1A* haploinsufficiency, a passive, noninvasive neuroimaging approach may help illuminate neuroendophenotypes that link the behavioral phenotype to the underlying neural mechanisms.

Exploring quantitative phenotype in UW-SNV participants illuminated phenotypic heterogeneity among individuals. While *DYRK1A* mutations significantly impact functioning in a number of domains, the severity of impairment varied among individuals. Family background may, in part, contribute to this variability. While still exploratory, variability in parental phenotype corresponded with variability observed in probands with *DYRK1A* haploinsufficiency. Most striking were familial patterns on measures of head circumference. Even with the range of microcephaly, probands with the smallest head sizes were related to parents with smaller head sizes compared to other parents within the UW-SNV group. Physiological characteristics are among the most highly correlated between parents and children in typically developing populations, ranging from 0.5 to 0.7 [52, 53]. Our findings suggest that, even in the presence of a de novo, disruptive *DYRK1A* mutation, parental phenotype may still impact their affected child's presentation. Of course, secondary genetic events, embryonic or early developmental influences, and treatment must also be considered as potential factors contributing to the variability.

Our findings must be considered in the context of limitations of this study. First, information available for

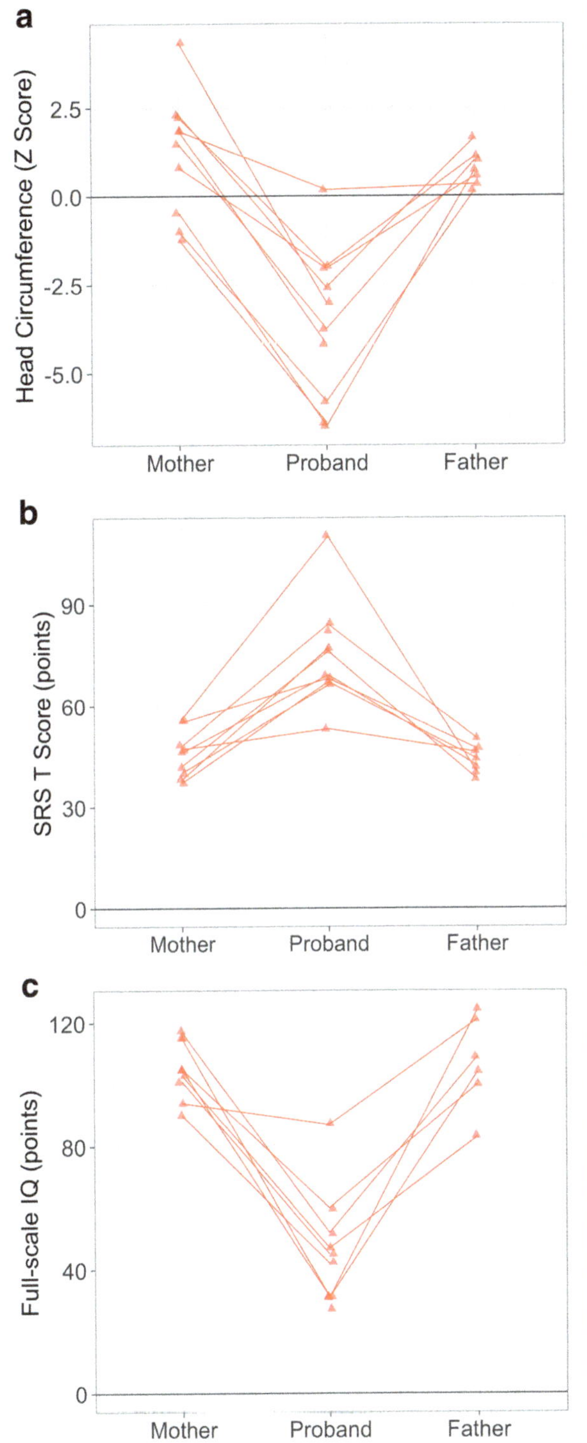

Fig. 5 Contribution of familial genetic background to head circumference, ASD symptoms, and IQ. UW-SNV cases are presented with their unaffected mothers and fathers on three phenotypic measures: **a** head circumference (*Z* score, SD), **b** ASD symptoms (Social Responsiveness Scale *T* score), and **c** IQ (full-scale standard score). Affected children presented with significantly more severe phenotypes compared to both unaffected mothers and fathers using Wilcoxon rank sum tests ($p < 0.001$). Variability in parental phenotype corresponds to proband variation. Probands with smaller head sizes relative to other UW-SNV cases correspond to parents who also have smaller head size and vice versa. There are similar patterns in cognition, perhaps more pronounced for fathers, such that fathers with higher IQ have probands with higher IQ relative to other *DYRK1A* cases. Related to social responsiveness, higher parental scores (i.e., greater social impairment) correspond to probands with greater social impairment. Also, note the apparent wider range of IQ variability for fathers ($SD = 14.99$) relative to mothers ($SD = 9.42$) and the wider range of head circumference variability for mothers ($SD = 1.81$) relative to fathers ($SD = 0.52$)

previously published cases varied widely. While some case reports provided detailed record of psychiatric history, others only included medical history, which also varied in its extensiveness. Full assessment history was unknown for previously published cases, raising questions whether phenotypic features left out of a case report were previously ruled out and confirmed absent or were not assessed. These variations highlight the importance of consistency in phenotypic assessment across future *DYRK1A* phenotype studies to ensure comprehensive and accurate phenotyping efforts. Second, those with *DYRK1A* mutations who participated in the same quantitative assessment battery remain small in number. Larger sample sizes are indeed needed to better understand the quantitative phenotype of *DYRK1A* haploinsufficiency and potential variability between affected individuals. Also, while comparison of *DYRK1A* mutation cases to idiopathic ASD provides important confirmation of distinct comorbidities within ASD, it is important to acknowledge that individuals in the idiopathic group may, with future advances in our understanding of the genetics of ASD, no longer be identified as idiopathic. The idiopathic group analyzed in this study likely represents a population with fewer syndromic features than populations with ASD and other genetic events. Thus, further studies and larger samples of other ASD-associated gene mutations are needed to further distinguish how the *DYRK1A* haploinsufficiency phenotype differs from that of other disruptive gene events. Future studies of this population should also aim for greater specificity in phenotypic characterization in efforts to better understand *DYRK1A* haploinsufficiency as a unique clinical profile. Continued study of ASD-associated genes, including *DYRK1A*, will allow for improved understanding of ASD subtypes and inform future approaches to personalized treatment.

Conclusions

DYRK1A haploinsufficiency results in a clinical phenotype which includes microcephaly, intellectual impairment, the presence of vision and motor difficulties, feeding difficulties, language delays, and ASD risk. The *DYRK1A* profile suggests a potential subtype of ASD. Despite a consistent profile, quantitative assessment highlights heterogeneity in the severity of impairments, with parental phenotype, reflecting genetic background, as a likely contributor to that variability among individuals.

Abbreviations

ASD: Autism spectrum disorder; CHR: Chromosomal rearrangement (including CNVs, translocations, and inversions); CNV: Copy number variation; Pub-CHR: Previously published chromosomal rearrangements; Pub-SNV: Previously published disruptive SNVs; SNV: Single nucleotide variant (disruptive variants include nonsense, frameshift, splice site, and missense mutations); UW-SNV: UW study participants with disruptive SNVs to *DYRK1A*

Acknowledgements

We would like to thank our funding sources and the families who took part in this study.

Funding

This research was supported by the National Institute for Mental Health, #R01MH100047 to R.A.B. and #R01MH101221 to E.E.E. E.E.E. is an investigator of the Howard Hughes Medical Institute.

Authors' contributions

RAB and EEE developed the study concept. EEE and TT performed genetic sequencing, and TT consulted on the presentation of gene variant data. Phenotypic data collection was carried out by RKE, HCM, and JG. RKE drafted the manuscript, and RAB, TT, JG, CMH, and EEE provided critical revisions. All authors approved the final version of the manuscript for submission.

Competing interests

The authors declare that they have no competing interests.

Author details

[1]Department of Psychiatry and Behavioral Sciences, University of Washington, CHDD Box 357920, Seattle, WA 98195, USA. [2]Department of Genome Sciences, University of Washington, Seattle, WA, USA. [3]School of Medicine, University of Washington, Seattle, WA, USA. [4]Howard Hughes Medical Institute, Seattle, WA, USA. [5]Center on Human Development and Disability, University of Washington, Seattle, WA, USA.

References

1. King BH, Navot N, Bernier R, Webb SJ. Update on diagnostic classification in autism. Current opinion in psychiatry. 2014;27(2):105–9. doi:10.1097/yco.0000000000000040. Epub 2014/03/04. PubMed PMID: 24441420
2. Lord C, Petkova E, Hus V, Gan W, Lu F, Martin DM, et al. A multisite study of the clinical diagnosis of different autism spectrum disorders. Arch Gen Psychiatry. 2012;69(3):306–13. doi:10.1001/archgenpsychiatry.2011.148. Epub 2011/11/09. PubMed PMID: 22065253; PubMed Central PMCID: PMCPMC3626112
3. Higdon R, Earl RK, Stanberry L, Hudac CM, Montague E, Stewart E, et al. The promise of multi-omics and clinical data integration to identify and target personalized healthcare approaches in autism spectrum disorders. Omics : a journal of integrative biology. 2015;19(4):197–208. doi:10.1089/omi.2015.0020. Epub 2015/04/02. PubMed PMID: 25831060; PubMed Central PMCID: PMCPMC4389910
4. Jeste SS, Geschwind DH. Disentangling the heterogeneity of autism spectrum disorder through genetic findings. Nat Rev Neurol. 2014;10(2):74–81. doi:10.1038/nrneurol.2013.278. Epub 2014/01/29. PubMed PMID: 24468882; PubMed Central PMCID: PMCPMC4125617
5. O'Roak BJ, Deriziotis P, Lee C, Vives L, Schwartz JJ, Girirajan S, et al. Exome sequencing in sporadic autism spectrum disorders identifies severe de novo mutations. Nat Genet. 2011;43(6):585–9. doi:10.1038/ng.835. Epub 2011/05/17. PubMed PMID: 21572417; PubMed Central PMCID: PMCPMC3115696
6. Iossifov I, O'Roak BJ, Sanders SJ, Ronemus M, Krumm N, Levy D, et al. The contribution of de novo coding mutations to autism spectrum disorder. Nature. 2014;515(7526):216–21. doi:10.1038/nature13908. Epub 2014/11/05. PubMed PMID: 25363768; PubMed Central PMCID: PMCPmc4313871
7. Pinto D, Pagnamenta AT, Klei L, Anney R, Merico D, Regan R, et al. Functional impact of global rare copy number variation in autism spectrum disorders. Nature. 2010;466(7304):368–72. doi:10.1038/nature09146. Epub 2010/06/10. PubMed PMID: 20531469; PubMed Central PMCID: PMCPMC3021798
8. Sanders SJ, He X, Willsey AJ, Ercan-Sencicek AG, Samocha KE, Cicek AE, et al. Insights into autism spectrum disorder genomic architecture and biology from 71 risk loci. Neuron. 2015;87(6):1215–33. doi:10.1016/j.neuron.2015.09.016. Epub 2015/09/25. PubMed PMID: 26402605; PubMed Central PMCID: PMCPMC4624267
9. Vorstman JA, Staal WG, van Daalen E, van Engeland H, Hochstenbach PF, Franke L. Identification of novel autism candidate regions through analysis of reported cytogenetic abnormalities associated with autism. Mol Psychiatry. 2006;11(1):1, 18-28. Epub 2005/10/06. PubMed PMID: 16205736. doi:10.1038/sj.mp.4001757.
10. Stessman HA, Bernier R, Eichler EE. A genotype-first approach to defining the subtypes of a complex disease. Cell. 2014;156(5):872–7. https://doi.org/10.1016/j.cell.2014.02.002. Epub 2014/03/04. PubMed PMID: 24581488; PubMed Central PMCID: PMCPMC4076166
11. Bernier R, Golzio C, Xiong B, Stessman HA, Coe BP, Penn O, et al. Disruptive CHD8 mutations define a subtype of autism early in development. Cell. 2014;158(2):263–76. doi:10.1016/j.cell.2014.06.017. Epub 2014/07/08. PubMed PMID: 24998929; PubMed Central PMCID: PMCPmc4136921
12. Helsmoortel C, Vulto-van Silfhout AT, Coe BP, Vandeweyer G, Rooms L, van den Ende J, et al. A SWI/SNF-related autism syndrome caused by de novo mutations in ADNP. Nat Genet. 2014;46(4):380–4. doi:10.1038/ng.2899. Epub 2014/02/18. PubMed PMID: 24531329; PubMed Central PMCID: PMCPmc3990853
13. van Bon BW, Coe BP, Bernier R, Green C, Gerdts J, Witherspoon K, et al. Disruptive de novo mutations of DYRK1A lead to a syndromic form of autism and ID. Mol Psychiatry. 2016;21(1):126–32. doi:10.1038/mp.2015.5. Epub 2015/02/25. PubMed PMID: 25707398; PubMed Central PMCID: PMCPMC4547916
14. O'Roak BJ, Vives L, Fu W, Egertson JD, Stanaway IB, Phelps IG, et al. Multiplex targeted sequencing identifies recurrently mutated genes in autism spectrum disorders. Science (New York, NY). 2012;338(6114):1619–22. doi:10.1126/science.1227764. Epub 2012/11/20. PubMed PMID: 23160955; PubMed Central PMCID: PMCPmc3528801
15. Bronicki LM, Redin C, Drunat S, Piton A, Lyons M, Passemard S, et al. Ten new cases further delineate the syndromic intellectual disability phenotype caused by mutations in DYRK1A. European journal of human genetics : EJHG. 2015;23(11):1482–7. doi:10.1038/ejhg.2015.29. Epub 2015/04/30. PubMed PMID: 25920557; PubMed Central PMCID: PMCPMC4613470
16. APA. Diagnostic and statistical manual of mental disorders. 5th ed. Washington, D.C: Author; 2013.
17. van Bon BW, Coe BP, BBA dV. In: Pagon RA, Adam MP, Ardinger HH, editors. DYRK1A-related intellectual disability syndrome. Seattle: University of Washington; 2015.
18. Tejedor F, Zhu XR, Kaltenbach E, Ackermann A, Baumann A, Canal I, et al. minibrain: a new protein kinase family involved in postembryonic neurogenesis in Drosophila. Neuron. 1995;14(2):287–301. Epub 1995/02/01. PubMed PMID: 7857639
19. Fotaki V, Dierssen M, Alcantara S, Martinez S, Marti E, Casas C, et al. Dyrk1A haploinsufficiency affects viability and causes developmental delay and abnormal brain morphology in mice. Mol Cell Biol. 2002;22(18):6636–47. Epub 2002/08/23. PubMed PMID: 12192061; PubMed Central PMCID: PMCPMC135639
20. Fotaki V, Martinez De Lagran M, Estivill X, Arbones M, Dierssen M. Haploinsufficiency of Dyrk1A in mice leads to specific alterations in the development and regulation of motor activity. Behav Neurosci. 2004;118(4):815–21. doi:10.1037/0735-7044.118.4.815. Epub 2004/08/11. PubMed PMID: 15301607

21. Ji J, Lee H, Argiropoulos B, Dorrani N, Mann J, Martinez-Agosto JA, et al. DYRK1A haploinsufficiency causes a new recognizable syndrome with microcephaly, intellectual disability, speech impairment, and distinct facies. European journal of human genetics : EJHG. 2015;23(11):1473–81. doi:10.1038/ejhg.2015.71. Epub 2015/05/07. PubMed PMID: 25944381; PubMed Central PMCID: PMCPMC4613469
22. Luco SM, Pohl D, Sell E, Wagner JD, Dyment DA, Daoud H. Case report of novel DYRK1A mutations in 2 individuals with syndromic intellectual disability and a review of the literature. BMC medical genetics. 2016;17:15. doi:10.1186/s12881-016-0276-4. Epub 2016/02/29. PubMed PMID: 26922654; PubMed Central PMCID: PMCPMC4769499
23. Moller RS, Kubart S, Hoeltzenbein M, Heye B, Vogel I, Hansen CP, et al. Truncation of the Down syndrome candidate gene DYRK1A in two unrelated patients with microcephaly. Am J Hum Genet. 2008;82(5):1165–70. doi:10.1016/j.ajhg.2008.03.001. Epub 2008/04/15. PubMed PMID: 18405873; PubMed Central PMCID: PMCPMC2427221
24. van Bon BW, Hoischen A, Hehir-Kwa J, de Brouwer AP, Ruivenkamp C, Gijsbers AC, et al. Intragenic deletion in DYRK1A leads to mental retardation and primary microcephaly. Clin Genet. 2011;79(3):296–9. doi:10.1111/j.1399-0004.2010.01544.x. Epub 2011/02/08. PubMed PMID: 21294719
25. Fraser FC, Sadovnick AD. Correlation of IQ in subjects with Down syndrome and their parents and sibs. J Ment Defic Res. 1976;20(3):179–82. Epub 1976/09/01. PubMed PMID: 135090
26. Malich S, Largo RH, Schinzel A, Molinari L, Eiholzer U. Phenotypic heterogeneity of growth and psychometric intelligence in Prader-Willi syndrome: variable expression of a contiguous gene syndrome or parent-child resemblance? Am J Med Genet. 2000;91(4):298–304. Epub 2000/04/15. PubMed PMID: 10766987
27. Moreno-De-Luca A, Evans DW, Boomer KB, Hanson E, Bernier R, Goin-Kochel RP, et al. The role of parental cognitive, behavioral, and motor profiles in clinical variability in individuals with chromosome 16p11.2 deletions. JAMA psychiatry. 2015;72(2):119–26. doi:10.1001/jamapsychiatry.2014.2147. Epub 2014/12/11. PubMed PMID: 25493922
28. Preece MA. The genetic contribution to stature. Horm Res. 1996;45(Suppl 2):56–8. Epub 1996/01/01. PubMed PMID: 8805046
29. Lonsdale J, Thomas J, Salvatore M, Phillips R, Lo E, Shad S, Foster B. The genotype-tissue expression (GTEx) project. Nat Genet. 2013;45(6):580-85. doi:10.1038/ng.2653.
30. Ruaud L, Mignot C, Guet A, Ohl C, Nava C, Heron D, et al. DYRK1A mutations in two unrelated patients. European journal of medical genetics. 2015;58(3):168–74. doi:10.1016/j.ejmg.2014.12.014. Epub 2015/02/03. PubMed PMID: 25641759
31. Iglesias A, Anyane-Yeboa K, Wynn J, Wilson A, Truitt Cho M, Guzman E, et al. The usefulness of whole-exome sequencing in routine clinical practice. Genetics in medicine : official journal of the American College of Medical Genetics. 2014;16(12):922–31. doi:10.1038/gim.2014.58. Epub 2014/06/06. PubMed PMID: 24901346
32. Okamoto N, Miya F, Tsunoda T, Kato M, Saitoh S, Yamasaki M, et al. Targeted next-generation sequencing in the diagnosis of neurodevelopmental disorders. Clin Genet. 2015;88(3):288–92. doi:10.1111/cge.12492. Epub 2014/08/27. PubMed PMID: 25156961
33. Bartsch O, Hinkel GK, Petersen MB, Konig U, Bugge M, Mikkelsen M, et al. A large family with subtelomeric translocation t (18;21)(q23;q22.1) and molecular breakpoint in the Down syndrome critical region. Hum Genet. 1997;100(5–6):669–75. Epub 1997/10/28. PubMed PMID: 9341890
34. Courcet JB, Faivre L, Malzac P, Masurel-Paulet A, Lopez E, Callier P, et al. The DYRK1A gene is a cause of syndromic intellectual disability with severe microcephaly and epilepsy. J Med Genet. 2012;49(12):731–6. doi:10.1136/jmedgenet-2012-101251. Epub 2012/10/27. PubMed PMID: 23099646
35. Fujita H, Torii C, Kosaki R, Yamaguchi S, Kudoh J, Hayashi K, et al. Microdeletion of the Down syndrome critical region at 21q22. Am J Med Genet A. 2010;152a(4):950–3. doi:10.1002/ajmg.a.33228. Epub 2010/04/02. PubMed PMID: 20358607
36. Matsumoto N, Ohashi H, Tsukahara M, Kim KC, Soeda E, Niikawa N. Possible narrowed assignment of the loci of monosomy 21-associated microcephaly and intrauterine growth retardation to a 1.2-Mb segment at 21q22.2. Am J Hum Genet. 1997;60(4):997–9. Epub 1997/04/01. PubMed PMID: 9106547; PubMed Central PMCID: PMCPMC1712454
37. Oegema R, de Klein A, Verkerk AJ, Schot R, Dumee B, Douben H, et al. Distinctive phenotypic abnormalities associated with submicroscopic 21q22 deletion including DYRK1A. Molecular syndromology. 2010;1(3):113–20. doi:10.1159/000320113. Epub 2010/10/30. PubMed PMID: 21031080; PubMed Central PMCID: PMCPMC2957846
38. Valetto A, Orsini A, Bertini V, Toschi B, Bonuccelli A, Simi F, et al. Molecular cytogenetic characterization of an interstitial deletion of chromosome 21 (21q22.13q22.3) in a patient with dysmorphic features, intellectual disability and severe generalized epilepsy. European journal of medical genetics. 2012;55(5):362–6. doi:10.1016/j.ejmg.2012.03.011. Epub 2012/05/03. PubMed PMID: 22548977
39. Yamamoto T, Shimojima K, Nishizawa T, Matsuo M, Ito M, Imai K. Clinical manifestations of the deletion of Down syndrome critical region including DYRK1A and KCNJ6. Am J Med Genet A. 2011;155a(1):113–9. doi:10.1002/ajmg.a.33735. Epub 2011/01/05. PubMed PMID: 21204217
40. Fischbach GD, Lord C. The Simons Simplex Collection: a resource for identification of autism genetic risk factors. Neuron. 2010;68(2):192–5. doi:10.1016/j.neuron.2010.10.006. Epub 2010/10/20. PubMed PMID: 20955926
41. Roche AF, Mukherjee D, Guo SM, Moore WM. Head circumference reference data: birth to 18 years. Pediatrics. 1987;79(5):706–12. Epub 1987/05/01. PubMed PMID: 3575026
42. Elliott CD. Differential Abilities Scales. 2nd ed. San Antonio: Harcourt Assessment; 2007.
43. Wechsler D, Hsiao-pin C. Wechsler abbreviated scale of intelligence. 2nd ed. San Antonio: Pearson; 2011.
44. Sparrow SS, Balla DA, Ciccheti DV, Doll EA. Vineland-II: Vineland adaptive behavior scales: survey forms manual. Circle Pines: AGS Publishing; 2005.
45. Lord C, Rutter M, DiLavore PC, Risi S. Autism Diagnostic Observation Schedule--WPS (ADOS-WPS). Los Angeles: Western Psychological Services; 1999.
46. Lord C, Rutter M, DiLavore PC, Risi S, Gotham K, Bishop SL. Autism Diagnostic Observation Schedule--Second Edition. 2nd ed. Los Angeles: Western Psychological Services; 2013.
47. Lord C, Rutter M, Le Couteur A. Autism Diagnostic Interview--Revised: a revised version of a diagnostic interview for caregivers of individuals with possible pervasive developmental disorders. J Autism Dev Disord. 1994;24(5):659–85. Epub 1994/10/01. PubMed PMID: 7814313
48. Constantino JN, Gruber CP. Social Responsiveness Scale. 2nd ed. Los Angeles: Western Psychological Services; 2012.
49. Christensen DL, Baio J, Van Naarden BK, Bilder D, Charles J, Constantino JN, et al. Prevalence and characteristics of autism spectrum disorder among children aged 8 years--Autism and Developmental Disabilities Monitoring Network, 11 Sites, United States, 2012. Morbidity and mortality weekly report Surveillance summaries (Washington, DC : 2002). 2016;65(3):1–23. 10.15585/mmwr.ss6503a1. Epub 2016/04/01. PubMed PMID: 27031587
50. Hudac CM, Kresse A, Aaronson B, DesChamps TD, Webb SJ, Bernier RA, et al. Modulation of mu attenuation to social stimuli in children and adults with 16p11.2 deletions and duplications Exploring the heterogeneity of neural social indices for genetically distinct etiologies of autism. (1866–1947 (Print)). D - NLM: PMC4514956 OTO - NOTNLM.
51. Hudac CM, Stessman HAF, DesChamps TD, Kresse A, Faja S, Neuhaus E, et al. Exploring the heterogeneity of neural social indices for genetically distinct etiologies of autism. (1866–1947 (Print)).
52. Clark PJ. The heritability of certain anthropometric characters as ascertained from measurements of twins. 1955(0002–9297 (Print)). D - CLML: 5630:10388 D - NLM: PMC1716621 OTO - NLM.

13

Basic and complex emotion recognition in children with autism

Shimrit Fridenson-Hayo[1], Steve Berggren[2,5], Amandine Lassalle[3,4], Shahar Tal[1], Delia Pigat[3], Sven Bölte[2,5], Simon Baron-Cohen[3] and Ofer Golan[1*]

Abstract

Background: Children with autism spectrum conditions (ASC) have emotion recognition deficits when tested in different expression modalities (face, voice, body). However, these findings usually focus on basic emotions, using one or two expression modalities. In addition, cultural similarities and differences in emotion recognition patterns in children with ASC have not been explored before. The current study examined the similarities and differences in the recognition of basic and complex emotions by children with ASC and typically developing (TD) controls across three cultures: Israel, Britain, and Sweden.

Methods: Fifty-five children with high-functioning ASC, aged 5–9, were compared to 58 TD children. On each site, groups were matched on age, sex, and IQ. Children were tested using four tasks, examining recognition of basic and complex emotions from voice recordings, videos of facial and bodily expressions, and emotional video scenarios including all modalities in context.

Results: Compared to their TD peers, children with ASC showed emotion recognition deficits in both basic and complex emotions on all three modalities and their integration in context. Complex emotions were harder to recognize, compared to basic emotions for the entire sample. Cross-cultural agreement was found for all major findings, with minor deviations on the face and body tasks.

Conclusions: Our findings highlight the multimodal nature of ER deficits in ASC, which exist for basic as well as complex emotions and are relatively stable cross-culturally. Cross-cultural research has the potential to reveal both autism-specific universal deficits and the role that specific cultures play in the way empathy operates in different countries.

Keywords: Autism spectrum condition, Emotion recognition, Basic emotions, Complex emotions, Cross-cultural research

Background

Autism spectrum conditions (ASC) are neurodevelopmental conditions characterized by social communication and interaction difficulties, circumscribed interests, and a preference for sameness and repetition. Individuals with ASC experience difficulties processing and interpreting socio-emotional cues [1–3]. These emotion recognition (ER) difficulties are recognized as part of the social communication challenge, characteristic of ASC [4] and predict adaptive socialization skills [5]. The recognition of others' emotions and mental states relies on the integration of emotional cues from various channels. These include facial expressions, vocal intonation, and body language, as well as contextual information [6].

Due to its centrality in emotional expression, the majority of ER research has focused on facial expression. In typical development (TD), the skills necessary to recognize and discriminate between emotional expressions are present from infancy [7, 8]. Throughout development, facial ER improves, with children gradually becoming "emotion experts" [9]. In contrast, children and adults with ASC show reduced attention to faces and facial expressions [10–13]. Altered attention, specifically to the eye region of the face [14, 15], has a significant effect on facial affect recognition in individuals with ASC [16]. In addition, children with ASC process faces in a piecemeal fashion rather than holistically [17–19]

* Correspondence: ofer.golan@biu.ac.il
[1]Department of Psychology, Bar-Ilan University, Ramat-Gan, Israel
Full list of author information is available at the end of the article

(see [20], for a different perspective). Consequently, children with ASC show reduced "face expertise" [11].

Some studies of facial ER have reported deficits in participants with ASC [21–24]. Other studies, however, have found facial emotion recognition skills in children with ASC to be equal to those in TD peers [25–28]. Recent review of facial expression in ASC had proposed that these differences in documented ER are dependent on participant demographics, task selection, and stimulus type [29]. Despite the extensive research on emotion recognition through facial expressions in ASC, most studies have either used still, rather than dynamic, stimuli [29, 30], allowed participants unlimited exposure to stimuli [31–33], or else limited their research to a narrow set of basic emotions [34, 35].

Another important channel of emotional information is prosody, which includes vocal intonation, stress, and rhythm [36]. Prosody plays an important role in linguistic functions as well as in emotional expression and comprehension [37, 38]. Whereas considerable research has documented the deficits children with ASC have in language production and comprehension, relatively few studies have examined the abilities of these children to recognize emotions through prosody [38, 39]. Studies on ER from prosody in individuals with ASC have yielded mixed results. Some studies have reported that adults or children with ASC experienced difficulties in using emotional prosody to identify the emotions of others [22, 36, 38, 40–43]. In contrast, several studies have reported that the emotional prosody perception in individuals with ASC is similar to that of TD controls [37, 44–47]. These mixed results could be due to methodological reasons [45], such as the use of cross-modal (e.g., face-voice) paradigms [48, 49] or the use of speech stimuli in which ER could rely on linguistic, rather than prosodic cues [3, 50].

A third channel of relevant emotional cues is body language, which includes gestures and postural changes. TD infants as young as 4 to 6 months show distinct attention to human biological motion [51]. At 2 years of age, children already rely on body language cues to predict the behavior of people they are watching [52], understand the goals of actions they observe [53], and anticipate people's intentions [54]. At 3 years of age, children can verbally interpret biological motion, an ability that peaks by about 5 years of age [55]. Finally, children as young as 4 years successfully use body language to recognize social interactions, an ability that peaks by the age of 7 to 8 years [56].

In ASC, studies demonstrate difficulties discriminating biological from non-biological motion [57–59] and no preference for biological motion over object motion [60, 61]. Studies of emotional body language comprehension in ASC are scarce. The existing ones reported difficulties recognizing emotional, but not non-emotional motion from point-light displays in individuals with ASC, compared to TD controls [62, 63]. Children with ASC can distinguish social from non-social scenes, solely based on whole-body movements presented in point-light and stick-figure displays [56], but fail to interpret the nature of the actions presented, especially in the case of social scenes [56, 64–66]. Hence, the body motion recognition deficit in ASC appears to be restricted to percepts requiring mentalization and emotional interpretation [67–69].

Most studies that examined the ability of people with ASC to understand body language have either used stimuli such as point-light displays [67–69] or stick figures [56] or limited their investigation to a narrow set of basic emotions [24, 70]. It is therefore important to investigate whether this documented deficit exists in full body video stimuli, demonstrating a wider range of emotions, including complex ones.

In addition to the unimodal emotion-processing deficits described above, individuals with ASC show problems integrating information across multiple modalities [71]. Many of the atypical perceptual experiences reported by people with ASC may stem from an inability to efficiently filter, process, and integrate information from different modalities, when presented simultaneously [72].

Most studies that examine multimodal processing focus on the integration of auditory and visual social stimuli linked to communication, such as speech and its corresponding lip movements [73, 74]. The results of most of these studies indicate that the ability to integrate audiovisual social stimuli is impaired in individuals with ASC [75–78]. On the other hand, there is little research on the integration of information from facial expressions and body language or from multiple modalities in context. Multimodal integration ER studies reveal that presenting emotional cues in different channels does not necessarily help, and may even hamper the ability of individuals with ASC to recognize emotions and mental states [79, 80]. Previous studies of multimodal ER in ASC have shown deficits in adults [81] and in children [82]. However, the stimuli presented in these studies included verbal content, in addition to the visual and auditory emotional cues. Since individuals with ASC rely on verbal content as a compensatory mechanism [25], an examination of multimodal ER in children with ASC, in which stimuli have no verbal content to rely on, is desirable. In the absence of a linguistic component, such stimuli could also be used for cross-cultural comparison of ER in ASC.

As described above, studies showing no ER differences between TD individuals and individuals with ASC focus mostly, if not solely, on basic emotions [24, 34, 35, 70]. The six emotions referred to as "basic" (happiness, sadness, fear, anger, surprise, and disgust) are suggested to be cross-culturally expressed and recognized [83] and are to some extent neurologically distinct [84]. Unlike basic emotions, complex emotions are considered more context and culture dependent [85, 86]. They involve attributing a cognitive state as well as an emotion and may be belief- rather than situation-based [87]. The examination of basic ER in children with ASC yielded mixed results, with some studies reporting basic ER deficit in this group [21, 49, 88], whereas others reporting no difficulties in recognition of the basic emotions in children with ASC [25, 26, 28]. In contrast, studies investigating recognition of complex emotions and other mental states by children with ASC, compared to TD children, have shown more conclusive deficits [3, 89]. However, no study so far has conducted a direct comparison of basic and complex ER in children with ASC and their TD peers.

In terms of cross-cultural ER differences, meta-analyses have documented evidence for an in-group advantage, in that emotional expressions are more accurately recognized by individuals within the same culture, versus other cultures [90, 91]. However, individuals with ASC have been found to have poorer understanding of emotional cues (as shown above), as well as lower sensitivity to social cues [10] and lower social conformity [92]. Since individuals with ASC are less socio-emotionally sensitive within their own cultures, it is possible that cross-cultural differences in ER, if found, would be smaller in the ASC groups than in the TD groups.

The current study aimed to compare the recognition of the six basic and 12 complex emotions by children with ASC and TD controls. We examined ER unimodally through faces, voices, and body language, as well as multimodally through integrative scenarios with no verbal content and tested basic and complex ER cross-culturally in three different countries: Israel, Britain, and Sweden. We assessed differences between 5 to 9-year-old children with autism in the average IQ range and TD controls, comparable for age, sex, and IQ. We predicted that (a) the ASC group would have lower scores on the different ER tasks, compared to controls; (b) basic emotions would be recognized more easily than complex emotions; (c) the group differences would be greater for complex ER than for basic ER; (d) cultural differences between the three sites would be greater for complex ER than for basic ER; and (e) cultural differences on ER would be greater in the TD groups than in the ASC groups.

Methods

Instruments

Intelligence

Two subtests from the Wechsler Intelligence Scales, *Vocabulary* and *Block Design*, were used, representing verbal and performance IQ. In Britain and Sweden, subtests were taken from the locally standardized versions of the second edition of the Wechsler Abbreviated Scales of Intelligence (WASI-2) [93]. In Israel, they were taken from the fourth edition of the Wechsler Intelligence Scale for Children [94] and the third edition of the Wechsler Primary and Preschool Scale of Intelligence (WPPSI-3) [95], used according to the child's age.

Autistic traits

The school-age form (4 to 18 years) of the Social Responsiveness Scale, second edition (SRS-2) [96], was used to assess the severity of autism traits. The SRS-2 measures social awareness, social communication, social motivation, social cognition, and inflexible behaviors applying a dimensional concept of autism. The SRS-2 includes 65 items, each scored on a four-point Likert scale, from 0 ("not true") to 3 ("almost always true"), yielding a maximum of 195. It has demonstrated with good to excellent reliability and validity [96] and with good intercultural validity [97].

Facial affect recognition

The Frankfurt Test and Training of Facial Affect Recognition (FEFA-2) [98, 99] is a computerized test, examining facial ER of the six basic emotions (and neutral). The normed FEFA-2 test module comprises a series of 50 items for faces, showing good to excellent internal consistency and stability. The FEFA-2 was used in this study as a convergent validator for the test battery.

Emotion recognition battery

Emotion recognition was tested using four tasks, comprising facial expression videos, decontextualized vocal utterances, body language videos, and integrative video clips, presenting all three modalities in context. The battery is based on stimuli from several sources: The face task comprised 5-s long video clips from *Mindreading* (www.jkp.com/mindreading) [100]. The voice and body tasks comprised 1- to 3-s long audio clips and 4- to 24-s long video clips from *The EU-Emotion Stimulus Set* [101, 102]. The integrative task used 3- to 19-s long sampled scenes from old television series, following Golan et al. [82].

The tasks assessed ER for the six basic emotions (*happy, sad, afraid, angry, disgusted, surprised*) and for 12 complex emotions (*interested, bored, excited, worried, disappointed, frustrated, proud, ashamed, kind, unfriendly, joking, hurt*). Clips representing each emotion in all modalities were sampled from the above sources. Audio clips used neutral utterances (e.g., "what's all this?"), spoken in appropriate emotional prosody. They were recorded in the native language on the three sites [101, 102]. In the body language clips, faces were masked, in order to prevent reliance on facial cues. In the integrative clips, the soundtrack was muffled, so that only paralinguistic information was available. Stimuli for the tasks were selected from an extended cross cultural ER survey, in which each stimulus was validated by 60 adults (20 from each site). In these surveys, participants had to recognize each stimulus by choosing the correct emotional label out of six options [101, 102]. Stimuli were considered valid if recognized correctly by at least 50% of the judges ($p < .00001$, binomial test). For each of the selected stimuli, the six-label scale was then reduced to four emotion labels—the target emotion label and three foils, in order to make it more suitable for children. One of the foils was always in the opposite valence to the target emotion (e.g., *afraid* as a foil for a *proud* target), and the other two were in the same valence as the target emotion (e.g., *excited* and *interested* as foils for a *proud* target). Label order was counterbalanced across items.

Next, item analysis was conducted with 20 TD children in Israel, 20 in Britain, and 10 in Sweden, aged 5 to 9 (half boys and half girls). Items were approved separately for each site, if the target answer was selected by at list 50% of the children in Israel and in Britain ($p < .01$, binomial test) and at least 60% in Sweden ($p < .02$, binomial test), and if none of the foils was selected by more than 40% of the children.

For the face task, 77.5% of the items met these criteria in Israel (with an average recognition rate of $M = 74.0\%$, s.d. = 12.1%), 86.5% met them in Britain (recognition rate: $M = 76.0\%$, s.d. = 12.4%), and 82.1% met them in Sweden (recognition rate: $M = 80.0\%$, s.d. = 12.7%). For the voice task, 78.8% of the items met the criteria in Israel (recognition rate: $M = 77.3\%$, s.d. = 13.6%), 91.7% in Britain (recognition rate: $M = 75.8\%$, s.d. = 14.6%), and 89.47% met them in Sweden (recognition rate: $M = 80.3\%$, s.d. = 10.7%). For the body task, 75.0% of the items met the criteria in Israel (recognition rate: $M = 76.7\%$, s.d. = 9.3%), 90.3% in Britain (recognition rate: $M = 81.3\%$, s.d. = 12.6%), and 85.3% met them in Sweden (recognition rate: $M = 86.6\%$, s.d. = 9.9%). For the integrative task, 88.6% of the items met the criteria in Israel (recognition rate: $M = 77.5\%$, s.d. = 12.2%), 95.5% in Britain (recognition rate: $M = 81.34\%$, s.d. = 14.0%), and 87.5% met them in Sweden (recognition rate: $M = 83.1\%$, s.d. = 13.7%).

Items that did not meet the inclusion criteria on the first item analysis round had their stimulus clip replaced, and the item analysis process was repeated until criteria were met. This resulted in slightly different stimuli being used in the face, body, and integrative tasks on the different sites (four items were different on the face task, one on the body task and one on the integrative task).

Following these steps, four ER tasks were created (face, voice, body, and integration). In the face, voice, and integrative tasks, each emotion was represented by two clips, with a total of 36 items (score range 0–36) per task. The body gesture task included only 24 items (score range 0–24), two per emotion, comprising the six basic emotions and six of the complex emotions (proud, worried, excited, disappointed, frustrated, bored). The other complex emotions were not represented in this task, as they required more than one individual to convey the emotion (e.g., unfriendly). Figure 1 presents screenshots of the three visual tasks.

The ER battery was validated through correlation analysis between the four ER task scores and participants' age, verbal and non-verbal abilities, level of autistic symptoms on the SRS-2, and FEFA-2 scores, as a convergent validator. Task intercorrelations were also computed. Bonferroni's correction for multiple correlations was used. The correlations are presented in Table 1.

As shown in the table, tasks were moderately intercorrelated (ranging between $r = .61$ and $.75$) and, in addition, had moderate positive correlations with participants' age (ranging between $r = .44$ and $.51$) and verbal ability (ranging between $r = .35$ and $.52$). Non-verbal ability was only correlated with the face task scores ($r = .26$, $p < .01$). All

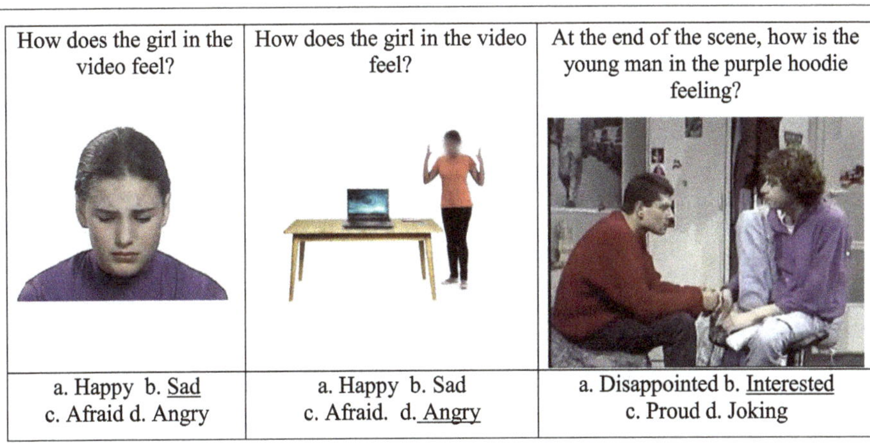

Fig. 1 Screenshots (left to right) of the Face, Body, and Integrative tasks

Table 1 Correlations of the emotion recognition tasks with background measures and with each other

	Face task	Voice task	Body task	Integrative task
Age	.48***	.51***	.44***	.47***
Vocabulary	.35***	.52***	.40***	.39***
Block design	.26**	0.12	0.14	0.17
SRS-2	−.41***	−.29**	−.38***	−.50***
FEFA-2	.54***	.49***	.46***	.49***
Voice task	.64***			
Body task	.61***	.68***		
Integrative task	.74***	.75***	.75***	

*$p < .05$, **$p < .01$, ***$p < .001$

tasks were negatively correlated with participants' level of autistic symptoms (ranging between $r = -.29$ and $-.50$) and positively correlated with the FEFA-2 (range: $r = .46$–$.54$).

Participants

The study was approved by the Psychology Research Ethics Committee at Cambridge University, by the Institutional Review Board at Bar-Ilan University, and by the Regional Board of Ethical Vetting Stockholm. Participants' assent and parents' informed consent were received before inclusion in the study. One hundred thirteen children, aged 5–9 years, took part in the study. The Israeli sample comprised 20 children in the ASC group and 22 in the TD group. The British sample comprised 16 children with ASC and 18 with TD. In Sweden, 19 children with ASC were compared to 18 children with TD. Participants with ASC had all been clinically diagnosed according to DSM-IV-TR or ICD-10 criteria [103, 104]. Diagnosis for children with ASC was corroborated by meeting ASC cutoff using the second edition of the *Autism Diagnostic Observation Schedule* (ADOS-2) [105]. Participants with ASC were recruited from volunteer databases, local clinics for children with ASC, special education classes and kindergartens, internet forums, and support organizations for individuals with ASC.

Participants in the TD groups were recruited from local primary schools and kindergartens. Parents reported their children had no psychiatric diagnoses or special educational needs, and none had a family member diagnosed with ASC. To screen out for ASC in the TD group, participants' parents filled in the Childhood Autism Spectrum Test (CAST) [106]. None of the TD group participants scored above the cutoff of 15. Groups were comparable locally on age, gender, and standard scores of two subtests from the Wechsler Abbreviated Scale of Intelligence (WASI-2) [93]: Vocabulary and Block design. ASC groups and TD groups, separately, were comparable on SRS scores. The groups' background data appears in Table 2.

Procedure

The research team met each child one to three times for assessment. In Israel, the meeting took place at the children's homes. In Britain, some meetings were held at children's homes and some at the Autism Research Centre in Cambridge. In Sweden, the meeting took place at the clinical research department KIND. All participants were tested individually. Parents filled out the SRS-2. The Wechsler subtests, the four ER computerized tasks, the FEFA-2, and ADOS-2 (children with ASC only) were administered to children.

The children were tested on the ER tasks in a counterbalanced form. Each task was preceded by two practice items. The experimenter read the instructions and the questions for all items, in order to avoid confounds due to reading difficulties. Optional answers were read out loud using neutral intonation, and the children were asked if they were familiar with all the possible answers. If the child was not familiar with a word, it was defined and demonstrated using a definition handout (e.g., *unfriendly: to be not nice to someone. John was unfriendly to Paul. He told him he didn't want to play with him*). There was no time limit to answer each item, but participants could watch or listen to each clip only once. Completion of the whole ER battery took 1.5–2.5 h, including breaks.

Table 2 Participant demographics

	Israel			Britain			Sweden		
	ASC ($n = 20$)	TD ($n = 22$)	t (40)	ASC ($n = 16$)	TD ($n = 18$)	t (32)	ASC ($n = 19$)	TD ($n = 18$)	t (35)
Age	7.45 (1.31)	7.50 (1.47)	0.13	8.58 (1.03)	7.80 (1.42)	1.86	6.97 (0.67)	7.36 (1.2)	1.21
Vocabulary	11.15 (4.26)	11.82 (2.99)	0.59	11.38 (3.56)	12.22 (2.71)	0.79	9.05 (1.90)	10.11 (1.74)	1.76
Block design	12.5 (2.96)	11.55 (2.3)	1.17	11.44 (2.48)	9.72 (3.12)	1.76	11.00 (2.79)	11.83 (2.7)	0.92
SRS-2	74.46 (8.34)	42.93 (3.58)	12.59**	82.19 (7.57)	43.00 (5.42)	17.17 **	79.32 (12.06)	39.53 (1.42)	14.26**
			χ^2 (1)			χ^2 (1)			χ^2 (1)
Sex (M:F)	18:2	19:3	0.13	15:1	13:5	2.70	15:4	15:3	0.12

**$p < .01$

Statistical analysis

In order to examine differences between basic and complex ER in the different tasks, since the number of basic and complex emotions included in each task differed, accuracy proportion scores of basic and complex ER in the different tasks were computed for each participant. Average proportions of basic and complex ER task scores for the groups in the three countries appear in Table 3. After confirming the assumptions for MANOVA are met, a multivariate analysis of covariance (MANCOVA) with repeated measures was computed, with accuracy proportion scores of the four tasks (face, voice, body, and integrative) as the dependent variables, complexity (basic, complex) as the within-subject factor and group (ASC, TD), and country (Israel, Britain, Sweden) as the between-group factors. Since participants in the three countries differed on age and verbal ability, these two factors were entered as covariates. Pairwise comparisons with Bonferroni's correction were used for further analysis of the interaction effects.

Results

Overall analysis

The MANCOVA yielded an overall main effect for group ($F[4,102] = 14.70$, $p < .001$, $\eta^2 = .37$) and for complexity ($F[4,102] = 10.49$, $p < .001$, $\eta^2 = .29$) but not for country ($F[8,204] = 1.73$, n.s.). Both age ($F[4,102] = 11.82$, $p < .001$, $\eta^2 = .32$) and verbal ability ($F[4,102] = 8.11$, $p < .001$, $\eta^2 = .24$) had significant overall effects as covariates. The three two-way interactions: group by country ($F[8,204] = 1.41$, n.s.), group by complexity ($F[4,102] = 1.56$, n.s.), and country by complexity ($F[8,204] = 1.90$, n.s.) were not significant, but a three-way interaction of group by country by complexity came out significant ($F[8,204] = 2.29$, $p < .05$, $\eta^2 = .08$). In addition, complexity had a significant interaction with age ($F[4,102] = 5.93$, $p < .001$, $\eta^2 = .19$).

Analysis per ER task

Effects of the analysis per ER task are detailed in Table 4. The analysis revealed the group, and complexity main effects found in the overall analysis were also significant for each and every task, with the TD group performing better than the ASC group over and above complexity and country, and with basic emotions recognized significantly better than complex emotions, over and above group and country. Age had a significant effect on all ER tasks, and verbal ability had a significant effect on all tasks but the face task. Similarly, the age by complexity interaction was significant for all ER tasks, with the exception of the face task. The three-way interaction of group by country by complexity came out significant only for the face task, suggesting this is the source for the interaction effect found in the overall analysis.

Pairwise comparisons revealed the TD group performed significantly better than the ASC group in Israel and in Britain both for basic (Israel: mean difference = .15, s.e. = .04, $p < .001$; Britain: mean difference = .17, s.e. = .05, $p < .001$) and for complex (Israel: mean difference = .11, s.e. = .04, $p < .01$; Britain: mean difference = .13, s.e. = .04, $p < .01$) emotions. However, in Sweden, group differences were found for complex emotions (mean difference = .13, s.e. = .04, $p < .01$) but not for basic emotions (mean difference = .02, s.e. = .04, n.s.). Figure 2 illustrates these effects in the three countries.

An examination of the age by complexity interaction in the different ER tasks revealed the interaction was significant for all tasks, with the exception of the voice task. In order to further examine the interaction, bivariate correlation analysis, with Bonferroni's correction, was conducted for age with basic and complex ER scores of each task, and the difference between the correlation of basic and complex emotions with age was compared for each task. The results, detailed in Table 5, show that, with the exception of the face task, age was more strongly correlated with complex ER than with basic ER for all tasks.

Additional findings

In addition to the effects found in the overall analysis, some additional interaction effects were found for

Table 3 Average proportions (s.d.) of basic and complex ER task scores for the ASC and TD groups in the three countries

	Israel				Britain				Sweden			
	Basic		Complex		Basic		Complex		Basic		Complex	
	ASC ($n = 20$)	TD ($n = 22$)	ASC ($n = 20$)	TD ($n = 22$)	ASC ($n = 16$)	TD ($n = 18$)	ASC ($n = 16$)	TD ($n = 18$)	ASC ($n = 19$)	TD ($n = 18$)	ASC ($n = 19$)	TD ($n = 18$)
Face task	.70 (.18)	.86 (.12)	.56 (.17)	.67 (.11)	.69 (.14)	.84 (.13)	.59 (.12)	.69 (.13)	.74 (.13)	.74 (.12)	.50 (.15)	.65 (.13)
Voice task	.68 (.22)	.73 (.13)	.57 (.24)	.72 (.15)	.64 (.14)	.74 (.16)	.68 (17)	.71 (.15)	.69 (.13)	.69 (.13)	.59 (.23)	.73 (.14)
Body task	.65 (.17)	.82 (.11)	.62 (.19)	.76 (.17)	.61 (.19)	.81 (.15)	.74 (20)	.80 (.18)	.69 (.17)	.76 (.16)	.57 (.23)	.67 (.19)
Integrative task	.72 (.20)	.85 (.14)	.59 (.20)	.77 (.11)	.71 (.20)	.84 (.11)	.61 (18)	.75 (.15)	.72 (.17)	.89 (.12)	.49 (.18)	.72 (.15)

Table 4 Main effects, interaction, and covariate effects, which were significant in the overall analysis, detailed by ER task

		Face task	Voice task	Body task	Integrative task
Group	*F* (1,105)	33.53***	9.11**	28.13***	47.38***
	η^2	.24	.80	.21	.31
Complexity	*F* (1,105)	8.50**	8.98**	8.58**	31.08***
	η^2	.08	.08	.08	.23
Group × country × complexity	*F* (2,105)	6.50**	2.31	1.36	.02
	η^2	.11	.04	.03	.00
Verbal ability	*F* (1,105)	2.86	32.87***	6.17**	4.96*
	η^2	.03	.24	.06	.05
Age	*F* (1,105)	32.40***	22.52***	24.04***	24.18***
	η^2	.24	.18	.19	.19
Age × complexity	*F* (1,105)	1.37	9.88**	6.50*	12.86***
	η^2	.01	.09	.06	.11

*$p < .05$, **$p < .01$, ***$p < .001$

specific tasks. These will be described here, since there were specific hypotheses about them, which were not found over and above tasks. A group by complexity interaction was found only for the voice task ($F[1,105] = 4.43$, $p < .05$, $\eta^2 = .04$). Pairwise comparisons revealed participants with ASC ($M = .61$, s.e. = .02) scored lower than TD participants ($M = .71$, s.e. = .02) on complex emotion scores (mean difference = .10, s.e. = .03, $p < .001$) but not on basic emotion scores (ASC: $M = .68$, s.e. = .02; TD: $M = .71$, s.e. = .02; mean difference = .03, s.e. = .03, n.s.). In addition, a country by complexity interaction effect was found significant only for the body task ($F[2,105] = 3.74$, $p < .05$, $\eta^2 = .07$). Pairwise comparisons revealed that in Sweden, the body task scores for basic emotions ($M = .75$, s.e. = .03) were higher than for complex emotions ($M = .64$, s.e. = .03; mean difference = .11, s.e. = .04, $p < .01$). No difference between basic and complex body task scores was found significant in Israel (mean difference = .04, s.e. = .03, n.s.) and in Britain (mean difference = .04, s.e. = .04, n.s.).

Discussion

The current study tested if there are differences in the recognition of basic and complex emotions between children with ASC and typically developing children across three countries: Israel, Britain, and Sweden. Emotion recognition (ER) was tested using dynamic facial expressions, body language, vocal expressions, and integrative scenarios. Children with ASC showed ER deficits in all three modalities and their integration in context. These deficits were found cross-culturally. Participants with ASC showed ER deficits in both basic

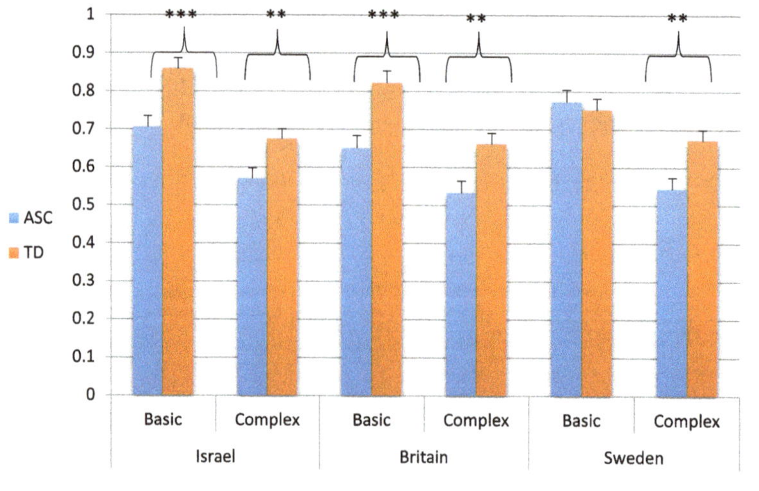

Note: **p<.01, *** p<.001

Fig. 2 Basic and complex emotion recognition group differences on the face task in the three countries

Table 5 Correlations of age with basic and with complex ER and the difference between them on the four tasks

	Basic	Complex	t (110)
Face task	.31**	.48**	2.12
Voice task	.25**	.50**	3.05**
Body task	.17	.51**	4.60***
Integrative task	.18	.52**	3.99***

$^{**}p < .01$ $^{***}p < .001$

and complex emotions. Cross-cultural agreement was found for all major findings, with minor deviations, reported below. Our findings highlight the multimodal nature of ER deficits in ASC, which exists for basic and complex emotions and is relatively stable cross-culturally.

As predicted, the ASC group had more difficulties in ER from facial expressions, body language, vocal expressions, and integrative scenarios, compared to the TD participants, even after controlling for age and verbal IQ. The significant group differences on task scores replicates previous findings of difficulties among individuals with ASC on emotion and mental state recognition from visual, auditory, and contextual stimuli [22, 24, 40, 43, 56, 66, 76–78]. These findings provide further support for ER and mentalizing deficits in children with ASC, which are evident cross-culturally.

As predicted, our findings show that basic emotions were recognized more easily than complex emotions on all modalities, regardless of child's diagnosis. However, contrary to our hypothesis, group differences for complex ER were not greater than those found on basic ER. With the exception of an interaction effect between complexity and group in the voice task, our findings showed ER deficits in 5–9-year olds with ASC exist over and above complexity level. These findings match some reports on basic ER deficits in high-functioning children with ASC [23, 24, 35, 41–43, 70] and reports on complex ER deficits in this group [3, 40, 82]. The deficit we describe in the ASC group in basic ER, which was not found in some other studies (e.g., [28, 46]), may result from the age group tested. Whereas in older age, children with ASC may develop compensatory mechanisms allowing them to recognize basic emotions [25], our examination reveals a comprehensive ER deficit in 5–9-year-old children with ASC.

Another finding of developmental importance was the age by complexity interaction found in the current study. This interaction, found over and above group, revealed moderate correlations between age and ER in complex emotions, across all modalities, suggesting 5–9-year olds are still developing their ability to recognize complex emotions, comprising mental, as well as situational, aspects. Weaker correlations were found for age with basic ER in the voice, body, and integrative tasks, but not on the face task, suggesting basic ER skills have matured for at least some of the children in the tested age group. Interestingly, our findings show that the facial ER skills of basic and complex emotions alike continue to develop in this age group. In view of the centrality of facial expressions in ER, these findings provide an interesting example of the continuing development of facial expertise [9].

It is important to note that all of our visual stimuli used video clips, rather than still pictures. It is possible that processing of dynamic stimuli, which are more ecological in nature, may be more challenging to children with ASC, in comparison to still images. Specific deficits in processing of dynamic stimuli [107] may explain why our paradigm, which employed only dynamic stimuli in the visual channel, had demonstrated ER deficits in basic, as well as in complex, emotions in the visual tasks, but only complex ER deficits in the auditory task.

A striking finding in our study was the lack of major cultural differences. Our hypotheses that complex ER would show greater cultural variability than basic ER and that TD children would show greater cultural variability than children with ASC were not supported. These findings stand in contrast with previous arguments about greater cultural diversity in complex ER [85, 86]. It is possible that such cultural differences would be more salient in older age groups, when the acquisition of culture-specific nuances has been completed.

However, some cultural differences were found on the face and body language tasks. For facial ER, children with ASC in Sweden had performed more poorly than TD controls only on complex emotions and not on basic ER. This was in contrast to the British and Israeli ASC groups, which showed facial ER deficits both for basic and complex emotions. In addition, a significant interaction was found between country and complexity in the body language task. The analysis revealed that regardless of diagnosis, participants in Sweden had more difficulties recognizing complex, compared to basic, emotions from body language. This difference was not found in Israel and Britain. It should be noted that the body task stimuli were filmed in Britain, comprising actors of various ethnicities. Whereas the basic, more automatic and cross-cultural emotions were easily recognized in Sweden, as they were in Britain and in Israel, the more subtle, complex manifestations of emotion in body language may have been more challenging for children in Sweden. An examination of body language emotions, performed by Scandinavian (in comparison to non-Scandinavian) actors should be conducted in order to support (or refute) this potential findings of an in-group advantage [108].

A few limitations of the study should be noted: The current study examined cultural differences in ER as part of a cross-cultural examination of differences between individuals with and without ASC. Whereas the sample size is sufficiently large for the main question of the study, a larger sample of TD individuals within each country may be needed in order to appropriately examine ER cultural differences in the general population. The examination of ER cultural differences (and ASC-TD differences) in the various modalities should also be extended to additional, non-western cultures, such as African, or Eastern cultures [90], as these may reveal greater cross-cultural differences than the ones reported here.

In the current study, we were unable to examine ER gender differences, due to the relatively small number of females in the ASC groups. Gender differences in ER were found among adult participants with ASC in some studies [35, 40] but not in others [109] A replication of the current study with larger samples could examine the existence of gender differences in children with ASC as well.

Another limitation lies in some methodological variability across the sites and more specifically to the administration of assessments at home vs. the lab. These differences had resulted from participants' difficulties to attend the lab in Israel and in Britain (due to distance and to parents' needs). Hence, the clinical teams traveled to children's homes. Despite the attempts to maintain a standardized testing environment (e.g., standardized protocol, individual assessment in a quiet room), it is possible that the different location for assessments had affected the results of this study. However, since the ASC and TD groups within each country were tested under similar conditions, it is unlikely that the different testing conditions have affected the group differences. Nonetheless, we recommend further studies to endorse more standardized structure if possible.

Conclusions

Our findings demonstrate a supra-modal emotion recognition deficit in children with ASC, cross-culturally, for basic and complex emotion alike. Although the ER skills of children with ASC improve with age, like their TD peers, this overall ER deficit persists and calls for interventions [110, 111] which might narrow the developmental ER gap between children with ASC and their TD peers at the earliest possible stage.

Abbreviations

ASC: Autism spectrum conditions; ER: Emotion recognition; TD: Typical development

Acknowledgements

We would like to thank the research participants and their families, as well as our dedicated research teams: in Britain: Kirsty Macmillan, Nisha Hickin, and Mathilde Matthews; in Sweden: Anna Råde and Nina Milenkovic; and in Israel: Tal Alfi, Hila Hakim, and Na'ama Amir.

Funding

The research leading to this work has received funding from the European Community's Seventh Framework Programme (FP7) under grant agreement no. [289021]. SvB was supported by the Swedish Research Council (Grant No. 523-2009-7054), and SBC was supported by the Autism Research Trust, the MRC, the Wellcome Trust, and the NIHR CLAHRC EoE during the period of this work.

Authors' contributions

SFH and ST collected the data in Israel. StB collected the data in Sweden. AL and DP collected the data in Britain. OG, SvB, and SBC obtained the funding and supervised the study in Israel, Sweden, and Britain, respectively. SFH and OG analyzed the data and wrote the manuscript. All authors read, commented, and approved the manuscript.

Competing interests

The authors declare that they have no competing interests.

Author details

[1]Department of Psychology, Bar-Ilan University, Ramat-Gan, Israel. [2]Center of Neurodevelopmental Disorders (KIND), Department of Women's and Children's Health, Karolinska Institutet, Stockholm, Sweden. [3]Autism Research Centre, Department of Psychiatry, University of Cambridge, Cambridge, UK. [4]Athinoula A. Martinos Center for Biomedical Imaging, Massachusetts General Hospital, Harvard Medical School, Charlestown, MA, USA. [5]Center of Psychiatry Research, Stockholm County Council, Stockholm, Sweden.

References

1. Kuusikko S, Haapsamo H, Jansson-Verkasalo E, Hurtig T, Mattila M-L, Ebeling H, Jussila K, Bölte S, Moilanen I. Emotion recognition in children and adolescents with autism spectrum disorders. J Autism Dev Disord. 2009;39:938–45.
2. Uljarevic M, Hamilton A. Recognition of emotions in autism: a formal meta-analysis. J Autism Dev Disord. 2013;43:1517–26.
3. Golan O, Sinai-Gavrilov Y, Baron-Cohen S. The Cambridge mindreading face-voice battery for children (CAM-C): complex emotion recognition in children with and without autism spectrum conditions. Mol Autism. 2015;6:22.
4. American Psychiatric Association. Diagnostic and statistical manual of mental disorders. 5th ed. VA: American Psychiatric Association; 2013.
5. Hudepohl MB, Robins DL, King TZ, Henrich CC. The role of emotion perception in adaptive functioning of people with autism spectrum disorders. Autism. 2015;19:107–12.
6. Foxe JJ, Molholm S. Ten years at the multisensory forum: musings on the evolution of a field. Brain Topogr. 2009;21:149–54.
7. Haviland JM, Lelwica M. The induced affect response: 10-week-old infants' responses to three emotion expressions. 1987, 23:97–104.
8. Leppänen JM, Moulson MC, Vogel-Farley VK, Nelson CA. An ERP study of emotional face processing in the adult and infant brain. Child Dev. 2007;78:232–45.
9. Herba C, Phillips M. Annotation: Development of facial expression recognition from childhood to adolescence: behavioural and neurological perspectives. J Child Psychol Psychiatry. 2004;45:1185–98.
10. Klin A, Jones W, Schultz R, Volkmar F, Cohen D. Visual fixation patterns during viewing of naturalistic social situations as predictors of social competence in individuals with autism. Arch Gen Psychiat. 2002;1(59(9)):809–16.
11. Dawson G, Webb SJ, McPartland J. Understanding the nature of face processing impairment in autism: insights from behavioral and electrophysiological studies. Dev Neuropsychol. 2005;27:403–24.
12. Papagiannopoulou EA, Chitty KM, Hermens DF, Hickie IB, Lagopoulos J. A systematic review and meta-analysis of eye-tracking studies in children with autism spectrum disorders. Soc Neurosci. 2014;9:610–32.
13. Guillon Q, Rogé B, Afzali MH, Baduel S, Kruck J, Hadjikhani N. Intact perception but abnormal orientation towards face-like objects in young children with ASD. Sci Rep. 2016;6:22119.
14. Baron-Cohen S, Wheelwright S, Jolliffe and T. Is there a "Language of the Eyes"? Evidence from normal adults, and adults with autism or asperger syndrome. Vis cogn 1997, 4:311–331.
15. Pelphrey KA, Sasson NJ, Reznick JS, Paul G, Goldman BD, Piven J. Visual scanning of faces in autism. J Autism Dev Disord. 2002;32:249–61.

16. Berggren S, Engström A-C, Bölte S. Facial affect recognition in autism, ADHD and typical development. Cogn Neuropsychiatry. 2016;21:213–27.
17. Happé F. Autism: cognitive deficit or cognitive style? Trends Cogn Sci. 1999;3:216–22.
18. Elgar K, Campbell R. Annotation: the cognitive neuroscience of face recognition: implications for developmental disorders. J Child Psychol Psychiatry. 2001;42:705–17.
19. van der Geest JN, Kemner C, Verbaten MN, van Engeland H. Gaze behavior of children with pervasive developmental disorder toward human faces: a fixation time study. J Child Psychol Psychiatry. 2002;43:669–78.
20. Tanaka JW, Sung A. The "Eye Avoidance" hypothesis of autism face processing. J Autism Dev Disord. 2016;46:1538–52.
21. Deruelle C, Rondan C, Gepner B, Tardif C. Spatial frequency and face processing in children with autism and Asperger syndrome. J Autism Dev Disord. 2004;34:199–210.
22. Diehl JJ, Bennetto L, Watson D, Gunlogson C, McDonough J. Resolving ambiguity: a psycholinguistic approach to understanding prosody processing in high-functioning autism. Brain Lang. 2008;106:144–52.
23. Grossman RB, Tager-Flusberg H. Reading faces for information about words and emotions in adolescents with autism. Res Autism Spectr Disord. 2008;2:681–95.
24. Philip RCM, Whalley HC, Stanfield a C, Sprengelmeyer R, Santos IM, Young a W, Atkinson a P, Calder a J, Johnstone EC, Lawrie SM, Hall J. Deficits in facial, body movement and vocal emotional processing in autism spectrum disorders. Psychol Med. 2010;40:1919–29.
25. Grossman JB, Klin A, Carter AS, Volkmar FR. Verbal bias in recognition of facial emotions in children with Asperger syndrome. J Child Psychol Psychiatry. 2000;41:369–79.
26. Castelli F. Understanding emotions from standardized facial expressions in autism and normal development. Autism. 2005;9:428–49.
27. Rosset DB, Rondan C, Da Fonseca D, Santos A, Assouline B, Deruelle C. Typical emotion processing for cartoon but not for real faces in children with autistic spectrum disorders. J Autism Dev Disord. 2008; 38:919–25.
28. Tracy JL, Robins RW, Schriber R a, Solomon M. Is emotion recognition impaired in individuals with autism spectrum disorders? J Autism Dev Disord. 2011;41:102–9.
29. Harms MB, Martin A, Wallace GL. Facial emotion recognition in autism spectrum disorders: a review of behavioral and neuroimaging studies. Neuropsychol Rev. 2010;20:290–322.
30. Wong N, Beidel DC, Sarver DE, Sims V. Facial emotion recognition in children with high functioning autism and children with social phobia. Child Psychiatry Hum Dev. 2012;43:775–94.
31. Macdonald H, Rutter M, Howlin P, Rios P, Conteur AL, Evered C, Folstein S. Recognition and expression of emotional cues by autistic and normal adults. J Child Psychol Psychiatry. 1989;30:865–77.
32. Humphreys K, Minshew N, Leonard GL, Behrmann M. A fine-grained analysis of facial expression processing in high-functioning adults with autism. Neuropsychologia. 2007;45:685–95.
33. Rump KM, Giovannelli JL, Minshew NJ, Strauss MS. The development of emotion recognition in individuals with autism. Child Dev. 2009;80: 1434–47.
34. Law Smith MJ, Montagne B, Perrett DI, Gill M, Gallagher L. Detecting subtle facial emotion recognition deficits in high-functioning autism using dynamic stimuli of varying intensities. Neuropsychologia. 2010;48:2777–81.
35. Sucksmith E, Allison C, Baron-Cohen S, Chakrabarti B, Hoekstra R a. Empathy and emotion recognition in people with autism, first-degree relatives, and controls. Neuropsychologia. 2013;51:98–105.
36. McCann J, Peppé S, Gibbon FE, O'Hare A, Rutherford M. Prosody and its relationship to language in school-aged children with high-functioning autism. Int J Lang Commun Disord. 2007;42:682–702.
37. Paul R, Augustyn A, Klin A, Volkmar FR. Perception and production of prosody by speakers with autism spectrum disorders. J Autism Dev Disord. 2005;35:205–20.
38. Lindner JL, Rosén L a. Decoding of emotion through facial expression, prosody and verbal content in children and adolescents with Asperger's syndrome. J Autism Dev Disord. 2006;36:769–77.
39. McCann J, Peppé S. Prosody in autism spectrum disorders: a critical review. Int J Lang Commun Disord. 2003;38:325–50.
40. Golan O, Baron-Cohen S, Hill JJ, Rutherford MD. The "Reading the Mind in the Voice" test-revised: a study of complex emotion recognition in adults with and without autism spectrum conditions. J Autism Dev Disord. 2007;37:1096–106.
41. Hubbard K, Trauner D a. Intonation and emotion in autistic spectrum disorders. J Psycholinguist Res. 2007;36:159–73.
42. Järvinen-Pasley A, Peppé S, King-Smith G, Heaton P. The relationship between form and function level receptive prosodic abilities in autism. J Autism Dev Disord. 2008;38:1328–40.
43. Globerson E, Amir N, Kishon-Rabin L, Golan O. Prosody recognition in adults with high-functioning autism spectrum disorders: from psychoacoustics to cognition. Autism Res. 2015;8:153–63.
44. Chevallier C, Noveck I, Happé F, Wilson D. What's in a voice? Prosody as a test case for the theory of mind account of autism. Neuropsychologia. 2011;49:507–17.
45. Grossman RB, Bemis RH, Plesa Skwerer D, Tager-Flusberg H. Lexical and affective prosody in children with high-functioning autism. J Speech Lang Hear Res. 2010;53:778.
46. Brennand R, Schepman A, Rodway P. Vocal emotion perception in pseudo-sentences by secondary-school children with autism spectrum disorder. Res Autism Spectr Disord. 2011;5:1567–73.
47. Brooks PJ, Ploog BO. Attention to emotional tone of voice in speech perception in children with autism. Res Autism Spectr Disord. 2013;7:845–57.
48. Grossman RB, Tager-Flusberg H. "Who said that?" Matching of low- and high-intensity emotional prosody to facial expressions by adolescents with ASD. J Autism Dev Disord. 2012;42:2546–57.
49. Hobson RP. The autistic child's appraisal of expressions of emotions. J Child Psychol Psychiatry. 1986;27:321–42.
50. Rutherford MD, Baron-Cohen S, Wheelwright S. Reading the mind in the voice: a study with normal adults and adults with Asperger syndrome and high functioning autism. J Autism Dev Disord. 2002;32:189–94.
51. Fox R, McDaniel C. The perception of biological motion by human infants. Science. 1982;218:486–7.
52. Onishi KH, Baillargeon R. Do 15-month-old infants understand false beliefs? Science. 2005;308:255–8.
53. Warneken F, Tomasello M. Altruistic helping in human infants and young chimpanzees. Science. 2006;311:1301–3.
54. Southgate V, Senju A, Csibra G. Action anticipation through attribution of false belief by 2-year-olds. Psychol Sci. 2007;18:587–92.
55. Pavlova M, Krägeloh-Mann I, Sokolov A, Birbaumer N. Recognition of point-light biological motion displays by young children. Perception. 2001;30:925–33.
56. Centelles L, Assaiante C, Etchegoyhen K, Bouvard M, Schmitz C. From action to interaction: exploring the contribution of body motion cues to social understanding in typical development and in autism spectrum disorders. J Autism Dev Disord. 2013;43:1140–50.
57. Blake R, Turner LM, Smoski MJ, Pozdol SL, Stone WL. Visual recognition of biological motion is impaired in children with autism. Psychol Sci. 2003;14:151–7.
58. Cook J, Saygin AP, Swain R, Blakemore S-J. Reduced sensitivity to minimum-jerk biological motion in autism spectrum conditions. Neuropsychologia. 2009;47:3275–8.
59. Falck-Ytter T, Rehnberg E, Bölte S. Lack of visual orienting to biological motion and audiovisual synchrony in 3-year-olds with autism. PLoS One. 2013;8:e68816.
60. Kaiser MD, Delmolino L, Tanaka JW, Shiffrar M. Comparison of visual sensitivity to human and object motion in autism spectrum disorder. Autism Res. 2010;3:191–5.
61. Annaz D, Campbell R, Coleman M, Milne E, Swettenham J. Young children with autism spectrum disorder do not preferentially attend to biological motion. J Autism Dev Disord. 2012;42:401–8.
62. Moore DG, Hobson RP, Lee A. Components of person perception: an investigation with autistic, non-autistic retarded and typically developing children and adolescents. Br J Dev Psychol. 1997;15:401–23.
63. Murphy P, Brady N, Fitzgerald M, Troje NF. No evidence for impaired perception of biological motion in adults with autistic spectrum disorders. Neuropsychologia. 2009;47:3225–35.
64. Bertone A, Mottron L, Jelenic P, Faubert J. Motion perception in autism: a "complex" issue. J Cogn Neurosci. 2003;15:218–25.
65. Pellicano E, Gibson L, Maybery M, Durkin K, Badcock DR. Abnormal global processing along the dorsal visual pathway in autism: a possible mechanism for weak visuospatial coherence? Neuropsychologia. 2005;43:1044–53.
66. Pellicano E, Gibson LY. Investigating the functional integrity of the dorsal visual pathway in autism and dyslexia. Neuropsychologia. 2008;46:2593–6.

67. Parron C, Da Fonseca D, Santos A, Moore DG, Monfardini E, Deruelle C. Recognition of biological motion in children with autistic spectrum disorders. Autism. 2008;12:261–74.
68. Atkinson AP. Impaired recognition of emotions from body movements is associated with elevated motion coherence thresholds in autism spectrum disorders. Neuropsychologia. 2009;47:3023–9.
69. Hubert B, Wicker B, Moore DG, Monfardini E, Duverger H, Fonséca D, Deruelle C. Brief report: Recognition of emotional and non-emotional biological motion in individuals with autistic spectrum disorders. J Autism Dev Disord. 2007;37:1393.
70. Grèzes J, Wicker B, Berthoz S, de Gelder B. A failure to grasp the affective meaning of actions in autism spectrum disorder subjects. Neuropsychologia. 2009;47:1816–25.
71. Marco EJ, Hinkley LBN, Hill SS, Nagarajan SS. Sensory processing in autism: a review of neurophysiologic findings. Pediatr Res. 2011;69(5 Part 2):48R–54R.
72. O'Neill M, Jones RSP. Sensory-perceptual abnormalities in autism: a case for more research? J Autism Dev Disord. 1997;27:283–93.
73. Brandwein AB, Foxe JJ, Butler JS, Russo NN, Altschuler TS, Gomes H, Molholm S. The development of multisensory integration in high-functioning autism: high-density electrical mapping and psychophysical measures reveal impairments in the processing of audiovisual inputs. Cereb Cortex. 2013;23:1329–41.
74. Grossman RB, Steinhart E, Mitchell T, McIlvane W. "Look who's talking!" Gaze patterns for implicit and explicit audio-visual speech synchrony detection in children with high-functioning autism. Autism Res. 2015;8:307–16.
75. Magnée MJ, de Gelder B, van Engeland H, Kemner C. Audiovisual speech integration in pervasive developmental disorder: evidence from event-related potentials. J Child Psychol Psychiatry. 2008;49:995–1000.
76. Mongillo EA, Irwin JR, Whalen DH, Klaiman C, Carter AS, Schultz RT. Audiovisual processing in children with and without autism spectrum disorders. J Autism Dev Disord. 2008;38:1349–58.
77. Taylor N, Isaac C, Milne E. A comparison of the development of audiovisual integration in children with autism spectrum disorders and typically developing children. J Autism Dev Disord. 2010;40:1403–11.
78. Irwin JR, Tornatore LA, Brancazio L, Whalen DH. Can children with autism spectrum disorders "Hear" a speaking face? Child Dev. 2011;82:1397–403.
79. Pierce K, Glad KS, Schreibman L. Social perception in children with autism: an attentional deficit? J Autism Dev Disord. 1997;27:265–82.
80. Hall GBC, Szechtman H, Nahmias C. Enhanced salience and emotion recognition in autism: a PET study. Am J Psychiatry. 2003;160:1439–41.
81. Golan O, Baron-Cohen S. Systemizing empathy: teaching adults with Asperger syndrome or high-functioning autism to recognize complex emotions using interactive multimedia. Dev Psychopathol. 2006;18:591–617.
82. Golan O, Baron-Cohen S, Golan Y. The "reading the mind in films" task [child version]: complex emotion and mental state recognition in children with and without autism spectrum conditions. J Autism Dev Disord. 2008;38:1534–41.
83. Ekman P. Facial expression and emotion. Am Psychol. 1993;48:384–92.
84. Wilson-Mendenhall CD, Barrett LF, Barsalou LW. Neural evidence that human emotions share core affective properties. Psychol Sci. 2013;24:947–56.
85. Griffiths PE. What emotions really are: the problem of psychological categories. Chicago: University of Chicago Press; 1997.
86. Izard C. Basic emotions, natural kinds, emotion schemas, and a new paradigm. Perspect Psychol Sci. 2007;2:260–80.
87. Harris PL. Children and emotion: the development of psychological understanding. Basil Blackwell; 1989.
88. Celani G, Battacchi MW, Arcidiacono L. The understanding of the emotional meaning of facial expressions in people with autism. J Autism Dev Disord. 1999;29:57–66.
89. Capps L, Yirmiya N, Sigman M. Understanding of simple and complex emotions in non-retarded children with autism.pdf. J child Psychol Psychiatry. 1992;35:1169–82.
90. Elfenbein HA, Ambady N. On the universality and cultural specificity of emotion recognition: a meta-analysis. Psychol Bull. 2002;128:203–35.
91. Juslin PN, Laukka P. Communication of emotions in vocal expression and music performance: different channels, same code? Psychol Bull. 2003;129:770–814.
92. Yafai A-F, Verrier D, Reidy L. Social conformity and autism spectrum disorder: a child-friendly take on a classic study. Autism. 2014;18:1007–13.
93. Wechsler D. Wechsler Abbreviated Scale of Intelligence. 2nd ed. San Antonio: Pearson; 2011.
94. Wechsler D. Wechsler Intelligence Scale for Children-Fourth Edition. San Antonio: Psychological Corporation; 2003.
95. Wechsler D. Wechsler primary and preschool scale of intelligence—third edition. San Antonio: Harcourt Assessment; 2002.
96. Constantino JN, Gruber C. The Social Responsiveness Scale—second edition (SRS-2). Torrance: Western Psychological Services; 2012.
97. Bölte S, Poustka F, Constantino JN. Assessing autistic traits: cross-cultural validation of the social responsiveness scale (SRS). Autism Res. 2008;1:354–63.
98. Bölte S, Hubl D, Feineis-Matthews S, Prvulovic D, Dierks T, Poustka F. Facial affect recognition training in autism: can we animate the fusiform gyrus? Behav Neurosci. 2006;120:211–6.
99. Bölte S, Ciaramidaro A, Schlitt S, Hainz D, Kliemann D, Beyer A, Poustka F, Freitag C, Walter H. Training-induced plasticity of the social brain in autism spectrum disorder. Br J Psychiatry. 2015;207:149–57.
100. Baron-Cohen S, Golan O, Wheelwright S, Hill JJ. Mind reading: the interactive guide to emotions. London: Jessica Kingsley Limited; 2004.
101. O'Reilly H, Pigat D, Fridenson S, Berggren S, Tal S, Golan O, Bölte S, Baron-Cohen S, Lundqvist D. The EU-emotion stimulus set: a validation study. Behav Res Methods. 2016;48:567–76.
102. Lassalle A, Pigat D, O'Reilly H, Berggen S, Fridenson-Hayo S, Tal S, Elfström S, Råde A, Golan O, Bölte S, Baron-Cohen S, Lundqvist D. The EU-Emotion Voice Database. 2016.
103. World Health Organisation. ICD-10—International Classification of Diseases (10th ed.). Geneva: World Health Organization; 1994.
104. American Psychiatric Association. Diagnostic and statistical manual of mental disorders, 4th edition. American Psychiatric Association; 2000.
105. Lord C, Rutter M, DiLavore P, Risi S, Gotham K, Bishop SL. Autism diagnostic observation schedule (2nd ed.). Los Angeles: CA: Western Psychological Services; 2012.
106. Scott FJ, Baron-Cohen S, Bolton P, Brayne C. The CAST (Childhood Asperger Syndrome Test): preliminary development of a UK screen for mainstream primary-school-age children. Autism. 2002;6:9–31.
107. Gepner B, Féron F. Autism: a world changing too fast for a mis-wired brain? Neurosci Biobehav Rev. 2009;33:1227–42.
108. Elfenbein HA, Beaupré M, Lévesque M, Hess U. Toward a dialect theory: cultural differences in the expression and recognition of posed facial expressions. Emotion. 2007;7:131–46.
109. Baron-Cohen S, Bowen DC, Holt RJ, Allison C, Auyeung B, Lombardo MV, Smith P, Lai M-C. The "reading the mind in the eyes" test: complete absence of typical sex difference in ~400 men and women with autism. PLoS One. 2015;10(8):e0136521.
110. Golan O, Ashwin E, Granader Y, McClintock S, Day K, Leggett V, Baron-Cohen S. Enhancing emotion recognition in children with autism spectrum conditions: an intervention using animated vehicles with real emotional faces. J Autism Dev Disord. 2010;40:269–79.
111. Kouo JL, Egel AL. The effectiveness of interventions in teaching emotion recognition to children with autism spectrum disorder. Rev J Autism Dev Disord. 2016;3:254–65.

14

Linguistic camouflage in girls with autism spectrum disorder

Julia Parish-Morris[1,2*], Mark Y. Liberman[3], Christopher Cieri[3], John D. Herrington[1,2], Benjamin E. Yerys[1,2], Leila Bateman[1], Joseph Donaher[4], Emily Ferguson[1], Juhi Pandey[1] and Robert T. Schultz[1,2]

Abstract

Background: Autism spectrum disorder (ASD) is diagnosed more frequently in boys than girls, even when girls are equally symptomatic. Cutting-edge behavioral imaging has detected "camouflaging" in girls with ASD, wherein social behaviors appear superficially typical, complicating diagnosis. The present study explores a new kind of camouflage based on language differences. Pauses during conversation can be filled with words like UM or UH, but research suggests that these two words are pragmatically distinct (e.g., UM is used to signal longer pauses, and may correlate with greater social communicative sophistication than UH). Large-scale research suggests that women and younger people produce higher rates of UM during conversational pauses than do men and older people, who produce relatively more UH. Although it has been argued that children and adolescents with ASD use UM less often than typical peers, prior research has not included sufficient numbers of girls to examine whether sex explains this effect. Here, we explore UM vs. UH in school-aged boys and girls with ASD, and ask whether filled pauses relate to dimensional measures of autism symptom severity.

Methods: Sixty-five verbal school-aged participants with ASD (49 boys, 16 girls, IQ estimates in the average range) participated, along with a small comparison group of typically developing children (8 boys, 9 girls). Speech samples from the Autism Diagnostic Observation Schedule were orthographically transcribed and time-aligned, with filled pauses marked. Parents completed the Social Communication Questionnaire and the Vineland Adaptive Behavior Scales.

Results: Girls used UH less often than boys across both diagnostic groups. UH suppression resulted in higher UM ratios for girls than boys, and overall filled pause rates were higher for typical children than for children with ASD. Higher UM ratios correlated with better socialization in boys with ASD, but this effect was driven by increased use of UH by boys with greater symptoms.

Conclusions: Pragmatic language markers distinguish girls and boys with ASD, mirroring sex differences in the general population. One implication of this finding is that typical-sounding disfluency patterns (i.e., reduced relative UH production leading to higher UM ratios) may normalize the way girls with ASD sound relative to other children, serving as "linguistic camouflage" for a naïve listener and distinguishing them from boys with ASD. This first-of-its-kind study highlights the importance of continued commitment to understanding how sex and gender change the way that ASD manifests, and illustrates the potential of natural language to contribute to objective "behavioral imaging" diagnostics for ASD.

Keywords: Autism, Language, Linguistic camouflage, Disfluency, Pragmatic communication, Sex differences, Gender differences, Filled pauses

* Correspondence: parishmorrisj@email.chop.edu
[1]Center for Autism Research, Children's Hospital of Philadelphia, Roberts Center for Pediatric Research, 2716 South Street, Philadelphia, PA 19146, USA
[2]Perelman School of Medicine, University of Pennsylvania, 3400 Civic Center Blvd, Philadelphia, PA 19104, USA
Full list of author information is available at the end of the article

N.B.: In this paper, our terminology is drawn from World Health Organization definitions [51]. The word "sex" refers to genetic makeup, and "gender" refers to a socio-cultural construct. Consistent with a recent review of sex differences in ASD [31], we explicitly acknowledge the significant and inevitable overlap between the two. Here, we use the words "girl" and "boy" to refer to biological sex.

Background

Autism spectrum disorder (ASD) is a behaviorally defined condition predominantly found in males [10, 19, 40, 49]. Recent research suggests that girls with ASD may "camouflage" real struggles with social communication by engaging in social mimicry and behaving in ways that are superficially typical, thus complicating diagnosis [7, 34]. For example, nonverbal communication (e.g., gesture) is broadly impaired in ASD [3]. Using 3D motion capture, a recent study showed that girls with ASD gesture in ways that are more vibrant and noticeable than boys with ASD, despite similar struggles with social communication [48]. In this way, girls effectively modified their behavior to mask a traditional area of weakness. In the present study, we use granular language-based analysis to explore another way in which girls with ASD achieve this social camouflage effect: by producing sex-typical filled pauses during naturalistic conversation.

Filled pauses

In the course of normal conversation, interlocutors pause, revise, and re-work their utterances, a process termed *disfluency* [11]. Disfluencies affect how speakers are perceived by others, and elevated rates of speech disfluencies have been linked to negative social perceptions of the speaker [8, 22, 45]. Pauses are disfluencies that occur during natural speech and can either remain unfilled (silent pauses) or be filled by words like *um*, *uh*, *like*, and *you know* (filled pauses). UM and UH, in particular, are thought to be social pragmatic hesitation markers with communicative value (e.g., facilitating comprehension by signaling to the listener that the speaker needs more time to finish communicating their current thought, or that they would like to hold/cede the floor [21]). However, there is growing evidence to suggest that UM and UH are not the same; UH is used to signal a short delay while UM may be used to signal more significant delays [11]. Large-scale cross-linguistic studies of spoken and written language show that these two markers are used with varying frequency by people from different demographic groups [1, 59]. For example, UM is used relatively more often by women, educated individuals, and younger generations than by men, less educated individuals, and older generations. In contrast, UH is used relatively more frequently by men, less educated individuals, and older generations than by women, more educated individuals, and younger generations (M. [37, 59]). This pattern is robust across American English, British English, Scottish English, Dutch, Norwegian, German, Danish, and Faroese [59].

Filled pauses in ASD

A significant body of research suggests that children and adults with ASD produce unusually high rates of various speech disfluencies [16, 35, 42, 50, 51, 54], but only three studies have specifically examined UM and UH. First, 4- to 8-year-olds with ASD use UM at lower rates than children without ASD [26]. This finding suggests that UM and UH may hinge on distinct cognitive processes, with UM more powerfully affected by the presence of autism [26]. Subsequent research showed that UM use by 8- to 21-year-olds normalizes when overall ASD symptoms drop off [28, 46], again lending support to the hypothesis that UM is associated with social competence. In a third study, language samples from children with ASD were compared to samples from children with specific language impairment, and individual variation in UM use was found to be a marker of pragmatic ability rather than a consequence of general language skill [24]. Taken together, these studies suggest that UM and UH are used differently by children with ASD, and that UM ratios [um/(um + uh)] associate with ASD symptoms.

One major limitation of this line of research is that sex differences in filled pause use have never been studied in individuals with ASD. If females have higher UM ratios than males [59], slight sex ratio differences across diagnostic groups could lead to erroneous results. For example, Gorman et al. [24] included 10% girls in their ASD group and 30% girls in their typical group. Elevated UM ratios in the typical group relative to the ASD group might thus be a consequence of sex ratio imbalances (because girls may produce higher UM ratios than boys)—and the TD group was enriched for girls. This observation, that slight differences in sex ratio by diagnostic group could change the results of scientific studies in a variety of domains, has implications for how we evaluate the presence and severity of ASD symptoms in girls and boys, and will influence the hunt for behavioral markers of ASD more broadly. In the case of UM and UH specifically, if girls with ASD exhibit gender-normative speech patterns, it could bias perception of their ASD symptoms. The current literature is unable to address this question, primarily out of an absence of speech data from females with ASD. Apart from Gorman et al. [24], the other two papers that explored UM vs. UH in children with ASD either did not report sample sex ratios at all [26], or included insufficient numbers of female participants with ASD to assess potential effects of sex on filler production (3 out of 24 or 12.5% in [28]).

The present study fills this gap with a large sample of children on the spectrum, including a representative proportion of girls (N = 65, 16 girls, 25%), along with a small comparison sample of typical children (N = 17, 9 girls, 53%). We hypothesized that girls and boys with ASD would show typical sex differences in filled pauses (i.e., girls would produce higher UM ratios than boys with ASD, driven by boys producing more UH than girls). We further hypothesized, based on prior research showing that scores on the Social Communication Questionnaire (SCQ; [46] higher scores indicate more lifetime ASD symptoms) decrease as UM ratio increases [24, 28], that higher UM ratios would be associated with fewer lifetime ASD symptoms. To address the possibility that girls in our ASD sample were more socially adept than boys, we compared parent reports of social communication ability by sex (using the Vineland Adaptive Behavior Scales-2nd edition, (VABS; [52]), and explored whether better social communication in girls explained sex differences in filled pause ratios. Finally, we analyzed subgroups of boys with ASD, and gauged the specificity of our UM/UH results by comparing boys and girls on seven additional linguistic features. Language samples were drawn from the interview section of the ADOS module 3 (requiring phrase speech; [41]). These samples provide a naturalistic back-and-forth conversation about social topics, and have been shown to contain meaningful rates of speech disfluencies in children with ASD [24, 26, 42].

Methods

Participants

Sixty-five children with ASD aged 6–17 contributed language samples during research visits to the Center for Autism Research at the Children's Hospital of Philadelphia (Table 1). Children were recruited from the larger Philadelphia area, and 85% of the sample was White according to parent report. Research-reliable clinical psychologists (100% female) used expert clinical judgment to make diagnoses of ASD according to DSM-IV-TR criteria [2] informed by the ADOS-2 Module 3 and the Autism Diagnostic Interview-Revised (ADI-R; [47]). Exclusion criteria included extreme prematurity (< 32 weeks) or low birth weight, genetic or medical history that explained ASD symptoms, uncorrected auditory or visual impairment, significant psychiatric conditions (e.g., active mood disorders or psychosis, but not common comorbidities like anxiety or ADHD), and contraindications for an MRI scan (e.g., braces). Inclusion criteria for the present subsample included the ability to use phrase speech, since all conversational data were drawn from Module 3 ADOS evaluations. Boys and girls did not differ significantly on age, General Conceptual Ability (GCA) using the Differential Abilities Scales-II (DAS-II; all participants had GCAs > 75), or ASD symptoms as measured by ADOS scores (Table 1). Despite statistically insignificant differences in chronological age, there were mean differences; we therefore included this variable in our analysis, to check for possible age influences on filled pauses. In addition, we recruited a small sample of typically developing children (N = 17; age in years: M = 11.32, SD = 2.21; GCA: M = 104, SD = 15) for the purposes of comparison.

Procedure

Research-reliable clinicians administered the ADOS to participants as part of 1- or 2-day study battery (rescored

Table 1 Demographics and clinical scores (mean (standard deviation)) for children with ASD

	Overall	Boys	Girls	Sex difference
Number	65	49	16	33 more boys
Age in years	9.96 (2.05)	9.73 (2.16)	10.66 (1.55)	Z = 1.60, p = 0.10
DAS-II GCA	105 (14)	106 (14)	104 (13)	Z = −0.07, p = 0.95
Verbal	107 (14)	107 (14)	106 (15)	Z = −0.35, p = 0.73
Nonverbal	106 (14)	106 (14)	105 (14)	Z = −0.24, p = 0.81
SCQ lifetime	19.82 (6.92)	19.49 (7.46)	20.81 (4.98)	Z = −1.01, p = 0.31
VABS composite	82.32 (13.22)	83.19 (13.26)	79.75 (13.18)	Z = −0.85, p = 0.39
Communication	87.75 (13.77)	88.21 (14.14)	86.38 (12.94)	Z = −0.31, p = 0.76
Socialization	77.95 (14.88)	79.36 (15.48)	73.81 (12.49)	Z = −1.74, p = 0.08
ADOS-2 overall[a]	6.49 (2.47)	6.55 (2.38)	6.31 (2.80)	Z = −0.18, p = 0.85
Social affect	6.29 (2.42)	6.29 (2.38)	6.31 (2.63)	Z = −0.008, p = 0.99
RRB	7.08 (2.54)	7.27 (2.32)	6.50 (3.14)	Z = −0.43, p = 0.67

Sex differences were assessed via nonparametric Mann-Whitney U tests. ADOS scores represent calibrated severity scores (comparison scores). Two male participants are missing Vineland Adaptive Behavior Scales (VABS) scores. *RRB* = repetitive behaviors and restricted interests

[a]Calibrated severity scores of 4 are equivalent to a raw score of 7 (ASD cut-off) and severity scores of 6 are equivalent to a raw score of at least 9 (autism cut-off) on the ADOS-2

as the ADOS-2, referred to as the ADOS-2 throughout this paper). The ADOS-2 was administered in a quiet room equipped with audio and video recording equipment. Parents consented to using these recordings for research purposes. Participant IQ was estimated using the DAS-II [18], and parents provided additional information via the ADI-R [47], the VABS [52], and the Social Communication Questionnaire (SCQ; [46] see the "Measures" section below). Families were compensated for time and travel. This research was conducted with approval and oversight from the Institutional Review Board of the Children's Hospital of Philadelphia.

Measures

All measures were administered in person, by telephone (for the ADI-R, if needed), or via US postal service (for parent questionnaires).

Autism Diagnostic Observation Schedule-2nd Edition (ADOS-2; [41]). The ADOS-2 is a semi-structured psychodiagnostic assessment for ASD, often used in combination with parent history (collected via ADI-R or SCQ combined with parent interview). ADOS-2 calibrated severity scores estimate the extent to which an individual is affected by ASD symptoms (0–10, with 0 representing least affected and 10 most affected [25]). Calibrated severity scores for the subdomains of social affect (0–10) and repetitive behaviors/restricted interests (0–10) were calculated as well [25, 27].

Differential Abilities Scales-II (DAS-II; [18]). The DAS-II is designed to estimate general intelligence in individuals aged 2–18 years. The DAS-II provides standard scores that are analogous with full-scale IQ (DAS-II General Conceptual Ability), verbal IQ (DAS-II verbal composite score), and performance IQ (DAS-II nonverbal composite score).

Social Communication Questionnaire (SCQ; [46]). The SCQ is a parent report questionnaire assessing current and lifetime autism symptoms. This study reports lifetime SCQ scores, with higher scores indicating greater lifetime autism symptomology.

Vineland Adaptive Behavior Scales (parent/caregiver rating form)-2nd edition (VABS; [52]). The VABS is a parent report measure of their child's adaptive behavior. It includes multiple domains of adaptive function, including socialization and communication. Higher scores indicate more proficient adaptive behavior.

Transcription

The largest continuous segment of the "interview questions" section of the ADOS-2 (in minutes) was orthographically transcribed using a specification developed in collaboration with the University of Pennsylvania's Linguistic Data Consortium (LDC). When possible, we transcribed the "Emotions," "Social Difficulties and Annoyance," "Friends, Relationships, and Marriage," and "Loneliness" sections. The "Break" section, which occurs within these sections, was not transcribed. Mean overall transcription length was 19.61 min per participant. Samples from boys (mean = 19.15 min) vs. girls (mean = 20.65) did not significantly differ in duration, Mann-Whitney $Z = -1.48$ $p = 0.14$. Each audio sample was segmented into utterances (separated by breath pauses) by an undergraduate student and checked by an experienced annotator. Speech segments were transcribed by a different undergraduate student, and adjudicated by a different experienced annotator. Segmentation, transcription, and adjudication were conducted using audio files only, blind to diagnosis. Nearly 50% of recordings were fully transcribed by two independent annotators, with pre-adjudication word-level agreement averaging 92%. Time-stamped textual transcriptions were aligned with audio files using a force-aligner developed at the LDC [60].

Variables

Word count was calculated by summing all words produced by each speaker (totwords). Instances of UM and UH were identified within each transcript, and summed. Three variables were calculated: average UM production (tot_um/totwords), average UH production (tot_uh/totwords), and um_ratio, which is the rate of UM produced relative to total filled pauses [tot_um/(tot_um + tot_uh)]. Total filled pause rate was calculated by dividing the sum of pauses filled by UM or UH by the total number of words produced by an individual [(tot_um + tot_uh)/totwords]. Average latency to respond to the ADOS-2 administrator was calculated by dividing the sum duration of all clinician-to-participant inter-turn pauses by the total number of pauses of that transition type. Speech rate was calculated by dividing the total number of words produced by each speaker by the summed duration of all segments for that speaker. An outlier-robust measure of dispersion in participants' fundamental frequency (F0) distribution (median absolute deviation from the median), captured pitch variation. All time variables are reported in milliseconds.

Statistical plan

Three generalized linear mixed effects logistic regression models assessed the relative effects of age, IQ, sex, and ASD symptoms on "tot_um," "tot_uh," and "um_ratio" in participants with ASD (software: R, package: lme4; [59]). In each case, the word of interest was coded as a "hit" while all other words were coded as "misses." Continuous variables were z-scored for interpretability, and participant identity was included with a random intercept. UM and UH variables were non-normal and contained outliers; analyses with and without outliers were found to yield the same pattern of results, so outliers were retained to capture the heterogeneity inherent in samples with ASD. Nonparametric Mann-Whitney *U* tests were used in place of standard *t* tests to account for non-normality (software: SPSS 23; Z is reported). Means and standard deviations are reported for the typically developing comparison group, but due to the small sample size, only nonparametric Mann-Whitney *U* tests were conducted. Spearman's Rho (ρ) was used to characterize correlational relationships between UM and UH variables and questionnaire scores for participants with ASD. Effect sizes for Mann-Whitney *U* tests are reported using $r = Z/[\text{sqrt}(N)]$ [20]. Following Cohen (1988), an *r* value of 0.1 is considered a small effect, 0.3 is a medium effect, and 0.5 is a large effect.

Results

Predictors of UM and UH in ASD

Generalized linear mixed effects logistic regression models revealed significant associations between sex, VABS socialization scores and average UH production in the ASD group, as well as UM ratio, but no association between sex and socialization and average UM production (Table 2). Age, GCA, SCQ, and VABS communication scores did not account for significant explanatory variance in the three filled pause variables, nor did interactions between any two variables. The pattern of results did not change when verbal and nonverbal composite scores were entered instead of DAS-II GCA.

Boys with ASD produced more UH relative to total words produced (mean = 0.0084, SD = 0.0077, 95% CI = 0.0062–0.0106) than girls with ASD (mean = 0.0044, SD = 0.0044, 95% CI = 0.0022–0.0066), mean difference = −0.004, 95% CI = −0.0081–0.00004, $Z = -1.98$, $p = 0.02$, $r = 0.29$. There was also a significant sex difference in UM ratio (mean difference = 19%, 95% CI = 0.04–0.34, $Z = -2.16$, $p = 0.03$, $r = 0.26$). Whereas girls produced UM during approximately 75% of pauses filled by UM or UH (SD = 17%; CI = 0.66–0.85), boys produced UM during an average of 56% of such pauses (SD = 29%, CI = 0.48–0.65). Average UM use did not differ in boys (mean = 0.0143, SD = 0.0156, 95% CI = 0.0098–0.0188) as compared to girls (mean = 0.0161, SD = 0.0125, 95% CI = 0.0094–0.0227), mean difference = 0.0017, 95% CI = −0.0069–0.0103, $Z = -1.19$, $p = 0.24$, $r = 0.15$, suggesting that greater UH use by boys (or reduced UH use by girls) drove the significant difference in the um/uh ratio.

UM and UH in typical controls

A similar pattern emerged in our sample of typically developing children. Typical boys produced more UH relative to total words produced (mean = 0.0083, SD = 0.0050, 95% CI = 0.0042–0.0124) than did typical girls (mean = 0.0032, SD = 0.0027, 95% CI = 0.0011–0.0053; mean difference = −0.0051, 95% CI = −0.0092–(−0.0010), $Z = -2.32$, $p = 0.02$, $r = 0.56$; Fig. 1). Similar to the ASD group, mean UM production relative to total words produced was comparable between typical boys (mean = 0.0301, SD = 0.0129, 95% CI = 0.0193–0.0408) and girls (mean = 0.0234, SD = 0.0184, 95% CI = 0.0011–0.0053; mean difference = −0.0067, 95% CI = −0.0233–0.0100, $Z = -1.06$, $p = 0.29$, $r = 0.26$). However, in contrast to the pattern seen in children with ASD, UM ratios were high for both typical girls (mean = 85%, SD = 14%, 95% CI = 74–95%) and boys (mean = 78%, SD = 15%, 95% CI = 65–91%; mean difference = 0.0673, 95% CI = −0.0827–0.2173, $Z = -0.87$, $p = 0.39$, $r = 0.21$.

Diagnostic group differences in UM and UH

Given our small TDC sample, we suggest that the following results be interpreted with caution. Overall, typical children filled more pauses than children with ASD (Table 3; $Z = -2.33$, $p = 0.02$, $r = 0.26$). Mann-Whitney *U* tests suggest that girls with ASD and typical girls used comparable levels of UM ($p = 0.34$) and UH ($p = 0.61$), and had similar UM ratios ($p = 0.16$; Fig. 1). In contrast,

Table 2 Generalized linear mixed effects regressions predicting average UM and UH relative to total words produced, and UM ratio (UM/(UM + UH))

	Average UM			Average UH			UM ratio		
	Est. (se)	*z*	*p*	Est. (se)	*z*	*p*	Est. (se)	*z*	*p*
Intercept	−4.33 (0.27)	−16.25	< 0.000	−5.98 (.23)	−26.51	< 0.000	−0.14 (.13)	−1.09	0.28
Age	−0.21 (0.16)	−1.38	0.17	−0.15 (0.12)	−1.21	0.23	0.05 (0.08)	−0.58	0.56
GCA	0.08 (0.16)	0.55	0.58	−0.11 (0.12)	−0.95	0.34	−0.04 (0.07)	0.53	0.59
Sex	−0.50 (0.30)	−1.68	0.09	0.82 (0.24)	3.36	< 0.001**	−0.46 (0.15)	−3.18	0.001**
SCQ	0.08 (0.21)	0.37	0.71	−0.02 (0.16)	−0.10	0.92	0.06 (0.11)	0.55	0.58
V Com	−0.12 (0.23)	−0.53	0.60	0.26 (0.17)	1.47	0.14	−0.08 (0.12)	−0.69	0.48
V Soc	0.16 (0.26)	0.62	0.54	−0.69 (0.20)	−3.48	< 0.001**	0.29 (0.13)	2.28	0.02*

Predictors associated with greater dependent variable values have positive log-odds (shown as estimate (Est.) with standard error (se) in parentheses). *V Com* Vineland Communication Domain scores, *V Soc* Vineland Socialization Domain scores, *Sex* 0 = girl, 1 = boy. * $p<.05$, ** $p<.01$

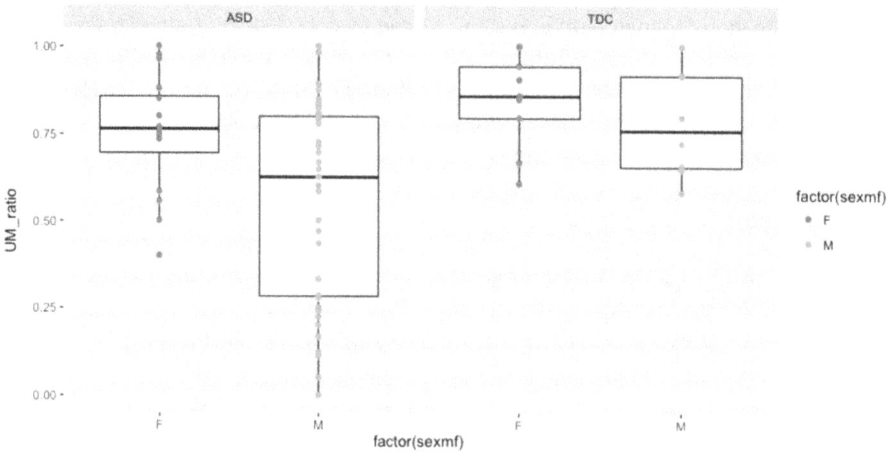

Fig. 1 UM ratio for girls (F) and boys (M) with and without ASD. *TDC* = typically developing control

boys with ASD produced significantly less UM (relative to total words produced) than typical boys (p = 0.002), and typical boys produced higher UM ratios than boys with ASD (p = 0.06). Boys in the ASD and TDC groups did not differ on average UH (p = 0.63).

Filled pauses and ASD symptoms

Generalized linear mixed effects logistic regression models revealed that UM ratio and average UH production are associated with VABS socialization scores in the ASD group. To rule out the possibility that slightly lower VABS scores in girls relative to boys in our sample unduly influenced the observed relationship between socialization and disfluency type, we explored whether relationships between filled pauses and VABS socialization scores held within boys and girls with ASD, separately (Fig. 2). Spearman's Rho correlations revealed a positive association between VABS socialization scores and UM ratio for boys (ρ = 0.30, p = 0.04) but not for girls (ρ = 0.007, p = 0.98; 2a). Increased UH use was associated with lower socialization scores for boys (ρ = −0.31, p = 0.04; 2b) and girls at similar strength (ρ = −0.32) but likely failed to reach significance in girls due to the smaller sample size. In contrast to similar relationships between average UH and socialization in boys and girls, opposite trends were observed in average UM; the relationship between UM and socialization scores was positive and insignificant in boys, and it was negative and insignificant in girls (2c). This pattern of results suggests that UM ratio and average UM are not sex-robust indicators of pragmatic ability or social impairment in ASD. UH, on the other hand, appears to be a promising indicator of poor socialization as reported by parents on the VABS, across both sexes.

Parsing heterogeneity in ASD

Every girl in the ASD group produced UM during at least 40% of filled pauses, and some produced UM during 100% of filled pauses. In contrast, boys with ASD ranged from 0 to 100% of pauses filled by UM vs. UH. This suggests the possibility of multiple subgroups of boys: primarily UMers and primarily UHers. We explored this heterogeneity among boys with ASD by splitting into three equal groups (by UM ratio) and comparing the top and bottom thirds of the boy group to girls. The bottom third of boys produced UH during filled pauses 60% of the time or more, and were

Table 3 UM use, UH use, and total filled pause rates, by sex and diagnostic group

	Average UM		Average UH		UM ratio		Filled pause rate	
	Mean (%)	SD (%)	Mean (%)	SD (%)	Mean (%)	SD (%)	Mean (%)	SD (%)
ASD								
Girls	1.6	1.2	0.44	0.44	75	17	2.0	1.5
Boys	1.4	1.6	0.84	0.77	56	29	2.3	1.7
TDC								
Girls	2.3	1.8	0.32	0.27	85	14	2.7	1.9
Boys	3.0	1.3	0.83	0.50	78	15	3.8	1.3

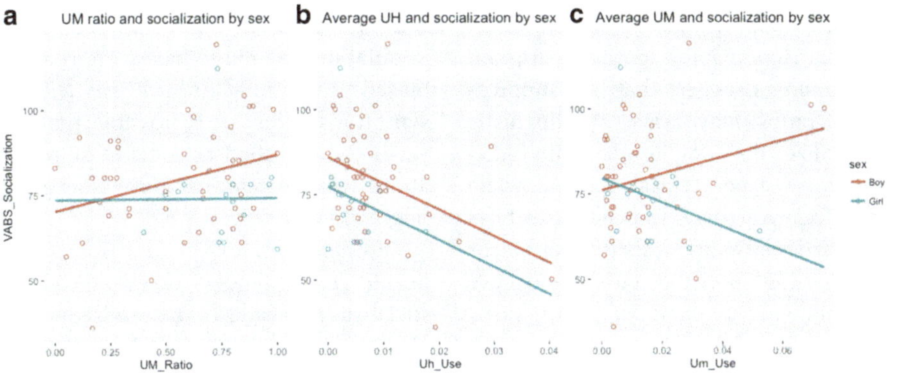

Fig. 2 Parent reported VABS socialization scores and UM ratio (**a**), average UH production relative to total words produced (**b**), and average UM production relative to total words produced (**c**) by boys and girls with ASD (female = *blue*; male = *red*). Correlations in **a** and **b** are significant for boys but not for girls; correlations in **c** are not significant, but are included to demonstrate opposite relationships between socialization and average UM production by sex

categorized as UHers. Boys that produced UM during 78% or more of filled pauses were categorized as UMers. No group differences survived correction for multiple comparisons in a multivariate ANOVA (all $ps > 0.21$; Table 4), indicating that the relationship between filled pause use and Vineland socialization is more dimensional than categorical and may be sensitive to sample size.

Specificity of filled pause differences

Finally, we considered the possibility that filled pauses represent just one of many low-level speech differences between boys and girls with ASD. To assess the specificity of variation in filled pause type, we conducted pairwise comparisons across a variety of other linguistic features. Results revealed that girls and boys with ASD did not differ on average total word count, filled pause rate, speech rate, number of turns, duration of turns, response latency, or pitch variation (Table 5).

Table 4 Subgroups of boys with ASD compared to girls with ASD

	Girls	Boy UHers	Boy UMers
Number	16	16	16
Age in years	10.66 (1.55)	10.05 (2.16)	10.04 (2.33)
IQ—full scale	104 (13)	105 (13)	107 (14)
Verbal	106 (15)	106 (13)	111 (15)
Nonverbal	105 (14)	106 (13)	105 (16)
SCQ current	20.81 (4.98)	19.00 (6.64)	18.81 (6.99)
Vineland ABC	79.75 (13.18)	80.06 (12.77)	86.93 (14.44)
Communication	86.38 (12.94)	86.81 (16.10)	90.80 (14.81)
Socialization	73.81 (12.49)	75.13 (14.82)	83.13 (14.53)
ADOS overall	6.31 (2.80)	7.25 (2.05)	5.56 (2.50)
Social affect	6.31 (2.63)	6.81 (2.48)	5.63 (2.42)
RRB	6.50 (3.14)	7.75 (2.11)	6.50 (2.68)

Discussion

Subtle linguistic markers influence how parents, teachers, clinicians, and peers perceive an individual's social skills during everyday conversation. For example, UM is a social pragmatic marker [21] used more often by younger people and women as compared to older people and men, and UH is used relatively more often by older people and men than by younger people and women [59]. Unusually low UM ratios have been reported in children/adolescents with ASD [28], and have been argued to mark difficulties with social communication [24]. In the present study, we asked whether a third variable not considered in prior research—speaker sex—might be important for understanding filled pause differences in children with ASD. Our results showed that girls with ASD and typical girls/boys exhibited higher UM ratios than boys with ASD, while girls in both diagnostic groups suppressed UH relative to their male counterparts. Importantly, filled pause differences in boys and girls with ASD in this study were not

Table 5 Pairwise comparisons between girls and boys with ASD on seven linguistic features (mean and standard deviation (SD))

	Girls	SD	Boys	SD	z	Sig.
Total word count	1116.69	533.25	1025.51	472.91	−0.61	$p = 0.54$
Filled pause rate	2.04%	1.5%	2.27%	1.7%	−0.20	$p = 0.84$
Speech rate	0.33	0.04	0.33	0.06	−0.50	$p = 0.62$
Num turns	141.56	45.09	138.08	58.16	−0.43	$p = 0.67$
Duration of turns	436.86	184.99	439.71	195.14	−0.20	$p = 0.84$
Latency to respond	0.83	0.45	0.88	0.33	−0.93	$p = 0.35$
Pitch variation	2.22	1.89	2.12	0.83	−0.81	$p = 0.42$

attributable to increased social pragmatic ability in girls, as girls and boys in our sample had equivalent social communication skills and comparable autism symptom severity. The present findings suggest that UH suppression and higher UM ratios may serve as "linguistic camouflage" to normalize the way a girl with ASD sounds relative to same-aged typical peers, while elevated rates of UH (relative to UM) may cause boys with ASD to sound particularly atypical. Intentional or not, overtly typical-sounding speech in girls could have some benefits (e.g., allowing a child to more easily "blend in" with classmates), while simultaneously complicating the detection of ASD, leading to missed or delayed diagnosis, and misdiagnoses that are more common in girls than boys [33].

Sex differences and UM Ratio

This is the first study to show that girls and boys with ASD show sex-specific patterns of filled pause use, and to compare these patterns in girls and boys without ASD. Importantly, girls with ASD in our study did not fill more pauses than boys; they filled them differently. Like typical children and children with specific language impairment [24], girls in the present study used UM during > 70% of all filled pauses. Boys with ASD, in contrast, used UM during only 55% of filled pauses. In contrast to prior research [28], we did not find relationships between ASD symptoms as measured by the SCQ and average UM production in the sample as a whole, nor did we find relationships between average UM and VABS socialization or communication scores. This indicates that even though girls are using typical-sounding speech patterns (as reflected by the UM ratio), it is not necessarily reflected in improved parental perceptions of their social communicative ability.

Why might girls with ASD fill conversational pauses with "typical-sounding" words, and suppress atypical words like UH, despite comparable social communication deficits to boys? One hypothesis is that girls are not using filled pauses as communicative tools, but rather produce higher UM ratios (and lower rates of UH) as a form of unconscious social mimicry or scripting [7, 30, 32, 33, 36]. According to this hypothesis, a girl with ASD might produce typical UM ratios to appear less atypical and improve her chances of successfully integrating during social situations. However, she may not necessarily understand the social meaning behind different filled pause types, and struggle with social communication as much as boys that do not "normalize" their UM ratios. Indeed, our results suggest that girls' linguistic camouflaging is more successful in some ways than others. Although girls with ASD produced higher UM ratios than boys with ASD due to UH suppression, their overall filled pause rate was still lower than typical participants, resulting in incomplete camouflage. This may be due to the nature of our sample; research-based ascertainment differs from population- or clinic-based approaches, and may have biased our sample toward girls with more pronounced symptoms. Thus, it is possible that girls who have not yet been identified as autistic or referred for an evaluation will engage in more successful (or complete) linguistic mimicry.

Another likely explanation for the sex differences reported here hinges on powerful forces of gender socialization. Indeed, research on typically developing children shows that parent perceptions, play practices, and styles of interaction differ systematically by child sex, with infant girls hearing more language, receiving more eye contact, and having more opportunities to engage in social-emotional interaction than infant boys [9]. These gendered caregiving differences have already been in full effect for 2 to 3 years before most ASD diagnoses are made [6, 9, 15, 17, 23], and may act as pressure on young girls to conform to "girl" expectations that include pragmatic competence. As Goldman [23] pointed out, "children (that are later diagnosed with ASD) are raised like any other children according to their sex. They are perceived as girls or boys and are taught to play, talk, and interact in accordance with the particular gender-based rules of their families." Thus, perhaps girls with ASD are not using filled pauses communicatively, but instead are responding to forces of gender socialization that expect girls to *sound* less pragmatically impaired, by suppressing UH and producing higher UM ratios. Since girls with ASD and typical girls are subject to the same gender-based influences during the first few years, it follows that their language might be similarly affected. Indeed, we found that typical girls also suppress UH and produce higher UM ratios than typical boys. This is only one possible hypothesis among a confluence of factors that likely relate to the differences observed in this study. Developmental research focused on younger children is needed to chart the causal pathways that lead to this type of linguistic variation in girls.

Sex differences and UH use

Consistent with prior research documenting UM and UH differences in adult men and women, our results suggest that sex differences in UH production are robust in children; boys in our sample produced more than twice as many UHs (0.84% for boys with ASD, 0.83% for TDC boys) as girls (0.44% for girls with ASD, 0.32% for TDC girls). In addition, we found negative relationships between UH production and perceived social ability across both sexes in ASD; this builds on a number of studies linking speech disfluencies to negative social perceptions of speakers [8, 22, 45].

What caused elevated UH in boys with ASD (and typical boys)? Unmeasured variation in basic cognition could explain this finding, since speakers tend to pause more often, and for longer, right before producing syntactically complex utterances or utterances that exceed their linguistic competency [4, 53]. Given that boys and girls in our sample did not differ significantly on IQ, however, basic cognitive differences are unlikely to have caused elevated UH use by boys (IQ was also not a significant predictor of any language variable in our models). Another possible explanation is language-based, since people with uneven language profiles tend to produce more disfluencies [5, 12, 39, 43, 55–57]. Our groups had comparable verbal IQ scores, but it is still possible that boys in our sample had slightly compromised or uneven language abilities relative to girls, who tend to have better language than boys in typical samples as well [44]. Future research is warranted to explore this possibility.

A third explanation, that poor coordination between motor and language systems results in greater UH use by boys with ASD relative to girls, stems from a growing body of research demonstrating subtle motor control differences in ASD [14]. For instance, people who produce high rates of stuttering-like disfluencies often struggle with speech- *and* non-speech motor tasks, suggesting a general deficiency in integrating sensory and motor control information (Smits Bandstraand De Nil, 2009; Webster, 1997; Smith et al., 2012; Louckset al., 2007; Max & Gracco, 2005). Elevated UH rates in boys with ASD may therefore indicate disrupted coordination across motor and language systems, and could provide clues about a global underlying motor-based pathobiology that partially accounts for social communication problems in ASD [14]. However, we know little about how the motor features of ASD may differ by sex; if UH is a marker of asynchrony across motor and language systems that disproportionately affects boys, and elevated UH production drives reduced UM ratios in boys, it could be that motor dysregulation leads to pragmatic problems even when the cognitive aspects of language are grossly intact. We did not measure motor ability in this study, leaving open the possibility that these differences explain some amount of variance, which may or may not vary by sex; future research will address this question.

Do sex-linked behavior differences necessitate sex-specific diagnostics and treatments for ASD?

Combined with a recent study showing gestural camouflaging in girls with ASD [48], the linguistic camouflage effect identified in this study suggests that subtle sex differences in behavioral domains relevant to ASD (e.g., language) could contribute to girls being missed—or misdiagnosed—due in part to a male-focused conceptualization of ASD and male-normed diagnostic tools. Computational approaches might be particularly useful as an objective way to "see through" various types of social camouflage in the context of screening and diagnosis, and could add to a battery of sex-normed diagnostic and characterization tools for ASD (at least one, the SRS-2, is already normed by sex [13, 31, 33]). In addition to sex-specific identification and characterization tools, behavior-dependent intervention outcome measures may also need to differ by sex. The goal of naturally and automatically integrating information about putative sex differences into the hunt for behavioral biomarkers could lead to creative new approaches that are more sensitive to the way ASD manifests in boys and girls. Notably, our results are consistent with recent large-scale research showing that sex differences in the cognitive and motor profiles of infant siblings of children with ASD are not unique to ASD risk, but rather reflect broader sex differences in the general population [44]. In their conclusion, Messinger and colleagues highlighted the need to compare girls with ASD to typically developing girls (and boys with ASD to typically developing boys). We echo this suggestion.

Limitations

This study differs from prior research in significant ways. Whereas some studies quantify a variety of disfluencies [42], the current research focused only on UM and UH. Unlike Gorman et al. [24], we counted multiple contiguous instances of UM and UH (i.e., if UM was repeated more than once during a filled pause, we counted it more than once. This allowed us to capture stuttering-like filled pauses). Our sample included the largest number of girls with ASD to date, reflecting a 4:1 ratio of boys-to-girls (close to the generally accepted average ratio in ASD). However, we did not include equal numbers of girls and boys with ASD, which led to power issues when examining variables within each sex separately, and we included only a small sample of typically developing control participants. As with some prior studies, we only focused on the interview section of the ADOS-2, and only used Module 3 recordings—future research should expand to new age ranges, ability levels, and ADOS-2 sections and modules.

An inherent limitation of analyzing language produced during semi-structured evaluations is that clinicians are free to ask questions in any order, or to skip questions completely if appropriate from a clinical perspective. Although all clinicians in the current study were research-reliable PhD-level psychologists administering the ADOS in a single center, it is likely that not all children were given probes in the same order. In addition, all clinicians in this study were female, which means that language samples from male participants may have included more

UM than if they had been interviewed by a male clinician [38]. Future research will systematically control for the sex of the interlocutor, to assess effects of sex match vs. mismatch on language variables in individuals with ASD. Finally, it is possible that clinicians differed in how often they asked questions vs. used open-ended comments to start conversations. These variations were limited to the extent possible, but are inherent in any research that relies on ADOS evaluations.

We did not examine the influence of co-occurring disorders or dimensions, such as anxiety, attention deficit/hyperactivity disorder, and executive dysfunction in ASD, on filled pause use. These nuances are ripe avenues for future research. Consistent with findings from other studies of children with ASD, our analyses revealed no relationships between age, IQ, and filled pause type. The lack of an age effect may be due to the age range of our sample (which does not extend into adulthood). Future research with older men and women with ASD is needed to elucidate how our findings change across the lifespan.

The present research represents a number of advances over prior studies. Our results are based on longer language samples than prior research (e.g., 20 min vs. 60 s in [28]). We analyzed UM/UH data from the largest group of individuals with ASD reported to date (65 in this study vs. 50 in [24] and 24 in [28]). Importantly, this is the very first study to examine sex differences in speech disfluencies in children with ASD, made possible by the inclusion of a relatively large number of girls with ASD (25% of our sample vs. 10% and 12.5% in prior work). This is also the first time UM and UH have been explored in typically developing boys and girls, who were found to produce even higher UM ratios than adult men and women [58–60]. Finally, the present research shows that the conclusions of past studies of UM and UH in children with ASD were not entirely wrong. Rather, they were correct for boys with ASD, and incorrect for girls.

Future directions

Prior research shows that children and adolescents with ASD produce more fillers when cognitive demands are high [28], which for individuals with social challenges, may occur more often when discussing social topics. Although others have shown that UM is used relatively less frequently by children with ASD across a variety of tasks [26], future research should specifically compare children's responses to highly social questions and less-social questions (e.g., about objects or interests). The discrepancy in UM and UH production between different question types that vary by social load may be even more informative than relative usage collapsed across an entire interaction. Due to constraints related to the semi-structured conversation format employed in the ADOS-2, we plan to conduct this subsequent experiment in a more controlled format.

Interestingly, Irvine and colleagues suggested that reduced UM use in ASD might contribute to the perception of speech as pedantic or stilted [28]. Based on our current findings, we propose that elevated UH during conversation might in fact drive the impression of pedantry, more so than reduced UM. In fact, high rates of UH (without corresponding increases in UM) might be so unusual in young people [59] that they contribute to some individuals with ASD sounding older than they appear (thus, the "little professor"). Future studies with older and larger samples of individuals with ASD, as well as human raters, are needed to test this hypothesis.

We found that filled pauses vary by sex in ASD, but the everyday consequences of these variations are unknown. Do typical-gendered language patterns in girls with ASD contribute to older age at diagnosis, missed diagnoses, or misdiagnosis? Given that early detection and early intervention are critical for maximizing functional outcomes in ASD [29], issues of under-referral and inadequate measurement for girls with ASD are not trivial. Outside of diagnostic issues, it is possible that suppressed UH and typical UM ratios in girls correlate with the perception of social normalcy by peers, thus helping to establish or maintain friendships. In addition, perhaps girls with ASD suppress UH more when talking to peers than when talking with adults, mimicking typical behavior and increasing their chances of social affiliation in classrooms or on playgrounds. Future studies in naturalistic settings, with a variety of interlocutors, are needed to answer these questions.

Conclusion

ASD experts make diagnostic decisions based on observable behavior, and subtle differences in how a child moves or talks will influence the way they are perceived. Gender socialization or social mimicry may lead to "camouflaged" behavior in girls with ASD, which, combined with widely held gender biases about how girls and boys *should behave* and true biological sex differences, likely complicate efforts to effectively identify and treat boys and girls with ASD. Recent attempts to reduce bias by directly sampling behavior and using objective, computational measurement tools hold promise over existing parent report and clinician rating scales [48], but even these new tools will likely be influenced by variables such as age, sex, gender socialization, socio-economic status, physical and mental health, and home and cultural environment. The findings reported here, identifying "linguistic camouflage" in girls with ASD, highlight the importance of continued commitment to understanding the complex web of biological and environmental factors that influence ASD emergence and presentation.

Abbreviations
ADOS-2: Autism Diagnostic Observation Schedule-2nd Edition; ASD: Autism spectrum disorder; DAS: Differential Abilities Scales-II–2nd Edition; SCQ: Social Communication Questionnaire; TDC: Typically developing control; VABS: Vineland Adaptive Behavior Scales

Acknowledgements
We gratefully acknowledge the children and families that participated in this research. We thank Katie Lowe, Tiffany Ryan, Joy Payton, and Ayana King Pointer from the Center for Autism Research, as well as all clinicians, staff, and students at CAR and LDC, particularly Caitlin Cieri.

Funding
This study was supported by an Autism Science Foundation Postdoctoral Fellowship to JPM; NICHD U54HD086984, NIMH RC1MH08879, Pfizer, and RWJ to RTS; NIMH (K23MH086111; PI: B.E. Yerys, R21MH092615; PI: B.E. Yerys), by the CHOP Clinical Translational Core and a New Program Development Award (to B.E. Yerys) through both the Intellectual and Developmental Disabilities Research Center funded by the National Institute of Child and Human Development (P30HD026979; PI: M. Yudkoff), and by a grant from the Philadelphia Foundation.

Authors' contributions
JPM, ML, CC, and RTS conceived of the idea, designed the study, conducted the analyses, and drafted the manuscript. JD provided critical expertise in the area of speech-language pathology and disfluencies. RTS, JH, JP, and BY collected participant data and revised the manuscript. LB and EF facilitated data processing, project management, idea refinement through excellent conversations with the first author, and manuscript revision. All authors read and approved the final manuscript.

Competing interests
The authors declare that they have no competing interests.

Author details
[1]Center for Autism Research, Children's Hospital of Philadelphia, Roberts Center for Pediatric Research, 2716 South Street, Philadelphia, PA 19146, USA. [2]Perelman School of Medicine, University of Pennsylvania, 3400 Civic Center Blvd, Philadelphia, PA 19104, USA. [3]Linguistic Data Consortium, University of Pennsylvania, 3600 Market St #810, Philadelphia, PA 19104, USA. [4]Center for Childhood Communication, Buerger Center for Advanced Pediatric Care, Children's Hospital of Philadelphia, 3500 Civic Center Blvd, Philadelphia, PA 19104, USA.

References
1. Acton EK. On gender differences in the distribution of um and uh. University of Pennsylvania Working Papers in Linguistics. 2011;17(2):2.
2. American Psychiatric Association. Diagnostic and statistical manual of mental disorders (4th ed., Text Revision). Washington, DC: American Psychiatric Association; 2000.
3. American Psychiatric Association. Diagnostic and statistical manual of mental disorders, 5th edition: DSM-5. 5th ed. Washington, D.C: American Psychiatric Publishing; 2013.
4. Anderson JD. Phonological neighborhood and word frequency effects in the stuttered disfluencies of children who stutter. J Speech Lang Hear Res. 2007;50(1):229–47. https://doi.org/10.1044/1092-4388 (2007/018).
5. Anderson JD, Pellowski MW & Conture EG. Childhood stuttering and dissociations across linguistic domains. Journal of Fluency Disorders. 2005; 30(3):219–253. https://doi.org/10.1016/j.jfludis.2005.05.006.
6. Anderson S, Ertac S, Gneezy U, List JA, Maximiano S. Gender, competitiveness, and socialization at a young age: evidence from a matrilineal and a patriarchal society. Rev Econ Stat. 2013;95(4):1438–43. https://doi.org/10.1162/REST_a_00309
7. Attwood T. The complete guide to Asperger's syndrome. London, England: Jessican Kingsley Publishers; 2006.
8. Boyle MP. Identifying correlates of self-stigma in adults who stutter: further establishing the construct validity of the Self-Stigma of Stuttering Scale (4S). J Fluen Disord. 2015;43:17–27. https://doi.org/10.1016/j.jfludis.2014.12.002
9. Cheslack-Postava K, Jordan-Young RM. Autism spectrum disorders: toward a gendered embodiment model. Soc Sci Med. 2012;74(11):1667–74. https://doi.org/10.1016/j.socscimed.2011.06.013
10. Christensen DL. Prevalence and characteristics of autism spectrum disorder among children aged 8 years—Autism and Developmental Disabilities Monitoring Network, 11 Sites, United States, 2012. MMWR. Surveillance Summaries, 65. 2016. Retrieved from http://www.cdc.gov/mmwr/volumes/65/ss/ss6503a1.htm.
11. Clark HH, Fox Tree JE. Using uh and um in spontaneous speaking. Cognition. 2002;84(1):73–111.
12. Clark CE, Conture EG, Walden TA & Lambert WE. Speech-Language Dissociations, Distractibility, and Childhood Stuttering. American Journal of Speech-Language Pathology. 2015:24(3)480. https://doi.org/10.1044/2015_AJSLP-14-0198.
13. Constantino JN, Charman T. Gender bias, female resilience, and the sex ratio in autism. J Am Acad Child Adolesc Psychiatry. 2012;51(8):756–8.
14. Cook J. From movement kinematics to social cognition: the case of autism. Philos Trans R Soc B. 2016;371(1693):20150372. https://doi.org/10.1098/rstb.2015.0372
15. Daniels AM, & Mandell DS. Explaining differences in age at autism spectrum disorder diagnosis: a critical review. Autism. 2013;1362361313480277.
16. De Marchena A, Eigsti I-M. The art of common ground: emergence of a complex pragmatic language skill in adolescents with autism spectrum disorders. J Child Lang. 2016;43(01):43–80. https://doi.org/10.1017/S0305000915000070
17. Eagly AH, Wood W. The origins of sex differences in human behavior: evolved dispositions versus social roles. Am Psychol. 1999;54(6):408–23. https://doi.org/10.1037/0003-066X.54.6.408
18. Elliott CD. Differential Ability Scales®-II-DAS-II. San Antonio: Harcourt Assessment; 2007. Retrieved from http://www.pearsonclinical.com/education/products/100000468/differential-ability-scales-ii-das-ii.html
19. Elsabbagh M, Divan G, Koh Y-J, Kim YS, Kauchali S, Marcín C, et al. Global prevalence of autism and other pervasive developmental disorders: global epidemiology of autism. Autism Res. 2012;5(3):160–79. https://doi.org/10.1002/aur.239
20. Field A. Discovering statistics using IBM SPSS statistics. 4th ed. London, England: SAGE Publications Inc.; 2005. Retrieved from https://us.sagepub.com/en-us/nam/discovering-statistics-using-ibm-spss-statistics/book238032%20.
21. Fox Tree JE. Listeners' uses of um and uh in speech comprehension. Mem Cogn. 2001;29(2):320–6. https://doi.org/10.3758/BF03194926
22. Gabel RM. Effects of stuttering severity and therapy involvement on attitudes towards people who stutter. J Fluen Disord. 2006;31(3):216–27. https://doi.org/10.1016/j.jfludis.2006.05.003
23. Goldman S. Opinion: sex, gender and the diagnosis of autism—a biosocial view of the male preponderance. Res Autism Spectrum Disord. 2013;7(6): 675–9. https://doi.org/10.1016/j.rasd.2013.02.006
24. Gorman K, Olson L, Hill AP, Lunsford R, Heeman PA, & van Santen JPH. "Uh" and "um" in children with autism spectrum disorders or language impairment. Autism Res. 2016, n/a-n/a. https://doi.org/10.1002/aur.1578.
25. Gotham K, Pickles A, Lord C. Standardizing ADOS scores for a measure of severity in autism spectrum disorders. J Autism Dev Disord. 2009;39(5):693–705. https://doi.org/10.1007/s10803-008-0674-3
26. Heeman PA, Lunsford R, Selfridge E, Black L, Van Santen J. Autism and interactional aspects of dialogue. In Proceedings of the 11th Annual Meeting of the Special Interest Group on Discourse and Dialogue. Association for Computational Linguistics. 2010. pp. 249–52. Retrieved from http://dl.acm.org/citation.cfm?id=1944551.
27. Hus V, Gotham K, & Lord C. Standardizing ADOS domain scores: separating severity of social affect and restricted and repetitive behaviors. J Autism Dev Disord. 2012. https://doi.org/10.1007/s10803-012-1719-1.
28. Irvine CA, Eigsti I-M, Fein DA. Uh, um, and autism: filler disfluencies as pragmatic markers in adolescents with optimal outcomes from autism spectrum disorder. J Autism Dev Disord. 2016;46(3):1061–70. https://doi.org/10.1007/s10803-015-2651-y
29. Kim SH, Lord C. The behavioral manifestations of autism spectrum disorders. In The neuroscience of autism spectrum disorders. Elsevier. 2013. pp. 25–37.

Retrieved from http://linkinghub.elsevier.com/retrieve/pii/B9780123919243000028.
30. Kopp S, Gillberg C. Girls with social deficits and learning problems: autism, atypical Asperger syndrome of a variant of these conditions. Eur Child Adolesc Psychiatry. 1992;1(2):89–99. https://doi.org/10.1007/BF02091791
31. Kopp S, Gillberg C. The Autism Spectrum Screening Questionnaire (ASSQ)-Revised Extended Version (ASSQ-REV): an instrument for better capturing the autism phenotype in girls? A preliminary study involving 191 clinical cases and community controls. Res Dev Disabil. 2011;32(6):2875–88. https://doi.org/10.1016/j.ridd.2011.05.017
32. Kreiser NL, White SW. ASD in females: are we overstating the gender difference in diagnosis? Clin Child Fam Psychol Rev. 2014;17(1):67–84. https://doi.org/10.1007/s10567-013-0148-9
33. Lai M-C, Lombardo MV, Auyeung B, Chakrabarti B, Baron-Cohen S. Sex/gender differences and autism: setting the scene for future research. J Am Acad Child Adolesc Psychiatry. 2015;54(1):11–24.
34. Lai M-C, Lombardo MV, Pasco G, Ruigrok ANV, Wheelwright SJ, Sadek SA, et al. A behavioral comparison of male and female adults with high functioning autism spectrum conditions. PLoS One. 2011;6(6):e20835. https://doi.org/10.1371/journal.pone.0020835
35. Lake JK, Humphreys KR, Cardy S. Listener vs. speaker-oriented aspects of speech: studying the disfluencies of individuals with autism spectrum disorders. Psychon Bull Rev. 2011;18(1):135–40. https://doi.org/10.3758/s13423-010-0037-x
36. Lehnhardt F-G, Falter CM, Gawronski A, Pfeiffer K, Tepest R, Franklin J, Vogeley K. Sex-related cognitive profile in autism spectrum disorders diagnosed late in life: implications for the female autistic phenotype. J Autism Dev Disord. 2016; 46(1):139–54. https://doi.org/10.1007/s10803-015-2558-7
37. Liberman M. Young men talk like old women. 2005. Retrieved August 3, 2016, from http://itre.cis.upenn.edu/~myl/languagelog/archives/002629.html.
38. Liberman M. More on UM and UH. 2014. Retrieved June 17, 2017, from http://languagelog.ldc.upenn.edu/nll/?p=13713.
39. Loucks TMJ, De Nil LF & Sasisekaran J. Jaw-phonatory coordination in chronic developmental stuttering. Journal of Communication Disorders. 2007;40(3):257–272. https://doi.org/10.1016/j.jcomdis.2006.06.016.
40. Loomes R, Hull L, Mandy WPL. What is the male-to-female ratio in autism spectrum disorder? A systematic review and meta-analysis. J Am Acad Child Adolesc Psychiatry. 2017;56(6):466–74. https://doi.org/10.1016/j.jaac.2017.03.013
41. Lord C, Rutter M, DiLavore PS, Risi S, Gotham K, Bishop SL. Autism diagnostic observation schedule, second edition (ADOS-2). Torrance: Western Psychological Services; 2012.
42. MacFarlane H, Gorman K, Ingham R, Presmanes Hill A, Papadakis K, Kiss G, van Santen J. Quantitative analysis of disfluency in children with autism spectrum disorder or language impairment. PLoS One. 2017;12(3):e0173936. https://doi.org/10.1371/journal.pone.0173936
43. Max L & Gracco VL. Coordination of Oral and Laryngeal Movements in the Perceptually Fluent Speech of Adults Who Stutter. Journal of Speech, Language, and Hearing Research 2005;48(3):524–542. https://doi.org/10.1044/1092-4388(2005/036).
44. Messinger DS, Young GS, Webb SJ, Ozonoff S, Bryson SE, Carter A, et al. Early sex differences are not autism-specific: a Baby Siblings Research Consortium (BSRC) study. Mol Autism. 2015;6(1):32. https://doi.org/10.1186/s13229-015-0027-y
45. Panico J, Healey EC, Brouwer K, Susca M. Listener perceptions of stuttering across two presentation modes: a quantitative and qualitative approach. J Fluen Disord. 2005;30(1):65–85. https://doi.org/10.1016/j.jfludis.2005.01.003
46. Rutter M, Bailey A, Lord C. SCQ: The Social Communication Questionnaire. Los Angeles: Western Psychological Services; 2003. Retrieved from https://www.wpspublish.com/store/Images/Downloads/Product/SCQ_Manual_Chapter_1.pdf.
47. Rutter M, Le Couteur A, Lord C. Autism diagnostic interview-revised. Los Angeles: Western Psychological Services; 2003.
48. Rynkiewicz A, Schuller B, Marchi E, Piana S, Camurri A, Lassalle A, Baron-Cohen S. An investigation of the 'female camouflage effect' in autism using a computerized ADOS-2 and a test of sex/gender differences. Molecular Autism. 2016;7(1) https://doi.org/10.1186/s13229-016-0073-0
49. Sandin S, Lichtenstein P, Kuja-Halkola R, Larsson H, Hultman C, Reichenberg A. The familial risk of autism. JAMA. 2014;311(17):1770–7. https://doi.org/10.1001/jama.2014.4144
50. Scaler Scott K, Tetnowski JA, Flaitz JR, Yaruss JS. Preliminary study of disfluency in school-aged children with autism: disfluency in autism. Int J Lang Commun Disord. 2014;49(1):75–89. https://doi.org/10.1111/1460-6984.12048
51. Shriberg LD, Paul R, McSweeny JL, Klin A, Cohen DJ, Volkmar FR. Speech and prosody characteristics of adolescents and adults with high-functioning autism and Asperger syndrome. J Speech Lang Hear Res. 2001;44(5):1097–115.
52. Sparrow SS, Cicchetti D, & Balla DA. Vineland Adaptive Behavior Scales, Second Edition (VinelandTM-II). Pearson. 2005.
53. Starkweather WC. Fluency and stuttering (Vol. xiv). Englewood Cliffs: Prentice-Hall, Inc.; 1987.
54. Suh J, Eigsti I-M, Naigles L, Barton M, Kelley E, Fein D. Narrative Performance of optimal outcome children and adolescents with a history of an autism spectrum disorder (ASD). J Autism Dev Disord. 2014;44(7):1681–94. https://doi.org/10.1007/s10803-014-2042-9
55. Smith, A., Goffman, L., Sasisekaran, J., & Weber-Fox, C. (2012). Language and motor abilities of preschool children who stutter: Evidence from behavioral and kinematic indices of nonword repetition performance. Journal of Fluency Disorders, 37(4), 344–358. https://doi.org/10.1016/j.jfludis.2012.06.001.
56. Smits-Bandstra S & De Nil L. Speech skill learning of persons who stutter and fluent speakers under single and dual task conditions. - PubMed - NCBI. Clinical Linguistics & Phonetics. 2009;23(1):38–57. https://doi.org/10.1080/02699200802394914.
57. Webster, WG. Principles of human brain organization related to lateralization of language and speech motor functions in normal speakers and stutterers. In: Hulstijn W, Peters HFM, van Lieshout PHHM, editors. Speech production: Motor control, brain research and fluency disorders. Amsterdam, The Netherlands: Elsevier; 1997. pp. 119–139.
58. WHO. Glossary of terms and tools. (n.d.). Retrieved July 5, 2016, from http://www.who.int/entity/gender-equity-rights/knowledge/glossary/en/index.html
59. Wieling M, Grieve J, Bouma G, Fruehwald J, Coleman J, Liberman M. Variation and change in the use of hesitation markers in Germanic languages. Lang Dyn Change. 2016;6(2):199–234.
60. Yuan J, Liberman M. Investigating consonant reduction in Mandarin Chinese with improved forced alignment. In INTERSPEECH. 2015. pp. 2675–8. Retrieved from https://www.ldc.upenn.edu/sites/www.ldc.upenn.edu/files/interspeech2015-mandarin-consonant-reduction.pdf

Critical region within 22q11.2 linked to higher rate of autism spectrum disorder

Caitlin C. Clements[1,2*†], Tara L. Wenger[1,3†], Alisa R. Zoltowski[1,4], Jennifer R. Bertollo[1], Judith S. Miller[1,5], Ashley B. de Marchena[1,6], Lauren M. Mitteer[7], John C. Carey[8], Benjamin E. Yerys[1,5], Elaine H. Zackai[7], Beverly S. Emanuel[7], Donna M. McDonald-McGinn[7] and Robert T. Schultz[1,5,7]

Abstract

Background: Previous studies have reported no clear critical region for medical comorbidities in children with deletions or duplications of 22q11.2. The purpose of this study was to evaluate whether individuals with small nested deletions or duplications of the LCR-A to B region of 22q11.2 show an elevated rate of autism spectrum disorder (ASD) compared to individuals with deletions or duplications that do not include this region.

Methods: We recruited 46 patients with nested deletions ($n = 33$) or duplications ($n = 13$) of 22q11.2, including LCR-A to B ($n_{del} = 11$), LCR-A to C ($n_{del} = 4$), LCR-B to D ($n_{del} = 14$; $n_{dup} = 8$), LCR-C to D ($n_{del} = 4$; $n_{dup} = 2$), and smaller nested regions ($n = 3$). Parent questionnaire, record review, and, for a subset, in-person evaluation were used for ASD diagnostic classification. Rates of ASD in individuals with involvement of LCR-B to LCR-D were compared with Fisher's exact test to LCR-A to LCR-B for deletions, and to a previously published sample of LCR-A to LCR-D for duplications. The rates of medical comorbidities and psychiatric diagnoses were determined from questionnaires and chart review. We also report group mean differences on psychiatric questionnaires.

Results: Individuals with deletions involving LCR-A to B showed a 39–44% rate of ASD compared to 0% in individuals whose deletions did not involve LCR-A to B. We observed similar rates of medical comorbidities in individuals with involvement of LCR-A to B and LCR-B to D for both duplications and deletions, consistent with prior studies.

Conclusions: Children with nested deletions of 22q11.2 may be at greater risk for autism spectrum disorder if the region includes LCR-A to LCR-B. Replication is needed.

Keywords: 22q11.2 deletion syndrome, 22q11.2 duplication syndrome, Autism spectrum disorder, *RANBP1*, Screening, Atypical, Nested, Syndromic autism, Prosopagnosia, Face processing

Background

22q11.2 deletion syndrome (22q11.2DS), also known as DiGeorge or velocardiofacial syndrome, is the most common microdeletion syndrome in humans. The 3 Mb region most frequently affected in 22q11.2DS can also be duplicated, resulting in 22q11.2 duplication syndrome (22q11.2DupS) [1]. Previous studies suggested a prevalence of 1 in 4000 live births for 22q11.2DS, but a recent study of consecutive pregnancies found an incidence of 1 in 992 live births––similar to that of trisomy 21 [2]. The incidence of 22q11.2DupS was found to be 1 in 850 [2].

The 22q11.2 region includes low copy repeats (LCRs or segmental duplication blocks) interspersed throughout the region that frequently result in "breakpoints" for a duplication or deletion. The most commonly duplicated or deleted region spans LCR-A to LCR-D (hereafter––"classic" deletion/duplication). However, smaller nested deletions occur in 15% of affected individuals and usually stretch from only LCR-A to LCR-B, or from LCR-B to LCR-D, but can also span LCR-A to LCR-C or LCR-C to LCR-D [3]. In other cases, deletions include the area upstream of LCR-A or extend past LCR-D (see Fig. 1). The diagnoses of 22q11.2DS or 22q11.2DupS can refer to patients with either a classic or nested deletion/duplication.

* Correspondence: Clements@sas.upenn.edu
†Equal contributors
[1]Center for Autism Research, The Children's Hospital of Philadelphia, 2716 South Street, Philadelphia, PA 19104, USA
[2]Department of Psychology, University of Pennsylvania, 3720 Walnut Street, Philadelphia, PA 19104, USA
Full list of author information is available at the end of the article

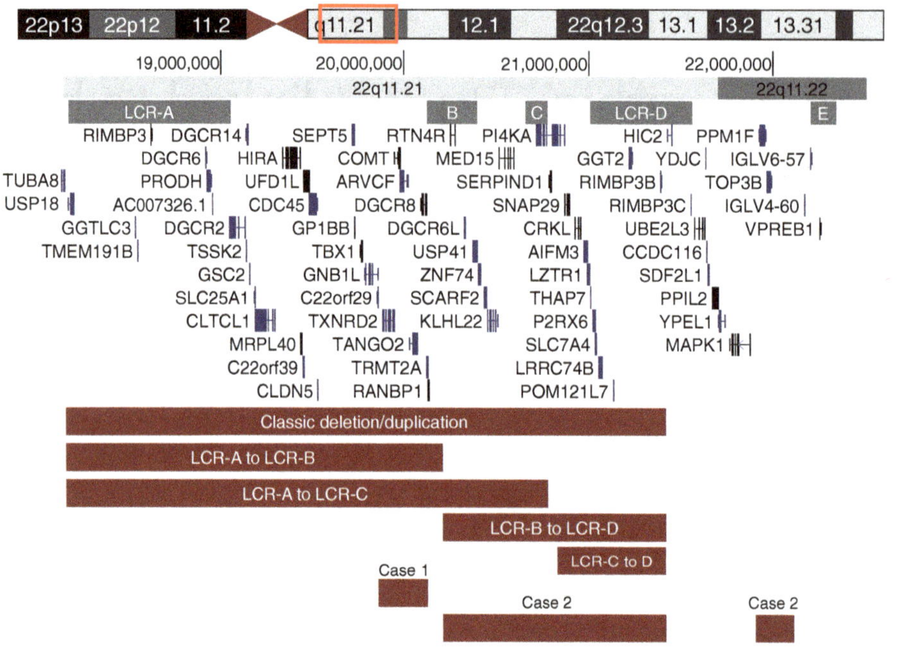

Fig. 1 22q11.2 diagram. Genes and low-copy repeat ("LCR") regions in the 22q11.2 region. Red bars depict deletions or duplications of participants. From GENCODE v24 genes in UCSC genome browser, December 2013 Assembly (genome.ucsc.edu)

The phenotypes of 22q11.2DS and 22q11.2DupS overlap with one another and show significant individual differences [4, 5]. The syndromes can affect almost any organ system, and individuals can present with diverse constellations of medical issues and structural malformations, as well as a wide range of severity. Common medical comorbidities include congenital heart disease, hypocalcemia, renal abnormalities, immune deficiencies, and neuropsychiatric differences [1]. There is a recognizable facial gestalt in 22q11.2DS, but no recognizable gestalt has been identified in 22q11.2DupS. The rate of medical problems is much lower in 22q11.2DupS [6].

The 22q11.2 region has also been associated with elevated rates of autism spectrum disorder (from now on referred to as "ASD"), attention deficit/hyperactivity disorder (ADHD), and most notably, schizophrenia. A recent large study of 22q11.2DS reported psychosis in 41% of adults and ADHD in 37% of children [7], although a psychiatric registry-based study found lower rates [8]. Interestingly, there are no reported individuals with 22q11.2DupS with schizophrenia, and one group even suggested that it may be protective for schizophrenia [9]. In contrast, an elevated risk of ASD is found in both 22q11.2DS and 22q11.2DupS. As many as 50% of individuals with 22q11.2DS and 38% with 22q11.2DupS have received community diagnoses of autism spectrum disorder; however, fewer meet strict diagnostic criteria in research settings with reported rates of 0–18% in 22q11.2DS [10–12] and 14–25% in 22q11.2DupS [6].

Despite significant heterogeneity in the 22q11.2 phenotype [13], little is known about critical regions that may confer risk for any specific part of the phenotype beyond schizophrenia, cleft palate, and cardiac anomalies. Prior reports point to *TBX1*, *CRKL*, and *MAPK1* as contributors to the cardiac [14–18] and cleft palate phenotypes [19] in 22q11.2DS. Other research linked schizophrenia risk in 22q11.2DS to hyperprolinemia associated with lowered expression of proline dehydrogenase (*PRODH*) [20, 21]. Some studies reported an association between schizophrenia risk in 22q11.2DS and the lower activity Met allele of catechol-O-methyltransferase (*COMT*) [20, 22, 23], but larger cohort studies found no evidence [24–26] (for review, see [27]). These risk genes span the 22q11.2 region, with *COMT*, *PRODH*, and *TBX1* lying between LCR-A and LCR-B, while *CRKL* lies between LCR-C and LCR-D, and *MAPK1* lies between LCR-D and LCR-E.

Recent research identified two genes as potential mediators of the ASD risk in 22q11.2DS. Radoeva et al. reported that in a sample of 87 individuals with 22q11.2DS, individuals with ASD were more likely to carry both the low-activity alleles of *COMT* and *PRODH* (leading to high levels of proline) than individuals without ASD [28]. Neither gene individually showed a significant direct relationship with ASD, although the pattern trended in that direction. Hidding et al. further demonstrated a quantitative relationship between ASD symptom severity and the combination of *COMT*-Met genotype and high proline levels in 45 individuals with

22q11.2DS with and without ASD [29]. Both results suggest that the interaction between *COMT* and *PRODH*, which lie in the LCR-A to B region, may increase ASD risk in individuals with 22q11.2DS.

The purpose of the present study was to leverage a novel study design to determine whether risk for autism can be narrowed to the LCR-A to LCR-B region within 22q11.2. Owing to the rarity of these nested structural variants, this is the first study to our knowledge that attempts to collect and phenotype large enough samples to test this hypothesis. We hypothesized that individuals harboring deleted LCR-A to LCR-B would show higher rates of ASD [30]; in addition to this region harboring *COMT* and *PRODH*, it also contains *RANBPI*, a gene involved in the metabotropic glutamate receptor (mGluR) gene network that we previously hypothesized could play a role in ASD in 22q11.2DS/DupS [30]. In addition, we describe two case studies (one from our cohort and one from the literature) with much smaller, atypical duplications within the LCR-A to B region to gain hints as to the role of specific genes.

Methods

Participants

Participants with nested 22q11.2 duplications or deletions

Participants included 43 individuals with a nested duplication (n = 13) or deletion (n = 30) of 22q11.2 that lay entirely within LCR-A to LCR-D but was not completely inclusive of LCR-A to LCR-D (see Table 1). The only exception to this was one participant who carried a duplication of LCR-B to LCR-D and also a very small duplication between LCR-E and LCR-F. Participants were recruited from a specialty clinic at The Children's Hospital of Philadelphia (CHOP) or were referred from a similar specialty clinic at another institution. The CHOP "22q and You" clinic represents the largest single-site 22q11.2 clinic in the world and maintains a large catchment area across the eastern US, with patients concentrated within a few hundred mile radius of CHOP. The sample includes probands who came to clinical attention, as well as their affected siblings (n = 2 with duplication and n = 3 with deletion) and parents (n = 2 with duplication and n = 2 with deletion) whose 22q11.2DS or 22q11.2DupS was identified after the proband's diagnostic process. The duplication or deletion was confirmed using single nucleotide polymorphism (SNP) microarray or Multiplex Ligation Probe Amplification (MLPA).

Samples whose copy number variations (CNVs) were tested by MLPA were examined using the SALSA P250 DiGeorge diagnostic probe kit (MRC-Holland, Amsterdam, The Netherlands). Commercially available software, Gene Marker from SoftGenetics (State College, PA), was used to analyze the data. Gene Marker has developed a completely integrated application for MLPA analysis with integrated functions specific for the analysis of data derived from MLPA reactions. Samples whose CNVs were identified by SNP array were analyzed using the Affymetrix SNP Array 6.0 platform following the manufacturer's instructions (Affymetrix, Santa Clara, CA, USA). Quality control values were calculated in Affymetrix Genotyping Console (Affymetrix), and any samples with contrast QC greater than 0.4 or mean absolute pairwise difference (MAPD) greater than 0.35 were excluded from further analysis. The B allele frequency and log R ratio plots were visualized using the Affymetrix Chromosome Analysis Suite to support CNV calls.

Table 1 Descriptive characteristics of all participants in study

Region	Number	% de novo[a]	Age mean (sd)	Age range (years)	% male
Total	46	60%	10.8(10.1)	0.8–39	52%
AB/AC deletion group	15	86%	8.9(4.2)	2–15	53%
A-B deletion	11	80%	7.8(3.8)	2–15	55%
A-C deletion	4	100%	11.8(4.4)	5–14	50%
BD/CD deletion group	18	69%	11.1(10.7)	1–38	50%
B-D deletion	14	77%	10.4(9.0)	1–38	43%
C-D deletion	4	33%	13.6(16.9)	0.8–36	75%
BD/CD duplication group	10	13%	14.5(15.2)	1–39	60%
B-D duplication	8	0%	16.5(16.6)	1–39	63%
C-D duplication	2	50%	6.5(2.0)	5–7	50%
A-B duplication[b]	1	Unknown	7.0	–	0%
E-F duplication[b]	2	0%	6.6(2.8)	4–8	50%

Participant characteristics for all individuals with a nested deletion or duplication of 22q11.2, including three case studies with atypical nested duplications noted with superscript *b*

[a]Percentage of individuals with known inheritance

[b]Case studies not included in statistical analysis, medical chart review, or AB/AC and BD/CD group totals

Three additional patients who carried very small and rare atypical duplications are included in this paper in a descriptive manner (in the case study sections), but are not combined with the other groups in tables, figures, or statistical analyses. One patient carried a very small duplication within LCR-A to LCR-B. The other two patients (who were related to three patients in the main LCR-B to D duplication group) carried a small duplication nested between LCR-E and LCR-F.

All 43 participants were included in the medical history chart review. Nine participants were excluded from the ASD and psychiatric symptom analyses (n = 34; see Fig. 2) for two types of reasons: (1) ASD classification could not be determined (n = 2; see below) or (2) if they presented with another medical issue likely to affect brain development (n = 2 extreme prematurity and/or birth weight < 5th centile, n = 2 with CEDNIK syndrome, n = 1 with 16p11.2 deletion which is independently associated with ASD, n = 2 history of hypoxic brain injury) [31–34]. Participant characteristics of the sample excluding these nine cases are described in Table 2. Please note that some ages differ from those in the medical record review (Table 1) because a review of updated records pertinent to ASD classification, when available, was conducted 3 years later to allow for infants to reach the age (3 years) at which ASD symptoms would be present.

Rates of autism were analyzed separately for individuals with nested deletions and duplications (see Table 3). Only one individual per family (the proband) was included to avoid confounding autism rates with risk factors shared by related individuals. In one family with B-D duplication, we included an affected family member instead of the proband because the proband harbored a 16p11.2 deletion. For deletions, 20 individuals were included after excluding five parents and younger siblings (2 B-D, 2 C-D, 1 A-B). For duplications, five individuals were included after excluding four parents and younger siblings (4 B-D). No individuals presented with nested duplications involving LCR-A to LCR-B or C.

Comparison cohorts

We compiled comparison questionnaire data from four cohorts. Detailed results of medical system chart review, neuropsychiatric questionnaires, ASD symptoms, and adaptive functioning of these four comparison groups have been published elsewhere [6]. Two cohorts were drawn from patients at the same clinic who had a

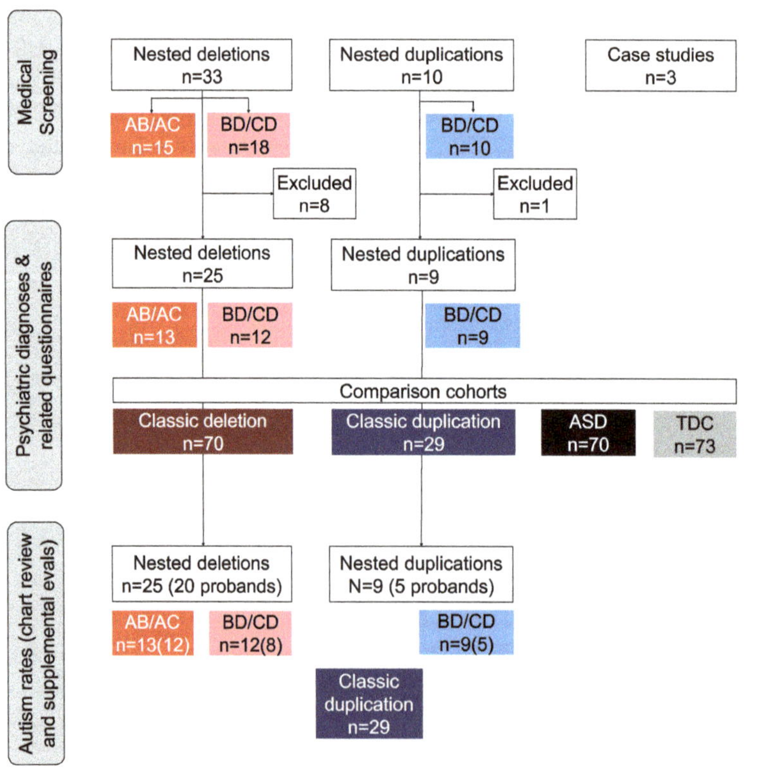

Fig. 2 Participant flow chart depicting the participants and comparisons included in each portion of the study. Group colors correspond to colors in Figs. 3 and 4 and Additional file 2. Abbreviations: *AB/AC* deletion or duplication spanning LCR-A to LCR-B or LCR-A to LCR-C, *ASD* non-syndromic autism spectrum disorder, *BD/CD* deletion or duplication spanning LCR-B to LCR-D or LCR-C to LCR-D, *classic deletion* typical 22q11.2 deletion syndrome involving LCR-A to D, *classic duplication* typical 22q11.2 duplication syndrome involving LCR-A to D, *LCR* low-copy repeat region, *TDC* typically developing controls

Table 2 Descriptive characteristics of participants included in psychiatric diagnosis rates

Region	Number	% de novo[a]	Age mean (sd)	Age range (years)	% male
AB/AC deletion group	13	83%	10 (4.2)	5–18	54%
A-B deletion	10	78%	8.9 (3.6)	5–15	60%
A-C deletion	3	100%	13.7 (4.8)	9–18	33%
BD/CD deletion group	12	50%	14.2 (12.7)	3–42	50%
B-D deletion	8	57%	13.4 (12.1)	4–42	38%
C-D deletion	4	33%	15.9 (15.5)	3–37	75%
BD/CD duplication group	9	14%	16.9 (14.7)	5–39	56%
B-D duplication	7	0%	19.4 (15.9)	5–39	57%
C-D duplication	2	50%	8 (4.1)	5–11	50%
Total	34	55%	13.3 (11.0)	3–42	53%

Participant characteristics for the subset of individuals with a nested deletion or duplication of 22q11.2 included in description of psychiatric diagnosis rates
[a]Percentage of individuals with known inheritance

confirmed classic (LCR-A to LCR-D) 22q11.2 duplication (n = 29) or deletion (n = 70). A non-syndromic ASD cohort (n = 70) and typically developing control cohort (n = 73) were drawn from other studies of neurodevelopment at the CHOP Center for Autism Research. These four cohorts were age- and sex-matched to one another but were not as well matched to either of the small nested samples described above to allow for inclusion of all eligible individuals with a nested CNV.

Informed consent was obtained for all 22q11.2 participants, as well as for all participants in the comparison cohorts (Institutional Review Board protocols #13-101307, #09-007275, #07-005689, and #10-007622).

Procedures

We collected data from record review, questionnaires administered remotely, and, for a subset, an autism-specific evaluation. Record review included the participant's electronic health record at CHOP whenever possible, as well as external medical and educational records (e.g., IEP evaluations) provided by families for individuals who did not receive routine medical care at our institution.

Medical record and developmental history review

Medical and developmental history was obtained from a questionnaire completed by the participant. A licensed pediatrician and medical geneticist (TLW) reviewed clinic notes, progress reports, radiology reports, laboratory reports, etc. in each participant's record to confirm key components reported by participants. Psychiatric and neurodevelopmental diagnostic history was documented in this process as it is routinely collected during clinical visits. Families were contacted by phone to resolve questions or discrepancies.

ASD diagnostic classification

Sources of diagnostic information Given that our hypotheses concerned rates of ASD, particular care was given to the ASD classification process. We assigned

Table 3 ASD rates among probands

Region	Number	n ASD (male)	% de novo[a]	Age mean (sd)	Age range (years)	% male
AB/AC deletion group	12	5(3)	90%	10.0 (4.4)	5–18	58%
A-B deletion	9	4(3)	90%	8.7 (3.7)	5–15	67%
A-C deletion	3	1(0)	100%	13.7 (4.8)	9–18	33%
BD/CD deletion group	8	0	60%	10.5 (4.8)	5–18	25%
B-D deletion	6	0	70%	10.2 (3.8)	6–17	17%
C-D deletion	2	0	0%	11.6 (9.1)	5–18	50%
Classic AD duplication	29	7(5)	67%	7.1 (3.4)	2–13	75%
BD/CD duplication group	5	1(0)	30%	12.7 (10.4)	5–31	60%
B-D duplication	3	1(0)	0%	15.8 (13.1)	7–31	67%
C-D duplication	2	0	50%	8.0 (4.1)	5–11	50%

Participant characteristics and autism diagnosis for all probands with a nested deletion of 22q11.2. Individuals harboring an AB or AC deletion presented with ASD at a rate of 41.6% (5 of 12). Case studies are excluded from this table
[a]Percentage of individuals with known inheritance

diagnostic status after a thorough record review of clinical, research, and educational records provided by families and available in the CHOP electronic health record. Participants differed in the frequency with which they received documented CHOP care. Continuous longitudinal data from CHOP developmental pediatricians and psychiatrists existed for individuals who lived locally, whereas records of individuals who lived further away or moved sometimes contained only the initial "22q and You" clinic evaluation. Participants were also asked to provide external medical and educational records.

All families were invited for an in-person ASD evaluation using the Autism Diagnostic Observation Schedule (ADOS and ADOS-2), parent interview, and IQ testing to complete a DSM-5 (*Diagnostic and Statistical Manual of Mental Illness*, 5th edition) checklist [35, 36]. However, since many of our families lived far away, this proved infeasible for a large percentage of the cases. Families who could not complete an in-person evaluation were invited for an hour-long parent phone interview with a clinician asking follow-up questions to Social Communication Questionnaire, Lifetime (SCQ) responses to complete an accurate DSM-5 checklist [35, 36].

"ASD" group We assigned participants to the "ASD" group if there was documentation of an ASD diagnosis (n = 5 deletions, n = 1 duplication). Five individuals had a diagnostic evaluation in their record; one did not, but had frequent references to the ASD diagnosis throughout the record. All participants scored above threshold (15) on the SCQ.

"No ASD" group We assigned "No ASD" (n = 20 deletions, n = 8 duplications) if ASD had been considered but specifically ruled out (n = 13 deletions, n = 3 duplications), or if there was no indication of ASD concerns in the available records (n = 7 deletions, n = 5 duplications). Two individuals (both LCR-B to D deletions) were excluded because a referral for an ASD evaluation had been recommended recently but not completed.

The *absence* of parental or professional concern about ASD is not routinely documented. Thus, we further investigated this group to determine whether there was a true absence of concern, or a lack of information. We studied parent/spouse report, provider report, behavioral descriptions, and referral history. The 22q clinic routinely refers to developmental behavioral pediatrics or psychiatry if parents indicate relevant concerns during intake, but parents without those concerns would not have had these appointments scheduled. The 22q clinic also routinely questions parents regarding developmental history and previous concern of psychiatric diagnoses from school or medical professionals, as this patient population is at high risk for psychosis and other psychiatric disorders. Any concerns and prior assessments are documented in detail. Therefore, we feel confident that families were routinely asked about developmental concerns and thus that a lack of referrals and text about concerns is a reasonably robust indicator of a lack of ASD concerns.

Neuropsychiatric questionnaires

We collected neuropsychiatric questionnaire data from participants under age 18. Questionnaires included a measure of adaptive functioning (Vineland Adaptive Behavior Scales–2nd Edition, "Vineland-II," completed for participants 0–18 years old [37]), a screener for psychiatric disorders based on DSM-IV checklists (Child and Adolescent Symptom Inventory-4R, "CASI-4R," completed for participants 5–18 years old depending on disorder [38]), and two measures of social behavior and autistic symptoms (Social Communication Questionnaire––Lifetime, "SCQ," completed for participants four and above [39], and the Social Responsiveness Scale or Social Responsiveness Scale, 2nd edition, "SRS-2" for participants 2.5–18 years old [40, 41]). Every questionnaire offers excellent psychometric properties, and all but the Social Communication Questionnaire provide standardized scores based on a large, representative norming sample. Please see Additional file 1 for characteristics of subsamples that completed each questionnaire.

Analysis

ASD rate To test our hypothesis that the LCR-A to LCR-B region might confer increased risk of ASD in 22q11.2 duplication and deletion syndromes, we compared ASD rates among individuals whose deletion affected the LCR-A to LCR-B region ("AB/AC group": LCR-A to B, or LCR-A to C) to individuals whose deletion did not affect the LCR-A to LCR-B region ("BD/CD group": LCR-B to D, and LCR-C to D). Thus, our first analysis compared the AB/AC group to the BD/CD group for deletions only. In a second, more conservative analysis, we compared only individuals with deletions of LCR-A to B to those with LCR-B to D (excluding cases with deleted LCR-A to C or LCR-C to D) to match the groups on approximate size and number of genes in the deletion.

Rates were compared using a one-tailed Fisher's exact test to account for cells with $n < 5$. An odds ratio (OR) cannot be computed when certain cells contain 0 observations; in these cases, we present 95% confidence intervals and p values from Fisher's exact test and effect sizes as chi-square statistics.

Our sample included no individuals with nested duplications involving LCR-A to B (i.e., no "AB/AC" group for duplications). Thus, we compared the BD/CD duplication group to individuals with the classic LCR-A to D duplication, which does involve LCR-A to B. These results are provided for descriptive purposes only due to the sample size of the nested duplications, which although is one of the largest reported, remains quite small .

Psychiatric symptoms (standardized questionnaires) In our dimensional analysis of psychiatric symptoms using questionnaire data, we analyzed raw scores on the SCQ, age-normed scores on the Vineland-II and SRS-2, and symptom composite scores on the CASI-4R. For deletions, we compared individuals in the "BD/CD" group to the AB/AC group . For duplications, we compared individual in the BD/CD group to the comparison cohort of classic duplications because our sample included no AB/AC duplications. We also compare the AB/AC deletion group to the classic deletion group as this information might prove directly useful clinically. Our interpretations focus on the size of the effect and its confidence interval, as opposed to inferential statistics, to avoid making overly strong statements based on a small sample, as suggested by many recent position papers, e.g., Button et al. [42] and Cumming et al. [43]. We present the effect sizes for each analysis and make our data available upon request so that the data generated here can be leveraged in any future meta-analyses to test our hypothesis directly.

Medical and psychiatric diagnoses We present rates of psychiatric and medical comorbidities by nested region separately for individuals who did and did not receive recommended screening. All analyses are descriptive and for characterization purposes only. Statistical significance was not tested due to small sample sizes within each nested region.

Results

Higher rates of ASD when LCR-A to B involved

We observed a trend toward a higher rate of ASD among probands with deletions in the AB/AC group (41.7%, or 5 in 12 individuals with LCR-A to B, or LCR-A to C) compared to the BD/CD group (0%, or 0 in 8 individuals with LCR-B to D, or LCR-C to D; $\chi = 4.4$, $p = 0.051$, CI 0.99, Inf; see Table 3). In a more conservative analysis that matched groups on approximate size of deleted region, we continued to observe similar rates of ASD within each group (44.4%, or 4 of 9 individuals with deletions of LCR-A to B, and 0%, or 0 in 6 individuals with deletions of LCR-B to D; $\chi = 3.64$, $p = 0.092$, CI 0.702, Inf). The rate of ASD did not change meaningfully when related individuals were included to increase sample size; the increased sample size provided more statistical power and revealed significant results ($n = 25$; 38.5% rate in AB/AC group, 0% in BD/CD group; $\chi = 5.77$, $p = 0.024$, CI 1.39, Inf). Thus, the LCR-A to B region may confer increased risk of ASD diagnosis, but a larger sample without related individuals is needed to confim.

Among duplications, individuals with the classic and BD/CD duplications showed similar rates of ASD (24.1% rate or 7 of 29 in classic group, 20% rate or 1 of 5 in BD/CD; OR = 0.79, $p = 0.764$, CI 0.03, Inf). Results did not change meaningfully when related individuals were included to increase sample size (21.4% rate in classic group, 11.1% rate or 1 of 9 in BD/CD; OR = 0.40, $p = 0.65$, CI 0.02, Inf), but this analysis in particular would benefit from a larger sample.

Our categorical analysis was supported by quantitative reports of autistic symptoms in the SRS-2 and SCQ (see Fig. 3). A subset of each group (BD/CD deletions, AB/AC deletions, BD/CD duplications, classic duplications, classic

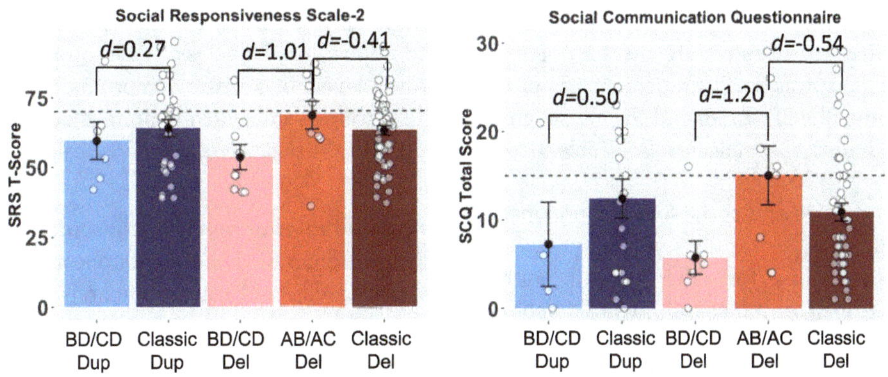

Fig. 3 Individuals with deleted LCR-A to B show higher levels of autistic symptoms. This figure depicts group means, standard errors, and the effect size of differences on two quantitative measures of autistic symptoms, the Social Responsiveness Scale-2 and the Social Communication Scale, Lifetime. Each point depicts one individual. Dashed lines indicate the threshold above which an individual is considered to screen positive for autism and warrant further evaluation. The groups with involvement of LCR-A to B show higher levels of social impairment, with large effect sizes for deletions and small to medium effect sizes for duplications. Effect sizes are not significant due to small samples (see Table 4). The AB/AC deletion group includes five individuals diagnosed with autism; the BD/CD deletion group includes zero. Abbreviations: *AB/AC* deletion spanning LCR-A to LCR-B or LCR-A to LCR-C; *BD/CD* deletion or duplication spanning LCR-B to LCR-D or LCR-C to LCR-D; *d* Cohen's *d* effect size; *del* deletion; *dup* duplication; *LCR* low-copy repeat region; *SCQ* Social Communication Questionnaire, Lifetime; *SRS* Social Responsiveness Scale

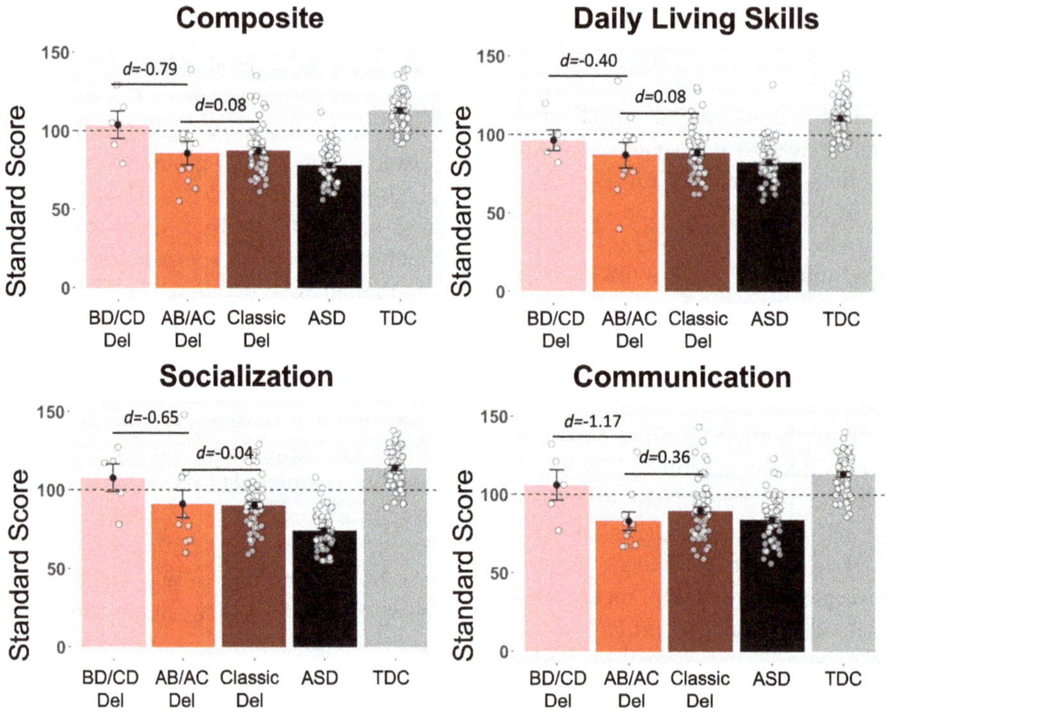

Fig. 4 Individuals with deleted LCR-A to B show modestly lower levels of adaptive functioning on the Vineland-II Adaptive Behavior Scales. This figure depicts group means, standard errors, and the effect size of differences on the Vineland-II, a measure of adaptive behavior. Each point depicts one individual). Higher scores on the Vineland-II indicate higher levels of functioning across the three domains and composite score, and standard scores are age-normed such that 100 (represented by the dashed line) indicates average. The AB/AC deletion group shows more impairment than the BD/CD nested deletions that do not involve LCR-A to B, with medium to large effect sizes; the AB/AC group also shows similar levels of impairment to the classic deletion group (deletion spanning LCR-A to D), with very small effect sizes. Abbreviations: *AB/AC* deletion spanning LCR-A to LCR-B or LCR-A to LCR-C, *ASD* individuals with non-syndromic autism spectrum disorder, *BD/CD* deletion spanning LCR-B to LCR-D or LCR-C to LCR-D, *d* Cohen's d effect size, *del* deletion, *LCR* low copy repeat region, *TDC* typically developing controls

deletions) completed the SCQ, including both individuals with and without ASD diagnoses. For deletions, the BD/CD group showed less autistic symptoms than the AB/CD group with large effect sizes (*d*'s of 1.01 and 1.20). For duplications, the difference was small-to-medium (*d*'s of 0.27 and 0.50) between the BD/CD group and the classic group. No effects reached statistical significance (see Table 4).

Moderately lower adaptive and social functioning when AB region involved

We computed effect sizes for differences in autistic symptoms, psychiatric symptoms, and adaptive behavior skills (see Figs. 3 and 4, Table 4, Additional file 2). For duplications, the differences were usually small between the BD/CD group and the classic duplication group (see Table 4, "Classic Duplication" rows). For deletions, the BD/CD group showed less impairment than the AB/AC group across most measures with medium or large effect sizes that did not reach statistical significance. We also calculated effect sizes for group differences between the AB/AC deletions and classic AD deletion groups and observed small or medium differences (see Table 4, "Classic Deletion" rows). We observed negligible differences between these two groups on most adaptive functioning scales. The classic deletion group showed slightly lower levels of autistic symptoms compared to the AB/AC group--small to medium effect sizes on the SRS-2 and SCQ--that were not statistically significant.

Increased rates of psychiatric disorders

In individuals with nested duplications or deletions, we observed elevated rates compared to population means in nearly every psychiatric disorder reported, including ADHD, OCD, ODD and related behaviors, depression, language disorders, global developmental delay, and intellectual disability. See Table 5 for observed rates of disorders by type of nested deletion or duplication.

Higher rates of medical comorbidities

We documented presence or absence of having received an appropriate screening test, and whether or not an

Table 4 Group means and effect sizes of group differences on neuropsychiatric questionnaires

	Number	Mean (SD)	*d*	95% confidence interval
SRS-2 T score		50 (10)		
BD/CD deletion	9	53.4 (13.6)		
AB/AC deletion	10	68.5 (15.7)	1.01	(− 0.07, 2.11)
Classic deletion	61	63.0 (12.6)	− 0.41	(− 1.11, 0.27)
BD/CD duplication	6	59.5 (16.6)		
Classic duplication	28	64.0 (16.3)	0.27	(− 0.67, 1.22)
SCQ raw total		Cutoff 15		
BD/CD deletion	7	5.7 (4.9)		
AB/AC deletion	8	15.0 (9.3)	1.20	(− 0.11, 2.52)
Classic deletion	52	10.8 (7.3)	− 0.54	(− 1.32, 0.23)
BD/CD duplication	4	7.2 (9.5)		
Classic duplication	22	12.4 (10.3)	0.50	(− 0.67, 1.68)
Vineland composite		100(15)		
BD/CD deletion	5	103.8 (19.6)		
AB/AC deletion	10	85.7 (24.0)	− 0.79	(− 2.11, 0.52)
Classic deletion	57	87.1 (15.9)	0.08	(− 0.61, 0.78)
BD/CD duplication	6	92.6 (18.7)		
Classic duplication	27	89.4 (19.4)	− 0.16	(− 1.11, 0.78)
Vineland communication		100(15)		
BD/CD deletion	5	106.0 (21.7)		
AB/AC deletion	10	83.0 (18.5)	− 1.17	(− 2.55, 0.20)
Classic deletion	58	89.7 (18.1)	0.36	(− 0.32, 1.06)
BD/CD duplication	6	92.1 (20.2)		
Classic duplication	27	91.2 (18.5)	− 0.04	(− 0.99, 0.90)
Vineland daily living		100(15)		
BD/CD deletion	5	96.4 (14.6)		
AB/AC deletion	10	86.9 (26.2)	− 0.40	(− 1.69, 0.87)
Classic deletion	57	88.4 (15.1)	0.08	(− 0.60, 0.78)
BD/CD duplication	6	91.8 (23.0)		
Classic duplication	28	93.6 (21.2)	0.08	(− 0.86, 1.02)
Vineland socialization		100(15)		
BD/CD deletion	5	107.6 (19.6)		
AB/AC deletion	10	91.0 (27.4)	− 0.65	(− 1.96, 0.65)
Classic deletion	57	90.1 (16.5)	− 0.04	(− 0.74, 0.64)
BD/CD duplication	6	98.1 (18.3)		
Classic duplication	27	90.8 (21.2)	− 0.35	(− 1.30, 0.60)
CASI ADHD				
BD/CD deletion	2	2.5 (1.3)		
AB/AC deletion	7	3.4 (1.4)	0.63	(− 1.56, 2.83)
Classic deletion	43	2.7 (1.2)	− 0.52	(− 1.36, 0.32)
BD/CD duplication	4	2.7 (2.1)		
Classic duplication	20	2.8 (1.3)	0.09	(− 1.09, 1.27)
CASI anxiety				
BD/CD deletion	2	1.3 (0.7)		
AB/AC deletion	7	1.9 (1.1)	0.49	(− 1.68, 2.67)
Classic deletion	43	2.3 (1.3)	0.30	(− 0.53, 1.14)
BD/CD duplication	4	1.9 (1.5)		
Classic duplication	20	1.8 (1.6)	− 0.05	(− 1.24, 1.12)
CASI ASD				
BD/CD deletion	1	n/a		
AB/AC deletion	4	1.0 (1.0)	n/a	n/a
Classic deletion	37	0.5 (0.4)	− 0.83	(− 1.94, 0.27)
BD/CD duplication	4	0.6 (0.4)		
Classic duplication	16	0.8 (0.8)	0.26	(− 0.98, 1.50)
CASI Schizoaffective				
BD/CD deletion	1	n/a		
AB/AC deletion	3	0.5(0.5)	n/a	n/a
Classic deletion	6	0.5(0.2)	− 0.09	(− 0.78, 0.61)
BD/CD duplication	0	n/a		
Classic duplication	4	0.5(0.2)	n/a	n/a
CASI behav. regulation				
BD/CD deletion	2	0.9 (0.4)		
AB/AC deletion	7	0.9 (0.6)	0.06	(− 2.08, 2.21)
Classic deletion	43	1.0 (0.6)	0.16	(− 0.67, 1.00)
BD/CD duplication	4	0.3 (0.3)		
Classic duplication	20	1.0 (0.8)	0.78	(− 0.42, 2.00)
CASI Depression				
BD/CD deletion	2	0.4 (0)		
AB/AC deletion	7	0.6 (0.7)	0.33	(− 1.82, 2.50)
Classic deletion	43	0.5 (0.7)	− 0.15	(− 0.99, 0.67)
BD/CD duplication	4	0.2 (0.4)		
Classic duplication	20	0.4 (0.4)	0.48	(− 0.70, 1.68)

Group means on neuropsychiatric questionnaires. We show 95% confidence intervals of effect sizes as Cohen's *d*, which can be interpreted as follows: 0.2 as small, 0.5 as medium, and 0.8 as large [54]. Means and standard deviations for each group are presented, as well as the mean and SD for each measure to aid in interpretation. We derived SRS T-scores using the updated SRS-2 norms for all participants, regardless of the version the participant completed. We averaged CASI-4R raw item scores on similar subscales into composites instead of using T-scores because we encountered a strong ceiling effect when using CASI-4R T-scores because CASI-4R norms collapse all high raw scores into a T-score of 70. Thus, population-normed means and standard deviations are not available for comparison for these averaged composites. For example, all items from the dysthymia subscale and major depression subscales were averaged into a "Depression" composite, after accounting for the number of items in each subscale so that both scales were weighted equally in the composite. The composites are interpreted as "3" indicating that on average, the parent endorsed symptoms in the domain as occurring "very often," 2 as "often," 1 as "sometimes," and 0 as "never"

Vineland Vineland Adaptive Behavior Scales, 2nd Edition; *CASI* Child and Adolescent Symptom Inventory-4R; *SCQ* Social Communication Questionnaire; *SRS-2* Social Responsiveness Scale, 2nd Edition; *n/a* not applicable

Table 5 Psychiatric disorder rates from parent and adult self-report and chart review

	Total (*n*)	No eval	Had eval	GDD	Lang Dx	ADHD	ID	ODD	OCD	Anxiety	MDD
AB/AC deletion	13	7.7%	92.3%	30.8%	0.0%	53.8%	0.0%	7.7%	23.1%	23.1%	0.0%
A-B deletion	10	10%	90%	30%	0%	50%	0%	10%	20%	20%	0%
< 3 yrs	1	1	0	0	0	0	0	0	0	0	0
3–14 yrs	8	0	8	2	0	4	0	0	1	1	0
15+ yrs	1	0	1	1	0	1	0	1	1	1	0
A-C deletion	3	0%	100%	33.3%	0%	66.7%	0%	0%	33.3%	33.3%	0%
3–14 yrs	1	0	1	1	0	0	0	0	0	0	0
15+ yrs	2	0	2	0	0	2	0	0	1	1	0
BD/CD deletion	12	33.3%	66.7%	16.7%	8.3%	8.3%	25%	8.3%	25%	25%	0%
B-D deletion	8	12.5%	87.5%	37.5%	0%	12.5%	12.5%	0%	0%	25%	25%
< 3 yrs	1	1	0	0	0	0	0	0	0	0	0
3–14 yrs	5	0	5	3	0	1	1	0	0	0	0
15+ yrs	2	0	2	0	0	0	0	0	0	2	2
C-D deletion	4	75%	25%	0%	0%	25%	0%	25%	25%	25%	25%
< 3 yrs	2	2	0	0	0	0	0	0	0	0	0
15+ yrs	2	1	1	0	0	1	0	1	1	1	1
BD/CD duplication	9	33.3%	66.6%	22.2%	0%	0%	44.4%	0%	11.1%	11.1%	11.1%
B-D duplication	7	42.9%	57.1%	28.6%	14.3%	28.6%	0%	0%	0%	14.3%	14.3%
< 3 yrs	1	1	0	0	0	0	0	0	0	0	0
3–14 yrs	3	0	3	2	1	1	0	0	0	1	0
15+ yrs	3	2	1	0	0	1	0	0	0	0	1
C-D duplication	2	0%	100%	100%	0%	0%	0%	0%	0%	0%	0%
3–14 yrs	2	0	2	2	0	0	0	0	0	0	0
Total sample	34	23.5%	76.5%	32.3%	2.9%	32.3%	2.9%	5.9%	11.8%	20.6%	11.8%

We observed elevated rates of psychiatric diagnoses among individuals with nested duplications or deletions relative to population base rates using parent- and self-report data confirmed in medical records. Among the full sample, 77% had received a psychiatric evaluation. The most commonly reported diagnoses in our sample included ADHD and Global Developmental Delay (GDD), which may reflect the sample's skew toward younger ages (see Table 2 for sample characteristics). We present rates for group totals, and we present *n*'s for age bins based roughly on when documentation of diagnosis would be expected (i.e., GDD and language disorders are frequently diagnosed before age 3, ADHD and ID are usually diagnosed in childhood after age 3, and depression and anxiety frequently onset during adolescence or adulthood) to facilitate interpretation of overall group rates because rates for disorders that frequently appear in adolescence (e.g., anxiety and depression) are likely underestimates

Abbreviations: *Eval* evaluation; *ADHD* attention deficit/hyperactivity disorder; *ID* intellectual disability; *OCD* obsessive compulsive disorder; *GDD* Global Developmental Delay; *Lang Dx* language disorder, receptive or expressive; *ODD* oppositional defiant disorder; *MDD* major depressive disorder; *Del* deletion; *Dup* duplication; *yrs* years

abnormality was identified, in individuals with nested deletions and duplications between LCR-A and D (see Table 6). In order to calculate conservative estimates for the prevalence of each medical comorbidity in each group, we report both the percentage of screened individuals and the percentage of total individuals.

Case study 1

Isolating specific genes: an individual with ASD and tiny duplication involving RANBP1 and COMT, not TBX1

One individual in our sample came to attention of clinical geneticists due to autism spectrum disorder and was found to have a small, 300 kb microduplication within the LCR-A to B region that included *RANBP1* and *COMT* but not *TBX1*. Detailed clinical evaluation and all recommended medical screening for individuals with 22q11.2-related disorders revealed none of the medical issues or dysmorphic features characteristic of the syndrome. However, the individual met diagnostic criteria for ASD, anxiety, and ADHD after evaluation by a neurodevelopmental pediatrician and standardized neuropsychiatric evaluation. The inheritance of this microduplication is unknown because parental testing was not possible. To our knowledge, no relatives carry an autism diagnosis but none have received formal evaluation. The individual's SNP array showed no other pathogenic variants. This individual was not included in group analyses because the duplication did not encompass the full LCR-A to B region.

Table 6 Medial comorbidities in individuals with nested deletion or duplication of 22q11.2

	A to B deletion ($n = 11$)	A to C deletion ($n = 4$)	B to D deletion ($n = 14$)	B to D duplication ($n = 8$)	C to D deletion ($n = 4$)	C to D duplication ($n = 2$)
Audiologic						
Audiogram	11	4	14	8	4	2
Abnormal	6	1	2	2	0	1
Abnormal Rate[a]	55%	25%	14%	25%	0%	50%
Abnormalities	CHL	CHL	SNHL	CHL, CSNHL	n/a	CHL
Cardiac						
Echocardiogram	9	4	11	5	2	1
Abnormal	7	3	7	1	1	0
Abnormal Rate[a]	64% (78%)	75%	50% (64%)	12% (20%)	25% (50%)	0%
Abnormalities	Enlarged PA, VR, PS, TOF with PS, IAA with ARSCA, TR, PDA	TA, RAA with ALSCA, dilated aortic root, VR, ASD/VSD	Aortic root dilation, aneurism of TV, ASD, PDA, PFO, TA, VSD	PFO	TOF with pulmonary valve stenosis	n/a
Endocrine						
Bloodwork	11	4	14	4	4	1
Abnormal	6	2	6	2	0	0
Abnormal Rate[a]	55%	50%	43%	25% (50%)	0%	0%
Abnormalities	Hypocalcemia hypothyroidism low vitamin D (each category $n = 2$)	Hypocalcemia	Hypocalcemia ($n = 2$), diabetes mellitus, borderline HbA1C, low growth factors, low vitamin D, hypothyroidism	Borderline abnormal thyroid function tests, neonatal hypoglycemia	n/a	n/a
GI						
Symptom screen	11	3	13	6	3	2
Abnormal	7	2	12	5	1	2
Abnormal rate[a]	64%	50% (67%)	86% (92%)	63% (83%)	25% (33%)	100%
Abnormalities	GERD ($n = 7$), constipation ($n = 4$), anal atresia ($n = 1$), feeding tube ($n = 2$)	Constipation ($n = 2$), GERD	GERD ($n = 11$), constipation ($n = 9$), feeding tube ($n = 4$)	GERD ($n = 4$), eosinophilic esophagitis, feeding tube	GERD, chronic constipation	GERD ($n = 2$), constipation, feeding tube
Hematologic						
CBC completed	11	4	14	8	4	2
Cytopenias	3	3	2	0	0	0
Abnormal Rate[a]	27%	75%	14%	0%	0%	0%
Immune						
Bloodwork	9	4	11	4	4	2
Abnormal	2	2	4	1	2	0

Table 6 Medial comorbidities in individuals with nested deletion or duplication of 22q11.2 *(Continued)*

	A to B deletion (n = 11)	A to C deletion (n = 4)	B to D deletion (n = 14)	B to D duplication (n = 8)	C to D deletion (n = 4)	C to D duplication (n = 2)
Abnormal Rate[a]	18% (22%)	50%	29% (36%)	13% (26%)	50%	0%
Abnormalities	Low Ig	Low Ig, T cell lymphopenia, inadequate vaccine titers	Low Ig (n = 2), absent thymus, inadequate vaccine response	Low Ig	Low Ig, recurrent MRSA infections, inadequate vaccine response	n/a
Neurologic						
Seizures	3	0	2	0	0	0
% reported	27%	0%	14%	0%	0%	0%
MRI	8	2	10	4	0	0
Abnormal MRI	3	1	3	2	n/a	n/a
Abnormal Rate[a]	27% (38%)	25% (50%)	21% (30%)	25% (50%)	0%	0%
MRI findings	Chiari 1, white matter lesions, pachygyria	Minimal bilateral congenital optic nerve hypoplasia	Chiari 1, hypoplastic corpus callosum, polymicrogyria	Prominent ventricles, subarachnoid spaces, choroid plexus cysts	n/a	n/a
Ophthalmologic						
Ophtho exam	9	4	11	3	4	1
Abnormal	3	2	5	1	0	0
Abnormal rate[a]	27% (33%)	50%	45%	13% (33%)	n/a	n/a
Abnormalities	Astigmatism, exophoria, nystagmus	Strabismus, minimal ONH	Anisocoria, iris coloboma, ONH nystagmus (n = 2), retinal detachment, strabismus (n = 3)	Amblyopia	n/a	n/a
Palate						
Clinical eval.	9	4	12	6	2	2
Abnormal	8	3	4	1	0	1
Abnormal rate[a]	89% (73%)	75% (27%)	33% (29%)	17% (13%)	0%	50%
Abnormalities	SMCP (n = 3) VPI (n = 8)	SMCP (n = 1), VPI (n = 3)	SMCP (n = 2), VPI (n = 4)	High arched palate with small uvula	n/a	VPI
Renal						
Ultrasound	9	2	9	6	2	1
Abnormal	3	0	1	4	1	0
Abnormal rate[a]	27% (33%)	0%	7% (11%)	50% (67%)	25% (50%)	0%
Abnormalities	Bilateral pelviectasis, nephrocalcinosis hydronephrosis	n/a	Medullary nephrocalcinosis	Duplicated collecting system, small kidneys (n = 3)	Solitary, low-lying kidney	n/a
Spine						
Screening x-rays	6	4	4	2	1	1

Table 6 Medial comorbidities in individuals with nested deletion or duplication of 22q11.2 *(Continued)*

	A to B deletion (n = 11)	A to C deletion (n = 4)	B to D deletion (n = 14)	B to D duplication (n = 8)	C to D deletion (n = 4)	C to D duplication (n = 2)
Abnormal	6	3	2	1	1	0
Abnormal Rate[a]	55% (100%)	38% (75%)	14% (50%)	13% (50%)	25% (100%)	0%
Abnormalities	Hypoplastic vertebra (n = 2), vertebral fusion (n = 4), extra lumbar vertebra	Fusion of C2-C3, kyphoscoliosis, thickened spinous process of C2	Scoliosis, C2-C3 fusion and dysmorphic dens, upswept C2	Hemivertebra at T9, absent rib	6 thoracic ribs and 6 lumbar vertebrae	n/a

The total number of patients in each group is designated in column headings. Each screened organ system is listed along with the number of patients who received the screening recommended for patients with classic 22q11.2 deletions and duplications. [a]We present the rate of patients with abnormal findings as a percentage of total patients. Many patients did not receive all recommended screening; when not all patients were screened, we use parentheses to note the percentage of patients with abnormal findings ofthose who received screening

Abbreviations: *ARSCA* aberrant right subclavian artery, *ALSCA* aberrant left subclavian artery, *ASD* atrial septal defect (in cardiac row only, in remainder of manuscript ASD refers to autism spectrum disorder), *CHL* conductive hearing loss, *C/SNHL* mixed conductive and sensorineural hearing loss, *GERD* gastroesophageal reflux disease, *HbA1C* hemoglobin A1C, *IAA* interrupted aortic arch, *Ig* immunoglobulins, *MRI* magnetic resonance imaging, *MRSA* methicillin-resistant *Staphylococcus aureus*, *ONH* optic nerve hypoplasia, *PA* pulmonary artery, *PDA* patent ductus arteriosus, *PFO* patent foramen ovale, *PS* pulmonic stenosis, *SMCP* submucous cleft palate, *SNHL* sensorineural hearing loss, *TA* truncus arteriosus, *TR* tricuspid regurgitation, *TOF* Tetralogy of Fallot, *TV* tricuspid valve, *VPI* velopharyngeal insufficiency, *VR* vascular ring, *VSD* ventricular septal defect, *n/a* not applicable

Case study 2

The role of background genetics: a family with LCR-B to D duplication and distal E-F duplication and autism and face processing deficits

The only individual in our analyses with autism in the BD/CD group carried a duplication of LCR-B to D. She had one sibling with the same LCR-B to D duplication and two siblings with a duplication of *TOP3B* (in a small region between LCR-E and F). One of the siblings with the *TOP3B* duplication had a history of an autism diagnosis but did not currently present with significant autism symptoms. Furthermore, the proband and the sibling with LCR-B to D duplication both showed decreased face processing abilities on the Benton Facial Recognition Test (mildly impaired in the proband, clinically impaired in the sibling). Face processing difficulties have not been reported in 22q syndromes before, and we do not posit that they are central to the syndromes, but rather that the family history of possible ASD and the genetic complexity of the family raises the question that other genetic factors may have contributed to the proband's autism. Future studies of autism in nested 22q11.2 should evaluate family members for ASD and prosopagnosia, and evaluate probands for phenotypes seen in other family members, to better understand the contribution of background genetics.

Discussion

To our knowledge, this study includes the largest group of individuals with nested deletions and duplications of 22q11.2 to be compared prospectively to classic deletions and duplications with standardized measures. These data suggest that individuals with deletion of the LCR-A to B region may have a higher rate of ASD (39–44%) than those without involvement (0%); the pattern was not replicated for duplications. Taken in conjunction with case study 1, these findings are consistent with our hypothesis that LCR-A to B may confer risk for ASD in 22q11.2 related disorders. However, we offer this evidence as preliminary support that requires further exploration with additional samples.

It is notable that the nested deletions of all individuals with ASD involved LCR-A to B and that we observed negligible differences between this group and the classic deletion spanning LCR-A to D in adaptive functioning. These results suggest that LCR-A to B could be contributing to the autistic phenotype in individuals with classic 22q11.2DS, as well as to decreased adaptive functioning. It is also notable that we observed no duplications of LCR-A to B or LCR-A to C in our full sample of 43 individuals, although such individuals are mentioned in much larger studies [44]. Thus, it remains to be tested in larger samples whether these individuals are as likely to present with ASD as those with the classic A-D duplication.

Implications for medical screening

Prior studies have suggested that individuals with nested deletions have similar types of medical problems to those with classic deletions and should receive similar clinical treatment. The medical chart review of our patients supported this hypothesis. It also suggested that our patients are representative of other previously reported patients with nested deletions with regard to the frequency and types of medical problems. It is notable that there appeared to be fewer medical problems in individuals with LCR-C to D. However, this region is much smaller, encompassing fewer genes than the other regions. In size and total number of genes, LCR-A to LCR-B and LCR-B to LCR-D are roughly equivalent, and the rates of medical comorbidities are similar. We also observed higher rates of some medical comorbidities in several of the nested groups as compared to individuals with full LCR-A to LCR-D deletions (e.g., cervical spine anomalies in 100% of screened individuals with LCR-A to LCR-B deletion), but our sample sizes are too small to determine if this is due to chance or truly represents a higher risk subgroup. We were somewhat surprised to find that many patients had not completed portions of the recommended medical screening for individuals with 22q11.2-related disorders. It is unclear if this is due to a perception by providers that individuals with nested deletions do not need as aggressive screening as those with full deletions or duplications. Overall, we observed rates of each of the medical comorbidities in the LCR-A to LCR-B and LCR-B to LCR-D subgroups that are comparable to rates in individuals with full LCR-A to LCR-D deletions or duplications. Although the rate of medical problems appears lower in the LCR-C to LCR-D deletion and duplication groups, the sample sizes are extremely small, and therefore, no strong conclusions can be made about the validity of an altered screening protocol for these patients.

RANBP1 as a potential ASD candidate gene

The LCR-A to B region associated with ASD risk in our sample involves approximately 25 genes, including *COMT*, *PRODH*, and *TBX1*. Prior research implicates the interaction of low activity *COMT* and *PRODH* alleles in ASD risk [28, 29]. Other genes in the region may also confer ASD risk, and indeed, the risk could be additive. We propose another possible candidate gene, Ran-binding protein 1 (*RANBP1*), which could not be examined given our study design with multiple candidate genes in the LCR-A to B region, warranting further investigations. We base this speculation on five circumstantial pieces of evidence.

First, we cite the involvement of *RANBP1* in the metabotropic glutamate receptor (mGluR) gene network [44], which is disrupted in two other syndromic forms of ASD, fragile X syndrome and tuberous sclerosis complex [45]. Second, we previously observed a 10-fold increase in ASD rate among individuals with 22q11.2DS with a "second hit" in an mGluR network gene compared to individuals without a "second hit" (5 affected in 25 individuals with 22q11.2 compared to 1 in 50) [30]. Third, two teratogens associated with increased rates of ASD––valproate and thalidomide––both decrease expression of *RANBP1* [46, 47, 48]. Fourth, the important link between *RANBP1* and expression in human brains was demonstrated by Meechan et al. [49], who showed higher *RANBP1* expression in developing fetal brains compared to adult brains during a peak in neurogenesis. Finally, several studies in the 22q11.2 animal literature highlight *RANBP1* as important for neural development in 22q11.2 (e.g., [49–51]). Taken together, these disparate pieces of literature converge on a role of *RANBP1* in brain development, and potentially in ASD. Like other genes and gene families recently associated with ASD, *RANBP1* serves a general function within the cell (metabolizing GTP and regulating material transport to the nucleus [52]). *RANBP1* has not been identified previously as an ASD candidate gene in large ASD studies; of the approximately 25 genes in the 22q11.2 LCR-A to LCR-B region, previous genome-wide association studies or whole exome sequencing studies have identified *PRODH* as a candidate gene with suggestive evidence and *TBX1* and *GNB1L* as candidate genes with minimal evidence at this time (SFARI gene database https://gene.sfari.org/database/human-gene/). It is not yet clear whether genes in this region modify ASD risk in the general population or in the context of 22q11.2 syndromes alone.

Insights from two case studies involving *TBX1* and *RANBP1*

Individuals with very small nested duplications and deletions offer a unique method of studying the associations between isolated regions or genes and individual features of the 22q11.2DS phenotype. In the present study, we could not tease apart the contributions of individual genes to portions of the phenotype, as the LCR-A to B region includes approximately 25 genes. Here, we contrast two case studies, case study 1 and a prior case study by Weisfeld-Adams and colleages [53], each with a very small duplication including either *TBX1* or *RANBP1*, but not both, to provide some insight into the possible relative contributions of *TBX1* and *RANBP1* to the phenotype in a descriptive fashion. Weisfeld-Adams et al. described a patient and sibling with duplication of six genes including *TBX1* but not *RANBP1*. This proband showed complex medical problems, but neither the 19-month-old proband nor the 3-year-old sibling showed any symptoms of autism or neurodevelopmental delay besides mild motor delay. (Although no concern for ASD was noted at 19 months of age, we caution against over-interpretation because ASD can be missed in toddlers when symptoms are not severe. However, by 19 months of age most children with 22q11.2DS show significant delays, little speech, and aloof social behavior, so the lack of delay suggests social development was on course.) In contrast, in case study 1, we described an individual with microduplication involving *RANBP1* but not *TBX1* who had ASD but no medical comorbidities. Both our patient, who had a purely psychiatric phenotype and duplication that *does* involve *RANBP1*, and the case presented by Weisfeld-Adams et al.––a purely medical phenotype that does *not* involve *RANBP1*––provide preliminary suggestive evidence that *RANBP1*, not *TBX1*, specifically might confer risk for ASD and other psychiatric diagnoses. Both microduplications include *COMT* and exclude *PRODH*, so we cannot speculate about the roles of these genes based on case studies.

Limitations

The two primary limitations of our study lie in the phenotyping and the sample size. This single-site study relied primarily on questionnaires and chart review, supplemented by in-person evaluation when feasible for the family. Thus, the phenotyping, while accurate, could be improved with systematic prospective evaluations. Our sample size was small, owing to the rarity of individuals with nested duplication or deletions in the 22q11.2 region. Our study would benefit from replication with a multi-site study that combines clinics around the world to improve statistical power.

Another limitation includes the unknown role of background genetics. We were unable to account for other contributors to ASD risk, such as common variants or known pathogenic variants occurring outside 22q11.2 that would be identified with whole-exome sequencing, not clinical genetic testing with MLPA and SNP arrays. However, this risk is likely to affect all groups equally. Furthermore, we believe this unknown potential risk is likely to be small compared to the known, larger ASD risk of carrying 22q11.2DS or DupS.

Future directions might involve whole-exome sequencing of 22q11.2 samples to identify other factors that contribute to ASD risk. Such a study should include an analysis leveraging the sequencing of *PRODH*, *COMT*, *RANBP1*, and *TBX1* in individuals with nested 22q11.2 deletions and duplications to isolate the influence of these mutations on the ASD phenotype.

Conclusions

We present data on medical and psychiatric issues in 44 individuals with nested duplications and deletions within the LCR-A to D region, along with two additional siblings with tiny duplication of *TOP3B*, the largest cohort of this type to be studied prospectively. We found increased rate of ASD among individuals with deleted LCR-A to B, compared to individuals whose nested deletions did not involve that region. We tentatively speculate that *RANBP1* could provide a potential mechanistic explanation for increased rates of ASD based on this finding, our reported case study, environmental ASD risk factors that also alter *RANBP1* expression, *RANBP1*'s role in the mGluR network, and the role of the mGluR network in other syndromic forms of ASD. We also conclude from our observation of the full spectrum of medical issues in each group that at this time, there is insufficient evidence to limit medical screening in individuals with nested duplications or deletions within the 22q11.2 region.

Abbreviations

22q11.2DS: 22q11.2 deletion syndrome; 22q11.2DupS: 22q11.2 duplication syndrome; ADHD: Attention-deficit/hyperactivity disorder; ADI-R: Autism Diagnostic Interview-Revised; ADOS: Autism Diagnostic Observation Schedule; ASD: Autism spectrum disorder; CASI-4R: Child and Adolescent Symptom Inventory-4R; CHOP: Children's Hospital of Philadelphia; CNV: Copy number variation; *COMT*: Catechol-O-methyltransferase; DSM: *Diagnostic and Statistical Manual of Mental Disorders*; FXS: Fragile X syndrome; LCR: Low-copy repeat; mGluR: Metabotropic glutamate receptor; MLPA: Multiplex ligation probe amplification; Ran: Ras-related nuclear protein; *RANBP1*: Ran-binding protein 1; SCQ: Social Communication Questionnaire; SNP: Single nucleotide polymorphism; SRS: Social Responsiveness Scale; TDC: Typically developing children; Vineland-II: Vineland Adaptive Behavior Scales-II

Acknowledgements

The authors wish to thank Katie Lowe, Karen Liao, Joy Payton, and all of the families who graciously offered their time to participate in the study, especially the families of patients highlighted in the case studies.

Funding

This study was funded by grants from the Simons Foundation Autism Research Initiative (275687), the National Institutes of Child and Human Development (U54 HD86984, R01 HD055741), the Pennsylvania Department of Health (SAP #4100042728, SAP #4100047863), the Robert Wood Johnson Foundation (#66727), and the National Institute of Mental Health (RC1MH08879, 5R01MH107431-02). This material is based upon work supported by the National Science Foundation Graduate Research Fellowship Program under grant no. DGE-1321851.

Authors' contributions

TW conceived of the study, assisted in identification of participants, performed medical chart review, and assisted in data interpretation and manuscript preparation. CCC was involved in project conception and design, performed psychological assessments on participants, performed psychological record review, provided all statistical analysis, interpreted results, and drafted the manuscript. AZ and JB recruited participants, administered questionnaires, collected data, and contributed to data analysis and editing of the manuscript. JSM was involved in experimental design, supervised and performed psychological assessments on participants, and edited the manuscript. AdM contributed to project design, performed assessments on participants, performed psychological record review, and edited the manuscript. JCC contributed to participant recruitment and edited the manuscript. BEY contributed to assessments of participants, consulted on statistical analysis approach, and edited the manuscript. LDP contributed to subject recruitment, administration of questionnaires, collected data, and reviewed the manuscript. BE, EZ, and DMM were involved in conception of the project, subject recruitment, confirmed cytogenetic diagnosis, and reviewed the manuscript. RTS contributed to all phases of the project including design, implementation, synthesis of results, analysis, and review of the manuscript. All authors approved the manuscript.

Competing interests

The authors declare that they have no competing interests.

Author details

[1]Center for Autism Research, The Children's Hospital of Philadelphia, 2716 South Street, Philadelphia, PA 19104, USA. [2]Department of Psychology, University of Pennsylvania, 3720 Walnut Street, Philadelphia, PA 19104, USA. [3]Department of Pediatrics, Seattle Children's Hospital, 4800 Sand Point Way NE, Seattle, WA 98105, USA. [4]Vanderbilt Brain Institute, Vanderbilt University School of Medicine, 465 21st Avenue South, Nashville, TN 37232, USA. [5]Department of Psychiatry, University of Pennsylvania, 3400 Civic Center Boulevard, Philadelphia, PA 19104, USA. [6]Department of Behavioral and Social Science, University of the Sciences, 600 South 43rd Street, Philadelphia, PA 19104, USA. [7]Department of Pediatrics, The Children's Hospital of Philadelphia, 3400 Civic Center Boulevard, Philadelphia, PA 19104, USA. [8]Department of Pediatrics, University of Utah, Salt Lake City, UT 84108, USA.

References

1. McDonald-McGinn DM, Emanuel BS, Zackai EH. 22q11.2 Deletion Syndrome. In: Pagon RA, Adam MP, Ardinger HH, Wallace SE, Amemiya A, Bean LJ, et al., editors. GeneReviews(®). Seattle (WA): University of Washington, Seattle; 1999. http://www.ncbi.nlm.nih.gov/books/NBK1523/.
2. Grati FR, Molina Gomes D, Ferreira JCPB, Dupont C, Alesi V, Gouas L, et al. Prevalence of recurrent pathogenic microdeletions and microduplications in over 9500 pregnancies. Prenat Diagn. 2015;35:801–9.
3. McDonald-McGinn DM, Kirschner R, Goldmuntz E, Sullivan K, Eicher P, Gerdes M, et al. The Philadelphia Story: the 22q11. 2 deletion: report on 250 patients. Genet Couns Geneva Switz. 1999;10:11–24.
4. Wentzel C, Fernström M, Öhrner Y, Annerén G, Thuresson A-C. Clinical variability of the 22q11. 2 duplication syndrome. Eur J Med Genet. 2008;51:501–10.
5. Kobrynski LJ, Sullivan KE. Velocardiofacial syndrome, DiGeorge syndrome: the chromosome 22q11.2 deletion syndromes. Lancet. 2007;370:1443–52.
6. Wenger TL, Miller JS, DePolo LM, de Marchena AB, Clements CC, Emanuel BS, et al. 22q11.2 duplication syndrome: elevated rate of autism spectrum disorder and need for medical screening. Mol Autism. 2016;7 doi:10.1186/s13229-016-0090-z.
7. Schneider M, Debbané M, Bassett AS, Chow EWC, Fung WLA, van den Bree M, et al. Psychiatric disorders from childhood to adulthood in 22q11.2 deletion syndrome: results from the International Consortium on Brain and Behavior in 22q11.2 Deletion Syndrome. Am J Psychiatry. 2014;171:627–39.
8. Hoeffding LK, Trabjerg BB, Olsen L, Mazin W, Sparsø T, Vangkilde A, et al. Risk of psychiatric disorders among individuals with the 22q11.2 deletion or duplication: a danish nationwide, register-based study. JAMA Psychiatry. 2017;74:282–90.
9. Rees E, Kirov G, Sanders A, Walters JTR, Chambert KD, Shi J, et al. Evidence that duplications of 22q11. 2 protect against schizophrenia. Mol Psychiatry. 2014;19:37.
10. Vorstman JAS, Morcus MEJ, Duijff SN, Klaassen PWJ, Heineman-de Boer JA, Beemer FA, et al. The 22q11.2 deletion in children: high rate of autistic disorders and early onset of psychotic symptoms. J Am Acad Child Adolesc Psychiatry. 2006;45:1104–13.
11. Ousley O, Evans AN, Fernandez-Carriba S, Smearman EL, Rockers K, Morrier MJ, et al. Examining the overlap between autism spectrum disorder and 22q11.2 deletion syndrome. Int J Mol Sci. 2017;18:1071.
12. Angkustsiri K, Goodlin-Jones B, Deprey L, Brahmbhatt K, Harris S, Simon TJ. Social impairments in chromosome 22q11.2 deletion syndrome (22q11.2DS): autism spectrum disorder or a different endophenotype? J Autism Dev Disord. 2014;44:739–46.
13. Michaelovsky E, Frisch A, Carmel M, Patya M, Zarchi O, Green T, et al. Genotype-phenotype correlation in 22q11. 2 deletion syndrome. BMC Med Genet. 2012;13:122.
14. Bengoa-Alonso A, Artigas-Lopez M, Moreno-Igoa M, Cattalli C, Hernandez-Charro B, Ramos-Arroyo MA. Delineation of a recognizable phenotype for the recurrent LCR22-C to D/E atypical 22q11.2 deletion. Am J Med Genet A. 2016;170:1485–94.

15. Guris DL, Fantes J, David T, Druker BJ, Imamoto A. Mice lacking the homologue of the human 22q11. 2 gene CRKL phenocopy neurocristopathies of DiGeorge syndrome. Nat Genet. 2001;27:293.
16. Lindsay EA, Vitelli F, Su H, Morishima M, et al. Tbx1 haploinsufficiency in the DiGeorge syndrome region causes aortic arch defects in mice. Nature. 2001;410:97.
17. Guo T, McDonald-McGinn D, Blonska A, Shanske A, Bassett AS, Chow E, et al. Genotype and cardiovascular phenotype correlations with TBX1 in 1,022 velo-cardio-facial/digeorge/22q11. 2 deletion syndrome patients. Hum Mutat. 2011;32:1278–89.
18. Jerome LA, Papaioannou VE. DiGeorge syndrome phenotype in mice mutant for the T-box gene, Tbx1. Nat Genet. 2001;27:286–91.
19. Herman SB, Guo T, McGinn DMM, Blonska A, Shanske AL, Bassett AS, et al. Overt cleft palate phenotype and TBX1 genotype correlations in velo-cardio-facial/DiGeorge/22q11. 2 deletion syndrome patients. Am J Med Genet A. 2012;158:2781–7.
20. Raux G, Bumsel E, Hecketsweiler B, van Amelsvoort T, Zinkstok J, Manouvrier-Hanu S, et al. Involvement of hyperprolinemia in cognitive and psychiatric features of the 22q11 deletion syndrome. Hum Mol Genet. 2006;16:83–91.
21. Jacquet H, Demily C, Houy E, Hecketsweiler B, Bou J, Raux G, et al. Hyperprolinemia is a risk factor for schizoaffective disorder. Mol Psychiatry. 2005;10:479.
22. Gothelf D, Eliez S, Thompson T, Hinard C, Penniman L, Feinstein C, et al. COMT genotype predicts longitudinal cognitive decline and psychosis in 22q11. 2 deletion syndrome. Nat Neurosci. 2005;8:1500.
23. Vorstman JA, Turetsky BI, Sijmens-Morcus ME, de Sain MG, Dorland B, Sprong M, et al. Proline affects brain function in 22q11DS children with the low activity COMT158 allele. Neuropsychopharmacology. 2009;34:739.
24. Bassett AS, Caluseriu O, Weksberg R, Young DA, Chow EW. Catechol-O-methyl transferase and expression of schizophrenia in 73 adults with 22q11 deletion syndrome. Biol Psychiatry. 2007;61:1135–40.
25. Baker K, Baldeweg T, Sivagnanasundaram S, Scambler P, Skuse D. COMT Val 108/158 Met modifies mismatch negativity and cognitive function in 22q11 deletion syndrome. Biol Psychiatry. 2005;58:23–31.
26. Murphy KC, Jones LA, Owen MJ. High rates of schizophrenia in adults with velo-cardio-facial syndrome. Arch Gen Psychiatry. 1999;56:940–5.
27. Bassett AS, Chow EW. Schizophrenia and 22q11. 2 deletion syndrome. Curr Psychiatry Rep. 2008;10:148.
28. Radoeva PD, Coman IL, Salazar CA, Gentile KL, Higgins AM, Middleton FA, et al. Association between autism spectrum disorder in individuals with velocardiofacial (22q11.2 deletion) syndrome and PRODH and COMT genotypes. Psychiatr Genet. 2014;24:269–72.
29. Hidding E, Swaab H, Sonneville LMJ, Engeland H, Vorstman J a S. The role of COMT and plasma proline in the variable penetrance of autistic spectrum symptoms in 22q11.2 deletion syndrome. Clin Genet. 2016;90:420–7.
30. Wenger TL, Kao C, McDonald-McGinn DM, Zackai EH, Bailey A, Schultz RT, et al. The role of mGluR copy number variation in genetic and environmental forms of syndromic autism spectrum disorder. Sci Rep. 2016;6:19372.
31. Snyder LG, D Angelo D, Chen Q, Bernier R, Goin-Kochel RP, Wallace AS, et al. Autism spectrum disorder, developmental and psychiatric features in 16p11. 2 duplication. J Autism Dev Disord. 2016;46:2734–48.
32. Fuchs-Telem D, Stewart H, Rapaport D, Nousbeck J, Gat A, Gini M, et al. CEDNIK syndrome results from loss-of-function mutations in SNAP29. Br J Dermatol. 2011;164:610–6.
33. D'Angelo D, Lebon S, Chen Q, Martin-Brevet S, Snyder LG, Hippolyte L, et al. Defining the effect of the 16p11. 2 duplication on cognition, behavior, and medical comorbidities. JAMA Psychiatry. 2016;73:20–30.
34. Dudova I, Markova D, Kasparova M, Zemankova J, Beranova S, Urbanek T, et al. Comparison of three screening tests for autism in preterm children with birth weights less than 1,500 grams. Neuropsychiatr Dis Treat. 2014;10:2201.
35. Lord C, Rutter M, DiLavore PC, Risi S. Autism diagnostic observation schedule (ADOS). Los Angeles, CA: Western Psychological Services; 1999.
36. American Psychiatric Association. Diagnostic and Statistical Manual. 5th ed. Arlington, VA: American Psychiatric Publishing; 2013.
37. Sparrow SS, Cicchetti DV, Balla DA. Vineland adaptive behavior scales, 2nd edition (Vineland II): survey interview form/caregiver rating form. Livonia, MN: Pearson Assessments; 2005.
38. Gadow KD, Sprafkin J. Child and adolescent symptom inventory-4R. Stony Brook, NY: Checkmate Plus; 2005.
39. Rutter M, Bailey A, Lord C. The Social Communication Questionnaire. Los Angeles, CA: Western Psychological Services; 2003.
40. Constantino JN, Gruber CP. Social Responsiveness Scale (SRS). Torrance, CA: Western Psychological Services; 2012.
41. Constantino JN, Gruber CP. Social Responsiveness Scale, 2nd edition (SRS-2). Los Angeles, CA: Western Psychological Services; 2012.
42. Button KS, Ioannidis JPA, Mokrysz C, Nosek BA, Flint J, Robinson ESJ, et al. Power failure: why small sample size undermines the reliability of neuroscience. Nat Rev Neurosci. 2013;14:365–76.
43. Cumming G. The new statistics: why and how. Psychol Sci. 2014;25:7–29.
44. Hadley D, Wu Z, Kao C, Kini A, Mohamed-Hadley A, Thomas K, et al. The impact of the metabotropic glutamate receptor and other gene family interaction networks on autism. Nat Commun. 2014;5 doi:10.1038/ncomms5074.
45. Auerbach BD, Osterweil EK, Bear MF. Mutations causing syndromic autism define an axis of synaptic pathophysiology. Nature. 2011;480:63–8.
46. Jennifer L Ingram, Stacey M Peckham, Barbara Tisdale, Patricia M Rodier, (2000) Prenatal exposure of rats to valproic acid reproduces the cerebellar anomalies associated with autism. Neurotoxicology and Teratology 22(3): 319-324.
47. Jakob Christensen, Therese Koops Grønborg, Merete Juul Sørensen, Diana Schendel, Erik Thorlund Parner, Lars Henning Pedersen, Mogens Vestergaard, (2013) Prenatal Valproate Exposure and Risk of Autism Spectrum Disorders and Childhood Autism. JAMA 309 (16):1696.
48. Kesavan Meganathan, Smita Jagtap, Vilas Wagh, Johannes Winkler, John Antonydas Gaspar, Diana Hildebrand, Maria Trusch, Karola Lehmann, Jürgen Hescheler, Hartmut Schlüter, Agapios Sachinidis, Yao Liang Tang, (2012) Identification of Thalidomide-Specific Transcriptomics and Proteomics Signatures during Differentiation of Human Embryonic Stem Cells. PLoS ONE 7 (8):e44228.
49. Meechan DW, Maynard TM, Wu Y, Gopalakrishna D, Lieberman JA, LaMantia A-S. Gene dosage in the developing and adult brain in a mouse model of 22q11 deletion syndrome. Mol Cell Neurosci. 2006;33:412–28.
50. Paronett EM, Meechan DW, Karpinski BA, LaMantia A-S, Maynard TM. Ranbp1, deleted in DiGeorge/22q11.2 deletion syndrome, is a microcephaly gene that selectively disrupts layer 2/3 cortical projection neuron generation. Cereb Cortex. 2015;25:3977–93.
51. Meechan DW, Tucker ES, Maynard TM, LaMantia A-S. Diminished dosage of 22q11 genes disrupts neurogenesis and cortical development in a mouse model of 22q11 deletion/DiGeorge syndrome. Proc Natl Acad Sci. 2009;106:16434–45.
52. Zhang MS, Arnaoutov A, Dasso M. RanBP1 governs spindle assembly by defining mitotic Ran-GTP production. Dev Cell. 2014;31:393–404.
53. Weisfeld-Adams JD, Edelmann L, Gadi IK, Mehta L. Phenotypic heterogeneity in a family with a small atypical microduplication of chromosome 22q11.2 involving TBX1. Eur J Med Genet. 2012;55:732–6.
54. Cohen J. The effect size. Stat Power Anal Behav Sci. 1988;2:284–8.

16

Urinary metabolomics of young Italian autistic children supports abnormal tryptophan and purine metabolism

Federica Gevi[1], Lello Zolla[1*], Stefano Gabriele[2] and Antonio M. Persico[3,4*]

Abstract

Background: Autism spectrum disorder (ASD) is still diagnosed through behavioral observation, due to a lack of laboratory biomarkers, which could greatly aid clinicians in providing earlier and more reliable diagnoses. Metabolomics on human biofluids provides a sensitive tool to identify metabolite profiles potentially usable as biomarkers for ASD. Initial metabolomic studies, analyzing urines and plasma of ASD and control individuals, suggested that autistic patients may share some metabolic abnormalities, despite several inconsistencies stemming from differences in technology, ethnicity, age range, and definition of "control" status.

Methods: ASD-specific urinary metabolomic patterns were explored at an early age in 30 ASD children and 30 matched controls (age range 2–7, M:F = 22:8) using hydrophilic interaction chromatography (HILIC)-UHPLC and mass spectrometry, a highly sensitive, accurate, and unbiased approach. Metabolites were then subjected to multivariate statistical analysis and grouped by metabolic pathway.

Results: Urinary metabolites displaying the largest differences between young ASD and control children belonged to the tryptophan and purine metabolic pathways. Also, vitamin B_6, riboflavin, phenylalanine-tyrosine-tryptophan biosynthesis, pantothenate and CoA, and pyrimidine metabolism differed significantly. ASD children preferentially transform tryptophan into xanthurenic acid and quinolinic acid (two catabolites of the kynurenine pathway), at the expense of kynurenic acid and especially of melatonin. Also, the gut microbiome contributes to altered tryptophan metabolism, yielding increased levels of indolyl 3-acetic acid and indolyl lactate.

Conclusions: The metabolic pathways most distinctive of young Italian autistic children largely overlap with those found in rodent models of ASD following maternal immune activation or genetic manipulations. These results are consistent with the proposal of a purine-driven cell danger response, accompanied by overproduction of epileptogenic and excitotoxic quinolinic acid, large reductions in melatonin synthesis, and gut dysbiosis. These metabolic abnormalities could underlie several comorbidities frequently associated to ASD, such as seizures, sleep disorders, and gastrointestinal symptoms, and could contribute to autism severity. Their diagnostic sensitivity, disease-specificity, and interethnic variability will merit further investigation.

Keywords: Autism, Autism spectrum disorder, Kynurenine, Melatonin, Metabolomics, Purinergic signaling, Quinolinic acid, Serotonin, Tryptophan

* Correspondence: zolla@unitus.it; apersico@unime.it
[1]Department of Ecological and Biological Sciences, University of Tuscia, Viterbo, Italy
[3]Unit of Child and Adolescent Neuropsychiatry, Interdepartmental Program "Autism 0-90", "Gaetano Martino" University Hospital, University of Messina, Messina, Italy
Full list of author information is available at the end of the article

Background

Autism spectrum disorder (ASD) represents a highly heterogeneous collection of neurodevelopmental conditions characterized by social and communication deficits, stereotypic and rigid patterns of behavior, restricted interests, and unusual sensory processing with onset in early childhood [1]. The prevalence of autism has increased significantly during the last two decades from 2–5/10,000 to 1:68 children [2, 3]. Changes in diagnostic criteria and increased attention by the medical community have certainly contributed to this trend [4]. Also, increasing parental age at conception has been shown to confer ASD risk [5], as well as some environmental factors, active especially during critical periods in prenatal/early postnatal neurodevelopment [6]. Finally, genetic susceptibility plays a prominent role in ASD pathogenesis through complex and heterogeneous underpinnings, ranging from rare variants endowed with full penetrance to common variants each explaining very small proportions of the overall phenotypic variance, either alone or through gene × environment interactions [7, 8].

Despite major advances in our understanding of the pathophysiology of ASD, this level of complexity and interindividual heterogeneity has largely hampered the translation of scientific knowledge into more effective clinical practices. ASD is still diagnosed exclusively through observation, standardized behavioral scales, and parental interviews; developmental trajectories of ASD children are periodically monitored but cannot be reliably predicted especially at an early age. Sensitive and specific quantitative biomarkers, measurable through laboratory, brain imaging, and/or electrophysiological techniques, could greatly aid clinicians in providing earlier diagnoses, more timely referrals to behavioral intervention programs, and evidence-based prognostic predictions [9].

Metabolomic technologies offer a sensitive means to search human biofluids for metabolite profiles potentially usable as biomarkers for neurodevelopmental disorders. A few studies have recently begun exploring the potential of urinary metabolomics in identifying ASD-specific metabolic patterns or in stratifying ASD patients into pathophysiologically meaningful subgroups [10–17]. Most studies have been performed on urines [10–16]; one study has explored blood plasma [17]. The analytical platforms most commonly used to identify and quantify metabolites are gas or liquid chromatography combined with mass spectroscopy (gas chromatography (GC)-mass spectroscopy (MS) and liquid chromatography (LC)-MS, respectively) [12, 16] and nuclear magnetic resonance spectroscopy (NMR) [10, 13, 14, 16, 18, 19]. In general, NMR displays greater speed and good reproducibility but also lower sensitivity compared to MS. Hence, MS- and NMR-based techniques should be viewed as complementary, not as superimposable approaches. An initial study, using 1H-NMR methods, showed an abnormal composition of urinary solutes indicative of perturbations in (a) the tryptophan/nicotinic acid metabolic pathway, (b) sulfur and amino acid metabolisms, and (c) gut microbiome, with an excess of several gut-derived co-metabolites [10]. Two other studies presumably assessing the same clinical sample with two different NMR-based technologies largely replicated these initial findings [13, 14]. Other studies using GC-MS, either alone [12, 15] or in combination with liquid chromatography [11], also identified perturbations in amino acid metabolism and gut microbial co-metabolites, as well as metabolic signatures of oxidative stress. Only one very recent study used both NMR and LC-MS, providing support for abnormalities in tryptophan metabolism, gut bacterial-derived compounds, purine and pyrimidine metabolism [16]. The only study exploring blood plasma reported metabolomic patterns compatible with (a) mitochondrial dysfunction, yielding reduced energy production and unbalanced redox status, (b) excess gut microbial co-metabolites, and (c) unbalances in various metabolic pathways, such as the Krebs cycle [17]. Collectively, metabolomic studies performed to this date suggest that autistic patients may share several metabolic abnormalities, especially involving some amino acid metabolisms, energy production, and oxidative stress, as well as the gut microbiome.

Moving from broad metabolic pathways to single compounds unveils inconsistencies between studies, which may stem from several potential confounds. Interethnic differences in the gut microbiota, stemming from differences in the nutrient composition of local diets, as well as age-related changes in both gut microbiota and human metabolism indeed require that case and control samples be tightly matched for these two variables. Age-related changes may be especially relevant to studies of ASD, where we have recently reported levels of urinary *p*-cresol to be elevated in autistic children compared to age-matched controls both in Italy and in France, but exclusively up until 8 years of age [20, 21]. Similar age-related changes in ASD have been previously described for other parameters, such as brain serotonin synthesis capacity [22, 23] and excessive head growth rates [24]. Finally, some studies have contrasted ASD patients with unrelated population controls [11, 14, 16, 17], while others have enrolled unaffected siblings as controls [15] and one study has used both [10]. These strategies are not equivalent, as first-degree relatives often fall within the broad autism spectrum (i.e., they display behavioral phenotypes intermediate between patients and population controls) [25]. In addition, siblings may carry protective gene variants with peculiar functional correlates, possibly distinct from the metabolic patterns of unrelated typically developing children.

Taking into consideration these methodological issues, in order to maximize the probability of reliably detecting differences in urinary metabolic patterns, we focused on autistic and unrelated typically developing children 2–8 years old, tightly matched by age, sex, Italian ancestry, and city of origin within the country [20]. To ensure broad metabolite detection coverage on urine samples, which comprise molecules generated both by human cells and by the gut microbiome, we employed hydrophilic interaction chromatography (HILIC)-LC-electrospray ionization (ESI)-MS, a technology particularly suitable to separate simple and complex mixtures of carbohydrates, amino acids, glycosides, and other natural polar products in biological fluids, such as human urine and plasma [26, 27]. Applying this experimental approach, urinary metabolites most significantly distinguishing autistic from typically developing children were found to primarily fall into the tryptophan and purine metabolic pathways.

Methods

Subjects

Thirty children with idiopathic ASD and thirty typically developing controls were recruited in Central and Northern Italy. These represent the vast majority of the 64 cases and controls aged 3–7 years assessed for urinary *p*-cresol in our previous study [20]. Their demographic and clinical characteristics are summarized in Additional file 1: Table S1. Diagnostic assessments and medical screening have been previously described [20] (also see Additional file 2 with Supplementary Methods). Tight sex- and age-matching (±1 year) was applied to recruit typically developing children devoid of any overt ASD symptomatology among the offspring of clinical/academic personnel [20]. Mean age (±SEM) of cases and controls was 4.83 ± 0.30 and 5.03 ± 0.32 years, respectively (Student's $t = -0.459$, 58 df, $P = 0.648$, n.s.), and the M:F ratio was 22:8. All cases and controls were of Italian descent and matched by geographical area or city of origin.

Urine collection and metabolite extraction

First-morning urines were collected at home by parents using sterile containers untreated with preservatives and were brought to each clinical center the same morning in wet ice. Urine samples were then frozen, shipped in dry ice, and stored at −80 °C continuously until analysis.

Urinary specific gravity was measured by refractometry following centrifugation at 13,000*g* for 10 min) using a digital refractometer (Euromex Clinical Digital Refractometer RD.5712, NL) previously calibrated with LC-MS grade water.

Urine aliquots (200 μl) were mixed with 200 μl of methanol:acetonitrile:water (50:30:20), vortexed for 30 min at max speed at 4 °C and then centrifuged at 16,000*g* for 15 min at 4 °C. Supernatants were collected for metabolomic analysis. Quality controls (QCs) were obtained from a pooled mixture of 10 μl aliquots of all urine samples and were analyzed every 15 samples.

HILIC-UHPLC

Metabolite separation was performed as previously described [28], by hydrophilic interaction chromatography (HILIC) using the Ultimate 3000 Rapid Resolution HPLC system (Dionex, Sunnyvale, CA), featuring a binary pump and vacuum degasser, well-plate autosampler with a six-port micro-switching valve, and a thermostated column compartment. A Phenomenex Luna 3 μm HILIC 200 A (150 × 2.0 mm) column, protected by a HILIC 4 × 2.0 mm ID guard column (Phenomenex, Torrance, CA), was used to perform metabolite separation over a phase B-to-phase A gradient lasting 35 min. For the HILIC separation, mobile phase "A" consisted in 50 mM ammonium acetate mixed with acetonitrile (95:5, *v*/*v*), while eluent "B" was composed of a mixture of 50 mM ammonium acetate:water plus acetonitrile (95:5, *v*/*v*). Acetonitrile, formic acid, and HPLC-grade water were purchased from Sigma-Aldrich (St. Louis, MO).

Mass spectrometry

MS analysis was carried out on an electrospray hybrid quadrupole time-of-flight instrument MicroTOF-Q (Bruker-Daltonik, Bremen, Germany) equipped with an ESI ion source, as previously described [29]. Mass spectra for metabolite-extracted samples were acquired both in positive and in negative ion modes; only data produced in negative mode are shown, because more powerful in analyzing urinary samples. ESI capillary voltage was set at 4500 V (−) ion mode. The liquid nebulizer was set at 27 psi, and the nitrogen drying gas was set to a flow rate of 6 L/min. Dry gas temperature was maintained at 200 °C. Data were stored in centroid mode and acquired with a stored mass range of 50–1200 *m*/*z*. Instrument calibration was performed externally every day with 10 mM sodium hydroxide in 50% isopropanol:water, 0.1% formic acid. Automated internal mass scale calibration was performed through direct automated injection of the calibration solution at the beginning and at the end of each run by a six-port divert valve.

Data elaboration and statistical analysis

Data were normalized by urinary specific gravity, because creatinine excretion may be abnormally reduced in ASD children [30]. Replicates were exported as mzXML files and processed through MAVEN.52 (available at http://genomics-pubs.princeton.edu/mzroll/

index.php?show=index) [31]. Mass spectrometry chromatograms were elaborated for peak alignment, matching and comparison of parent and fragment ions, and tentative metabolite identification (within a 10-ppm mass deviation range between observed and expected results against the imported Kyoto Encyclopedia of Genes and Genomes (KEGG) database). Representative examples of mass determination and MS/MS fragmentation graphs are presented for kynurenine, melatonin, and tryptophan in Additional file 3: Figure S1. Multivariate statistical analyses were performed on the entire metabolomics data set using the MetaboAnalyst 3.0 software (http://www.metaboanalyst.ca) [32], which also overviewed data variance structure in an unsupervised manner and produced scatter plots.

Orthogonal partial least squares discriminant analysis (OPLS-DA), which defines a predictive model that describes the direction of the maximum covariance between a dataset (X) and class membership (Y), was then used to maximize the difference in metabolic profiles between cases and controls [33, 34]. OPLS-DA was performed using the Excel add-in Multibase package (Numerical Dynamics, Japan; http://www.numericaldynamics.com/) by applying orthogonal signal correction on the metabolite concentrations shifted, $\log_{10}$ transformed, centered, and scaled to unit variance.

Performance of the optimal model was tested by a receiver operating characteristic (ROC) curve analysis and the validation data set, as performed using MetaboAnalyst 3.0 software (http://www.metaboanalyst.ca) [32].

For case-control contrasts of single urinary metabolites, significance threshold was held at a nominal $P < 0.05$ with no correction for multiple testing, because (a) differences in single metabolite concentrations were tested only following significant differences in pathway enrichment were detected, (b) intra-pathway variability of single metabolites is non-independent, and (c) also different metabolic pathways are not fully independent, as some metabolites fall into more than one pathway. Detailed and summary statistics are provided in Additional files 4 and 5.

Results

The urinary metabolomes of young autistic and typically developing children are largely distinguishable on the three-dimensional OPLS-DA plot depicting the first three principal components (PC), which together explain 31.4% of the total variance (Fig. 1; accuracy, Q2 and R2 data are shown in Additional file 6). Approximately 10,000 peaks per sample were obtained referring to the KEGG database; among them, 202 metabolites were analyzed more precisely and identified. The top 25 most discriminating metabolites between cases and controls were further defined based on "variable influence on the projection" (VIP) scores >1 (Fig. 2). ROC analysis using this set of 25 metabolites yielded an AUC = 0.893 (95% CI 0.72–0.96), as shown in Additional file 7. The "metabolome overview" obtained through metabolic pathway analysis (MetPA) shows tryptophan metabolism, purine metabolism, vitamin B_6 metabolism, and phenylalanine-tyrosine-tryptophan biosynthesis as the four most perturbed metabolic pathways in ASD (Fig. 3).

Given the relevance of tryptophan-derived compounds in many neural functions, tryptophan metabolism was assessed in greater detail at the level of specific intermediates (Fig. 4):

- The kynurenine pathway displays increases in xanthurenic acid and especially in quinolinic acid, paralleled by a considerable decrease in kynurenic acid (Fig. 4, path A).
- The serotonin pathway shows a significant decrease in melatonin and its catabolite N-acetyl-5-methoxy-tryptamine, which have the same molecular weight and thus fall under the same MS peak (Fig. 4, path B).
- Bacterial degradation of tryptophan yields in ASD, compared to controls, prominently larger urinary concentrations of indoxyl sulfate and other indole derivatives, including indolyl-3-acetic acid and especially indolyl lactate (Fig. 4, paths C and D).

Also, purine metabolism was found to convey sizable discriminative power, because ASD cases display higher urinary concentrations of many purine metabolites compared to controls, including, among others, inosine, hypoxanthine, and xanthosine (Fig. 5).

Discussion

The present study reports significant urinary metabolomic differences between young children with idiopathic ASD and typically developing controls. At least some of the metabolic perturbations described here may reflect pathophysiologically meaningful abnormalities, possibly bearing functional consequences at the clinical level. Three strengths of the experimental design may have contributed to this positive outcome: (a) a focus on early infancy, by recruiting children within a relatively narrow age window precisely defined on the basis of previous urinary metabolic data [20, 21]; (b) the use of UHPLC-MS paired with HILIC, a very sensitive and reliable method ensuring maximum accuracy in the separation of small urinary solutes [26, 27]; (b) a pathway-centered approach, moving beyond the identification of single urinary ASD markers [10–17], as beautifully exemplified by urinary metabolomic studies of rodent models of ASD [35–37]. In particular, our recruitment strategy substantially differs from previous case-control study designs, minimizing age-dependent heterogeneity by

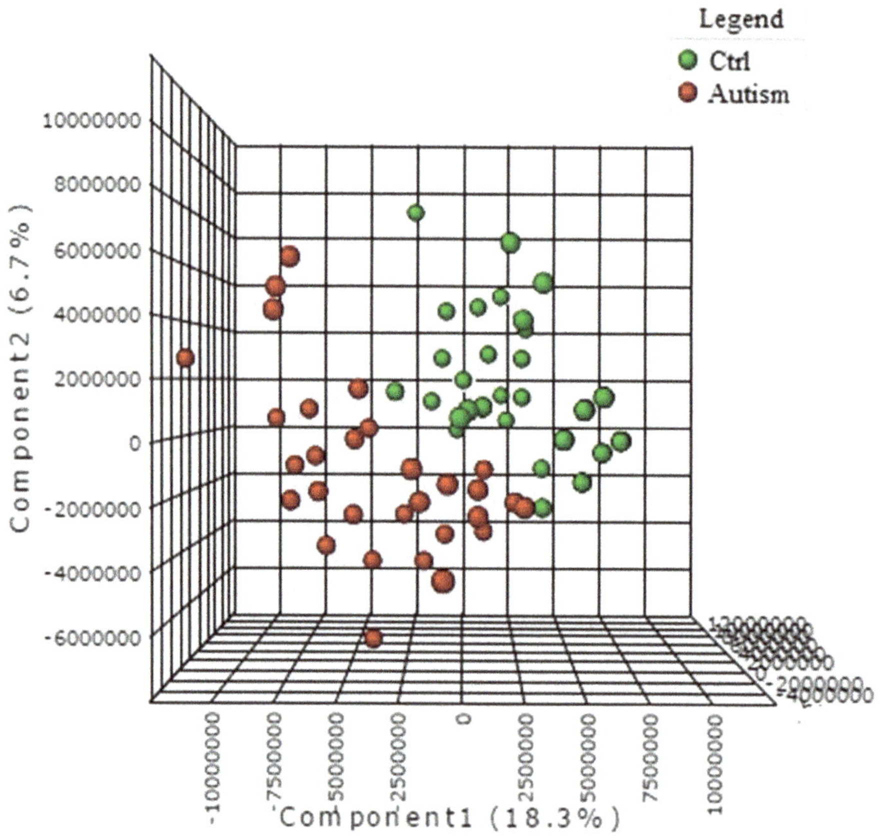

Fig. 1 OPLS-DA 3D plot based on normalized and mean-centered data. Each data point represents the metabolome of a single individual. Some data points may be superimposed to each other

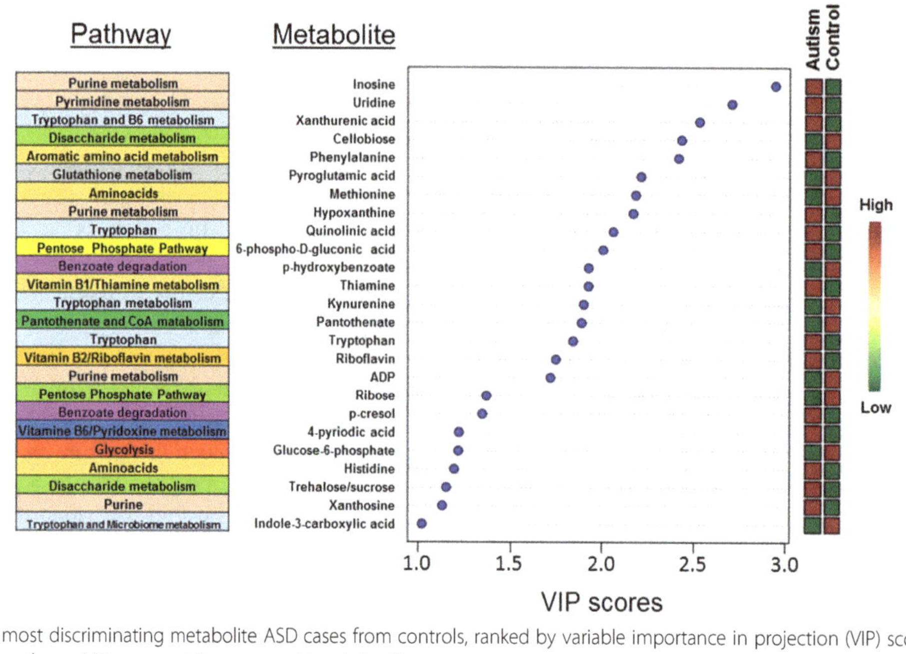

Fig. 2 The top 25 most discriminating metabolite ASD cases from controls, ranked by variable importance in projection (VIP) scores, and their KEGG biochemical pathway. VIP scores >1.0 were considered significant

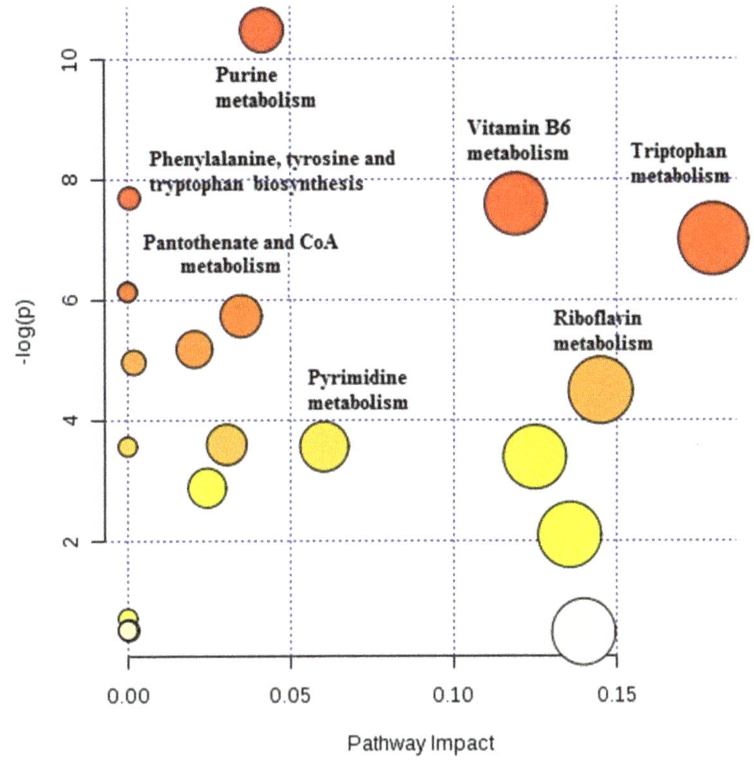

Fig. 3 Metabolic pathway analysis plot. Color intensity (*white* to *red*) reflects increasing statistical significance, while *circle diameter* covaries with pathway impact. The graph was obtained plotting on the *y-axis* the –log of *p* values from the pathway enrichment analysis and on the *x-axis* the pathway impact values derived from the pathway topology analysis

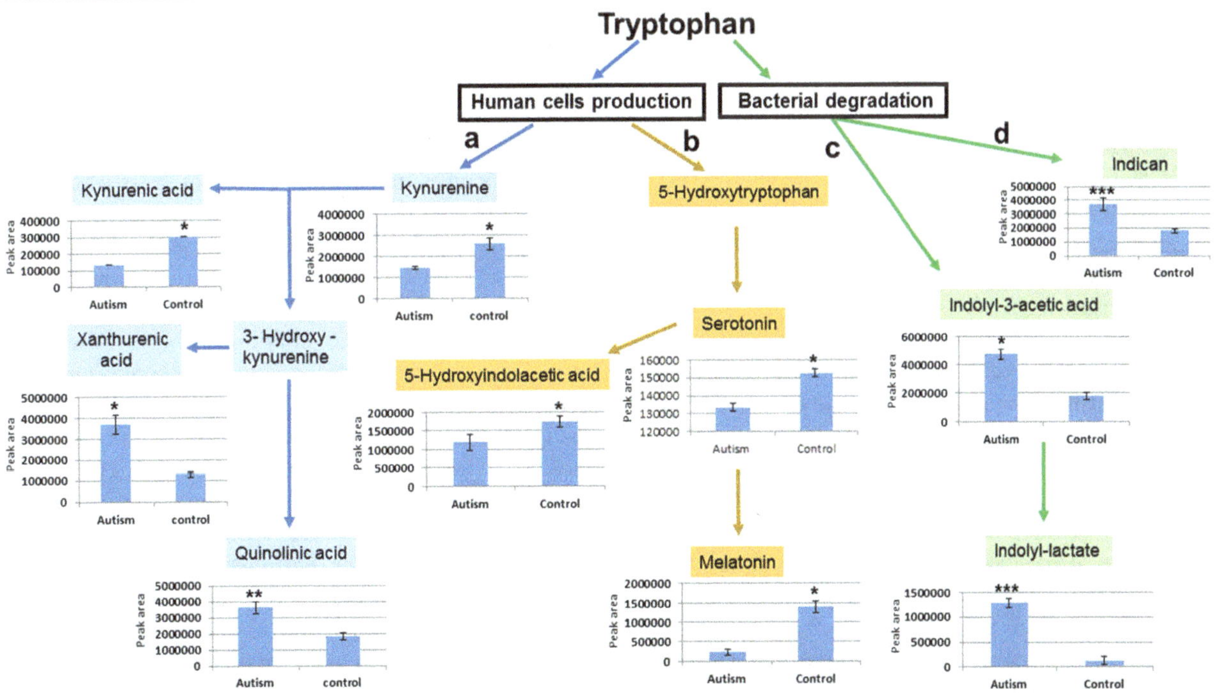

Fig. 4 Quantification of tryptophan metabolites: **a** kynurenine pathway; **b** serotonin/melatonin pathway; **c**–**d** bacterial degradation products. *Peak areas* for each metabolite were normalized by urinary specific gravity. Nominal *P* values: $^{*}P < 0.05$, $^{**}P < 0.0.1$, $^{***}P < 0.001$

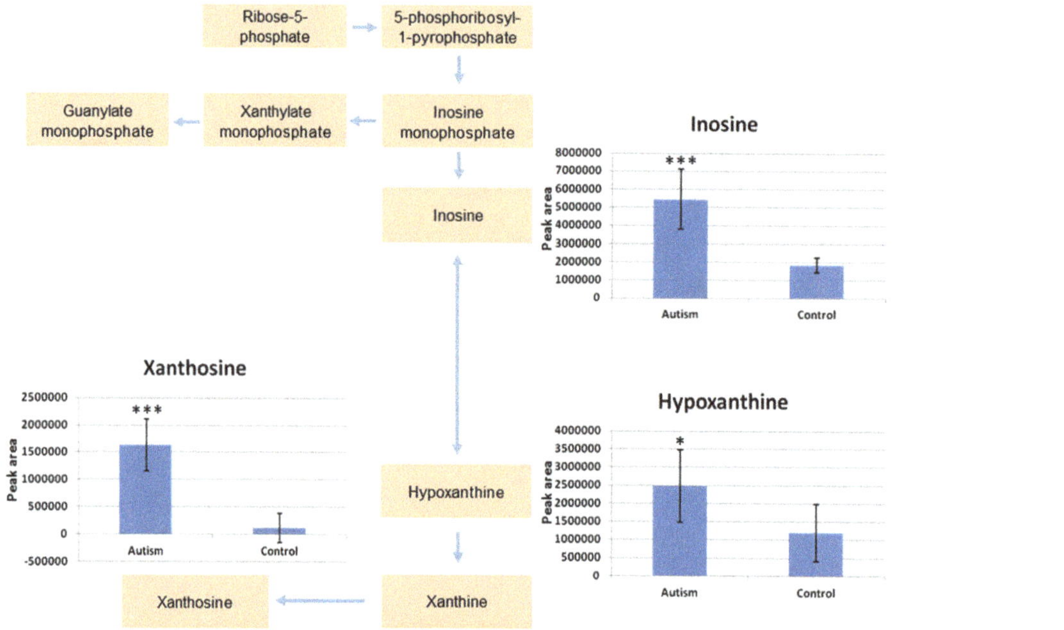

Fig. 5 Quantification of purine metabolites. *Peak areas* for each metabolite were normalized by urinary specific gravity. Nominal P values: $^{*}P < 0.05$, $^{**}P < 0.0.1$, $^{***}P < 0.001$

setting data-driven age thresholds (i.e., 2–8 years old) [20, 21], and applying tight age and sex matching between cases and controls. This strategy seemingly circumvents sample size limitations which would apply to an unfocused and unmatched case-control design. Future replications obtained applying similar recruitment criteria will enhance confidence in the pathophysiological relevance and the interethnic generalizability of our findings.

The tryptophan metabolic pathway collectively displays the largest perturbations in ASD (Fig. 3). Over 90–95% of dietary L-tryptophan is usually metabolized along the kynurenine pathway, 1–2% is converted to serotonin, and approximately 4–6% undergoes bacterial degradation prior to gut absorption through the Na^+-amino acid co-transporter B^0AT1 (Slc6a19) [38, 39]. The latter pathway yields indole derivatives not produced by mammalian metabolism, such as indoxyl sulfate [40]. Hence, changes in urinary amounts of multiple metabolites provide more reliable evidence of perturbed tryptophan metabolism, as compared to determinations of single metabolites or tryptophan itself, which also suffer from reduced statistical power due to control for multiple testing (Figs. 4 and 5). In the urines of young autistic children, we have indeed observed a substantial increase of xanthurenic acid and especially of quinolinic acid, paralleled by a decrease in kynurenine and kynurenic acid (Fig. 4, path A). This pattern is extremely interesting but must be interpreted with some caution in the absence of parallel assessments of the cerebrospinal fluid (CSF). On the one hand, the enzymes responsible for the synthesis of quinolinic acid and xanthurenic acid are primarily expressed in the microglia and in macrophages, whereas the path leading to kynurenic acid is functional in astrocytes [41]. Hence, it would be tempting to speculate that these opposite trends between cases and controls reflect an abnormal activation of microglia, which has been repeatedly seen in ASD postmortem brains [42–44], even as early as at 4 years of age [45]. On the other hand, urinary levels of quinolinic acid and kynurenic acid reflect peripheral production of these compounds, which do not pass the blood-brain barrier [41]. However, 3-hydroxykynurenine does pass the blood-brain barrier [41]. Interestingly, urinary concentrations of metabolite downstream of this compound (quinolinic acid and xanthurenic acid) are elevated in autistic children, whereas metabolite upstream of 3-hydroxykinurenine (kynurenine and kynurenic acid) are higher among controls (Fig. 4, path A). Conceivably, these trends could reflect an outflow of 3-hydroxykynurenine from the central nervous system (CNS) into the systemic circulation, where macrophage activation presumably at the level of the gut or in other peripheral organs, can transform this compound into quinolinic acid and xanthurenic acid, as well as into nicotinic acid (NAD), in agreement with previous data [10]. It will thus be important to verify this metabolomic scenario in the CSF, because it could have at least two important clinical implications: (a) quinolinic acid acts as gliotoxin, proinflammatory mediator, and pro-oxidant molecule, boosting oxidative stress by stimulating microglia to release large amounts of NO and superoxide; (b) quinolinic acid exerts excitotoxic effects by acting as an *N*-methyl-D-aspartate (NMDA) receptor agonist, stimulating glutamate release, blocking glutamate reuptake into astrocytes, and reducing the activity of glutamine synthase; instead, kynurenic acid exerts neuroprotection via NMDA antagonism at the glycine binding site, as well as antioxidant effects [41, 46, 47]. In summary, the urinary metabolic imbalance documented here, if present also in the CNS, could favor enhanced oxidative stress and the well-known excitation>inhibition imbalance present in ASD, fostering seizures in as many as 20% of autistic individuals [48].

Another consequence of the preferential metabolization of tryptophan along the main branch of the kynurenine pathway is the relative decrease in the production of serotonin and melatonin (Fig. 4, path B). The serotonin pathway sees tryptophan being converted into 5-hydroxytryptophan (5-HTP) by tryptophan hydroxylase and onwards to 5-hydroxytryptamine (5-HT) or serotonin by 5-HTP decarboxylase. Serotonin can then be catabolized to 5-hydroxyindoleacetic acid (5-HIAA) or transformed into N-acetylserotonin by arylalkylamine N-acetyltransferase (AANAT). N-acetylserotonin is further methylated by N-acetylserotonin O-methyltransferase (ASMT) to generate the neurohormone 5-methyl-5-methoxy-N-tryptamine or melatonin. Decreases in the serotonin metabolite 5-HIAA are only modest, while urinary melatonin and its catabolite N-acetyl-5-methoxytryptamine display a more pronounced mean reduction (both share the same molecular weight and fall under the same MS peak, labeled in Fig. 4, path B, as “melatonin” only). This confirms previous assessments performed in plasma or urine [10, 49–52], while lending further support to blunted melatonin synthesis possibly due to reduced ASMT enzyme activity in ASD [53, 54]. Melatonin is synthesized and released by the pineal gland into the systemic circulation and readily passes the blood-brain barrier [55]. Its well-known role in circadian rhythmicity makes it an ideal candidate to explain the frequent occurrence, especially at the onset of ASD and during early infancy, of sleep disorders highly responsive to melatonin as a pharmacological therapy [56].

Metabolites produced by gut bacteria are well-represented also in our ASD sample, as in previous studies [10–17]. In addition to urinary *p*-cresol, found elevated in these same urine samples both here (Fig. 3) and previously using a different technology [20], we also detect a significant increase in indole derivatives of bacterial tryptophan including indolyl 3-acetic acid, indoxyl sulfate, and most prominently, indolyl lactate (Fig. 4, path C). Bacterial species expressing tryptophanase, the enzyme responsible for transforming tryptophan into indole derivatives, include *Escherichia coli*, *Proteus vulgaris*, *Paracolobactrum coliform*, *Achromobacter liquefaciens*, and *Bacteroides* spp. [40]. Once produced in the gut lumen, indole is absorbed, oxidized to indoxyl, conjugated with sulfate, and excreted as urinary indoxyl sulfate. About 3% of tryptophan entered with the diet is excreted as indoxyl sulfate [37]. Additional small amounts of tryptophan are converted into other indole derivatives found elevated here in ASD children, such as indolyl-3-acetic acid and indolyl lactate (Fig. 4, path C). The latter compound and indolyl 3-acetic acid are direct precursors of indolylacrylol glycine, found elevated in ASD by some [57] but not all studies [58, 59]. Predictably, the exact urinary bacterial compounds found elevated in ASD do differ in distinct metabolomic studies. This is not surprising since, in addition to differences in sample demographics and sensitivity of available technologies, ethnicity also exerts profound influences on the microbiome, reflecting dietary, genetic, and immunological specificities involved in the host-microbiome interactions [60]. Despite these discrepancies at the level of single compounds, urinary metabolomic studies consistently report an excess of microbiome-derived urinary metabolites, collectively supporting gut dysbiosis in ASD. These results point toward possible negative effects on CNS function exerted by microbiome-derived metabolites. At least three examples are available, albeit with different degrees of support: (a) urinary *p*-cresol amounts were found correlated with ASD severity [20] or with the intensity of stereotypic behaviors in young autistic children [21]; (b) i.c.v. injection of propionic acid, an enteric-derived short chain fatty acid, produces ASD-like behaviors in the rat [61]; (c) indoxyl sulfate is a known risk factor for cognitive impairment in chronic renal disease [62]: its influx across the blood-brain barrier using the organic anion transporter 3 significantly reduces the efflux of various neurotransmitter metabolites through the same transporter, leading to their accumulation [63]. Importantly, sizable improvements in behavioral and serum metabolome abnormalities were recorded using the maternal immune activation (MIA) rodent model of ASD following the correction of gut dysbiosis using *Bacteroides fragilis* [64].

Purine metabolites are also well represented in the urines of ASD children, which display a large excess of inosine, hypoxanthine, and xanthosine (Figs. 3 and 5). This pattern bears an interesting resemblance to the excess of urinary inosine and hypoxanthine detected in *Fmr1* knock-out mice, an animal model of fragile-X syndrome [35]. Also, mice exposed prenatally to MIA triggered by poly(I:C) injected at E12.5 and E17.5 show an excess of urinary inosine [36]. This excess of urinary purinergic metabolites has been interpreted as part of a "cell danger metabolic response" involving mitochondrial dysfunction, adenosine triphosphate (ATP), and adenosine diphosphate (ADP) release, activation of a variety of purinergic receptors yielding microglial activation, innate, and adaptive immunity responses and leukocyte chemotactics [65]. Inborn errors of purine metabolism are associated with behavioral abnormalities including autistic features [66]. Strikingly, inhibition of purine metabolism by suramin, a competitive antagonist at P2X and P2Y purinergic receptors, reverses behavioral, neurochemical, transcriptional, and metabolomics abnormalities both in the *Fmr1* knock-out mouse and in MIA mice exposed to poly(I:C) during pregnancy [35–37]. Conceivably, this metabolic abnormality, shared between human ASD and genetic/immunological rodent models could thus represent a valuable biomarker to help guide therapeutic interventions. In addition, the cell danger response also yields relative vitamin B_6 deficiency and the enzyme kynureninase is B_6 dependent [65]; hence, a cell danger metabolic response in the presence of adequate tryptophan intake could also explain the decreased kynurenine and increased xanthurenic and quinolinic acid observed here (Fig. 4). Interestingly, these abnormalities have been sometimes overcome with vitamin B_6 supplementation [67], a therapeutic approach initially proposed for ASD in conjunction with magnesium supplementation [68]. In light of the present data, B_6-Mg^{++} supplementation in ASD may deserve further scrutiny in urinary biomarker-driven therapeutic trials, as no firm conclusion on its potential efficacy has yet been reached [69].

Conclusions

Targeting young autistic children and tightly matched controls, using the sensitive approach HILIC UHPLC-MS, and applying metabolic pathway analysis, we identified several urinary metabolic pathways significantly altered in ASD: tryptophan, purine, and vitamin B_6 metabolisms; phenylalanine, and tyrosine biosynthesis; and to a lesser extent, pantothenate and CoA, riboflavin, and pyrimidine metabolisms. Several of these same pathways, especially tryptophan, purine, and gut microbiome metabolisms, are also abnormal in animal models of ASD and provide very interesting leads toward possible pathophysiological explanations for specific symptoms present in many autistic children, such as seizures and sleep disorders. These metabolic abnormalities may apply to young children only, as suggested by studies of urinary *p*-cresol [20, 21]. It will indeed be very important to now perform a similar metabolomic assessment on ASD individuals and controls older than 8 years of age. Investigations of CSF metabolomics will be necessary to verify to what extent peripheral results reflect CNS pathophysiology. Finally, studies involving other diagnostic groups bordering with ASD, such as ADHD, intellectual disability, expressive language disorder, and obsessive-compulsive disorder, will be required to assess the disease specificity of the metabolomic abnormalities reported here and to determine their potential value as ASD-specific biomarkers, possibly able to aid clinicians in providing more reliable diagnoses in early infancy.

Abbreviations

5-HIAA: 5-hydroxyindoleacetic acid; 5-HT: 5-hydroxytryptamine; 5-HTTP: 5-hydroxytryptophan; AANAT: N-acetylserotonin by arylalkylamine N-acetyltransferase; ADHD: attention deficit hyperactivity disorder; ADP: adenosine diphosphate; ASD: autism spectrum disorder; ASMT: N-acetylserotonin O-methyltransferase; ATP: adenosine triphosphate; CNS: central nervous system; CSF: cerebrospinal fluid; ESI: electrospray ionization; GC: gas chromatography; HILIC: hydrophilic interaction chromatography; KEGG: Kyoto Encyclopedia of Genes and Genomes; LC: liquid chromatography; MetPA: metabolic pathway analysis; MIA: maternal immune activation; MS: mass spectroscopy; NAD: nicotinic acid; NMDA: *N*-methyl-D-aspartate; NMR: nuclear magnetic resonance; OPLS-DA: orthogonal partial least squares discriminant analysis; TOF: time of flight; VIP: variable influence on the projection

Acknowledgements

We gratefully acknowledge the patients, controls, and family members who participated in this study and the clinicians who contributed to patient recruitment within the framework of the 2011 collaborative *p*-cresol project.

Funding

This work was supported by the Italian Ministry for University, Scientific Research and Technology (PRIN n.2006058195), the Italian Ministry of Health (CCM2012), the Fondazione Gaetano e Mafalda Luce (Milan, Italy), the Autism Research Institute (San Diego, CA), and the Innovative Medicines Initiative Joint Undertaking (EU-AIMS, n. 115300). LZ and FG are supported by mobility studentship funds and post-doctoral research grant by the Interuniversity Consortium for Biotechnologies (CIB).

Authors' contributions

FG and LZ conducted the metabolomics analyses, analyzed and interpreted the biochemical data, and drafted the manuscript. SG collected the urine samples, interpreted the data, and drafted the manuscript. AMP designed the study, was responsible for clinical assessments, interpreted the data, and wrote the manuscript. All authors read and approved the manuscript.

Competing interests

The authors declare that they have no competing interests.

Author details

[1]Department of Ecological and Biological Sciences, University of Tuscia, Viterbo, Italy. [2]Unit of Child and Adolescent Neuropsychiatry, Laboratory of Molecular Psychiatry and Neurogenetics, University Campus Bio-Medico, Rome, Italy. [3]Unit of Child and Adolescent Neuropsychiatry, Interdepartmental Program "Autism 0-90", "Gaetano Martino" University Hospital, University of Messina, Messina, Italy. [4]Mafalda Luce Center for Pervasive Developmental Disorders, Milan, Italy.

References

1. American Psychiatric Association. Diagnostic and Statistical Manual of Mental Disorders. 5th ed. Washington, DC; 2013.
2. Fombonne E. Epidemiology of pervasive developmental disorders. Pediatr Res. 2009;65:591–8.
3. Developmental Disabilities Monitoring Network Surveillance Year 2010 Principal Investigators, Centers for Disease Control and Prevention (CDC). Prevalence of autism spectrum disorder among children aged 8

years—autism and developmental disabilities monitoring network, 11 sites, United States, 2010. MMWR Surveill Summ. 2014;63:1–21.
4. Rutter M. Incidence of autism spectrum disorders: changes over time and their meaning. Acta Paediatr. 2005;94:2–15.
5. Frans EM, Sandin S, Reichenberg A, Långström N, Lichtenstein P, McGrath JJ, Hultman CM. Autism risk across generations: a population-based study of advancing grandpaternal and paternal age. JAMA Psychiat. 2013;70:516–21.
6. Persico AM, Merelli S. Environmental factors and autism spectrum disorder. In: Leboyer M, Chaste P, editors. Autism spectrum disorders: phenotypes, mechanisms and treatments. vol. 180. Basilea: Karger; 2015. p. 113–34.
7. Persico AM, Napolioni V. Autism genetics. Behav Brain Res. 2013;251:95–112.
8. Berg JM, Geschwind DH. Autism genetics: searching for specificity and convergence. Genome Biol. 2012;13:247.
9. Ruggeri B, Sarkans U, Schumann G, Persico AM. Biomarkers in autism spectrum disorder: the old and the new. Psychopharmacology (Berl). 2014;231:1201–16.
10. Yap IK, Angley M, Veselkov KA, Holmes E, Lindon JC, Nicholson JK. Urinary metabolic phenotyping differentiates children with autism from their unaffected siblings and age-matched controls. J Proteome Res. 2010;9:2996–3004.
11. Ming X, Stein TP, Barnes V, Rhodes N, Guo L. Metabolic perturbance in autism spectrum disorders: a metabolomics study. J Proteome Res. 2012;11:5856–62.
12. Emond P, Mavel S, Aidoud N, Nadal-Desbarats L, Montigny F, Bonnet-Brilhault F, Barthélémy C, Merten M, Sarda P, Laumonnier F, Vourc'h P, Blasco H, Andres CR. GC-MS-based urine metabolic profiling of autism spectrum disorders. Anal Bioanal Chem. 2013;15:5291–300.
13. Mavel S, Nadal-Desbarats L, Blasco H, Bonnet-Brilhault F, Barthélémy C, Montigny F, Sarda P, Laumonnier F, Vourc'h P, Andres CR, Emond P. 1H-13C NMR-based urine metabolic profiling in autism spectrum disorders. Talanta. 2013;114:95–102.
14. Nadal-Desbarats L, Aïdoud N, Emond P, Blasco H, Filipiak I, Sarda P, Bonnet-Brilhault F, Mavel S, Andres CR. Combined 1H-NMR and 1H-13C HSQC-NMR to improve urinary screening in autism spectrum disorders. Analyst. 2014;139:3460–8.
15. Noto A, Fanos V, Barberini L, Grapov D, Fattuoni C, Zaffanello M, Casanova A, Fenu G, De Giacomo A, De Angelis M, Moretti C, Papoff P, Ditonno R, Francavilla R. The urinary metabolomics profile of an Italian autistic children population and their unaffected siblings. J Matern Fetal Neonatal Med. 2014;2:46–52.
16. Diémé B, Mavel S, Blasco H, Tripi G, Bonnet-Brilhault F, Malvy J, Bocca C, Andres CR, Nadal-Desbarats L, Emond P. Metabolomics study of urine in autism spectrum disorders using a multiplatform analytical methodology. J Proteome Res. 2015;14:5273–82.
17. West PR, Amaral DG, Bais P, Smith AM, Egnash LA, Ross ME, Palmer JA, Fontaine BR, Conard KR, Corbett BA, Cezar GG, Donley EL, Burrier RE. Metabolomics as a tool for discovery of biomarkers of autism spectrum disorder in the blood plasma of children. PLoS One. 2014;9:e112445.
18. Nicholson G, Rantalainen M, Li JV, Maher AD, Malmodin D, Ahmadi KR, Faber JH, Barrett A, Min JL, Rayner NW, Toft H, Krestyaninova M, Viksna J, Neogi SG, Dumas ME, Sarkans U, MolPAGE Consortium, Donnelly P, Illig T, Adamski J, Suhre K, Allen M, Zondervan KT, Spector TD, Nicholson JK, Lindon JC, Baunsgaard D, Holmes E, McCarthy MI, Holmes CC. A genome-wide metabolic QTL analysis in Europeans identifies functional effects of two loci shaped by recent positive selection. PLoS Genet. 2011;7:1002270.
19. Gebregiworgis T, Powers R. Application of NMR metabolomics to search for human disease biomarkers. Comb Chem High Throughput Screen. 2012;15:595–610.
20. Altieri L, Neri C, Sacco R, Curatolo P, Benvenuto A, Muratori F, Santocchi E, Bravaccio C, Lenti C, Saccani M, Rigardetto R, Gandione M, Urbani A, Persico AM. Urinary *p*-cresol is elevated in small children with autism spectrum disorder. Biomarkers. 2011;16:252–60.
21. Gabriele S, Sacco R, Cerullo S, Neri C, Urbani A, Tripi G, Malvy J, Barthelemy C, Bonnet-Brihault F, Persico AM. Urinary *p*-cresol is elevated in young French children with autism spectrum disorder: a replication study. Biomarkers. 2014;19:463–70.
22. Chugani DC, Muzik O, Behen M, Rothermel R, Janisse JJ, Lee J, Chugani HT. Developmental changes in brain serotonin synthesis capacity in autistic and nonautistic children. Ann Neurol. 1999;45:287–95.
23. Chandana SR, Behen ME, Juhász C, Muzik O, Rothermel RD, Mangner TJ, Chakraborty PK, Chugani HT, Chugani DC. Significance of abnormalities in developmental trajectory and asymmetry of cortical serotonin synthesis in autism. Int J Dev Neurosci. 2005;23:171–82.
24. Courchesne E, Pierce K, Schumann CM, Redcay E, Buckwalter JA, Kennedy DP, Morgan J. Mapping early brain development in autism. Neuron. 2007;56:399–413.
25. Piven J, Palmer P, Jacobi D, Childress D, Arndt S. Broader autism phenotype: evidence from a family history study of multiple-incidence autism families. Am J Psychiatry. 1997;154:185–90.
26. Hemstrom P, Irgum K. Hydrophilic interaction chromatography. J Sep Sci. 2006;29:1784–821.
27. Alpert AJ. Electrostatic repulsion hydrophilic interaction chromatography for isocratic separation of charged solutes and selective isolation of phosphopeptides. Anal Chem. 2008;80:62–76.
28. D'Alessandro A, Gevi F, Zolla L. A robust high resolution reversed-phase HPLC strategy to investigate various metabolic species in different biological models. Mol Biosyst. 2011;7:1024–32.
29. Gevi F, D'Alessandro A, Rinalducci S, Zolla L. Alterations of red blood cell metabolome during cold liquid storage of erythrocyte concentrates in CPD–SAGM. J Proteomics. 2012;76 Spec No:168–80.
30. Whiteley P, Waring R, Williams L, Klovrza L, Nolan F, Smith S, Farrow M, Dodou K, Lough WJ, Shattock P. Spot urinary creatinine excretion in pervasive developmental disorders. Pediatr Int. 2006;48:292–7.
31. Melamud E, Vastag L, Rabinowitz JD. Metabolomic analysis and visualization engine for LC-MS data. Anal Chem. 2010;82:9818–26.
32. Xia J, Mandal R, Sinelnikov I, Broadhurst D, Wishart DS. MetaboAnalyst 2. 0—a comprehensive server for metabolomic data analysis. Nucleic Acids Res. 2012;40:W127–33.
33. Dettmer K, Aronov PA, Hammock BD. Mass spectrometry based metabolomics. Mass Spectrom Rev. 2007;26:51–78.
34. Ellis DI, Goodacre R. Metabolic fingerprinting in disease diagnosis: biomedical applications of infrared and Raman spectroscopy. Analyst. 2006;131:875–85.
35. Naviaux JC, Wang L, Li K, Bright AT, Alaynick WA, Williams KR, Powell SB, Naviaux RK. Antipurinergic therapy corrects the autism-like features in the fragile X (Fmr1 knockout) mouse model. Mol Autism. 2015;6:1.
36. Naviaux JC, Schuchbauer MA, Li K, Wang L, Risbrough VB, Powell SB, Naviaux RK. Reversal of autism-like behaviors and metabolism in adult mice with single-dose antipurinergic therapy. Transl Psychiatry. 2014;4:e400.
37. Naviaux RK, Zolkipli Z, Wang L, Nakayama T, Naviaux JC, Le TP, Schuchbauer MA, Rogac M, Tang Q, Dugan LL, Powell SB. Antipurinergic therapy corrects the autism-like features in the poly(IC) mouse model. PLoS One. 2013;8:e57380.
38. Böhmer C, Bröer A, Munzinger M, Kowalczuk S, Rasko JE, Lang F, Bröer S. Characterization of mouse amino acid transporter B0AT1 (slc6a19). Biochem J. 2005;389(Pt 3):745–51.
39. Singer D, Camargo SM, Ramadan T, Schäfer M, Mariotta L, Herzog B, Huggel K, Wolfer D, Werner S, Penninger JM, Verrey F. Defective intestinal amino acid absorption in Ace2 null mice. Am J Physiol Gastrointest Liver Physiol. 2012;303:G686–95.
40. Keszthelyi D, Troost FJ, Masclee AA. Understanding the role of tryptophan and serotonin metabolism in gastrointestinal function. Neurogastroenterol Motil. 2009;21:1239–49.
41. Maddison DC, Giorgini F. The kynurenine pathway and neurodegenerative disease. Semin Cell Dev Biol. 2015;40:134–41.
42. Vargas DL, Nascimbene C, Krishnan C, Zimmerman AW, Pardo CA. Neuroglial activation and neuroinflammation in the brain of patients with autism. Ann Neurol. 2004;57:67–8.
43. Suzuki K, Sugihara G, Ouchi Y, Nakamura K, Futatsubashi M, Takebayashi K, Yoshihara Y, Omata K, Matsumoto K, Tsuchiya KJ, Iwata Y, Tsujii M, Sugiyama T, Mori N. Microglial activation in young adults with autism spectrum disorder. JAMA Psychiat. 2013;70:49–58.
44. Gupta S, Ellis SE, Ashar FN, Moes A, Bader JS, Zhan J, West AB, Arking DE. Transcriptome analysis reveals dysregulation of innate immune response genes and neuronal activity-dependent genes in autism. Nat Commun. 2014;5:5748.
45. Morgan JT, Chana G, Pardo CA, Achim C, Semendeferi K, Buckwalter J, Courchesne E, Everall IP. Microglial activation and increased microglial density observed in the dorsolateral prefrontal cortex in autism. Biol Psychiatry. 2010;68:368–76.

46. Guillemin G, Smith DG, Smythe GA, Armati PJ, Brew GJ. Expression of the kynurenine pathway enzymes in human microglia and macrophages. Adv Exp Med Biol. 2003;527:105–12.
47. Guillemin GJ. Quinolinic acid: neurotoxicity. FEBS J. 2012;279:1355.
48. Kohane IS, McMurry A, Weber G, MacFadden D, Rappaport L, Kunkel L, Bickel J, Wattanasin N, Spence S, Murphy S, Churchill S. The co-morbidity burden of children and young adults with autism spectrum disorders. PLoS One. 2012;7:e33224.
49. Nir I, Meir D, Zilber N, Knobler H, Hadjez J, Lerner Y. Brief report: circadian melatonin, thyroid-stimulating hormone, prolactin, and cortisol levels in serum of young adults with autism. J Autism Dev Disord. 1995;25:641–54.
50. Kulman G, Lissoni P, Rovelli F, Roselli MG, Brivio F, Sequeri P. Evidence of pineal endocrine hypofunction in autistic children. Neuroendocrinol Lett. 2000;21:31–4.
51. Tordjman S, Anderson GM, Pichard N, Charbuy H, Touitou Y. Nocturnal excretion of 6-sulphatoxymelatonin in children and adolescents with autistic disorder. Biol Psychiatry. 2005;57:134–8.
52. Tordjman S, Anderson GM, Bellissant E, Botbol M, Charbuy H, Camus F, Graignic R, Kermarrec S, Fougerou C, Cohen D, Touitou Y. Day and nighttime excretion of 6-sulphatoxymelatonin in adolescents and young adults with autistic disorder. Psychoneuroendocrinology. 2012;37:1990–7.
53. Melke J, Goubran Botros H, Chaste P, Betancur C, Nygren G, Anckarsäter H, Rastam M, Ståhlberg O, Gillberg IC, Delorme R, Chabane N, Mouren-Simeoni MC, Fauchereau F, Durand CM, Chevalier F, Drouot X, Collet C, Launay JM, Leboyer M, Gillberg C, Bourgeron T. Abnormal melatonin synthesis in autism spectrum disorders. Mol Psychiatry. 2008;13:90–8.
54. Pagan C, Delorme R, Callebert J, Goubran-Botros H, Amsellem F, Drouot X, Boudebesse C, Le Dudal K, Ngo-Nguyen N, Laouamri H, Gillberg C, Leboyer M, Bourgeron T, Launay JM. The serotonin-N-acetylserotonin–melatonin pathway as a biomarker for autism spectrum disorders. Transl Psychiatry. 2014;4:e479.
55. Vitte PA, Harthe C, Lestage P, Claustrat B, Bobillier P. Plasma, cerebrospinal fluid, and brain distribution of 14C-melatonin in rat: a biochemical and autoradiographic study. J Pineal Res. 1988;5:437–53.
56. Rossignol DA, Frye RE. Melatonin in autism spectrum disorders: a systematic review and meta-analysis. Dev Med Child Neurol. 2011;53:783–92.
57. Bull G, Shattock P, Whiteley P, Anderson R, Groundwater P, Lough JW, Lees G. Indolyl-3- acryloylglycine (IAG) is a putative diagnostic urinary marker for autism spectrum disorders. Med Sci Monit. 2003;9:CR422–5.
58. Wang L, Angley MT, Gerber JP, Young RL, Abarno DV, McKinnon RA, Sorich MJ. Is urinary indolyl-3-acryloylglycine a biomarker for autism with gastrointestinal symptoms? Biomarkers. 2009;14:596–603.
59. Wright B, Brzozowski AM, Calvert E, Farnworth H, Goodall DM, Holbrook I, Imrie G, Jordan J, Kelly A, Miles J, Smith R, Town J. Is the presence of urinary indolyl-3-acryloylglycine associated with autism spectrum disorder? Dev Med Child Neurol. 2005;47:190–2.
60. Li M, Wang B, Zhang M, Rantalainen M, Wang S, Zhou H, Zhang Y, Shen J, Pang X, Zhang M, Wei H, Chen Y, Lu H, Zuo J, Su M, Qiu Y, Jia W, Xiao C, Smith LM, Yang S, Holmes E, Tang H, Zhao G, Nicholson JK, Li L, Zhao L. Symbiotic gut microbes modulate human metabolic phenotypes. Proc Natl Acad Sci U S A. 2008;105:2117–22.
61. Thomas RH, Meeking MM, Mepham JR, Tichenoff L, Possmayer F, Liu S, MacFabe DF. The enteric bacterial metabolite propionic acid alters brain and plasma phospholipid molecular species: further development of a rodent model of autism spectrum disorders. J Neuroinflammation. 2012;9:153.
62. Watanabe K, Watanabe T, Nakayama M. Cerebro-renal interactions: impact of uremic toxins on cognitive function. Neurotoxicology. 2014;44:184–93.
63. Ohtsuki S, Asaba H, Takanaga H, Deguchi T, Hosoya K, Otagiri M, Terasaki T. Role of blood-brain barrier organic anion transporter 3 (OAT3) in the efflux of indoxyl sulfate, a uremic toxin: its involvement in neurotransmitter metabolite clearance from the brain. J Neurochem. 2002;83:57–66.
64. Hsiao EY, McBride SW, Hsien S, Sharon G, Hyde ER, McCue T, Codelli JA, Chow J, Reisman SE, Petrosino JF, Patterson PH, Mazmanian SK. Microbiota modulate behavioral and physiological abnormalities associated with neurodevelopmental disorders. Cell. 2013;155:1451 63.
65. Naviaux RK. Metabolic features of the cell danger response. Mitochondrion. 2014;16:7–17.
66. Nyhan WL, James JA, Teberg AJ, Sweetman L, Nelson LG. A new disorder of purine metabolism with behavioral manifestations. J Pediatr. 1969;74:20–7.
67. Tada K, Yokoyama Y, Nakagawa H, Yoshida T, Arakawa T. Vitamin B6 dependent xanthurenic aciduria. Tohoku J Exp Med. 1967;93:115–24.
68. Martineau J, Barthelemy C, Garreau B, Lelord G. Vitamin B6, magnesium, and combined B6-Mg: therapeutic effects in childhood autism. Biol Psychiatry. 1985;20:467–78.
69. Nye C, Brice A. Combined vitamin B6-magnesium treatment in autism spectrum disorder. Cochrane Database Syst Rev. 2005;4:CD003497.

17

A randomized placebo-controlled pilot study of *N*-acetylcysteine in youth with autism spectrum disorder

Logan K. Wink[1], Ryan Adams[1], Zemin Wang[2], James E. Klaunig[2], Martin H. Plawecki[3], David J. Posey[4], Christopher J. McDougle[5] and Craig A. Erickson[1*]

Abstract

Background: Social impairment is a defining feature of autism spectrum disorder (ASD) with no demonstrated effective pharmacologic treatments. The goal of this study was to evaluate efficacy, safety, and tolerability of oral *N*-acetylcysteine (NAC), an antioxidant whose function overlaps with proposed mechanisms of ASD pathophysiology, targeting core social impairment in youth with ASD.

Methods: This study was a 12-week randomized, double-blind, placebo-controlled trial of oral NAC in youth with ASD. Study participants were medically healthy youth age 4 to 12 years with ASD, weighing ≥15 kg, and judged to be moderately ill based on the Clinical Global Impressions Severity scale. The participants were randomized via computer to active drug or placebo in a 1:1 ratio, with the target dose of NAC being 60 mg/kg/day in three divided doses. The primary outcome measure of efficacy was the Clinical Global Impressions Improvement (CGI-I) scale anchored to core social impairment. To investigate the impact of NAC on oxidative stress markers in peripheral blood, venous blood samples were collected at screen and week 12.

Results: Thirty-one patients were enrolled (NAC = 16, placebo = 15). Three participants were lost to follow-up, and three left the trial due to adverse effects. The average daily dose of NAC at week 12 was 56.2 mg/kg ($SD = 9.7$) with dose ranging from 33.6 to 64.3 mg/kg. The frequency of adverse events was so low that comparisons between groups could not be conducted. At week 12, there was no statistically significant difference between the NAC and placebo groups on the CGI-I ($p > 0.69$) but the glutathione (GSH) level in blood was significantly higher in the NAC group ($p < 0.05$). The oxidative glutathione disulfide (GSSG) level increased in the NAC group, however only at a trend level of significance ($p = 0.09$). There was no significant difference between the NAC and placebo groups in the GSH/GSSG ratio, DNA strand break and oxidative damage, and blood homocysteine levels at week 12 ($ps > 0.16$).

Conclusions: The results of this trial indicate that NAC treatment was well tolerated, had the expected effect of boosting GSH production, but had no significant impact on social impairment in youth with ASD.

Keywords: Autism, Autism spectrum disorder, Social impairment, *N*-acetylcysteine, Oxidative stress

* Correspondence: Craig.erickson@cchmc.org
[1]Cincinnati Children's Hospital Medical Center, University of Cincinnati College of Medicine, 3333 Burnet Avenue MLC 4002, Cincinnati, OH 45229, USA
Full list of author information is available at the end of the article

Background

Social and communication impairments are the defining features and key predictors of long-term outcome in autism spectrum disorder (ASD) [1, 2]. To date, no medication has demonstrated significant impact on these core deficits in controlled trials. In 2014, the United States Center for Disease Control reported that one in 68 children in the USA is diagnosed with ASD, highlighting the critical need for targeted treatment development in this disorder [3]. Growing neurobiologic understanding of ASD has identified glutamatergic neurotransmission and metabolic pathways impacting oxidative stress levels as potential targets of drug development in this complex disorder [4]. Glutamatergic dysfunction appears to play a significant role in ASD pathology, as studies have identified abnormal peripheral glutamate levels, aberrant glutamate expression in the postmortem brain, and genetic abnormalities in glutamate signaling genes in individuals with ASD [5]. Excessive oxidative stress also has been identified as playing a potential role in ASD pathophysiology. Increased peripheral oxidative biomarkers, evidence of oxidative stress in the postmortem brain, and abnormalities in genes encoding for antioxidant enzymes have been reported in individuals with ASD [4, 6, 7].

N-acetylcysteine (NAC) is a unique antioxidant whose function overlaps with both the glutamatergic and oxidative stress hypotheses proposed to contribute to the pathophysiology of ASD. NAC is the *N*-acetyl derivative of L-cysteine used for decades in treatment of acetaminophen overdose, as a mucolytic in chronic obstructive pulmonary disease, and as a renal protectant in contrast-induced nephropathy [8]. NAC is rapidly absorbed via oral dosing, though total oral bioavailability of NAC is quite low (~9 %) [9]. NAC crosses the blood-brain barrier (BBB), though its efficiency may depend upon dose, administration, and formulation [10]. In the brain, NAC is oxidized from L-cysteine to cystine which is ultimately involved in regulation of extracellular glutamate levels [11]. NAC is cell membrane permeable and is reduced to cysteine intracellularly, which is a key component of the antioxidant glutathione (GSH) [10]. NAC's involvement in both extracellular glutamate modulation and intracellular restoration of antioxidant GSH levels, coupled to its long history of human safety data, make NAC an intriguing substance in ASD-targeted treatment development.

Placebo-controlled studies of NAC in ASD have previously focused on treatment of ASD-associated irritability marked by physical aggression, self-injurious behavior, and severe tantrums. A pilot placebo-controlled study by Hardan et al. (2012) demonstrated a significant reduction in irritability symptoms as measured by the Aberrant Behavior Checklist Irritability subscale [12] (ABC-I) in 29 youth aged 3.2–10.7 years with ASD [13]. Additionally, two small double-blind, placebo-controlled studies of NAC in conjunction with risperidone for treatment of irritability in youth with ASD also showed a significant reduction in ABC-I subscale scores in the NAC-treated groups [14, 15]. Furthermore, case studies have demonstrated improvement of core ASD features including social communication and repetitive behaviors with NAC treatment; however, this effect has not been confirmed in controlled trials [16, 17].

To date, no study of NAC in ASD has evaluated the impact of NAC on markers of oxidative stress in peripheral blood. Individuals with ASD are believed to have decreased total GSH levels and elevated levels of oxidative glutathione disulfide (GSSG) [4]. These abnormalities lead to a reduction in the ratio of active GSH to inactive GSSH resulting in increased intracellular oxidative stress which may impact on individual's capacity to maintain cellular methylation and increase vulnerability to oxidative damage [18]. This change has the potential to decrease an individual's ability to resist infection, resolve inflammation, and respond to environmental exposures. Correction of these abnormalities with NAC treatment could have substantial impact on the health of individuals with ASD.

The goal of this randomized, double-blind, placebo-controlled pilot study of NAC in youth with ASD was to evaluate the efficacy of oral NAC targeting core social impairment of ASD and evaluate the safety and tolerability of NAC in this population. Additionally, this project incorporated measures of oxidative stress that may be impacted by NAC treatment, including measures of pre- and post-treatment peripheral whole blood levels of GSH and GSSG. We hypothesized that treatment with NAC in this population would result in improvement in core social impairment of ASD as measured by the Clinical Global Impression Improvement (CGI-I) scale [19], and that NAC treatment would result in increased GSH and GSSH levels.

Methods

Study design

This study was a 12-week randomized, double-blind, placebo-controlled pilot trial of oral NAC in youth with ASD. The study was conducted at Indiana University School of Medicine (IUSM) between December 2006 and November 2009. The study was approved by the IUSM institutional review board. Guardians of all participants provided written informed consent prior to study enrollment. Assent was obtained from enrolled youth when possible.

Study participants were youth ages 4 to 12 years with a diagnosis of autistic disorder, Asperger's disorder, or pervasive developmental disorder not otherwise specified (PDD NOS). Subjects with known genetic syndromes associated with autism were excluded (for example, fragile X syndrome, tuberous sclerosis). Participants were diagnosed via clinical interview completed by study physician with expertise in ASD (DJP, CJM, CAE), based on the Diagnostic and Statistical Manual of Mental Disorders, Fourth Edition (DSM-IV) [20] diagnostic criteria, and corroborated by administration of the Autism Diagnostic Interview-Revised [21] (ADI-R). Participants diagnosed with PDD NOS demonstrated pervasive impairment in social interaction and/or communication skills as well as stereotyped behaviors and restricted interests, but did not meet full criteria for diagnosis of autistic disorder or Asperger's disorder. All participants weighed ≥15 kg and were medically healthy based on physical exam and review of medical history completed by study physicians. Participants were judged by study physician as being at least "moderately ill" as measured by the Clinical Global Impression Severity [19] (CGI-S) scale rating at baseline. The CGI-S is a clinician-rated global assessment of symptom severity scale ranging from 1 to 7 (1 = normal, not at all ill; 2 = borderline ill; 3 = mildly ill; 4 = moderately ill; 5 = markedly ill; 6 = severely ill; 7 = among the most extremely ill patients). Concomitant medications were permitted if doses were stable for at least 60 days prior to study initiation and remained stable throughout the study. Participants taking known glutamatergic modulators such as dextromethorphan, D-cycloserine, amantadine, memantine, lamotrigine, or riluzole were excluded. Patients taking daily acetaminophen, daily nonsteroidal anti-inflammatory medications, daily antioxidant medications such as high-dose vitamin supplements, and medications with known drug-interactions (i.e., carbamazepine) within 30 days of baseline were also excluded. Subjects were required to be able to swallow capsules. Potential subjects with profound cognitive impairment (mental functioning below 18 months of age) as measured by the Leiter International Test of Intelligence-Revised [22] were excluded.

Following screening and baseline measures, participants were randomized 1:1 via computer—by the investigational pharmacy. All participants, guardians, and investigators remained blind to study assignment. NAC and matching placebo were prepared by CustomMed Apothecary. Participants randomized to active drug were administered capsules containing 300 or 600 mg of NAC, with a target dose of 60 mg/kg/day in three divided doses and a maximum dose of 4200 mg/day. Patients weighing 15 to 30 kg began treatment with a starting dose of 300 mg/day; those weighing above 30 kg started with 600 mg/day. Patients were required to tolerate a minimum dose of 300 mg/day to continue in the trial. Dose was titrated to the target dose over the first 3 weeks of study participation. Dose then remained stable for all subjects in the last 9 weeks of the study, although reductions due to adverse effects were permitted at any time. Subjects were evaluated in person at screen and baseline, by phone at week 2, and in person at weeks 4, 8, and 12. Assessment for adverse effects was completed during each interaction. Vital signs including height, weight, blood pressure, and heart rate were measured at every in-person study visit. Safety labs including complete blood cell count (CBC) and comprehensive metabolic panel (CMP) were collected at screen and week 12.

The primary outcome measure of efficacy was the CGI-I scale anchored to study physician (DJP, CJM, CAE) assessment of core social impairment considering the individuals' overall level of cognitive, adaptive, and social functioning. The CGI-I is a clinician-rated global assessment of symptom change rated on a scale from 1 to 7 (1 = very much improved; 2 = much improved; 3 = minimally improved; 4 = no change; 5 = minimally worse; 6 = much worse; 7 = very much worse). In this study, a positive response to NAC treatment was defined as scoring a 1 "very much improved "or 2 "much improved" on the CGI-I. Study physicians completed annual CGI training to ensure internal consistency with this outcome measure. Secondary outcome measures included the CGI-S, ABC, Social Responsiveness Scale [23] (SRS) raw score, and Vineland Adaptive Behavior Scales 2nd Edition [24] (VABS-II) survey edition raw score. The SRS is a standardized, caregiver reported measure of the core symptoms of ASD [23]. The ABC is a parent questionnaire measuring five behavioral domains including irritability, social withdrawal, stereotypy, hyperactivity, and inappropriate speech [12]. The VABS-II is a semi-structured caregiver interview which provides a measure of an individual's overall adaptive functioning [24]. All measures have been used extensively in ASD research [25–27]. The CGI-I was completed at weeks 4, 8, and 12. The ABC and SRS were completed at baseline and weeks 4, 8, and 12. The CGI-S and VABS-II were completed only at baseline and week 12.

Early morning, fasting, venous blood samples for measurement of oxidative stress biomarkers GSH, GSSH, total homocysteine, strand breakage, and oxidative DNA damage were collected in EDTA containing Vacutainers at screen and week 12.

Measurement of reduced and oxidized glutathione

Concentrations of reduced and oxidized glutathione (GSH and GSSG) in whole blood samples were analyzed simultaneously using HPLC-electrochemical detection as described previously [28]. Briefly, 1 ml of blood sample was added to 0.5 ml precipitating solution containing 0.2 M perchloric acid and 100 μM EDTA, and vortexed briefly. After incubation at room temperature for 45 min, samples were centrifuged at 10,000*g* for 3 minutes. The resulting supernatants were filtered and injected into high-performance liquid chromatography (HPLC; Waters 2690) for analysis immediately or frozen in liquid nitrogen and stored at −80 °C before analysis. The separation of analytes was achieved on a reverse phase Symmetry C-18 column (5 μm, 150 × 4.6 mm; Waters). GSH and GSSG were detected using an ESA Coulochem II (ESA Inc. Chelmsford, MA) equipped with a guard cell. The potential settings for the detector were E1 450 mV, E2 900 mV, and guard cell 1000 mV. The amount of GSH and GSSG was calculated from the respective calibration curves, and the ratio of GSH/GSSG for each sample was also calculated.

Measurement of blood homocysteine

Total homocysteine in whole blood sample was determined using an HPLC method as described previously with minor modifications [29, 30]. Briefly, 1 ml EDTA blood samples were lysed by vigorously shaking for at least 10 s after adding 10 μl Nonidet P40 (pure) and 10 μl citric acid monohydrate (2.5 M). The lysates were then centrifuged at 10,000*g* for 3 minutes at room temperature. Following reduction of the sample with tri-n-butylphosphine, precipitation of protein with perchloric acid and derivatization with ammonium 7-fluorobenzo-2-oxa-1,3-diazole-4-sulfonate, the samples were then analyzed using reversed-phase high-performance liquid chromatography (Waters Alliance 2695 separation module) followed by fluorescence detection (Waters 474 fluorescence detector) (Waters Corporation, Milford, MA).

Direct and oxidative DNA damage: comet assay

Immediately after blood collection, whole blood (10 μl) was mixed with 0.5 ml RPMI 1640 containing 10 % FBS, 10 % DMSO, 1 mM deferoxamine, step-frozen and stored at −80 °C until analysis. The comet assay was performed as described previously [31, 32]. Briefly, 6 μl of blood was mixed with 70 μl 1 % low-melting-point agarose and applied onto comet slides (Trevigen Inc, Gaithersburg, MD). Cells were lysed, placed in alkali buffer, and then electrophoresed. Slides were stained with ethidium bromide, and 100 randomly selected nuclei/sample were evaluated (Komet 5.5; Kinetic Imaging Ltd., Liverpool, UK). For the assessment of oxidative DNA damage, a modified alkaline comet assay was performed that included enzymatic digestion with formamidopyrimidine-DNA glycosylase (fpg) prior to electrophoresis. DNA damage was expressed as Comet (Olive) tail moment [(tail mean − head mean) × tail%DNA/100].

Statistical analysis

Our sample size (goal 32 participants) was chosen based on recommendation for sampling in pilot studies where little is known about treatment response rates [33]. Baseline demographic data including age, sex, race, level of intellectual quotient (IQ), ASD diagnostic sub-type, concomitant medications, and clinical ratings (CGI-S, ABC, SRS, and VABS-II scores) was compiled, and means and percentages were calculated to describe the NAC and placebo groups. Baseline demographic differences between groups were tested using chi-square tests (categorical data) and independent sample t test (continuous data) using a two-tailed p value of 0.05 for the alpha.

For the CGI-I primary outcome measure, differences between the two treatment groups were tested at weeks 4, 8, 12 using chi-square tests. For the CGI-S secondary outcome measure, a chi-square test was employed to examine change from baseline to week 12 by creating two CGI-S categories: (1) those subjects whose severity score decreased (i.e., clinically improved) by at least one point from baseline to week 12 and (2) those subjects whose scores remained the same during the same period. For the ABC, SRS, VABS-II, and oxidative stress biomarkers, differences between the groups for change in each outcome measure over the course of the study were tested using multi-level modeling (i.e., we examined if there were differences between the two groups in terms of change in the outcome scores over the course of the study). For each outcome, time was modeled at level-one as a random effect with treatment group entered as a level-two fixed effect. The cross-level interaction between group and time tested the differences between the two groups in the change over time using maximum likelihood estimation with robust standard errors with Mplus 5.21 [34] (baseline, week 4, week 8, and week 12 data was used for the ABC and SRS; baseline and week 12 data was used for the VABS-II and oxidative stress biomarkers). Since there is no method to directly calculate the effect size of the between-subject effects on the within-subject effects for multilevel modeling, we calculated an effect size of the difference between the groups on the mean differences between baseline and week 12 for the groups. Specifically, a Cohen's d was calculated by subtracting the mean score at week 12 from the score at baseline for each group, and a difference score was calculated by subtracting the change scores between the groups. This difference score was then divided by the pooled standard deviation of the change scores. Independent sample t tests were used to compare the levels of oxidative markers between NAC and placebo groups at baseline and week 12. For all types of tests, a one-tailed p value of 0.05 was used as the alpha. A one-tailed test was used based on the a priori hypothesis that the NAC group would have greater change in clinical ratings and oxidative stress markers over the course of the study than the placebo group. We did not correct for multiple comparisons given the pilot nature of the work.

Adverse event data was compiled to describe the NAC and placebo groups. Separate analyses were conducted for the vital sign measurements, CMP, and CBC employing the same method as the treatment analyses, though only two time points, screen and week 12, were evaluated.

Results

Thirty-one participants initially enrolled in the trial; however, six participants did not complete the study. Three participants were lost to follow-up after week 4 (two NAC and one placebo), and three withdrew due to irritability (NAC), diarrhea and encopresis (placebo), and defiant and self-injurious behavior (placebo), respectively. At baseline, data for all 31 enrolled subjects was employed in the analysis. Post-baseline, only data for the 25 completers was analyzed, as there is no method for imputing data for multi-level models.

At baseline, participants ranged in age from 4 to 12 years. The average age was 7.6 years ($SD = 2.5$, $n = 16$) for the NAC group and 8.2 years ($SD = 2.9$, $n = 15$) for the placebo group (Table 1). The majority of the participants were male (>75 %), white (>90 %), and had an IQ above 85. For the NAC group, the ASD diagnostic sub-types were primarily autistic disorder (43.8 %) and PDD-NOS (43.8 %) while the placebo group included primarily those with autistic disorder (46.7 %) and Asperger's disorder (33.3 %). On the CGI-S scale, the majority of the participants in both groups (>85 %) were rated as either 5 "markedly" or 6 "severely ill". There was no statistically significant baseline difference between groups for any clinical ratings (ABC, SRS, VABS-II), with the exception of a trend toward significantly higher score on the ABC stereotypy subscale in the placebo group (t value = 1.85, 0.07; NAC $M = 4.75$, $SD = 3.3$; placebo $M = 7.00$, $SD = 4.9$). Additionally, there was no significant difference in type or number of baseline concomitant medications between groups (all $ps > 0.11$).

The average daily dose of NAC at week 12 was 56.2 mg/kg ($SD = 9.7$) with dose ranging from 33.6 to 64.3 mg/kg. Overall, NAC was well tolerated by study participants. The majority of adverse events occurred only once, and the frequency of adverse events was so low that comparisons between groups could not be conducted (Table 2). Overall, upper respiratory symptoms were the most commonly reported event for both groups (NAC $n = 10$, 62.5 %; placebo $n = 6$, 40.0 %). The next

Table 1 Demographic data and baseline characteristics

	Groups				Test of differences
	NAC		Placebo		
Characteristics	*n*/total	%	*n*/total	%	Chi-square[a]
Gender—male	12/16	75.0	12/15	80.0	0.11
Race—White	16/16	100.0	14/15	93.3	1.01
Diagnosis					
Autistic disorder	7/16	43.8	7/15	46.7	0.03
Asperger's disorder	2/16	12.5	5/15	33.3	1.92
PDD-NOS	7/15	43.8	3/15	20.0	1.98
CGI-S					
Marked (5)	6/16	37.5	9/15	60.0	1.57
Severe (6)	9/16	56.3	6/15	40.0	0.82
Extreme (7)	1/16	6.3	0/15	0.0	0.97
Concomitant medication (y/n)	6/16	37.5	10/15	66.7	2.64
Medication types					
Psychostimulants	3/16	18.7	3/15	20.0	0.01
Alpha 2 agonists	1/16	6.2	2/15	13.3	0.44
Antipsychotics	4/15	25.0	5/15	33.3	0.26
Sleep aids	6/16	37.5	2/15	13.3	2.36
Antidepressants	1/16	6.2	3/15	20.0	1.30
Antiepileptic medication	2/16	12.5	0/15	0.0	2.01
	Mean	*SD*	Mean	*SD*	*t* test[b]
Age	7.63	2.5	8.20	2.9	0.59
Full scale IQ	86.27	21.8	87.43	11.7	0.18
Number of concomitant medications per participant	1.20	1.8	0.94	1.0	0.51

[a]Two-tailed significance $^{+}p < .10$; $^{*}p < .05$. No p values for these chi-squares reached significance at .05 and ranged from .11 to .87

[b]Two-tailed significance $^{+}p < .10$; $^{*}p < .05$ and ps ranged from .56 to .94

NAC N-acetylcysteine, *PDD-NOS* pervasive developmental disorder not otherwise specified, *CGI-S* clinical global impression severity scale

Table 2 Frequency of adverse effects

	NAC ($n = 16$)			Placebo ($n = 15$)		
Adverse effects	Mild	Mod	Severe	Mild	Mod	Severe
URI	9	1	0	5	1	0
Headache	3	0	0	2	1	0
Stomachache	2	0	0	2	0	0
Fever	2	1	0	0	0	0
Irritability	2	0	0	1	0	0
Insomnia	2	0	0	0	0	0
Otitis media	1	1	0	1	0	0
Increased enuresis	1	0	0	1	0	0
Interrupted sleep	1	0	0	1	0	0
Localized rash	1	0	0	1	0	0
Nausea	1	0	0	1	0	0
Stereotypy	0	0	0	2	0	0

The table only lists adverse effects occurring ≥2 times across the samples
Placebo group reported one moderate case of the following adverse effects: defiant behavior, hives, itchy skin, and threats to hurt self
Placebo group reported one mild case of the following adverse effects: accidental injury (arm), constipation, diarrhea, dry mouth, emotional outburst, encopresis, increased hyperactivity, self-injurious behavior (skin picking), sinus infection, skin infection, sore throat, urinary tract infection, and weight gain
NAC group reported one mild case of the following adverse effects: aggression, appetite increase, behavior worse, change in speech, early morning awakening, edema, medical or surgical procedure, swollen neck/lymph nodes, and tic
NAC N-acetylcysteine, *Mod* moderate, *URI* upper respiratory infection

most frequent events were headaches (NAC $n = 3$, 18.7 %; placebo $n = 3$, 20.0 %), stomachache (NAC $n = 2$, 12.5 %; placebo $n = 2$, 13.3 %), and fever (NAC $n = 3$, 18.7 %; placebo $n = 1$, 6.7 %). The majority of reported adverse events were mild, with only five (6.7 %) reported as moderate. No severe adverse events were reported. There were no significant differences found between the groups for changes from screen to week 12 on vital signs or safety lab values (all $p > 0.10$).

Primary and secondary outcomes

There was no statistically significant difference between the NAC and the placebo groups at week 4 ($p > 0.60$), week 8 ($p > 0.79$), or week 12 ($p > 0.69$) on the CGI-I primary outcome measure (Table 3). At each time period, at least half of all participants (≥50 %) were rated as having no change. On the CGI-S secondary outcome measure, no participants were noted to have increased scores suggesting clinical worsening of symptoms. There were also no differences between the NAC and placebo groups for those whose severity scores decreased from baseline to week 12 ($\chi^2 = 0.43$, $p = 0.40$; NAC 46.2 %, $n = 6$; placebo 33.3 %, $n = 4$). On the ABC, SRS, and VABS-II secondary outcome measures, the employed models found no significant differences between groups in change from baseline to week 12 (all *ps* > 0.13 (Table 4)). Using the cutoff of a Cohen's *d* of 0.25 for small, 0.50 for medium, and 0.80 for large, 100 % of the effects were ≤ the small effect size [35]. For all of the models that had a small effect size, the placebo group consistently had the larger average decrease in score.

Table 3 Clinical Global Impression-Improvement scale score, NAC vs. placebo

	Groups				Test of differences
	NAC		Placebo		
	n/total	%	*n*/total	%	Chi-square[a]
Week 4					0.28
Response	4/15	26.7	5/14	35.7	
No response	11/15	73.3	9/14	64.3	
Week 8					0.07
Response	5/13	38.5	4/12	33.3	
No response	8/13	61.5	8/12	66.7	
Week 12					0.15
Response	6/12	50.0	5/11	45.5	
No response	6/12	50.0	6/11	54.5	

[a]One-tailed significance $^+p < .10$; $^*p < .05$. No *p* values for these chi-squares reached significance at .05 and ranged from .60 to .79
Response = very much improved (1) or much improved (2); no response = minimally improved (3), no change (4), minimally worse (5); no participants scored much worse (6) or very much worse (7)
NAC N-acetylcysteine

Oxidative stress biomarkers

Baseline (pre-treatment) levels of the oxidative markers including GSH, GSSG, GSH/GSSG ratio, DNA strand break and oxidative damage, and blood homocysteine were not significantly different between the NAC and placebo groups ($p > 0.05$ for all). At week 12, the GSH level in blood was significantly higher in the NAC group compared to placebo (780.3 vs. 640.4 μM; $p < 0.05$, Table 4). The GSSG level increased in the NAC treatment group, however with only marginal significance in comparison with the placebo group (16.7 vs. 12.5 μM; $p = 0.09$, Table 4). Using the Cohen's *d* cutoff employed above for effect sizes, the size of the differences for the significant and the marginally significant effects were large- and medium-sized effects, respectively. For the GSH/GSSG ratio, strand break and oxidative damage of DNA, as well as blood homocysteine, there were no significant differences between the NAC and placebo groups from baseline to week 12 (*ps* > 0.16).

Discussion

This study was designed to evaluate the safety and efficacy of NAC targeting core social impairment in youth with ASD. The results of this randomized, placebo-controlled trial indicate that NAC treatment was well tolerated by study participants, had the expected effect of boosting GSH production in peripheral blood, but had no significant impact on the core social impairment

Table 4 Means, standard deviations, and differences in change scores between NAC and Placebo groups

	NAC				Placebo						
	Baseline		12 Weeks		Baseline		12 Weeks			Group with largest change[b]	Cohen's *d*
	M	SD	M	SD	M	SD	M	SD	*z* test[a]		
ABC											
Hyperactivity	20.6	12.4	17.4	16.4	22.6	10.5	15.1	10.8	1.04	PLB	0.34
Speech	3.9	2.8	4.1	3.9	5.7	2.9	5.14	3.5	0.66	PLB	0.24
Irritability	17.0	11.8	14.9	14.0	18.3	9.2	12.0	7.3	1.09	PLB	0.40
Lethargy	13.8	8.1	10.0	7.1	14.0	10.5	7.9	4.7	1.15	PLB	0.31
Stereotypy	4.8	3.3	3.9	5.1	7.0	4.9	5.8	4.0	0.56	PLB	0.09
SRS											
Total score	108.5	20.7	85.8	34.9	109.1	16.5	89.1	26.3	0.32	NAC	0.11
VABS-II											
Comm	85.9	32.1	88.5	32.5	89.4	32.2	95.0	30.3	0.85	PLB	0.09
Daily Liv. Sk.	93.1	33.7	99.0	37.1	87.6	28.1	98.6	33.4	0.17	PLB	0.16
Socialization	66.8	18.8	71.7	18.7	68.3	20.7	75.9	21.0	0.87	PLB	0.14
Composite	61.3	19.4	62.9	17.1	53.6	15.1	60.5	18.8	1.08	PLB	0.30
Levels in whole blood (uM)											
GSH	484.8	212.7	780.3	220.6	474.5	191.6	640.4	190.9	1.74*	NAC	0.64
GSSG	12.0	2.5	16.7	10.5	12.8	5.0	12.5	4.4	1.37⁺	NAC	0.88
GSH/GSSG	43.4	25.6	53.5	16.8	45.2	31.8	59.6	27.0	0.34	PLB	0.17
Homocysteine	4.3	6.1	9.9	13.7	1.9	1.2	5.6	6.8	0.41	NAC	0.27
DNA damage											
DNA strand breakage	0.7	0.1	0.7	0.3	0.6	0.2	0.6	0.1	0.38	EVEN	0.00
Oxidative DNA damage	0.9	0.2	1.2	0.4	1.1	0.5	1.2	0.6	0.95	NAC	0.45

[a]One-tailed significance ⁺$p < .10$; *$p < .05$. *Z* test of the effect of between level variable of group on the within-level variable of time testing if the change from baseline to week 12 is different between groups. No one-tailed *p* values for these *z* tests reached significance at .05 and ranged from .13 to .50
[b]Identifies which group had the largest change from baseline to week 12
NAC N-acetylcysteine, *M* mean, *SD* standard deviation, *ABC* Aberrant Behavior Checklist, *PLB* placebo, *SRS* social responsiveness scale, *VABS-II* Vineland adaptive behavior scale 2nd edition, *Comm* communication, *Liv. Sk.* living skills, *GSH* glutathione, *GSSG* oxidative glutathione disulfide

of ASD when compared to placebo treatment. The results of this study do not support the use of NAC for treatment of core social impairment of ASD, though the health impact of the resultant increase on GSH remains unclear. In addition, the study did not note other behavioral improvements with NAC use such as the reduction in irritability reported by Harden et al. (2012) [13].

Interpretation of these results must be taken in context of the study's limitations. Participant diagnoses were made by study physicians with expertise in ASD corroborated by the ADI-R similar to methods employed in other ASD drug studies [36]. Nevertheless, administration of a research reliable Autism Diagnostic Observation Schedule would have added to the validity of diagnoses in this study. Furthermore, limitation of the study to just participants with diagnosis of autistic disorder would have lessened the heterogeneity of our sample. Our study population was potentially biased toward individuals with higher level of functioning, as the majority of participants had IQ above 85. This limits the generalizability of these study results to the broader population of individuals with ASD. This higher functioning study population may have also contributed to lack of improvement in irritability noted in this study. The baseline ABC-I of study participants was 17.0 (*SD* 11.8) in the NAC group and 18.3 (*SD* 9.2) in the placebo group, which is slightly below the standard cutoff ABC-I score of 18 used in drug studies targeting ASD-associated irritability [36]. However, the baseline ABC-I scores in our study are higher than those in the Hardan study which demonstrated improvement irritability with NAC treatment [13], so the impact this had on our study outcome is unclear. Additionally, the small sample size combined with the inherent significant placebo response rates in ASD core symptom trials enhances type II error potential thus rendering the project potentially underpowered to detect meaningful change. The small sample size also reduces the ability to effectively correlate treatment response with baseline oxidative stress markers or with change in such markers with treatment.

The NAC formulation employed in this study was a powder which was encapsulated by the investigative pharmacy and stored under normal pharmacy conditions. No studies of impurity were completed on this compound, and no analyses were completed to assess its stability. Furthermore, this packaging was different than the method employed by Hardan et al. (2012) who utilized an individual foil packaging method to protect the integrity of the active ingredient against oxidation [13]. While this difference could have in theory reduced the potency of our formulation, the biologic impact of our treatment was clear given the significant NAC-associated increase in GSH levels at week 12. It is unclear; however, if the change in oxidative markers and potential clinical impact may have differed had we employed an individual foil packaging method. Further, whether an increase in peripheral blood GSH levels, and the NAC formulation employed in our study, translates to clinically significant CNS antioxidant activity is unclear as there remains debate in the field regarding the ability of NAC to efficiently cross the BBB [10]. In future studies, alterations to NAC formulation including esterification of the carboxyl group producing *N*-acetylcysteine ethyl ester or creation of the amide derivative *N*-acetylcysteine amide may increase this medication's oral bioavailability, BBB permeability, and therefore therapeutic potential [10].

Conclusions

The results of this study suggest that NAC treatment does not have significant impact on the core social impairment of ASD. However, the small study size limits interpretation of these results. Additional larger-scale study powered to predict treatment response based on baseline peripheral oxidative markers may be indicated. Future studies may also wish to consider the use of a NAC formulation with improved bioavailability and BBB permeability.

Abbreviations

ABC: Aberrant Behavior Checklist; ADI-R: Autism Diagnostic Inventory Revised; ASD: autism spectrum disorder; BBB: blood-brain barrier; CBC: complete blood cell count; CGI-I: Clinical Global Impression Improvement; CGI-S: Clinical Global Impression Severity; CMP: comprehensive metabolic panel; GSH: glutathione; GSSG: glutathione disulfide; HPLC: high-performance liquid chromatography; IQ: intellectual quotient; IUSM: Indiana University School of Medicine; M: mean; N: number; NAC: *N*-acetylcysteine; PDD NOS: pervasive developmental disorder not otherwise specified; SD: standard deviations; SRS: Social Responsiveness Scale; VABS-II: Vineland Adaptive Behavior Scale 2nd Edition.

Competing interests

The authors declare that they have no interests that compete directly with this work, though Dr. Wink and Dr. Erickson do receive research support from various sources for other work. Dr. Wink's current research is supported by the Simons Research Foundation, Autism Speaks, Riovant Sciences Ltd, and Cures Within Reach. Dr. Wink has also served as a past consultant for Otsuka. Dr. Erickson is a past consultant to Alcobra Pharmaceuticals, the Roche Group, and Novartis. Dr. Erickson holds non-related IP held by CCHMC and Indiana University. Dr. Erickson receives research grant support from the John Merck Fund, Cincinnati Children's Hospital Medical Center, Autism Speaks, the National Fragile X Foundation, The Roche Group, Neuren Pharmaceuticals, and Riovant Sciences Ltd. Dr. Adams, Dr. Wang, Dr. Klaunig, Dr. Plawecki, Dr. Posey, and Dr. McDougle report no potential conflicts of interest. This study was funded by the Autism Speaks.

Authors' contributions

LKW drafted the manuscript. RA completed the statistical analysis and assisted with drafting the statistical portion of the manuscript. ZW and JEK completed the oxidative stress biomarker analysis and drafted the portion of the manuscript describing this work. MHP assisted in drafting the manuscript and reviewed the data analysis. DJP and CJM designed and executed the study and reviewed the manuscript. CAE participated in study design, study execution, and oversaw all aspects of manuscript development. All authors read and approved the final manuscript.

Acknowledgements

We would like to acknowledge the contributions of Arlen Kohn MA and Lauren Mathieu-Frasier MA for their assistance with study coordination and data collection.

Funding

Autism Speaks Treatment Grant.

Author details

[1]Cincinnati Children's Hospital Medical Center, University of Cincinnati College of Medicine, 3333 Burnet Avenue MLC 4002, Cincinnati, OH 45229, USA. [2]Investigative Toxicology and Pathology, School of Public Health, Indiana University, Bloomington, IN, USA. [3]Department of Psychiatry, Christian Sarkine Autism Treatment Center, Riley Hospital for Children at Indiana University Health, Indiana University School of Medicine, Indianapolis, IN, USA. [4]Indianapolis, IN, USA. [5]Lurie Center for Autism, Departments of Psychiatry and Pediatrics, Massachusetts General Hospital and MassGeneral Hospital for Children, Harvard Medical School, Boston, MA, USA.

References

1. Kanner L. Autistic disturbances of affective contact. Nerv Child. 1943;2:217–50.
2. Reichow B, Steiner AM, Volkmar F. Cochrane review: social skills groups for people aged 6 to 21 with autism spectrum disorders (ASD). Evidence-based child health : a Cochrane review journal. 2013;8(2):266–315.
3. Autism Spectrum Disorder, Data and Statistics [http://www.cdc.gov/ncbddd/autism/data.html]. Accessed 4/3/2016.
4. James SJ, Melnyk S, Jernigan S, Cleves MA, Halsted CH, Wong DH, et al. Metabolic endophenotype and related genotypes are associated with oxidative stress in children with autism. Am J Med Genet B Neuropsychiatr Genet. 2006;141B(8):947–56.
5. Erickson CA, Posey DJ, Stigler KA, McDougle CJ. Glutamatergic function in autism. In: Heresco-Levy U, editor. Glutamate in Neuropsychiatric Disorders. Trivandrum: Research Signpost; 2008. p. 197–212.
6. Kern JK, Jones AM. Evidence of toxicity, oxidative stress, and neuronal insult in autism. J Toxicol Environ Health B Crit Rev. 2006;9(6):485–99.
7. James SJ, Rose S, Melnyk S, Jernigan S, Blossom S, Pavliv O, et al. Cellular and mitochondrial glutathione redox imbalance in lymphoblastoid cells derived from children with autism. FASEB J. 2009;23(8):2374–83.
8. Deepmala, Slattery J, Kumar N, Delhey L, Berk M, Dean O, et al. Clinical trials of N-acetylcysteine in psychiatry and neurology: a systematic review. Neurosci Biobehav Rev. 2015;55:294–321.
9. Olsson B, Johansson M, Gabrielsson J, Bolme P. Pharmacokinetics and bioavailability of reduced and oxidized N-acetylcysteine. Eur J Clin Pharmacol. 1988;34(1):77–82.
10. Bavarsad Shahripour R, Harrigan MR, Alexandrov AV. N-acetylcysteine (NAC) in neurological disorders: mechanisms of action and therapeutic opportunities. Brain Behav. 2014;4(2):108–22.
11. Berk M, Malhi GS, Gray LJ, Dean OM. The promise of N-acetylcysteine in neuropsychiatry. Trends Pharmacol Sci. 2013;34(3):167–77.
12. Aman MG, Singh NN, Stewart AW, Field CJ. The Aberrant Behavior Checklist: a behavior rating scale for the assessment of treatment effects. Am J Ment Defic. 1985;5:485–91.

13. Hardan AY, Fung LK, Libove RA, Obukhanych TV, Nair S, Herzenberg LA, et al. A randomized controlled pilot trial of oral N-acetylcysteine in children with autism. Biol Psychiatry. 2012;71(11):956–61.
14. Ghanizadeh A, Moghimi-Sarani E. A randomized double blind placebo controlled clinical trial of N-Acetylcysteine added to risperidone for treating autistic disorders. BMC Psychiatry. 2013;13:196.
15. Nikoo M, Radnia H, Farokhnia M, Mohammadi MR, Akhondzadeh S. N-acetylcysteine as an adjunctive therapy to risperidone for treatment of irritability in autism: a randomized, double-blind, placebo-controlled clinical trial of efficacy and safety. Clin Neuropharmacol. 2015;38(1):11–7.
16. Ghanizadeh A, Derakhshan N. N-acetylcysteine for treatment of autism, a case report. J Res Med Sci. 2012;17(10):985–7.
17. Marler S, Sanders KB, Veenstra-VanderWeele J. N-acetylcysteine as treatment for self-injurious behavior in a child with autism. J Child Adolesc Psychopharmacol. 2014;24(4):231–4.
18. Melnyk S, Fuchs GJ, Schulz E, Lopez M, Kahler SG, Fussell JJ, et al. Metabolic imbalance associated with methylation dysregulation and oxidative damage in children with autism. J Autism Dev Disord. 2012;42(3):367–77.
19. Guy W. ECDEU assessment manual for psychopharmacology, Publication No. 76-338. Washington: U.S. DHEW, NIMH; 1976.
20. American, Psychiatric Association. Diagnostic and Statistical Manual of Mental Disorders. Washington: American Psychiatric Press; 1994.
21. Lord C, Rutter M, Le Couteur A. Autism Diagnostic Interview-Revised: a revised version of a diagnostic interview for caregivers of individuals with possible pervasive developmental disorders. J Autism Dev Disord. 1994;24(5):659–85.
22. Roid G, Miller L. Leiter International Performance Scale—revised. Wood Dale: Stoelting Company; 1997.
23. Constantino J, Gruber C. Social Responsiveness Scale. 2005.
24. Sparrow S, Cicchetti D, Balla DA. Vineland Adaptive Behaviors Scales. 2008.
25. Research Units on Pediatric Psychopharmacology Autism N. Risperidone in children with autism and serious behavioral problems. N Engl J Med. 2002; 347(5):314–21.
26. McDougle CJ, Scahill L, Aman MG, McCracken JT, Tierney E, Davies M, et al. Risperidone for the core symptom domains of autism: results from the study by the autism network of the research units on pediatric psychopharmacology. Am J Psychiatry. 2005;162(6):1142–8.
27. Buxbaum JD, Bolshakova N, Brownfeld JM, Anney RJ, Bender P, Bernier R, et al. The Autism Simplex Collection: an international, expertly phenotyped autism sample for genetic and phenotypic analyses. Molecular autism. 2014;5:34.
28. Melnyk S, Pogribna M, Pogribny I, Hine RJ, James SJ. A new HPLC method for the simultaneous determination of oxidized and reduced plasma aminothiols using coulometric electrochemical detection. J Nutr Biochem. 1999;10(8):490–7.
29. Vester B, Rasmussen K. High performance liquid chromatography method for rapid and accurate determination of homocysteine in plasma and serum. Eur J Clin Chem Clin Biochem. 1991;29(9):549–54.
30. Probst R, Brandl R, Blumke M, Neumeier D. Stabilization of homocysteine concentration in whole blood. Clin Chem. 1998;44(7):1567–9.
31. Collins AR, Dobson VL, Dusinska M, Kennedy G, Stetina R. The comet assay: what can it really tell us? Mutat Res. 1997;375(2):183–93.
32. Singh NP, McCoy MT, Tice RR, Schneider EL. A simple technique for quantitation of low levels of DNA damage in individual cells. Exp Cell Res. 1988;175(1):184–91.
33. Julious S. Sample size of 12 per group rue of thumb for a pilot study. Pharm Stat. 2005;4:287–91.
34. Muthen LK, Muthen BO. Mplus User's Guide 6th Edition. Los Angeles: Muthen and Muthen; 1998.
35. Cohen J. Statistical power analysis for the behavioral sciences. 2nd ed. Hillsdale: L. Erlbaum Associates; 1988.
36. McCracken JT, McGough J, Shah B, Cronin P, Hong D, Aman MG, et al. Risperidone in children with autism and serious behavioral problems. N Engl J Med. 2002;347(5):314–21.

18

Altered functional organization within the insular cortex in adult males with high-functioning autism spectrum disorder: evidence from connectivity-based parcellation

Takashi Yamada[1,2†], Takashi Itahashi[1†], Motoaki Nakamura[1,3], Hiromi Watanabe[1], Miho Kuroda[1,4,5], Haruhisa Ohta[1], Chieko Kanai[1], Nobumasa Kato[1] and Ryu-ichiro Hashimoto[1,2,6,7*]

Abstract

Background: The insular cortex comprises multiple functionally differentiated sub-regions, each of which has different patterns of connectivity with other brain regions. Such diverse connectivity patterns are thought to underlie a wide range of insular functions, including cognitive, affective, and sensorimotor processing, many of which are abnormal in autism spectrum disorder (ASD). Although past neuroimaging studies of ASD have shown structural and functional abnormalities in the insula, possible alterations in the sub-regional organization of the insula and the functional characteristics of each sub-region have not been examined in the ASD brain.

Methods: Resting-state functional magnetic resonance imaging (rs-fMRI) data were acquired from 36 adult males with ASD and 38 matched typically developed (TD) controls. A data-driven clustering analysis was applied to rs-fMRI data of voxels in the left and right insula to automatically group voxels with similar intrinsic connectivity pattern into a cluster. After determining the optimal number of clusters based on information theoretic measures of variation of information and mutual information, functional parcellation patterns in both the left and the right insula were compared between the TD and ASD groups. Furthermore, functional profiles of each sub-region were meta-analytically decoded using Neurosynth and were compared between the groups.

Results: We observed notable alterations in the anterior sector of the left insula and the middle ventral sub-region of the right insula in the ASD brain. Meta-analytic decoding revealed that whereas the anterior sector of the left insula contained two functionally differentiated sub-regions for cognitive, sensorimotor, and emotional/affective functions in TD brain, only a single functional cluster for cognitive and sensorimotor functions was identified in the anterior sector in the ASD brain. In the right insula, the middle ventral sub-region, which is primarily specialized for sensory- and auditory-related functions, showed a significant volumetric increase in the ASD brain compared with the TD brain.

(Continued on next page)

* Correspondence: dbridges50@gmail.com
†Equal contributors
[1]Medical Institute of Developmental Disabilities Research, Showa University, 6-11-11 Kita-karasuyama, Setagaya-ku, Tokyo, Japan
[2]ATR Brain Information Communication Research Laboratory Group, 2-2-2 Hikaridai, Seika-cho, Sorakugun, Kyoto, Japan
Full list of author information is available at the end of the article

(Continued from previous page)

Conclusions: The results indicate an altered organization of sub-regions in specific parts of the left and right insula of the ASD brain. The alterations in the left and right insula may constitute neural substrates underlying abnormalities in emotional/affective and sensory functions in ASD.

Keywords: Autism spectrum disorder, Resting-state functional magnetic resonance imaging, Insula, Connectivity-based functional parcellation

Background

Autism spectrum disorder (ASD) has been increasingly conceptualized as a disease of large-scale brain networks [1]. Among multiple nodes that constitute the brain's networks, several brain regions have emerged as key structures that particularly contribute to abnormal functionalities in the ASD brain. The insular cortex is one such brain region, whose structural and functional abnormalities are frequently reported in the neuroimaging literature of ASD. Structurally, alterations of the gray matter (GM) volume have been identified in the anterior and posterior parts of the right insula in adult ASD [2–4]. Functionally, a comprehensive meta-analysis of functional imaging studies has revealed hypoactivation in the right anterior insula during various social tasks including face recognition and mentalizing [5]. Regarding connectivity, previous resting-state fMRI studies of adolescent and adult ASD have shown reduced functional connectivity (FC) of the anterior, middle, and posterior insula with distant brain regions, including the amygdala and the somatosensory cortex [6–8]. Convergent evidence from these structural, functional, and FC studies strongly prompts more detailed investigations of the insula to advance our understanding of the neural substrates of ASD.

Recent progress in anatomical studies has enabled more finely grained investigations into the neural organization of the insula. Traditionally, the insula has been divided into the following three regions: (1) anterior agranular, (2) posterior granular, and (3) precentral dysgranular [9–11]. However, a recent histological study has identified at least three distinct regions within the posterior insula alone [12], indicating the presence of a more fine-grained subdivision of this brain region. Similarly, FC analysis using fMRI data has led to recent progress in understanding the functional anatomy of the insular cortex. The rationale behind the FC approach is that the connectivity pattern of a brain region is a significant determinant of its functional role [13, 14]. FC patterns of the insular cortex have been mainly investigated using resting-state FC analyses or meta-analyses of co-activation patterns obtained in task-based fMRI studies. Using data-driven clustering methods in which voxels with similar FC patterns were grouped into a functional unit (parcel), Cauda and colleagues have identified two sub-regions of the ventral-anterior and dorsal-posterior insula based on resting-state FC [15] and co-activation patterns obtained in task-based fMRI studies [16]. On the other hand, a more recent study using data-driven clustering analysis of resting-state FC data supported the tripartite subdivision into dorsal-anterior, ventral-anterior, and posterior regions [17]. Based on the fact that each sub-region has a distinct FC pattern, this study used a meta-analytic co-activation tool (Neurosynth) and succeeded in decoding the functional profiles of insular sub-regions using reverse inference from the FC patterns seeded from each sub-region [18]. These studies demonstrate the utility of data-driven FC-based clustering methods in the study of insular functional organization, particularly when they are used in combination with meta-analytical tools such as the Neurosynth framework.

The aforementioned studies reporting a functional parcellation of the insula confirm the traditional cytoarchitecture-based subdivision scheme of this brain region. However, given more recent evidence indicating an even finer subdivision within the posterior insula, the data-driven FC clustering approach is expected to lead to a more finely grained functional parcellation of this brain region. Indeed, Kelly and colleagues gradually increased the number of parcels in the insula starting at two and examined changes in functional parcellation patterns using resting-state FC data, gray matter structural images, and a task-based fMRI co-activation map [19]. They observed consistent patterns of fine-scale functional parcellation across these three different modalities when using up to nine parcels. Comparing parcellation patterns at multiple scale levels (coarse vs. fine subdivisions) revealed that insular sub-regions are organized in a pseudo-hierarchical fashion, such that an increment in the number of subdivisions results in a finer division of an already existing cluster rather than generating a completely new parcellation pattern. These results indicate that the insular cortex is organized at multiple spatial scales and that finer parcellation patterns may offer additional insights into the functional organization of this structure.

In the present fMRI study, we examined the functional organization of the insula in adult males with ASD by applying the data-driven clustering method to resting-state FC data. Although localized alterations in insular gray matter volume, cortical activation, and FC have previously been reported in neuroimaging studies of ASD [6–8], to our knowledge, no study has examined the possibility of an altered organization of functionally heterogeneous insular sub-regions in the ASD brain. In this study, we first examined whether the functional organization of the insula is altered in subjects with ASD compared with typically developed (TD) controls. When we detected significant alterations, we then attempted to identify functions of the affected sub-regions by applying a meta-analytical decoding tool [18] to FC patterns of insular sub-regions. In this series of analyses, we needed to determine the optimal number of clusters for parcellation. Given previous findings indicating multiple spatial scales of insular organization [19], we expected that finer parcellation schemes would be more sensitive to subtle but significant functional alteration than coarser subdivisions adopted by traditional bi- or tripartite schemes.

Methods

Participants

Thirty-six high-functioning adult males with ASD and 38 age-matched TD males participated in this study. The diagnostic procedure to identify patients with ASD was the same as in our previous studies [20–22]. Briefly, an experienced psychiatrist and a clinical psychologist independently interviewed the patients (together with their caregivers when available) for approximately 3 h regarding their developmental history, present illness, life history, and family history. The diagnosis of ASD was made only when there was a consensus between the psychiatrist and clinical psychologist based on the criteria of the Diagnostic and Statistical Manual of Mental Disorders, Fourth Edition (DSM-IV-TR) (American Psychiatric, 2000). In addition, the diagnosis was reconfirmed after at least a 2-month of follow-up period. TD subjects were recruited through advertisements and acquaintances. None of the TD participants reported any severe medical problems or a neurological or psychiatric history. Except for six TD participants, participants completed the Japanese version of the autism spectrum quotient (AQ) test [23]. Table 1 shows detailed demographic information for the study participants.

We confirmed that all of the participants were right-handed using the Edinburgh Handedness Inventory [24]. The intelligence quotient (IQ) scores of all participants with ASD were evaluated using either the Wechsler Adult Intelligence Scale-Third Edition (WAIS-III) or the WAIS-Revised (WAIS-R), while those of TD subjects were estimated using a Japanese version of the National Adult Reading Test (JART) [25]. There were no significant differences between the two groups in age or IQ scores (both $p > 0.1$). Out of 36 participants with ASD, 24 individuals underwent either (1) Diagnostic Interview for Social and Communicative Disorders (DISCO) only ($n = 5$), or (2) Autism Diagnostic Observation Schedule (ADOS) only ($n = 11$), or (3) both ($n = 8$). The remaining 12 ASD participants did not undergo either of the auxiliary diagnostic tool of DISCO or ADOS. All of the five participants who underwent only the DISCO satisfied the DISCO diagnostic criteria for ASD. Out of the 11 participants who underwent only the ADOS, ten satisfied the ADOS diagnostic criteria for ASD, while one participant had a total ADOS score that was lower than the cut-off score ($6 < 7$); however, the same subject satisfied the cut-off scores for the "communication" and "social reciprocity" subscales of the ADOS ("communication": $2 \geq 2$, "social reciprocity": $4 \geq 4$), and therefore he was regarded as an individual with ASD. All of the eight participants who underwent the DISCO and ADOS satisfied the criteria for ASD for both measures. All participants provided written informed consent. This study was conducted in accordance with the principles of the Declaration of Helsinki and was approved by the Ethics Committee of the Faculty of Medicine of Showa University.

Table 1 The demographic data for the participants

	TD ($n = 38$)			ASD ($n = 36$)			Statistics	
	Mean	SD	Range	Mean	SD	Range	df	*P* value
Age (years)	32.5	7.3	19–47	29.9	7.1	19–46	72	0.14
Full-scale IQ	109.5	8.4	87.5–119.8	106.2	13.9	83–134	72	0.23
Handedness	92.7	20.3	5.3–100	87.9	24.5	5.9–100	72	0.37
AQ score	15.5	5.6	7–30	36.3	4.9	23–43	66	<0.001
ADOS								
Total				12.8	3.8	5–21		
Communication				4.2	1.7	2–8		
Social reciprocity				8.6	2.8	3–12		

Note: WAIS-III or -R was administrated to all participants with ASD, and the IQ score was estimated for all TDs based on JART. The AQ score was collected from 32 TDs and all participants with ASD

Data acquisition

All scans were acquired using a 1.5T GE Signa system (General Electric, Milwaukee, WI, USA). The resting-state functional images were acquired using a gradient echo-planar imaging sequence (in-plane resolution: 3.4375 × 3.4375 mm, echo time (TE): 40 ms, repetition time (TR): 2000 ms, flip angle: 90°, slice thickness: 4 mm with a 1-mm slice gap, matrix size: 64 × 64, 27 axial slices). Two-hundred and eight volumes were acquired in a single run, and the first four volumes were discarded to allow for T1 equilibration. We also obtained a high-resolution T1-weighted spoiled gradient recalled 3D MRI image (in-plane resolution: 0.9375 × 0.9375 mm, 1.4 mm slice thickness, TR: 25 ms, TE: 9.2 ms, matrix size: 256 × 256, 128 sagittal slices). Each participant was instructed to lie still with his eyes closed and to not think of anything in particular, yet stay awake in the dim scanner room.

Data preprocessing

With the exception of the pinpoint use of Analysis of Functional NeuroImages (AFNI) [26], we mainly used the Statistical Parametric Mapping software (SPM 8) (Wellcome Department of Cognitive Neurology, London, UK) to preprocess the resting-state functional magnetic resonance imaging (rs-fMRI) data. Unless otherwise specified, rs-fMRI data were preprocessed using functions implemented in the SPM software. First, functional images were adjusted for slice timing and then were corrected for head motion. None of the participants moved translationally more than 2 mm (x, y, and z) or rotated more than 2° (roll, pitch, and yaw) in relation to the first volume. We next skull-stripped the functional images using 3dAutomask and 3dcalc and despiked the time series using 3dDespike in AFNI to account for the impact of outliers. The functional images were then co-registered to each participant's T1 image and normalized to the Montreal Neurological Institute (MNI) template, resampled to a resolution of 2 × 2 × 2 mm. Finally, the images were smoothed using a 6-mm Gaussian kernel.

We calculated covariates from the segmented white matter and cerebrospinal fluid using the "aCompCor" method [27] in order to remove artefactual components from the fMRI time series. These covariates, together with 12 head motion parameters (6 motion parameters and their first-order temporal derivatives), were then regressed out from the smoothed rs-fMRI data. To further remove possible effects of sub-millimeter motion on estimations of functional connectivity, we applied the scrubbing method in the following manner [28, 29]: (1) the framewise displacement (FD) and frame-by-frame signal intensity change (DVARS) indices were calculated immediately after head motion correction; (2) we regarded a volume as a motion-contaminated volume either when its FD value was greater than 0.5 mm or when its DVARS value was greater than the 75th percentile plus 1.5 times the interquartile range; (3) the signal values of the motion-contaminated volumes were interpolated by applying the cubic spline function [28]; (4) a band-pass filter (0.009–0.08 Hz) was applied to further reduce the effects of low-frequency drifts and high-frequency physiological noise; (5) finally, the interpolated volumes were deleted. There were no significant differences between the two groups either in the mean (± standard deviation [SD]) FD (0.115 ± 0.042 in TD, 0.107 ± 0.049 in ASD; $p = 0.495$) or in the mean (± SD) DVARS (TD: 12.94 ± 2.05, ASD: 12.86 ± 1.83, $p = 0.863$). The number of deleted volumes after the scrubbing procedures was 5.24 ± 4.90 for the TD group and 4.25 ± 4.23 for the ASD group. No significance difference was found between groups ($p = 0.36$).

Connectivity-based functional parcellation

Figure 1 illustrates the processing scheme for the connectivity-based parcellation of the insula. Briefly, we generated a group of functional connectivity maps for each participant using every voxel in the insula as a seed. We then applied a clustering method to the resulting groups of connectivity maps for the left and the right insula separately and identified a set of voxel clusters such that each voxel in the same cluster had a similar connectivity pattern. After calculating the cluster map for each individual, we again applied the clustering method to matrices that represent patterns of similarity of clustering either within the TD or the ASD group to obtain separate group-level functional parcellation maps for the TD and ASD groups.

Specifically, we first identified all of the voxels included in the insula as follows: (1) voxels in the standard spaces of the left and the right insula were defined using the Harvard-Oxford probabilistic atlas thresholded at 25 % probability; (2) voxels in the insula from both hemispheres were further constrained by conjunction with a study-specific GM mask, which represented voxels that survived the threshold of 40 % GM probability in every participant. This method of generating the study-specific GM masks was based on previous studies [30, 31]. This procedure resulted in the inclusion of 1161 voxels in the left insula and 1179 voxels in the right insula.

Next, we generated a group of voxel-based functional connectivity maps by calculating temporal correlations between time series of each individual voxel in the insula and those of all voxels within the study-specific GM mask, except for the voxels in the insula. This procedure resulted in the generation of 1161 maps for the left insula and 1179 maps for the right insula in each participant. Connectivity maps of the Pearson's correlation coefficients were then converted to Z-scores using the Fisher's r-to-z transformation.

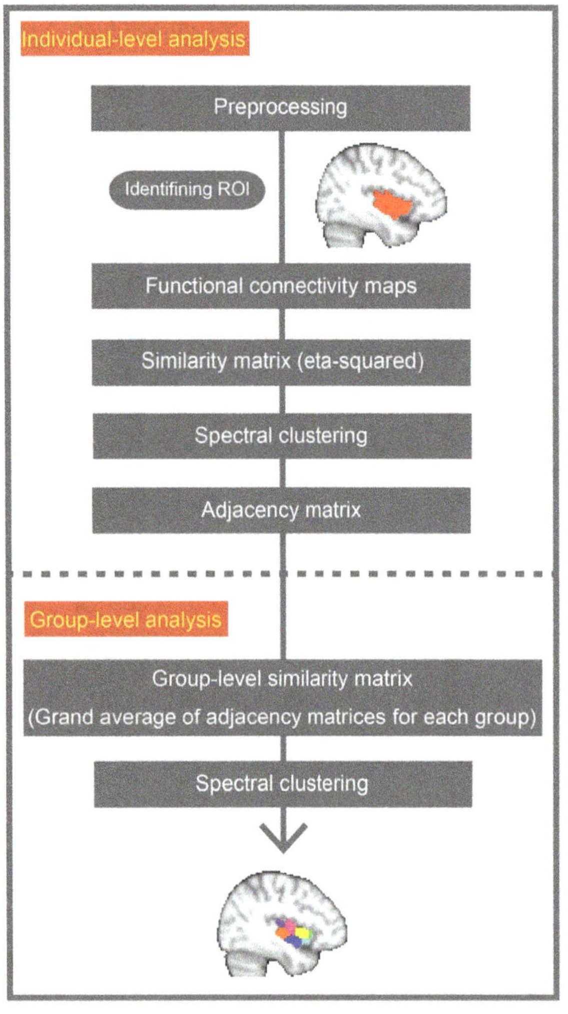

Fig. 1 The procedure for the functional connectivity-based parcellation of the insula. We first identified voxels in the left and right insula of each participant and generated a set of functional connectivity maps by correlating the resting-state time-series of each voxel with voxels in a whole gray matter mask (excluding the insula) for each hemisphere. Following a Fisher's z-transformation for functional connectivity maps, we constructed the individual-level similarity matrix using eta-squared, which is a measure of similarity between a pair of functional connectivity maps (see the "Connectivity-based functional parcellation" section). We applied the spectral clustering algorithm to the set of individual-level similarity matrices in order to cluster voxels with similar time-series of the resting-state signal fluctuations. For group-level analysis, we first calculated a binary adjacency matrix for each participant. Adjacency matrices of all participants were averaged separately for TD and ASD individuals to generate a group-level similarity matrix. Finally, we applied the spectral clustering algorithm to the group-level similarity matrix to assign a *k* clustering label to each voxel (see the "Connectivity-based functional parcellation" section)

For the functional parcellation, we evaluated the similarities of functional connectivity patterns among the 1161 maps for the left insula and the 1179 maps for the right insula. Following previously described methods [19, 32–34], we calculated the eta-squared value as a measure of similarity between a pair of connectivity maps as follows:

$$\text{eta squared} = 1 - \frac{\sum_{i=1}^{n}\left\{(a_i - m_i)^2 + (b_i - m_i)^2\right\}}{\sum_{i=1}^{n}\left\{(a_i - X)^2 + (b_i - X)^2\right\}}$$

where a_i and b_i are the Z-scored connectivity values at voxel i in connectivity maps a and b, respectively. m_i is the mean of the two connectivity map values at voxel i, and X is the mean of all voxels of the two connectivity maps. Using the eta-squared values between all pairs of connectivity maps, we constructed the individual-level similarity matrix for the left and the right insula separately (1161 × 1161 matrix for the left insula and 1179 × 1179 matrix for the right insula). After determining the optimal number of clusters (k, see the "Estimation of optimal number of clusters" section), we applied the spectral clustering algorithm to each of the individual-level similarity matrices and parcellated either the left or the right insula into k clusters based on similarities in functional connectivity patterns.

After performing functional parcellation at the individual-level, we next performed group-level functional parcellation as follows [33]: (1) we generated a binary adjacency matrix whose value was 1 if a pair of voxels belonged to the same cluster and zero otherwise for each participant, (2) we then generated a group-level similarity matrix by averaging the adjacency matrices of all individuals within each group, and (3) we applied the spectral clustering algorithm to the group-level similarity matrix to assign one of the k clustering labels to each voxel.

The spectral clustering algorithm arbitrarily assigns one of the k clustering labels to each voxel. To compare the parcellation results of the two groups, we first fixed the configuration of labels in the TD group as a reference. Then, for each of the possible instantiation of the k labels in the ASD group, we calculated the ratio of the voxels having the same label to those having different labels in the two groups. We selected the configuration of labels that maximized this ratio.

Estimation of the optimal number of clusters

Before applying the spectral clustering method, we determined the optimal number of clusters (k) using two complementary indices that evaluate the goodness of clustering solutions: variation of information (VI) and mutual information (MI) [35]. VI is an information-theoretic measure that quantifies the information lost and gained in changing clustering solution A to clustering solution B. This measure can thus be used as an index of dissimilarity [19]. On the other hand, MI is an information-theoretic measure that represents the similarity between clustering solutions. We examined the VI and MI values from 2 to 10 for each k value for the left and the right insula and for the TD and ASD groups separately and selected the optimal k value. A k value with a low VI and a high MI indicates a good solution in terms of similarity.

To calculate VI and MI, we used a split-half procedure, as described previously [36, 37]. First, in order to determine an optimal k value not biased toward the TD or ASD groups, all of the participants were randomly assigned to one of two groups (group A and group B). We then applied the aforementioned spectral clustering algorithm to each group for each k ($k = 2, 3, \ldots, 10$) and obtained group-level parcellation maps for each group. Finally, we compared the clustering of the two groups by calculating VI and MI for each k. We repeated this procedure 100 times, as in previous studies. A previous functional connectivity-based parcellation study on the insula demonstrated that the stability of the solutions substantially decreases when the number of clusters (k) exceeds 10 [19]. Therefore, we explored k values ranging from 2 to 10 in the present study.

In order to determine the optimal k value, we first identified a set of "good solutions" using VI and MI independently and then determined the optimal values using the logical product of the two solutions. Since VI is a measure of dissimilarity, we identified points (k values) of "local minimal" VI as good solutions. Similarly, since MI is a measure of similarity, we identified points (k values) of "local maximal" MI as good solutions. Here, a local minimum of VI is defined as a range of points with a significantly smaller value than its two adjacent points. The local maximum MI value was determined in a similar manner. We determined the optimal k value as the point where local minimal VI and local maximal MI values converge.

We also performed another split-half procedure within the TD group by randomly assigning participants with TD into one of two groups (group 1 or group 2) while changing k from 2 to 10. We did this to ensure that the optimal k value determined by our procedure was not biased due to contamination from the ASD group.

Comparison of functional parcellation patterns between the TD and ASD groups

After the parcellation of the insula in each participant, we examined between-group differences in the volumes of specific sub-regions by performing a permutation test, as previously described [33]. Briefly, we randomly assigned participants to one of the two groups by permuting the diagnostic labels of all of the participants and then applied our clustering algorithm to each of the permuted groups. The sub-regions in each group were re-labeled following the aforementioned procedure, which used the labels from the original TD group as references (see the "Connectivity-based functional parcellation" section). This procedure was repeated 5000 times to obtain the null distribution of volumetric differences between the groups. We deemed between-group volumetric differences statistically significant when the difference between the TD and ASD groups fell above the 95th percentile of the null distribution.

Meta-analytic decoding of the sub-regions' connectivity maps

In addition to analyzing sub-regional volumes, we also examined whether there are significant alterations in functional characteristics of insular sub-regions in ASD. We thus examined the functional profiles of each sub-region in the TD and ASD groups separately using a recently developed meta-analytic tool called "Neurosynth" [18]. Given a pattern of functional connectivity as an input, the tool allows us to decode the relevant psychological and physiological functions (e.g., "cognitive control," "emotion," and "perception") strongly associated with that pattern.

As a first step, we performed functional connectivity analysis using each of the insular sub-regions as a region of interest (ROI). We generated maps of the Pearson's correlation coefficients between the averaged time series of a sub-region and those of all voxels within the GM mask for each individual. After transformation into z-maps, the maps of all participants in the TD and ASD groups were separately subjected to a one-sample t test using age as a nuisance covariate to obtain the connectivity pattern at the group level. The resulting t-statistic maps were converted to z-statistic maps and then fed into Neurosynth as inputs for meta-analytic decoding.

In order to characterize the functional properties of each functional connectivity map, we determined the top 5 terms that showed the strongest correlations with each functional connectivity map. Related terms (e.g., "emotion" and "emotional") were merged into a single term of the base form. This procedure yielded a total of 14 terms, as some of the same terms were repeatedly selected across all sub-regions for both hemispheres. Finally, we drew a radar chart consisting of these 14 terms to visually assess the potential psychological and physiological functions of each sub-region as functional fingerprints. To visualize the similarities (and dissimilarities) of these functional fingerprints, we constructed a 14-dimensional feature vector whose elements were the correlation coefficients of the 14 terms for each sub-region. We then calculated the Pearson's correlation coefficient between pairs of feature vectors to represent the similarities between sub-regions in terms of functional fingerprints.

Connectivity-based parcellation of the intracalcalrine cortex as a control region

The functional parcellations of the insula resulted in different patterns between the TD and ASD groups (see the "Visual inspection of functional connectivity-based parcellation" section). To examine whether group differences in the parcellation patterns have any regional selectivity, we applied the same clustering analysis to the intracalcarine cortex as a control region.

The intracalcarine cortex as defined in the Harvard-Oxford probabilistic atlas (thresholded at 25 probability) roughly corresponds to the primary visual cortex and its neighboring regions. Given the evidence of alterations in vision-related functions in some ASD individuals (e.g., enhanced visual search ability [38, 39]), it may not be possible to strongly assert that functional organizations within the lower-order visual cortices are unaltered in the ASD brain. However, we propose that the intracalcarine cortex may serve as a control for the insula for the following reasons: (1) the region is thought to be dedicated to visual processing (in contrast to the multiple distinct functions of the insula) and (2) the size of the region (1405 voxels) is comparable to those of the left and right insula (left: 1161 voxels, right: 1179 voxels).

We estimated the optimal cluster number in the intracalcarine cortex using MI and VI in the same manner as that for the left and right insula (see the "Estimation of the optimal number of clusters" section). After determining the optimal number of clusters of this region, the parcellation patterns were visually inspected and compared between groups. Furthermore, a possible volumetric alteration was examined using a permutation test for each sub-region (see the "Comparison of functional parcellation patterns between the TD and ASD groups" section).

Assessment for the replicability of functional parcellation patterns

To assess the stability of the functional parcellation patterns, we performed a replication analysis using subsets of the data. First, we divided the participants of each group into six folds (in the case of the ASD group, 6 participants per fold [36 participants in total]). The stability of the parcellation pattern was examined using the leave-one-fold-out method. In other words, we applied the clustering method to the data for the remaining five folds and repeated the procedure for six times until all six folds were excluded. This procedure resulted in six parcellation patterns. We then examined the similarity between the parcellation pattern using all participants in the group and each of the six parcellation patterns that were generated using the leave-one-fold-out method. We used the MI as an index of similarity of the two patterns.

Results

Optimal number of clusters

Figure 2 shows the means and standard errors of the mean (SEM) of VI and MI for the left and the right insula for each clustering solution. In the left insula, VI had local minima at $k = 5$ and 8 (VI: 0.167 ± 0.0031 [mean $\pm$ SEM] for $k = 5$ and VI: 0.151 ± 0.0026 for $k = 8$), while MI had a local maximum at $k = 8$ (MI: 0.740 ± 0.0046) (Fig. 2a). Following the criteria for the selection of the optimal number of clusters using VI and MI (see the "Estimation of optimal number of clusters" section), we determined an optimal k of 8 for the left insula. In the right insula, VI had local minima at $k = 7$ and 8 (VI: 0.154 ± 0.0024 for $k = 7$ and VI: 0.155 ± 0.0022 for $k = 8$), while MI had a local maximum at $k = 8$ (MI: 0.732 ± 0.0039) (Fig. 2b). We determined an optimal k of 8 for the right insula using the information that we obtained from VI and MI.

Visual inspection of functional connectivity-based parcellation

Figure 3 illustrates the functional parcellation patterns of the left and right insula in the TD and ASD groups when $k = 8$. We named the eight sub-regions based on their locations along the anterior-posterior and dorsal-ventral axes. Figure 4 shows the magnified picture of the parcellation pattern of the left insula of the TD group (Fig. 3a). We first divided the whole region anterior, middle, posterior, and posterior-most sectors along the anterior-posterior axis (Fig. 4a). Each of the anterior and posterior sectors was further divided into dorsal and ventral sub-regions. The 3 sub-regions in the middle sector were labeled as middle dorsal, center, and middle ventral sub-regions (Fig. 4b). We thus obtained eight sub-regions as follows: (1) anterior sector: anterior dorsal (AD) and ventral (AV) sub-regions; (2) middle sector: middle dorsal (MD), central (C), and middle ventral (MV) sub-regions; (3) posterior sector: posterior dorsal (PD) and ventral (PV) sub-regions; and (4) posterior-most sub-region. Note that this labeling is similarly applicable to the parcellation pattern in the right insula (Fig. 3b). We also note that our parcellation patterns were highly similar to previously identified patterns based on resting-state FC studies of a neurotypical population [19]. Most notably, the parcellation patterns in our study and those in the previous study were consistent in that the anterior and posterior sectors were divided into two sub-regions and the middle sector was divided into three sub-regions.

In comparison to the parcellation patterns of the TD group, we observed notable localized alterations in both the left and the right insula in the ASD group. Specifically, we observed that the left anterior sector, which was divided into two sub-regions in the TD group, contained only a single sub-region in the ASD group (Fig. 3c).

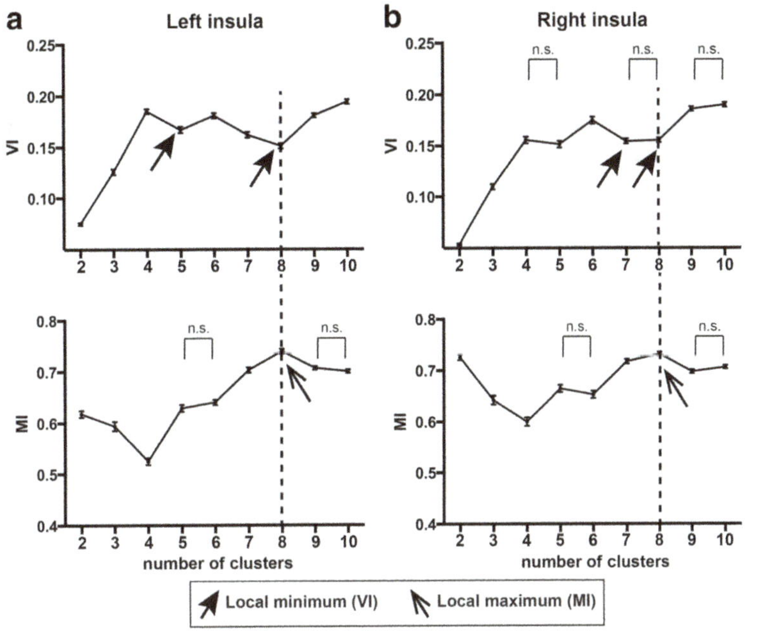

Fig. 2 Determination of the optimal number of clusters based on VI and MI. The VI and MI values are shown for every clustering solution for *k* values ranging from 2 to 10 for each side of the insula (**a** Left insula, **b** Right insula). *Arrows* indicate either local minima of VI or local maxima of MI. *Dashed lines* denote the optimal number of solutions as determined using both VI and MI. The *error bars* denote standard errors of the mean for 100 repetitions of the split-half procedure (see the "Estimation of the optimal number of clusters" section). *n.s.* indicates no statistically significant difference between points

Moreover, the left PV sub-region, which was a single region in the TD group, was divided into two sub-regions in the ASD group. On the other hand, the parcellation patterns of the middle and posterior-most sectors in the ASD group were largely unchanged from those of the TD group. In the right insula, the MV sub-region was expanded and the central sub-region was shifted in the posterior direction in the ASD group (Fig. 3d). Aside from localized alterations, the parcellation patterns in the anterior and posterior-most sectors were largely the same in the two groups. These observations indicate that the organization of functional sub-regions may be altered in specific parts of the left and right insula in ASD.

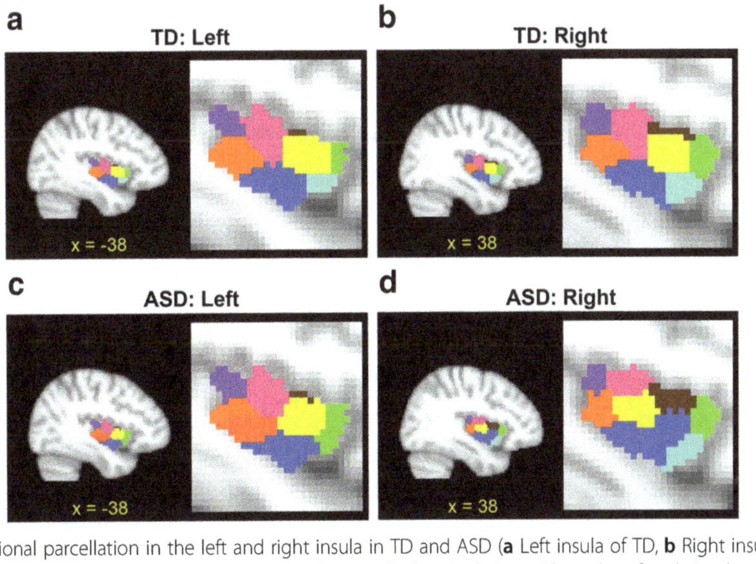

Fig. 3 The patterns of functional parcellation in the left and right insula in TD and ASD (**a** Left insula of TD, **b** Right insula of TD, **c** Left insula of ASD, **d** Right insula of ASD). Each figure is presented in sagittal and magnified sagittal views. The color of each insular sub-region reflects the color of the corresponding sub-region in the TD and ASD groups

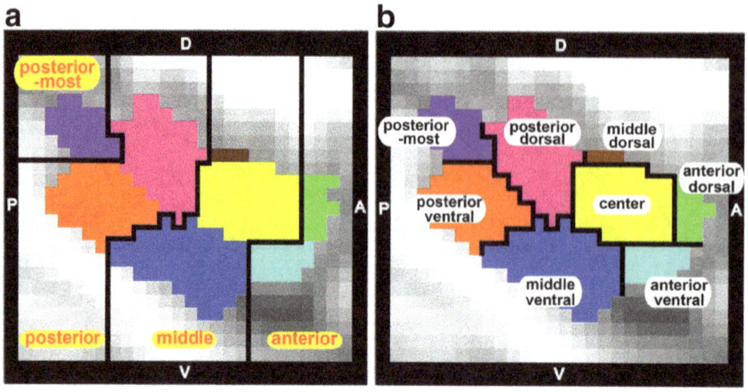

Fig. 4 Spatial configurations and labels for the insular sub-regions. The parcellation pattern of the left insula of the TD group is magnified. We divided the whole region anterior, middle, posterior, and posterior-most sectors along the anterior-posterior axis (**a**). Further subdivision along the dorsal-ventral axis in each sector resulted in eight sub-regions in total (**b**): (1) anterior sector: anterior dorsal (AD) and ventral (AV) sub-regions (*green* and *cyan*), (2) middle sector: middle dorsal (MD), central (C), and middle ventral (MV) sub-regions (*brown*, *yellow*, and *blue*), (3) posterior sector: posterior dorsal (PD) and ventral (PV) sub-regions (*magenta* and *orange*), and (4) posterior-most sub-region (*purple*). *D* dorsal, *V* ventral, *A* anterior, *P* posterior

Meta-analytical decoding of the left insular sub-regions

We investigated the functional profiles of the anterior sub-regions and the PV sub-region in the left insula, where the functional parcellations were visually different between the TD and ASD groups. First, we performed a meta-analytic decoding of the functions of the two anterior sub-regions (AD and AV) in the TD group and of the anterior sub-region in the ASD group. The results are presented as a radar chart in Fig. 5. The functional profile of the anterior sub-region in the ASD group showed an almost identical pattern to that of the AD sub-region in the TD group ($r = 0.97$). Although the profile of the ASD anterior sub-region also significantly correlated with that of the AV sub-region in the TD group ($r = 0.86$), the profile of the anterior sub-region in the ASD group was clearly more similar to that of the AD sub-region in the TD group. Therefore, the alterations of the anterior sector in the ASD group may be characterized as the absence of the AV sub-region together with the volumetric expansion of the AD sub-region. The volumetric increase was statistically confirmed by the permutation test (ASD anterior sub-region > TD AD sub-region, $p = 0.024$) (Additional file 1: Figure S1a). When the functional profiles were compared between the AD and AV sub-regions, the AV sub-region was more highly associated with terms related to affection and emotion, such as "reward," "fear," "anxiety," and "affective," whereas the AD sub-region was more

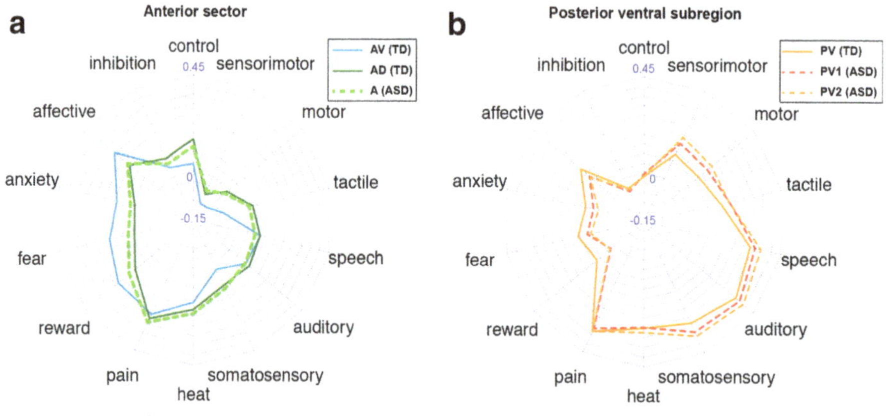

Fig. 5 The meta-analytic decoding of sub-regions in the left anterior sector and posterior ventral sub-regions. **a** The radar chart that shows the correlation of left anterior ventral (AV) and anterior dorsal (AD) sub-regions in the TD group and the anterior section in the ASD group with the 14 terms of interest. Note that the profile of the ASD anterior sector is more similar to that of the AD sub-region rather than the AV sub-region in the TD group. **b** The radar chart that shows the correlation of left posterior ventral (PV) sub-region in the TD group and the two parcels within the PV sub-region (PV1 and PV2) with the 14 terms of interest. The profiles of these three sub-regions were highly similar

preferably associated with a cognitive terms ("control" and "inhibition") and sensorimotor terms ("sensorimotor," "motor," "tactile," and "somatosensory").

We next performed a meta-analytic decoding of the function of the PV sub-region in the TD group and functions of the two PV sub-regions in the ASD group. For simplicity, we will label the anterior portion of the PV sub-region in the ASD group as PV1 and the posterior PV as PV2. When comparing the PV sub-region in the TD group with the two PV sub-regions in the ASD group, we observed almost identical functional profiles among these sub-regions (TD PV and ASD PV1: $r = 0.96$; TD PV and ASD PV2: $r = 0.95$; ASD PV1 and ASD PV2: $r = 1.00$).

Meta-analytical decoding of the right insular sub-regions

We next examined functional alterations in the right insular sub-regions of the ASD group. We previously noted the visual observation suggesting the extension of the MV sub-region into the more dorsal part of the insula (see the "Visual inspection of functional connectivity-based parcellation" section). We statistically confirmed this observation by using the permutation test and finding a significant group difference (ASD > TD, $p = 0.003$) (Additional file 1: Figure S1b). Meta-analytic decoding of the MV sub-region revealed that the region was strongly associated with terms related to perceptual processes such as "pain," "somatosensory," "auditory," "speech," and "heat," and that such functional profiles were almost identical between the TD and ASD groups ($r = 0.99$) (Fig. 6a). In addition to the spatial expansion of the MV sub-region, our visual inspection indicated that the position of the C sub-region had shifted in the posterior direction in the ASD group. In order to examine possible functional alterations in this region, we performed meta-analytic decoding of the C sub-region in the two groups and found highly dissimilar patterns ($r = 0.45$). However, we observed that the C sub-region in the ASD group was functionally similar to the PV sub-region in the TD group ($r = 0.98$), which was strongly associated with terms largely related to perceptual ("somatosensory," "tactile," and "auditory") and motor processes. The results are consistent with the observation of the spatial shift of the C sub-region toward the posterior direction in the ASD group.

Group differences in individual variability in insula parcellation

Our analysis showed significant differences in functional parcellation patterns between the TD and ASD groups. However, recent studies have suggested that the ASD brain is highly idiosyncratic, indicating that each individual ASD brain may be greatly discrepant from the group mean [40]. Therefore, it may be argued that the inter-individual variability in the insula parcellation patterns is larger in the ASD than in the TD and that such enhanced variability might have played a role in the altered parcellation pattern in the ASD. To test this possibility, we calculated the MIs between each individual adjacency matrix of the ASD participants and the group-level similarity matrix (see the "Connectivity-based functional parcellation" section) of the ASD group when the cluster number (k) was optimally set to 8 (eight sub-regions). Similarly, the MIs were also calculated for the TD individuals using the TD group-level similarity matrix. If the parcellation pattern in each individual brain is more idiosyncratic in the ASD group, then the MI should be significantly reduced in the ASD group than in the TD group. However, we did not observe a significant difference in MIs between the ASD and TD groups in either the left or right insula (left insula: $t = -1.54$, $p = 0.13$, right insula: $t = 0.038$, $p = 0.97$).

We also reasoned that the degree of idiosyncrasy in the insular parcellation pattern of an individual might be associated with his or her severity of the ASD symptoms.

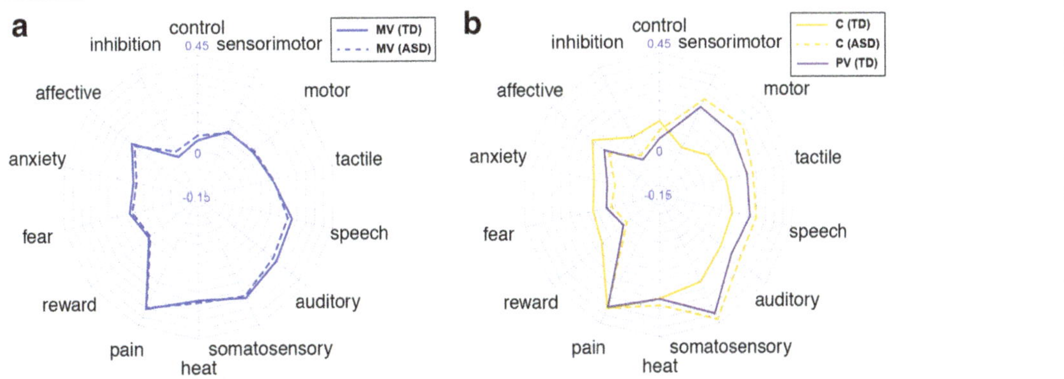

Fig. 6 The meta-analytic decoding in the right middle ventral, central, and posterior ventral sub-regions. **a** The radar chart that shows the correlation of the middle ventral (MV) sub-region in both groups with the 14 terms of interest. **b** The radar chart shows the correlation of the central (C) and posterior ventral (PV) sub-regions in both groups with the 14 terms of interest

To explore this possibility, we first evaluated the degree of idiosyncrasy using the MI values between the adjacency matrix of each ASD individual and the group-level similarity matrix of ASD individuals. These MIs represented the discrepancy from the mean ASD parcellation pattern. Then we computed the correlation between the AQ scores and the MI values, but the correlation was not significant (left insula: $r = 0.03$, $p = 0.85$, right insula: $r = -0.02$, $p = 0.90$). We also calculated the individual MIs using the group-level similarity matrix of TD individuals, as indices for the discrepancy from the typical (mean TD) parcellation pattern. However, no significant correlation with the total AQ score was found in either the left or right insula (left insula: $r = 0.04$, $p = 0.83$, right insula: $r = -0.02$, $p = 0.90$).

Functional parcellation in the intracalcarine cortex

The same clustering methods as those used for the insula were applied to the control region of the intracalcarine cortex. MI reached the local maximum at $k = 7$, 8, 9, and 10, and VI reached the local minimum at $k = 6$ and 7 (Additional file 2: Figure S2). Following the same criteria as that for the insula, we determined an optimal k of 7. Based on visual inspection, the functional parcellation patterns at $k = 7$ were highly comparable between the TD and ASD groups (Additional file 3: Figure S3). Permutation tests for the volume of each sub-region revealed no significant group differences in any of the seven sub-regions (light blue region: $p = 0.36$, green region: $p = 0.67$, orange region: $p = 0.55$, yellow region: $p = 0.58$, magenta region: $p = 0.55$, blue region: $p = 0.52$, violet region: $p = 0.31$). The comparable parcellation pattern between groups in the control region indicates that group differences that were identified by our connectivity-based parcellation may be selective to parts of brain regions, including the left and right insula.

Replicability of the functional parcellation patterns in the insula

We examined the replicability of the functional parcellation patterns using the leave-one-fold-out method (six folds in each group) (see the "Assessment for the replicability of functional parcellation patterns" section). The means and SEM of MIs between the parcellation pattern for all participants in a group and each of the six parcellation patterns that were generated using the leave-one-fold-out method were as follows: TD: 0.88 ± 0.02 (mean $\pm$ SEM), ASD: 0.81 ± 0.01 for the left insula; TD: 0.90 ± 0.02, ASD: 0.79 ± 0.01 for the right insula. These high MI values indicate good stability for the parcellation patterns of the left and right insula in both groups.

We also examined the replicability of the group differences in the sub-regional volumes that were identified in the left and right insula. In the left insula, the anterior sub-region of the ASD group was significantly larger than the AD sub-region of the TD group (see the "Meta-analytical decoding of the left insular sub-regions" section). In the right insula, the MV sub-region was significantly larger for the ASD group than the TD group (see the "Meta-analytical decoding of the right insular sub-regions" section). For these two sub-regions, we subtracted the volume of the ASD group from that of the TD group for each of the six leave-one-fold-out steps. Because the aim of this analysis was to test whether the subtracted value is significantly lower than 0, we performed a one-sample, one-tailed t test using the six samples. As a result, we observed a significant difference for both sub-regions (the left sub-region: $t = -2.88$, $p = 0.017$; the right sub-region: $t = -2.64$, $p = 0.023$). Therefore, the group differences in the sub-regional volumes were also replicable.

Discussion

In this study, we performed an automatic functional parcellation of the insular cortex in adult male ASD by adopting a data-driven clustering method based on resting-state FC patterns of voxels. In the comparison with matched TD brain, we observed notable alterations in specific sub-regions in the left and right insular cortices of ASD brain. These alterations were localized to the anterior sub-regions of the left insula and the middle ventral sub-region of the right insula. In the left insula, whereas the anterior sector contained two functionally differentiated sub-regions in TD brain, only a single functional cluster was identified in the anterior sector in the ASD group. No clear group-difference was observed in the control region of the intracalcarine cortex using the same resting-state FC-based parcellation method. Additional analyses using subsets of the entire dataset confirmed the high stability of the insular parcellation patterns in both groups. Meta-analytical decoding revealed the absence of sub-region specialized for emotional and affective functions in the anterior sector in the ASD brain. The middle ventral sub-region of the right insula, which is primarily specialized for sensory and auditory-related functions, extended into the more dorsal parts of the insula and its volume was significantly enlarged compared with the same region in the TD brain. We thus observe alterations in the functional organization of the left and right insular sub-regions, which may underlie abnormalities in emotional/affective and sensory domains in ASD.

The left insula lacks an emotion-related sector in ASD

We found a notable difference in the anterior sector of the left insula when we carried out a group comparison of functional parcellation patterns. Specifically, whereas the anterior sector was parceled into dorsal and ventral sub-regions in the TD group, only a single cluster was identified in the anterior sector in the ASD group. Analysis of the functional profiles of the two sub-regions indicate a functional differentiation in the TD brain, such that the ventral sub-region is characterized by selective involvement in emotional and affective processes, fear, anxiety, and reward, whereas the dorsal sub-region is more strongly involved in cognitive and sensorimotor functions compared with the ventral sub-region. On the other hand, the functional profile of the single anterior cluster in the ASD brain closely matched that of the dorsal rather than the ventral sub-region in the TD brain. Therefore, we report that the left anterior insula in ASD is functionally altered and is characterized by the absence of the sub-region for emotional and affective functions.

It is notable that such an alteration in functional parcellation was observed in the left insula. Based on anatomical evidence of left-to-right asymmetry in peripheral autonomic efferent neurons and homeostatic afferent neurons, as well as a review of neuroimaging literature, an influential model of the insula posits that the left insula is associated with parasympathetic ("affiliative") functions, while the right side is associated with sympathetic ("aroused") functions. This idea provides the neurobiological foundation for the functional laterality of emotion. According to this model, the left anterior insula is more strongly involved in "positive (energy enrichment)" emotions. Consistent with this view, previous fMRI studies of neurotypical populations demonstrated the left-lateralized activation of the anterior insula during the viewing of pleased facial expressions [41] and when mothers viewed their own child [42] and experienced maternal and romantic love [43]. These observations indicate a dichotomy of emotion, so that the left anterior insula may be viewed as critical for group-oriented (affiliative) emotions as opposed to individual-oriented emotions.

Our observation of the absence of the anterior sub-region for emotional and affective functions in ASD may predict abnormalities in group-oriented emotions. Consistently, a recent model of ASD focused on the concept of "social motivation" and proposed that the core problems of ASD may be explained by extremely diminished social motivation [44]. According to previous surveys, half of the adults with ASD report having no particular friends [45] and score significantly lower on items in the friendship questionnaire that concern attitudes toward interpersonal relationships, such as pleasure in close friendship and interest in people [46]. Therefore, the functional alteration in the anterior section of the left anterior insula may provide a neurological basis for the lack of group-oriented emotion and behavior in ASD.

The right insula has an enlarged sensory and auditory-related section in ASD

We identified a significant alteration of functional parcellation patterns in the right insula. Specifically, we observed an increase in the volume of the middle ventral sub-region, which is specialized for auditory-related and other sensory functions. Convergent evidence from anatomical, electrophysiological, brain lesion, and neuroimaging studies indicate that the insular cortex is involved in multimodal sensory functions, including somatosensory, olfactory, visceral, and auditory functions [47]. In particular, previous reports have highlighted a critical role for the insula in various aspects of auditory function, including auditory attention, music, the processing of novel auditory stimuli, temporal processing, and visual-auditory integration [47]. Our analyses of the functional profiles of insular sub-regions indicate that the middle ventral sub-region is specifically associated with such auditory and sensory functions.

Given the functional profiles of the above insular sub-regions, it is plausible that the volumetric expansion of the right middle ventral sub-region is associated with sensory abnormalities in ASD, including those in the auditory domain. Indeed, atypical sensory reactivity, including altered auditory sensitivity, has recently been recognized as a core symptom of ASD under the new diagnostic criteria of DSM-5 [48]. In addition to evidence for auditory hypersensitivity revealed by clinical questionnaires [49, 50], recent behavioral experiments have revealed a more detailed picture of the altered auditory processing in ASD. Although individuals with ASD have been shown to be impaired in some auditory functions, such as auditory attention reorienting and the modulation of auditory perception [51], it is notable that they outperform TD subjects in a number of auditory functions, such as auditory stream segregation [52] and the perception of pitch [53] and time [54]. Abnormalities in sensations other than audition have been also reported in the previous literature [55, 56]. Although we acknowledge the need for further investigation to establish the functional significance of the volumetric enlargement of the right middle ventral sub-region, our observations raise the interesting possibility that this alteration may involve parts of the neural mechanisms underlying altered sensation in ASD.

Limitations

We acknowledge a few limitations of the present study. Firstly, the present study restricted recruitment to adult males. This restriction was made because several studies have reported effects of age [57] and sex [58] on functional connectivity, at least for neurotypical populations. Given the possibility that age and sex may be critical factors for the etiological and phenotypic heterogeneity of ASD [59], we need to carry out further studies targeting specific populations excluded in the present study.

Secondly, we determined the optimal cluster number k by the combined use of VI and MI. However, the choice of the optimal k may be an inherent problem in any data-driven clustering analysis, given that the gold standard for the selection of this value has not yet been established. Indeed, previous studies have adopted a variety of methods for determining the optimal k value, such as using a combination of percent agreement and VI [19], VI only [36], validation indicator [17], and Dice's coefficient between test and re-test data [33]. Among all of the possible measures, we selected MI and VI, because the combined use of the two measures allows for the estimation of the three critical features of clustering solutions: similarity, dissimilarity, and stability. Although we acknowledge some uncertainty in our analysis, we note that our method unequivocally determined the optimal k for each hemisphere and that the $k = 8$ was optimal even when the TD data was used (Additional file 4: Figure S4). These results indicate the validity and robustness of our method, at least for the current dataset.

Thirdly, in contrast to the task-related fMRI design, it may be argued that the resting-state FC study alone does not allow us to directly test hypotheses about the relationship between particular brain regions and their functions. To overcome this general limitation of the resting-state FC study, we have adopted the meta-analytical decoding method of Neurosynth, which uses meta-analysis of co-activation data in the fMRI literature and performs a reverse inference regarding the functions of the sub-region of interest from an FC pattern seeding that sub-region. Although this approach has been gaining credibility in recent fMRI studies [17, 60], we still acknowledge the need of the hypothesis-driven approaches, such as task-related fMRI studies, to establish the links between alterations in specific insular sub-regions and abnormal functions in the ASD brain. The present findings based on data-driven approaches are expected to provide specific hypotheses in designing such hypothesis-driven studies in the future.

Fourthly, only one control region was used to show that the functional alterations that we observed in the organization of the insula are not present in functionally intact brain regions in individuals with ASD. Although this remains a limitation of the study, at least in the intracalcarine cortex, we were able to show that the functional parcellation pattern in the ASD group was highly comparable to that of the TD group in visual inspection and in volumes of the corresponding sub-regions that were revealed using permutation test. Although more control regions may be needed, using the intracalcarine cortex as a control region has raised the specificity of our findings for the insula.

Conclusions

To conclude, the present study uses data-driven clustering analysis of the multi-voxel resting state FC data to reveal altered functional parcellation in the insular cortex of the ASD brain. With the combined use of meta-analytic decoding analysis, we observed localized alterations in sub-regional organization in each side of the insula in ASD. In the left insula, two anterior sub-regions were merged into a single sub-region in which selective involvement in affective and emotional functions was absent. In the right insula, the middle ventral sub-region for auditory-related and sensory functions was significantly increased in volume. Such alterations in functional organization in the insular cortex may constitute neural abnormalities that underlie emotional/affective and sensory problems in ASD.

Additional files

Additional file 1: Figure S1. The statistical test for between-group difference in the sub-regional volume using the permutation procedure. The histograms illustrate the null distribution of volume differences between groups (in voxels) induced by the permutation procedure in the left anterior dorsal (AD) sub-region (the anterior sector in ASD) (a) and in the right middle ventral (MV) sub-region (b). The red dashed vertical line indicates the observed volume differences between correctly labeled TD and ASD groups. The negative values indicate that the sub-region is smaller in TD brain compared to the corresponding sub-region in ASD.

Additional file 2: Figure S2. Determination of the optimal number of clusters based on VI and MI in intracalcarine cortex. The intracalcarine cortex was selected as a control region. The VI and MI values are shown for every clustering solution for k values ranging from 2 to 10. Arrows indicate either local minima of VI or local maxima of MI. Dashed lines denote the optimal number of solutions as determined using both VI and MI. The error bars denote standard errors of the mean for 100 repetitions of the split-half procedure (see the "Estimation of the optimal number of clusters" section). "n.s." indicates no statistically significant difference between points.

Additional file 3: Figure S3. The patterns of functional parcellation in the intracalcarine cortex in TD and ASD. Figures show the parcellation patterns at the optimal cluster number (k) of 7. Each figure is presented in axial and magnified axial views. The color of each intracalcarine sub-region reflects the color of the corresponding sub-region in the TD and ASD groups. Note the highly comparable parcellation patterns between groups.

Additional file 4: Figure S4. VI and MI values for clustering solutions ($k = 2$ to 10) using only TD participants. The dashed line denotes the optimal number of solutions based on the same criteria as in Fig. 2. The error bars are standard errors of the mean. Each kind of arrows points to the optimal number of solutions based on "similarity" and "dissimilarity" criteria. "n.s." indicates that the MI or VI values are not significantly different between the 2 bracketed points.

Abbreviations

AD: Anterior dorsal; ADOS: Autism Diagnostic Observation Schedule; AFNI: Analysis of Functional NeuroImages; AQ: Autism spectrum quotient; ASD: Autism spectrum disorder; AV: Anterior ventral; C: Center; DISCO: Diagnostic Interview for Social and Communicative Disorders; DSM: Diagnostic and Statistical Manual of Mental Disorders; DVARS: D referring temporal derivative and VARS referring the root mean squared; FC: Functional connectivity; FD: Framewise displacement; fMRI: Functional magnetic resonance imaging; GM: Gray matter; IQ: Intelligence quotient; JART: Japanese version of the National Adult Reading Test; MD: Middle dorsal; MI: Mutual information; MNI: Montreal Neurological Institute;

MV: Middle ventral; PD: Posterior dorsal; PV: Posterior ventral; ROI: Region of interest; rs-fMRI: Resting-state functional magnetic resonance imaging; SD: Standard deviation; SPM: Statistical Parametric Mapping; TE: Echo time; TD: Typically developed; TR: Repetition time; VI: Variation of information; WAIS: Wechsler Adult Intelligence Scale

Acknowledgements
This study is the result of "Development of BMI Technologies for Clinical Application" carried out under the Strategic Research Program for Brain Sciences by the Ministry of Education, Culture, Sports, Science and Technology of Japan. This work was also supported by the Japan Society for the Promotion of Science (JSPS) Grant-in-Aid for Scientific Research (C) (16K10236 to T.Y.), a Grant-in-Aid for Young Scientists (B) (16K17363 to T.I.), and a Grant-in-Aid for Scientific Research on Innovative Areas (23118003; Adolescent Mind & Self-Regulation to R.H.) from the Ministry of Education, Culture, Sports, Science, and Technology of Japan.

Authors' contributions
TY and TI conceived of the study, performed the analysis, and drafted and revised the manuscript. TY, TI, MN, HW, HO, CK, and RH participated in the data acquisition. MK, TY, MN, HW, HO, and CK were in charge of the clinical assessment. NK participated in the design of the study and supervised the study. MN, MK, HW, HO, CK, and NK revised the manuscript for important intellectual content. RH participated in its design, coordination, and analysis and helped to write and revise the manuscript. All authors read and approved the final manuscript.

Competing interests
The authors declare that they have no competing interests.

Author details
[1]Medical Institute of Developmental Disabilities Research, Showa University, 6-11-11 Kita-karasuyama, Setagaya-ku, Tokyo, Japan. [2]ATR Brain Information Communication Research Laboratory Group, 2-2-2 Hikaridai, Seika-cho, Sorakugun, Kyoto, Japan. [3]Kinko Hospital, Kanagawa Psychiatric Center, 2-5-1 Serigaya, Yokohama, Kanagawa, Japan. [4]Child Mental Health-care Center, Fukushima University, 1 Kanayagawa, Fukusima-shi, Fukushima, Japan. [5]Department of Child Neuropsychiatry, Graduate School of Medicine, The University of Tokyo, 7-3-1 Hongou, Bunkyo-ku, Tokyo, Japan. [6]Department of Language Sciences, Graduate School of Humanities, Tokyo Metropolitan University, 1-1 Minami-Osawa, Hachioji-shi, Tokyo, Japan. [7]Research Center for Language, Brain and Genetics, Tokyo Metropolitan University, 1-1 Minami-Osawa, Hachioji-shi, Tokyo, Japan.

References

1. Menon V. Large-scale brain networks and psychopathology: a unifying triple network model. Trends Cogn Sci. 2011;15:483–506.
2. Cauda F, Geda E, Sacco K, D'Agata F, Duca S, Geminiani G, Keller R. Grey matter abnormality in autism spectrum disorder: an activation likelihood estimation meta-analysis study. J Neurol Neurosurg Psychiatry. 2011;82:1304–13.
3. Ecker C, Suckling J, Deoni SC, Lombardo MV, Bullmore ET, Baron-Cohen S, Catani M, Jezzard P, Barnes A, Bailey AJ, et al. Brain anatomy and its relationship to behavior in adults with autism spectrum disorder: a multicenter magnetic resonance imaging study. Arch Gen Psychiatry. 2012; 69:195–209.
4. Kosaka H, Omori M, Munesue T, Ishitobi M, Matsumura Y, Takahashi T, Narita K, Murata T, Saito DN, Uchiyama H, et al. Smaller insula and inferior frontal volumes in young adults with pervasive developmental disorders. Neuroimage. 2010;50:1357–63.
5. Di Martino A, Ross K, Uddin LQ, Sklar AB, Castellanos FX, Milham MP. Functional brain correlates of social and nonsocial processes in autism spectrum disorders: an activation likelihood estimation meta-analysis. Biol Psychiatry. 2009;65:63–74.
6. Di Martino A, Yan CG, Li Q, Denio E, Castellanos FX, Alaerts K, Anderson JS, Assaf M, Bookheimer SY, Dapretto M, et al. The autism brain imaging data exchange: towards a large-scale evaluation of the intrinsic brain architecture in autism. Mol Psychiatry. 2014;19:659–67.
7. Ebisch SJ, Gallese V, Willems RM, Mantini D, Groen WB, Romani GL, Buitelaar JK, Bekkering H. Altered intrinsic functional connectivity of anterior and posterior insula regions in high-functioning participants with autism spectrum disorder. Hum Brain Mapp. 2011;32:1013–28.
8. von dem Hagen EA, Stoyanova RS, Baron-Cohen S, Calder AJ. Reduced functional connectivity within and between 'social' resting state networks in autism spectrum conditions. Soc Cogn Affect Neurosci. 2013;8:694–701.
9. Augustine JR. The insular lobe in primates including humans. Neurol Res. 1985;7:2–10.
10. Augustine JR. Circuitry and functional aspects of the insular lobe in primates including humans. Brain Res Brain Res Rev. 1996;22:229–44.
11. Mesulam MM, Mufson EJ. Insula of the old world monkey. I. Architectonics in the insulo-orbito-temporal component of the paralimbic brain. J Comp Neurol. 1982;212:1–22.
12. Kurth F, Eickhoff SB, Schleicher A, Hoemke L, Zilles K, Amunts K. Cytoarchitecture and probabilistic maps of the human posterior insular cortex. Cereb Cortex. 2010;20:1448–61.
13. Passingham RE, Stephan KE, Kotter R. The anatomical basis of functional localization in the cortex. Nat Rev Neurosci. 2002;3:606–16.
14. Uddin LQ, Kinnison J, Pessoa L, Anderson ML. Beyond the tripartite cognition-emotion-interoception model of the human insular cortex. J Cogn Neurosci. 2014;26:16–27.
15. Cauda F, D'Agata F, Sacco K, Duca S, Geminiani G, Vercelli A. Functional connectivity of the insula in the resting brain. Neuroimage. 2011;55:8–23.
16. Cauda F, Costa T, Torta DM, Sacco K, D'Agata F, Duca S, Geminiani G, Fox PT, Vercelli A. Meta-analytic clustering of the insular cortex: characterizing the meta-analytic connectivity of the insula when involved in active tasks. Neuroimage. 2012;62:343–55.
17. Chang LJ, Yarkoni T, Khaw MW, Sanfey AG. Decoding the role of the insula in human cognition: functional parcellation and large-scale reverse inference. Cereb Cortex. 2013;23:739–49.
18. Yarkoni T, Poldrack RA, Nichols TE, Van Essen DC, Wager TD. Large-scale automated synthesis of human functional neuroimaging data. Nat Methods. 2011;8:665–70.
19. Kelly C, Toro R, Di Martino A, Cox CL, Bellec P, Castellanos FX, Milham MP. A convergent functional architecture of the insula emerges across imaging modalities. Neuroimage. 2012;61:1129–42.
20. Itahashi T, Yamada T, Watanabe H, Nakamura M, Jimbo D, Shioda S, Toriizuka K, Kato N, Hashimoto R. Altered network topologies and hub organization in adults with autism: a resting-state fMRI study. PLoS One. 2014;9:e94115.
21. Watanabe H, Nakamura M, Ohno T, Itahashi T, Tanaka E, Ohta H, Yamada T, Kanai C, Iwanami A, Kato N, Hashimoto R. Altered orbitofrontal sulcogyral patterns in adult males with high-functioning autism spectrum disorders. Soc Cogn Affect Neurosci. 2014;9:520–8.
22. Yamada T, Ohta H, Watanabe H, Kanai C, Tani M, Ohno T, Takayama Y, Iwanami A, Kato N, Hashimoto R. Functional alterations in neural substrates of geometric reasoning in adults with high-functioning autism. PLoS One. 2012;7:e43220.
23. Wakabayashi A, Baron-Cohen S, Wheelwright S, Tojo Y. The autism-spectrum quotient (AQ) in Japan: a cross-cultural comparison. J Autism Dev Disord. 2006;36:263–70.
24. Oldfield RC. The assessment and analysis of handedness: the Edinburgh inventory. Neuropsychologia. 1971;9:97–113.
25. Matsuoka K, Uno M, Kasai K, Koyama K, Kim Y. Estimation of premorbid IQ in individuals with Alzheimer's disease using Japanese ideographic script (Kanji) compound words: Japanese version of National Adult Reading Test. Psychiatry Clin Neurosci. 2006;60:332–9.
26. Cox RW. AFNI: software for analysis and visualization of functional magnetic resonance neuroimages. Comput Biomed Res. 1996;29:162–73.
27. Behzadi Y, Restom K, Liau J, Liu TT. A component based noise correction method (CompCor) for BOLD and perfusion based fMRI. Neuroimage. 2007;37:90–101.
28. Carp J. Optimizing the order of operations for movement scrubbing: comment on Power et al. Neuroimage. 2013;76:436–8.
29. Power JD, Barnes KA, Snyder AZ, Schlaggar BL, Petersen SE. Spurious but systematic correlations in functional connectivity MRI networks arise from subject motion. Neuroimage. 2012;59:2142–54.
30. Di Martino A, Zuo XN, Kelly C, Grzadzinski R, Mennes M, Schvarcz A, Rodman J, Lord C, Castellanos FX, Milham MP. Shared and distinct intrinsic functional network centrality in autism and attention-deficit/hyperactivity disorder. Biol Psychiatry. 2013;74:623–32.

31. Zuo XN, Ehmke R, Mennes M, Imperati D, Castellanos FX, Sporns O, Milham MP. Network centrality in the human functional connectome. Cereb Cortex. 2012;22:1862–75.
32. Barnes KA, Nelson SM, Cohen AL, Power JD, Coalson RS, Miezin FM, Vogel AC, Dubis JW, Church JA, Petersen SE, Schlaggar BL. Parcellation in left lateral parietal cortex is similar in adults and children. Cereb Cortex. 2012;22:1148–58.
33. Nebel MB, Joel SE, Muschelli J, Barber AD, Caffo BS, Pekar JJ, Mostofsky SH. Disruption of functional organization within the primary motor cortex in children with autism. Hum Brain Mapp. 2014;35:567–80.
34. Nelson SM, Cohen AL, Power JD, Wig GS, Miezin FM, Wheeler ME, Velanova K, Donaldson DI, Phillips JS, Schlaggar BL, Petersen SE. A parcellation scheme for human left lateral parietal cortex. Neuron. 2010;67:156–70.
35. Meilă M. Comparing clusterings—an information based distance. J Multivar Anal. 2007;98:873–95.
36. Kahnt T, Chang LJ, Park SQ, Heinzle J, Haynes JD. Connectivity-based parcellation of the human orbitofrontal cortex. J Neurosci. 2012;32:6240–50.
37. Kelly C, Uddin LQ, Shehzad Z, Margulies DS, Castellanos FX, Milham MP, Petrides M. Broca's region: linking human brain functional connectivity data and non-human primate tracing anatomy studies. Eur J Neurosci. 2010;32:383–98.
38. Dakin S, Frith U. Vagaries of visual perception in autism. Neuron. 2005;48: 497–507.
39. Gliga T, Bedford R, Charman T, Johnson MH, Team B. Enhanced visual search in infancy predicts emerging autism symptoms. Curr Biol. 2015;25: 1727–30.
40. Hahamy A, Behrmann M, Malach R. The idiosyncratic brain: distortion of spontaneous connectivity patterns in autism spectrum disorder. Nat Neurosci. 2015;18(2):302–9.
41. Jabbi M, Swart M, Keysers C. Empathy for positive and negative emotions in the gustatory cortex. Neuroimage. 2007;34:1744–53.
42. Leibenluft E, Gobbini MI, Harrison T, Haxby JV. Mothers' neural activation in response to pictures of their children and other children. Biol Psychiatry. 2004;56:225–32.
43. Bartels A, Zeki S. The neural correlates of maternal and romantic love. Neuroimage. 2004;21:1155–66.
44. Chevallier C, Kohls G, Troiani V, Brodkin ES, Schultz RT. The social motivation theory of autism. Trends Cogn Sci. 2012;16:231–9.
45. Howlin P, Goode S, Hutton J, Rutter M. Adult outcome for children with autism. J Child Psychol Psychiatry. 2004;45:212–29.
46. Baron-Cohen S, Wheelwright S. The Friendship Questionnaire: an investigation of adults with Asperger syndrome or high-functioning autism, and normal sex differences. J Autism Dev Disord. 2003;33:509–17.
47. Bamiou D-E, Musiek FE, Luxon LM. The insula (Island of Reil) and its role in auditory processing. Brain Res Rev. 2003;42:143–54.
48. American Psychiatric Association. Diagnostic and statistical manual of mental disorders. 5th ed. Washington: American Psychiatric Publisher; 2013.
49. Takayama Y, Hashimoto R, Tani M, Kanai C, Yamada T, Watanabe H, Ono T, Kato N, Iwanami A. Standardization of the Japanese version of the Glasgow Sensory Questionnaire (GSQ). Res Autism Spectr Disord. 2014;8:347–53.
50. Tavassoli T, Hoekstra RA, Baron-Cohen S. The Sensory Perception Quotient (SPQ): development and validation of a new sensory questionnaire for adults with and without autism. Mol Autism. 2014;5:29.
51. Orekhova EV, Stroganova TA. Arousal and attention re-orienting in autism spectrum disorders: evidence from auditory event-related potentials. Front Hum Neurosci. 2014;8:34.
52. Lin IF, Yamada T, Komine Y, Kato N, Kashino M. Enhanced segregation of concurrent sounds with similar spectral uncertainties in individuals with autism spectrum disorder. Sci Rep. 2015;5:10524.
53. Bonnel A, Mottron L, Peretz I, Trudel M, Gallun E, Bonnel A-M. Enhanced pitch sensitivity in individuals with autism: a signal detection analysis. J Cogn Neurosci. 2003;2:226–35.
54. Stewart ME, Griffiths TD, Grube M. Autistic traits and enhanced perceptual representation of pitch and time. J Autism Dev Disord. 2015. epub ahead of print. PMID: 26189179.
55. Duerden EG, Taylor MJ, Lee M, McGrath PA, Davis KD, Roberts SW. Decreased sensitivity to thermal stimuli in adolescents with autism spectrum disorder: relation to symptomatology and cognitive ability. J Pain. 2015;16:463–71.
56. Yasuda Y, Hashimoto R, Nakae A, Kang H, Ohi K, Yamamori H, Fujimoto M, Hagihira S, Takeda M. Sensory cognitive abnormalities of pain in autism spectrum disorder: a case-control study. Ann Gen Psychiatry. 2016;15:8.
57. Dosenbach NU, Nardos B, Cohen AL, Fair DA, Power JD, Church JA, Nelson SM, Wig GS, Vogel AC, Lessov-Schlaggar CN, et al. Prediction of individual brain maturity using fMRI. Science. 2010;329:1358–61.
58. Filippi M, Valsasina P, Misci P, Falini A, Comi G, Rocca MA. The organization of intrinsic brain activity differs between genders: a resting-state fMRI study in a large cohort of young healthy subjects. Hum Brain Mapp. 2013;34:1330–43.
59. Ecker C, Murphy D. Neuroimaging in autism—from basic science to translational research. Nat Rev Neurol. 2014;10:82–91.
60. Pauli WM, O'Reilly RC, Tal Y, Wager TD. Regional specialization within the human striatum for diverse psychological functions. Proc Natl Acad Sci U S A. 2016;113:1907–12.

19

Blood–brain barrier and intestinal epithelial barrier alterations in autism spectrum disorders

Maria Fiorentino[1,4*], Anna Sapone[1,2], Stefania Senger[1,4], Stephanie S. Camhi[1,3], Sarah M. Kadzielski[4], Timothy M. Buie[4], Deanna L. Kelly[5], Nicola Cascella[6] and Alessio Fasano[1,3,4]

Abstract

Background: Autism spectrum disorders (ASD) are complex conditions whose pathogenesis may be attributed to gene–environment interactions. There are no definitive mechanisms explaining how environmental triggers can lead to ASD although the involvement of inflammation and immunity has been suggested. Inappropriate antigen trafficking through an impaired intestinal barrier, followed by passage of these antigens or immune-activated complexes through a permissive blood–brain barrier (BBB), can be part of the chain of events leading to these disorders. Our goal was to investigate whether an altered BBB and gut permeability is part of the pathophysiology of ASD.

Methods: *Postmortem* cerebral cortex and cerebellum tissues from ASD, schizophrenia (SCZ), and healthy subjects (HC) and duodenal biopsies from ASD and HC were analyzed for gene and protein expression profiles. Tight junctions and other key molecules associated with the neurovascular unit integrity and function and neuroinflammation were investigated.

Results: Claudin (*CLDN*)-5 and -12 were increased in the ASD cortex and cerebellum. *CLDN-3*, *tricellulin*, and *MMP-9* were higher in the ASD cortex. *IL-8*, *tPA*, and *IBA-1* were downregulated in SCZ cortex; *IL-1b* was increased in the SCZ cerebellum. Differences between SCZ and ASD were observed for most of the genes analyzed in both brain areas. CLDN-5 protein was increased in ASD cortex and cerebellum, while CLDN-12 appeared reduced in both ASD and SCZ cortexes. In the intestine, 75% of the ASD samples analyzed had reduced expression of barrier-forming TJ components (*CLDN-1*, *OCLN*, *TRIC*), whereas 66% had increased pore-forming CLDNs (*CLDN-2*, *-10*, *-15*) compared to controls.

Conclusions: In the ASD brain, there is an altered expression of genes associated with BBB integrity coupled with increased neuroinflammation and possibly impaired gut barrier integrity. While these findings seem to be specific for ASD, the possibility of more distinct SCZ subgroups should be explored with additional studies.

Keywords: Blood–brain barrier, Autism spectrum disorders, Gut–brain axis, Gut permeability, Schizophrenia, Neuroinflammation, Postmortem brain, Duodenal biopsies

* Correspondence: mrfiorentino@mgh.harvard.edu
[1]Mucosal Immunology and Biology Research Center, Massachusetts General Hospital for Children, Boston, MA, USA
[4]Department of Pediatrics, Harvard Medical School, Boston, MA, USA
Full list of author information is available at the end of the article

Background

Autism spectrum disorders (ASD) are neurodevelopmental diseases with complex symptoms and whose neurobiological basis remains poorly understood. Research suggests that a combination of genetic, autoimmune, environmental, and perhaps in utero risk factors leading to neuroinflammation can contribute to the pathogenesis of ASD [1–6] as well as other neurobehavioral and/or neuropsychiatric disorders including schizophrenia (SCZ) [7–13]. Over-expression of acute phase proteins in the serum, brain, and cerebrospinal fluid of ASD as well as SCZ individuals suggests that inflammation is involved in the pathophysiology of these diseases [4, 6, 14–21]. Autoimmune diseases have been associated with increased risk of ASD and SCZ [10, 22–28] suggesting altered or inappropriate immune responses.

Furthermore, many ASD patients experience gastrointestinal (GI) symptoms and/or dysfunctions [29–38]. Clinical observations describe increased intestinal permeability in ASD [39–42], and permeability to food antigens derived from the partial digestion of wheat (gliadorphins) and cow's milk (casomorphins) has been reported in both ASD and SCZ [41, 43–46].

Despite research efforts, there are no defined explanations of how environmental triggers can lead to these neurobehavioral conditions. One hypothesis, based on the interconnectivity of the gut–brain axis, suggests that inappropriate antigen trafficking through an impaired intestinal barrier, followed by passage of antigens or activated immune complexes through a permissive blood–brain barrier (BBB), can be part of the chain of events leading to neuroinflammation and thereby subsequent disease.

Table 1 List of primers used for RT-qPCR

Gene	Accession number	5′ OLIGO	3′ OLIGO	Gene function in the brain/gut context
CLDN-1	NM_021101	GTGATAGCAATCTTTGTGGC	ACTAAAATAGCCAGACCTGC	Barrier-forming claudin
CLDN-5	NM_001130861	GAACTTCCTGAAGTGGTGTC	CCAGACCTCTCAATCTTCAC	Barrier-forming claudin; endothelial cell-specific
CLDN-12	NM_001185072	GAGAAGCAGGCTCAGATTAT	AGATTCAGAACTTCCCTGTG	Function at BBB unknown
OCLN	U53823	CACACCACACCTACACTC	TCCAAGATAAACCAATCTGCT	Barrier-forming component of the TJs
VE-Cad	X79981	AGTTCTTCCGAGTCACAAAA	TCAGGTTATACCAGGGGTAG	Main integral membrane protein of endothelial AJs; controls endothelial cell survival, stabilization of blood vessel assembly, and vascular permeability
MMP-9	NM_004994	TGTACCGCTATGGTTACACTCG	GGCAGGGACAGTTGCTTCT	Metalloprotease involved in local proteolysis of the extracellular matrix and in leukocyte migration
MMP-2	NM_004530	TACAGGATCATTGGCTACACACC	GGTCACATCGCTCCAGACT	Metalloprotease involved in local proteolysis of the extracellular matrix and in leukocyte migration
tPA	NM_001319189	CCGGCTACGGCAAGCA	AGCGGCTGGATGGGTACA	Serine protease involved in the synthesis of MMPs and BBB damage
18S	X03205	AGAAACGGCTACCACATCCA	CCCTCCAATGGATCCTCGTT	Ribosomal RNA (control gene for qPCR)
CLDN-2	NM_001171092	QIAGEN		Pore-forming claudin; regulates paracellular ion and water flow
CLDN-3	NM_001306	QIAGEN		Barrier-forming component of the TJs
CLDN-10	NM_001160100	QIAGEN		Pore-forming claudin; regulates paracellular ion flow
CLDN-15	NM_001185080 NM_014343 NM_138429	QIAGEN		Pore-forming claudin; regulates paracellular ion flow
TRIC	NM_001038603	QIAGEN		Barrier-forming component of the TJs
IL-1b	NM_000576	QIAGEN		Pro-inflammatory cytokine involved in increased BBB permeability
IL-6	NM_000600	QIAGEN		Pro-inflammatory cytokine
IL-8	NM_000584	QIAGEN		Pro-inflammatory cytokine
IL-10	NM_000572	QIAGEN		Anti-inflammatory cytokine
TSPO	NM_000714	QIAGEN		Mitochondrial protein expressed on reactive glial cells; biomarker for inflammation in the brain
tTG6	NM_001254734	QIAGEN		Marker of gluten-related neuroinflammation
MSFD2A	NM_001136493	QIAGEN		Key regulator of BBB function; required for the establishment of a functional BBB
IBA-1	NM_001623	QIAGEN		Marker of microglia activation

Table 2 Demographic and clinical characteristics of subjects analyzed in this study

						Cortex and CBL	
MBC #	Age	Race	Sex	Diagnosis	PMI	Cause of death	Additional clinical information
585	42	AA	M	SCZ	16	Pulmonary embolism	Tox (at death): doxepin
612	45	W	M	SCZ	24	Suicide, doxepin intoxication	N/A
628	59	W	M	SCZ	13	Pulmonary thromboembolia	Tox (at death): ETOH, diphenhydramine
664	53	W	M	SCZ	11	ASCVD	Tox (at death): olanzapine
705	47	W	M	SCZ	16	Deep vein thrombosis	N/A
737	55	W	M	SCZ	12	ASCVD	N/A
741	40	W	M	SCZ	14	Motor vehicle accident	Tox (at death): cocaine
751	28	W	M	SCZ	34	Suicide, GSW to chest	Tox (at death): olanzapine
783	53	W	M	SCZ	19	Manner undetermined	N/A
831	53	W	M	SCZ	14	ASCVD	N/A
4334	11	H	M	ASD	27	Acute hemorrhagic tracheobronchitis	History of epilepsy. Brain edema, acute, mild. Otherwise normal brain
4999	20	W	M	ASD	14	Cardiac arrythmia	PDD, autism, and severe mental retardation. Naltrexone
5027	37	AA	M	ASD	26	Obstruction of bowel due to adhesion	Risperdal and Luvox
5115	46	W	M	ASD	29	Complications of pseudomyxoma peritonei	Adult brain with moderate atherosclerosis
5144	7	W	M	ASD	3	Cancer, complication of	Rhabdomyosarcoma
5176	22	AA	M	ASD	18	Subdural hemorrhage	Risperdal
5308	4	W	M	ASD	21	Skull fractures	Struck by a car. Multifocal subarachnoid hemorrhage
5403	16	W	M	ASD	35	Cardiac arrhythmia	Developmental delays. GI evaluations
1464	42	W	M	Control	19	Pulmonary embolism	Chest and abdominal pain, pale, and diaphoretic
1829	25	W	M	Control	21	Electrocution	N/A
1831	44	W	M	Control	17	CO_2 inhalation complicating ASCVD	History of hypertension. Complained of headaches
1936	46	W	M	Control	13	ASCVD	History of HBP. Had been experiencing chest pain
5024	56	W	M	Control	10	ASCVD; diabetes mellitus	Smoker, no drinking of ETOH. History of prescription drug abuse. On insulin, metformin, oxycodone, Levaquin, and Lyrica
5185	21	W	M	Control	26	Car accident	Drink ETOH prior to death
5189	40	W	M	Control	14	Cardiac arrhythmia complicated by drowning	Severe stomach pains, chest palpitations, and nausea
5276	22	W	M	Control	18	Heroin intoxication	Asthma and drug abuse; smoker
5237	52	W	M	Control	13	HASCVD	ETOH and cocaine abuse. Clean for 30 days and not feeling well
5349	24	W	M	Control	16	Combined drug intoxication	Drug use
5553	54	W	M	Control	17	Hypertensive atherosclerosis heart disease	History of HTN and daily ETOH intake
5615	50	W	M	Control	19	N/A	N/A
4337	8	AA	M	Control	16	Blunt force neck injury. Car accident	Asthma. Brain petechiae, fresh
4670	4	W	M	Control	17	Commotio cordis (struck by a ball in the sternum)	N/A
5334	12	H	M	Control	15	Hanging/suicide	N/A

					Duodenum (biopsies)	
Study #	Age	Race	Sex	Diagnosis	GI symptoms	Additional clinical information
GBA #2	8	W	M	ASD	Non-apparent	Food allergies, GFCF diet, probiotics
GBA #3	11	W	M	ASD	GERD, vomiting, bloating	Asperger's. No milk diet
GBA #6	19	W	M	ASD	Regurgitation after each meal, constipation	History of aggressive behaviors

Table 2 Demographic and clinical characteristics of subjects analyzed in this study *(Continued)*

GBA #7	21	W	F	ASD	GERD, erosive esophagitis, IBS, severe constipation, occasional diarrhea	GFCF diet
GBA #10	9	W	M	ASD	EoE, GERD, constipation, vomiting	Asthma, somewhat loose stools. Dairy-free diet
GBA #12	6	AA	M	ASD	Non-apparent	Eats only pureed food
GBA #13	5	AA	M	ASD	Severe constipation, GERD, abdominal pain, runny stools	Asthma, food allergies
GBA #14	3	W	M	ASD	Chronic constipation	History of obesity, restricted diet (yogurt, milk, juice)
GBA #15	11	W	F	ASD	GERD, constipation	Macrocephaly, sleep disorder
GBA #16	6	W	M	ASD	Gastroesophageal reflux, constipation	Food and seasonal allergies, asthma
GBA #18	16	W	F	ASD	Constipation, abdominal pain, heartburn, regurgitation	Acute mono, weight loss
GBA #20	6	AA	F	ASD	GERD with esophagitis, constipation	ADHD, asthma. Vegetarian
GBA #5	10	HL	M	HC	Abdominal pain, nausea, vomiting, sometimes diarrhea	Lactose-free diet
GBA #8	16	W	F	HC	Constipation, abdominal pain, burping, bloating	GFCG diet, some FODMAP diet
GBA #9	16	W	F	HC	Dysphagia, abdominal pain, regurgitation	
GBA #11	15	W	F	HC	Abdominal pain, GERD	Seasonal allergies, lactose intolerance, dairy-free and nut-free diet, ADHD, obesity
GBA #17	21	W	F	HC	Nausea, vomiting, upset stomach, GERD. Abdominal pain	Previous duodenitis and gastritis, hepatic adenoma
GBA #19	6.5	N/A	M	HC	GERD, constipation	Hydronephrosis, nephrocalcinosis, clubfoot, seasonal allergies, asthma
GBA #21	15	W	M	HC	Dysphagia, esophagitis	Asthma
GBA #23	15	W	M	HC	Abdominal pain, IBS-like constipation	N/A
GBA #24	4	W	M	HC	Reflux	History of constipation. Dairy-free diet

W white, *AA* African-American, *HL* Hispanic-Latino, *M* male, *F* female, *HC* healthy control, *ASD* autism spectrum disorder, *GBA* gut–brain axis study; *GERD* gastroesophageal reflux disease, *GFCF* gluten-free casein-free, *PMI* postmortem interval, *ADD/ADHD* attention-deficit/hyperactivity disorder, *ASCVD* atherosclerotic cardiovascular disease, *HASCVD* hypertensive arteriosclerotic cardiovascular disease, *PDD/PDD-NOS* pervasive developmental disorder/not otherwise specified, *OCD* obsessive-compulsive disorder

The BBB plays a critical role in the central nervous system (CNS) defense through limiting the access of circulating solutes, macromolecules, and cells that could negatively impact neuronal activity. Dysfunctions of the BBB have been associated with numerous neurological disorders, such as stroke, epilepsy, multiple sclerosis, and Parkinson's and Alzheimer's disease [47–56].

The overall goal of this study was to assess whether a dysfunctional BBB or gut barrier could contribute pathophysiologically to ASD. To address this, we conducted an in-depth molecular analysis of the components associated with the BBB and gut barrier integrity in postmortem brain tissue and small intestinal biopsies obtained from ASD subjects. In addition, we assessed changes in the BBB integrity of patients with SCZ as SCZ is a psychiatric illness in which the involvement of inflammation, immunity and altered BBB integrity have been postulated [22, 23, 57, 58].

Methods

Postmortem tissues

Human frozen postmortem brain tissue blocks (1 to 2 cm^3) from the frontal cortex (Brodmann's area 45) and cerebellum (CBL) of 15 HC and eight ASD subjects were obtained from the NICHD Brain and Tissue Bank for Developmental Disorders at the University of Maryland, Baltimore, MD, USA, which is a Brain and Tissue Repository of the NIH NeuroBioBank. Additionally, the Maryland Brain Collection of the Maryland Psychiatric Research Center at the University of Maryland School of Medicine, Baltimore, USA, provided ten SCZ samples from each of the two aforementioned brain areas of interest.

Duodenal biopsies

Biopsy specimens were taken from the second portion of the duodenum from ASD ($n = 12$) and control ($n = 9$) patients with GI symptoms undergoing esophagogastroduodenoscopy (EGD) for clinically indicated reasons. All study subjects provided written informed consent for the collection of additional biopsies, for the purpose of this study, during the procedure. This study was approved by the Partners Human Research Committee (PHRC) at Massachusetts General Hospital and performed in accordance with the ethical standards and regulatory requirements set forth by the Declaration of Helsinki.

Gene expression profile analysis

Total RNA was isolated from samples (~100 mg) using Trizol (Life Technologies, Carlsbad, CA) and/or Direct-zol RNA miniprep spin columns (Zymo Research, Irvine, CA) following the manufacturers' instructions. RNA concentrations and A260/A280 and A260/A230 ratios were measured with the NanoDrop spectrophotometer (Thermo Scientific) before 2 μg total RNA were reverse transcribed using random hexamer primers and Maxima universal first strand cDNA synthesis kit #1661 (Thermo Fisher Scientific, Waltham, MA). Real-time quantitative PCR (qPCR) was used to measure gene expression levels and was performed in an iCycler96X detection system (Bio-Rad, Hercules, CA) according to the manufacturer's protocol. In brain tissues, we analyzed the expression level of genes associated with the formation, integrity, and function of the BBB and neuroinflammation, as follows: Claudin(*CLDN)*-1, *CLDN-3*, *CLDN-5*, and *CLDN-12*; occludin (*OCLN*); tricellulin (*TRIC*); vascular endothelial cadherin (*VE-Cad*); interleukin (*IL*)-1b, *IL-6*, *IL-8*, and *IL-10*; the microglia activation marker ionized calcium-binding adaptor molecule (*IBA*)-1; the translocator protein 18 kDa (*TSPO*); matrix metalloprotease (*MMP*)-2 and *MMP-9*; tissue transglutaminase (*tTG*)-6; tissue plasminogen activator (*tPA*); and the major facilitator super family domain containing 2A (*MFSD2A*). Duodenal biopsies were evaluated for the expression of *CLDN-1, CLDN-2, CLDN-10, CLDN-15, TRIC*, and *OCLN. 18S* housekeeping gene was chosen as internal control. *CLDN-2, CLDN-3, CLDN-10, CLDN-15, TRIC, IL-1b, IL-6, IL-8, IL-10, tTG-6, IBA-1, TSPO*, and *MSFD2A* primers were purchased from Qiagen (RT^2 qPCR or Quantitect Primer Assay). The other primer sets used were purchased by IDT (Integrated DNA Technologies, Coralville, IA), and their sequences together with gene function in the context of the BBB and/or gut are listed in Table 1. The sequence specificity of synthesized primers (IDT) were determined by the online Blast program from the National Center for Biotechnology Information website (http://www.ncbi.nlm.nih.gov/blast/Blast.cgi) and compared with the GenBank database. Differences in gene expression profiles were evaluated applying the $2^{(-ddCT)}$ method [59].

Protein detection

Western blot analysis was performed as routinely described. Brain tissues (~100 mg) were homogenized on ice in lysis buffer [RIPA Buffer (Sigma, S. Louis, MO)] containing protease inhibitor cocktail (Complete Mini,

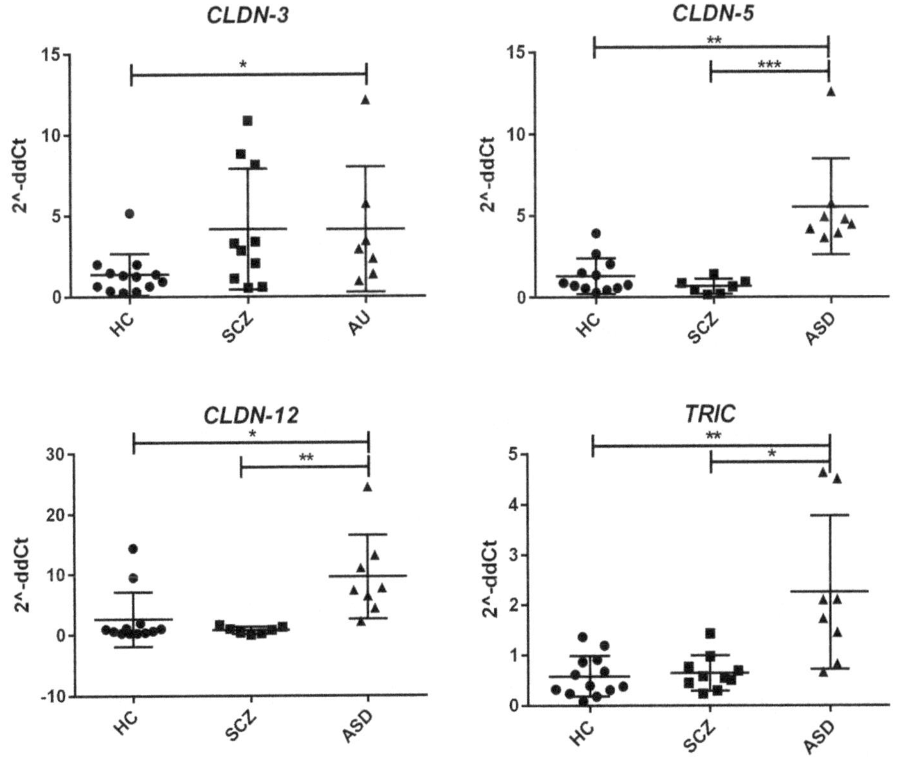

Fig. 1 Altered gene expression level of TJ components in the cortex of ASD subjects. Each *dot* represents data from a single subject. Gene expression level is reported as 2^{-ddCT} with normalization of mRNA expression to the endogenous control *18S*. Mean ± SEM are reported for each group. One-way ANOVA test has been used to evaluate statistical significance. *$p < 0.05$; **$p < 0.01$; ***$p < 0.001$

Roche). Homogenates were centrifuged at 14 K rpm for 30 min at 4 °C in a benchtop centrifuge. The supernatant, representing total protein lysate, was collected, and protein concentration was determined by Lowry protein assay (DC, BioRad, Hercules, CA) using bovine serum albumin (BSA) as a protein standard. Protein lysates were mixed with loading buffer and reducing agent (both from Life Technologies, Carlsbad, CA) and heated at 99 °C for 5 min. The lysates were then loaded on 4–20% Tris-Glycine gels (Life Technologies, Carlsbad, CA) and after gel electrophoresis transferred onto PVDF membranes. The membranes were blocked with 5% BSA in Tris buffered saline with 0.1% Tween 20 (TBST), and incubated with primary antibody overnight at 4 °C. Actin was used as loading control while ACTA2, also known as alpha-smooth muscle actin (in this paper reported as SMA), was used for quantitative analysis normalization for tight junction (TJ) proteins. The membranes were washed three times with TBST and incubated with secondary antibody (diluted 1:5000 in 5% BSA-TBST) for 1 h at room temperature. Western blot signal was visualized using a LI-COR Odyssey infrared scan (LI-COR Biosciences, Lincoln, NE). Results were quantified with the ImageJ 1.47 software (NIH). The protein levels were

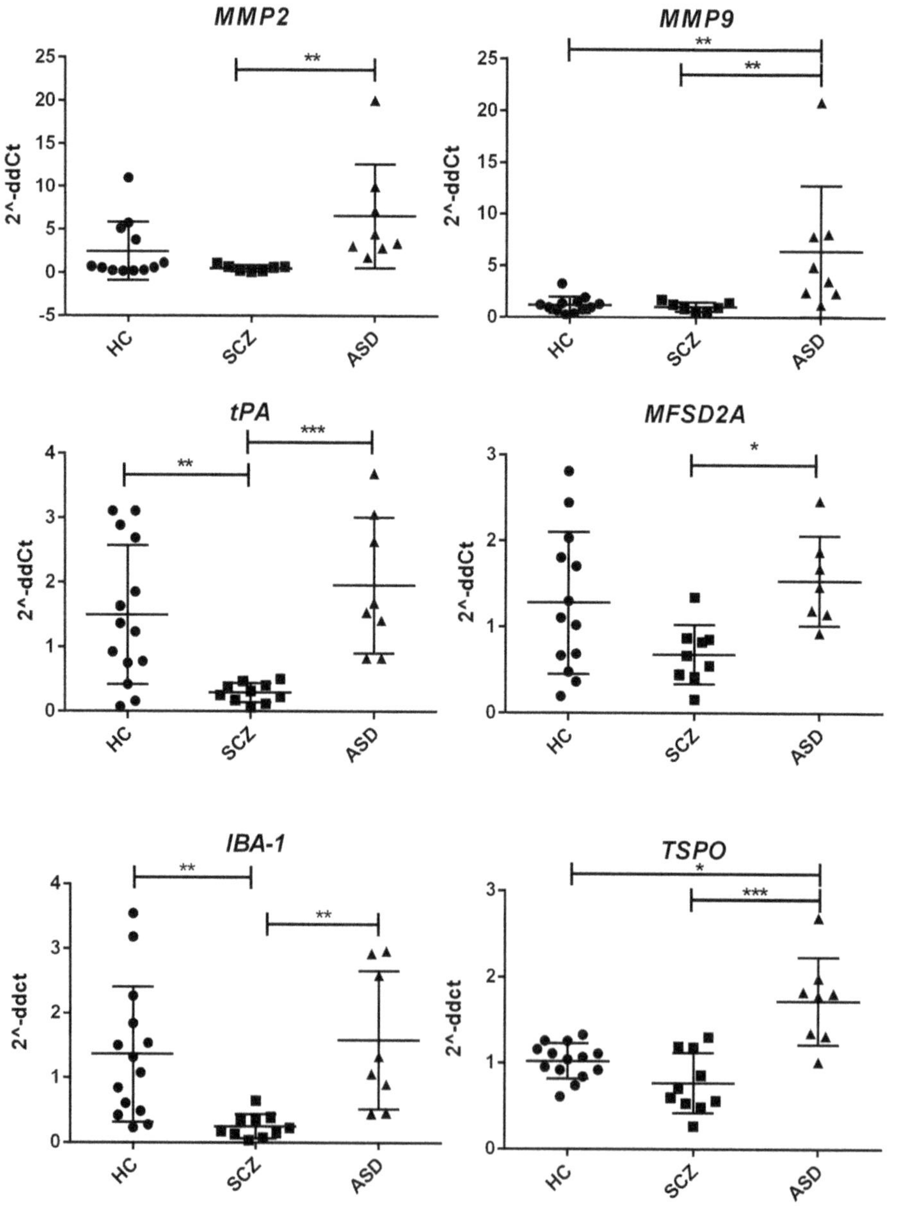

Fig. 2 Gene expression profile of BBB function associated components in the cortex of HC, ASD, and SCZ subjects. Each *dot* represents data from a single subject. Gene expression level is reported as 2^{-ddCT} with normalization of mRNA expression to the endogenous control *18S*. Mean ± SEM are reported for each group. One-way ANOVA test has been used to evaluate statistical significance. *$p < 0.05$; **$p < 0.01$; ***$p < 0.001$

normalized as ratio to actin or SMA, as internal controls. Data represent the average of a minimum of two independent experiments.

Antibodies

Mouse anti-claudin-5 (cat # 35–2500; 1:500) antibody was purchased from Life Technologies, (Carlsbad, CA). Mouse anti-actin protein antibody (cat # 82353; 1:2000) was purchased from Thermo Fisher Scientific (Waltham, MA). Rabbit anti-claudin-12 (cat # NBP1-87450; 1:500) was purchased from Novus Biologicals (Littleton, CO). Rabbit anti-alpha-smooth muscle actin (SMA) antibody (#Ab5694; 1:1000) was purchased from Abcam (Cambridge, MA). LI-COR IRDye800 anti-rabbit (LI-COR Biosciences, Lincoln, NE; cat # 92632211) and Alexa Fluor 680 goat anti-mouse (Thermo Fisher Scientific, Waltham, MA; cat # A21057) were used as secondary antibodies in WB analysis.

Statistics

Data were analyzed by using the GraphPad (San Diego, CA) software. Comparisons among groups were made by the one-way ANOVA (Kruskal–Wallis *H* test; Dunn's test for multiple comparisons). Differences between two groups were calculated by the unpaired *t* test (Mann–Whitney). All data with $p < 0.05$ were considered significant.

Results

Subjects

A total of 33 brain sections from the three subject groups were studied. No drug abuse or gunshot wounds were reported for ASD subjects. Two of the ASD individuals were on therapy with one antipsychotic and/or antidepressant. Those ASD cases whose cause of death was drowning were not considered for the brain study to eliminate the damaging effects on brain and vasculature caused by hypoxia/anoxia [60, 61]. Of the ten SCZ individuals, no medical records were available. The only existing information was collected at autopsy: the post-mortem toxicological analysis showed that three had used antipsychotics and/or antidepressants, one had used cocaine and one had ingested alcohol prior to death. Similar to ASD patients, no gunshot wounds at the head region were reported for SCZ subjects. The control cases had no known neurological disorder or known neuropathology. Three HC out of 15 had a history of drugs and/or alcohol abuse. Biopsies from the second portion of the duodenum were collected from the ASD ($n = 12$) and control ($n = 8$) patients with gastrointestinal symptoms. The available clinical characteristics of the analyzed subjects, together with demographic data are summarized in Table 2.

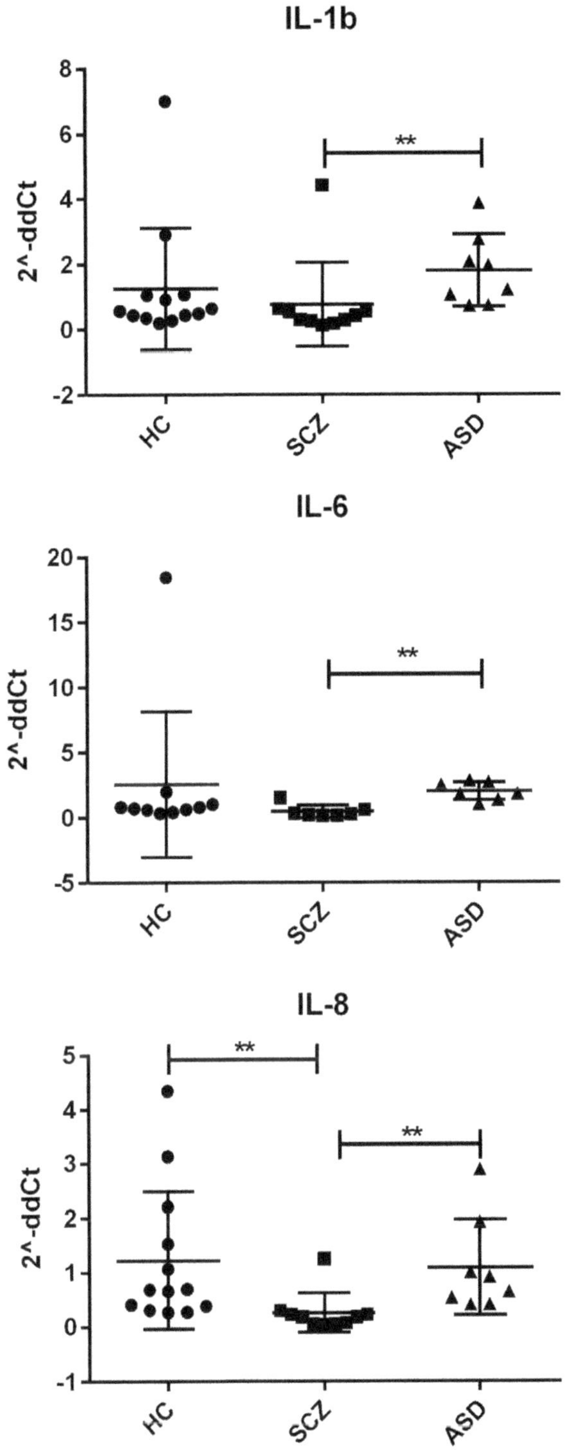

Fig. 3 Gene expression profile of some pro-inflammatory cytokines in the cortex of HC, ASD, and SCZ subjects. Each *dot* represents data from a single subject. Gene expression level is reported as 2^{-ddCT} with normalization of mRNA expression to the endogenous control *18S*. Mean ± SEM are reported for each group. One-way ANOVA test has been used to evaluate statistical significance. $^{**}p < 0.01$

Genes associated with BBB integrity and function are differentially regulated in the brain of ASD subjects

To assess the integrity of the BBB, we measured the gene expression levels of the major components of the brain microvascular endothelial tight junctions (TJs) by qRT-PCR, in the cortex and CBL of HC ($n = 15$), ASD ($n = 8$), and SCZ ($n = 10$) subjects. In the cortex, *CLDN-3, -5,* and *-12* and *TRIC* were upregulated in ASD subjects compared to controls (Fig. 1). Neither *CLDN-1, OCLN,* nor *VE-Cad* were differentially expressed in the cortex in any of the groups analyzed (not shown). Gene expression profiles of *tPA, IBA-1, TSPO, MFSD2A,* pro-inflammatory cytokines, and members of the matrix metalloprotease (MMP) family, described to be linked to BBB function disruption and/or neuroinflammation, were also analyzed. Results showed that in the cortex of ASD subjects, *MMP-9* and *TSPO* were significantly upregulated compared to those of the HC, whereas *tPA* and *IBA-1* appeared downregulated in SCZ compared in HC (Fig. 2). None of the pro-inflammatory cytokines analyzed were differentially regulated in ASD compared in HC. While *IL-8* appeared significantly reduced in SCZ vs. HC, all cytokines evaluated were expressed at a lower level in SCZ compared to ASD (Fig. 3). *IL-10* and *tTG6* expressions were below detection levels. In the CBL, similar to our findings in the cortex, *CLDN-5, −12* and *TSPO* were found to be elevated in ASD subjects when compared to HC (Fig. 4). Among the other genes analyzed, *IL-1b* appeared significantly higher in SCZ vs. HC (Fig. 4). As a general observation, unlike ASD, SCZ subjects clustered well together for most of the genes analyzed in both brain areas. The gene expression fold changes relative to HC (=1) and the corresponding *p* values are summarized in Table 3.

BBB tight junction proteins are altered in ASD and SCZ subjects

To understand whether our gene expression results correlated with levels of protein produced, we performed western blotting analysis of tissue lysates using commercially available antibodies against some TJ components in both the cortex and CBL of HC, ASD, and SCZ subjects. Consistent with the gene expression profile, we observed a significant higher level of CLDN-5 in the cortex of ASD subjects, compared in HC (Fig. 5). Interestingly and in this case in opposition to gene expression results, CLDN-12 was reduced in the cortex of ASD and also showed a reduced trend in SCZ subjects (Fig. 5).

In the CBL (Fig. 6), the production of CLDN-5 in ASD appeared slightly higher than in HC ($p = 0.1$), whereas its level in SCZ was reduced compared to

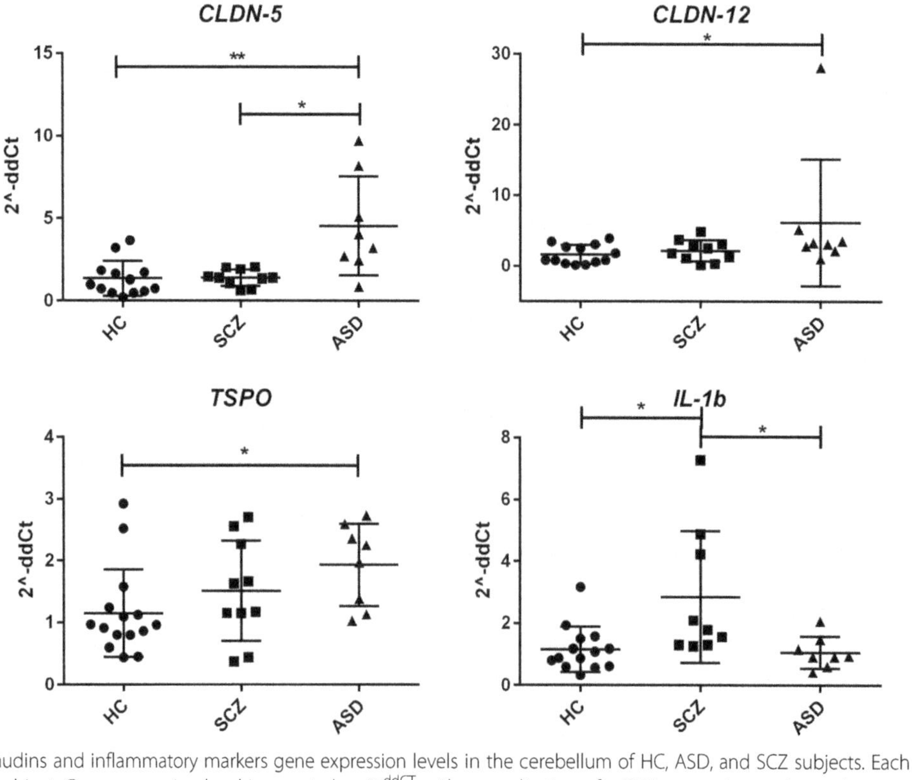

Fig. 4 Increased claudins and inflammatory markers gene expression levels in the cerebellum of HC, ASD, and SCZ subjects. Each *dot* represents data from a single subject. Gene expression level is reported as 2^{-ddCT} with normalization of mRNA expression to the endogenous control *18S*. Mean ± SEM are reported for each group. One-way ANOVA test has been used to evaluate statistical significance. *$p < 0.05$; **$p < 0.01$

Table 3 Summary of gene expression profiling by RT-qPCR

Gene	Fold change		*p* values		
			Cortex		
	SCZ	ASD	HC vs. SCZ	HC vs. ASD	ASD vs. SCZ
CLDN-1	0.7	2.3	ns	ns	ns
CLDN-3	2.7	3.0	<0.05	<0.05	ns
CLDN-5	0.5	5.1	ns	<0.0001	<0.0001
CLDN-12	0.5	7.7	ns	<0.01	<0.001
IBA-1	0.2	1.2	<0.01	ns	<0.01
IL-1b	0.4	1.5	ns	ns	<0.01
IL-6	0.3	1.9	ns	ns	<0.01
IL-8	0.2	1.1	<0.01	ns	<0.01
IL-10	0.5	3.9	ns	ns	ns
MMP-9	0.9	4.5	ns	<0.001	<0.001
MMP-2	0.4	4.9	ns	<0.05	<0.001
MSFD2A	0.6	1.5	ns	ns	ns
OCLN	1.2	1.4	ns	ns	ns
tPA	0.2	1.7	<0.001	ns	<0.01
TRIC	1.3	1.8	ns	<0.001	<0.01
TSPO	0.7	1.7	ns	<0.05	<0.001
VE-Cad	0.8	1.3	ns	ns	ns
			Cerebellum		
CLDN-1	1.3	1.8	ns	ns	ns
CLDN-3	0.6	1.2	ns	ns	ns
CLDN-5	1.3	3.6	ns	0.01	<0.05
CLDN-12	1.5	3.7	ns	<0.05	ns
IBA-1	1.0	1.2	ns	ns	ns
IL-1b	2.3	1.0	0.01	ns	<0.05
IL-6	1.1	0.3	ns	ns	ns
IL-8	1.8	0.9	ns	ns	ns
IL-10	1.3	0.9	ns	ns	ns
MMP-9	1.0	1.9	ns	ns	ns
MMP-2	0.7	2.8	ns	ns	ns
OCLN	1.2	1.5	ns	ns	ns
tPA	1.2	1.5	ns	ns	ns
TRIC	0.6	0.9	ns	ns	ns
TSPO	1.3	1.8	ns	<0.05	ns
VE-Cad	1.4	1.3	ns	ns	ns
			Duodenum (biopsies)		
CLDN-1	N/A	1.7	N/A	ns	N/A
CLDN-2	N/A	2.3	N/A	ns	N/A
CLDN-10	N/A	4.0	N/A	ns	N/A
CLDN-15	N/A	1.6	N/A	ns	N/A
OCLN	N/A	1.2	N/A	ns	N/A
TRIC	N/A	1.6	N/A	ns	N/A

Gene expression levels are presented as fold change vs. HC (=1) using the formula 2(−ΔΔCt). Statistical difference among groups is calculated by the one-way ANOVA (Kruskal–Wallis *H* test). Differences between two groups are calculated by the Mann–Whitney unpaired *t* test. All data with $p < 0.05$ were considered significant

ns non-significant, *N/A* not applicable

that in HC ($p = 0.07$), although data did not reach statistical significance. No differences were observed for CLDN-12 among the groups.

Increased pore-forming CLDNs and decreased barrier-forming TJ components expression in the intestine of ASD patients

To corroborate our hypothesis of a possible involvement of a dysfunctional intestinal barrier in the pathogenesis of ASD, we analyzed small intestinal biopsies of ASD and HC subjects for TJ defects (Fig. 7). Our results showed that 75% (9 out of 12) of the samples analyzed had a decreased expression of at least one barrier-forming TJ component (*CLDN-1, OCLN, TRIC*), whereas about 66% (eight out of 12) showed increased levels of pore-forming CLDNs, described to increase intestinal permeability (*CLDN-2, CLDN-10, CLDN-15*) ([62–65]).

Discussion

To the best of our knowledge, this is the first study addressing the molecular signature of BBB dysfunctions in ASD and SCZ in human samples. In spite of the obvious small sample number, due to the nature of the samples and the consequent procurement difficulty, we observed statistically significant differences among the study groups. However, it is also worthwhile to acknowledge that the small sample number may have affected some otherwise possibly significant results, which could have emerged if a larger number of tissues had been available.

Our molecular analysis of the BBB integrity and function shows an altered BBB in the ASD subjects evaluated. Indeed, the increased gene expression of MMP-9 we detected in ASD subjects supports our hypothesis of an impaired BBB, most likely associated with neuroinflammation. Several pieces of evidence indicate that MMP-9 secretion induces BBB disruption and this is an important step in the development of inflammatory diseases of the nervous system [66–74]. Although we did not observe elevated gene expression levels of pro-inflammatory cytokines in the ASD subjects analyzed in this study, we found a significantly high expression of *TSPO* in the ASD brain. *TSPO* increased expression level in activated microglia and reactive astrocytes [75–81] is

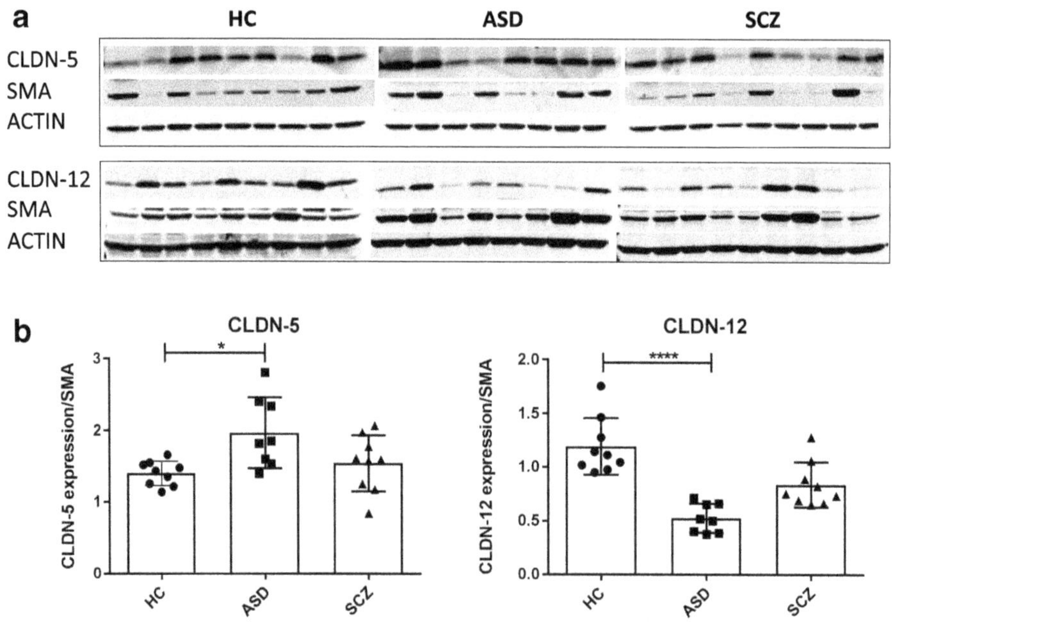

Fig. 5 Increased CLDN-5 and decreased CLDN-12 expression in the cortex of ASD subjects. **a** Brain tissues were lysed and immunoblotted with anti-claudin-5, anti-claudin-12, SMA or actin antibody. **b** Densitometry analysis of the results from the western blots is shown, where the data are normalized against SMA expression and are expressed as the mean ± standard error. Quantitative results represent the average of three independent experiments.$^{*}p < 0.05$; $^{****}p < 0.0001$

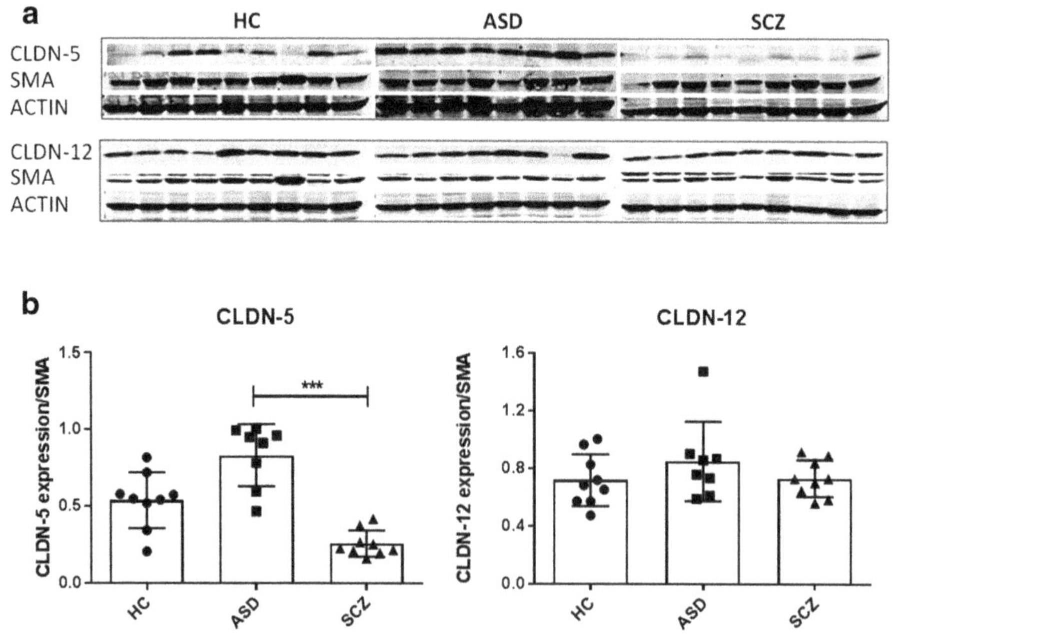

Fig. 6 Increased CLDN-5 expression in the cerebellum of ASD subjects. **a** Western blots of brain lysates immunoblotted with anti-claudin-5, anti-claudin-12, SMA or actin antibody. **b** Densitometry analysis of the results from the western blots is shown, where the data are normalized against SMA expression and are expressed as the mean ± standard error. Quantitative results represent the average of three independent experiments. $^{***}p < 0.001$

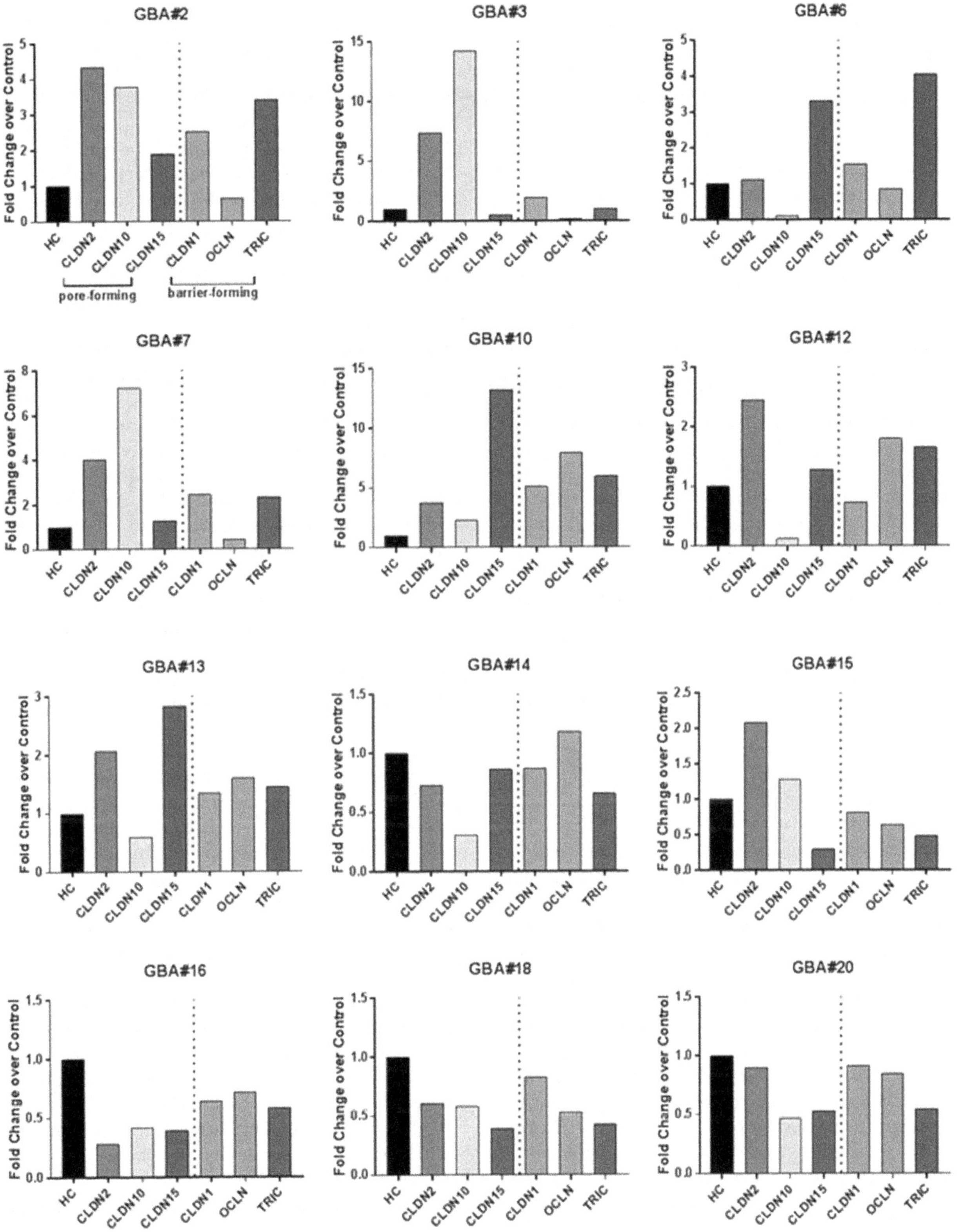

Fig. 7 (See legend on next page.)

(See figure on previous page.)
Fig. 7 Increased pore-forming claudins and decreased barrier-forming TJ components expression in the small intestine of HC and ASD subjects. Gene expression levels of TJ components in duodenal biopsies from HC ($n = 9$) and ASD patients ($n = 12$). *CLDN-2, -10* and/or *-15* levels are higher in eight out of 12 ASD samples, compared in controls. *CLDN-1, OCLN,* and/or *TRIC* levels are decreased in nine out of 12 ASD samples over controls. Each graph represents single patient results. Data are expressed as fold change over the averaged controls

associated with brain injury and neuroinflammation, making TSPO a reliable marker of brain inflammation.

Of the four claudins (i.e., *CLDN-1*, *-3*, *-5* and *-12*) that to date are thought to be incorporated in the BBB [82–85], we found that two were significantly more expressed in the ASD brain as compared in HC. *CLDN-5*, the major and more abundant cell adhesion molecule of TJs in brain endothelial cells, is expressed 5.1 and 3.6 times higher in the cortex and CBL of ASD subjects, respectively, than in those of HC (Table 3). Similarly, *CLDN-12* is expressed about 7.7 and 3.6 times more in the ASD cortex and CBL, respectively, than in the control group. *CLDN-3*, on the other hand, appears elevated by about 2.7 and 3.0 times in the cortex of both SCZ and ASD subjects, respectively, compared in that of HC. *TRIC*, another component of the TJs associated with increased epithelial tightness and decreased permeability to macromolecules [86], appears significantly elevated in the ASD cortex, suggesting either a more competent BBB or a compensatory mechanism for disrupted endothelial barrier integrity.

At the protein level, CLDN-5 is elevated in the ASD cortex, consistent with its mRNA expression, whereas, on the other hand, CLDN-12 is significantly reduced. An increased gene expression of sealing TJ components (*CLDN-5*, *-12*, and *-3* and *TRIC*) should imply a tighter BBB and a better control in the diffusion of macromolecules. However, our data on *MMP9* and *TSPO* expression compatible with ongoing neuroinflammation suggest a compensatory mechanism to repair a compromised BBB. Another plausible explanation for the CLDN-5 data is that, once produced, the protein is not capable of being incorporated into the TJ complex because of impaired trafficking to the endothelial cell–cell interface or because the protein has some mutations that prevent it from establishing homophilic and/or heterophilic protein–protein interactions, leading to a sustained compensatory gene expression and protein accumulation. On the other hand, the discrepancy between gene upregulation and decreased protein expression observed for CLDN-12 might suggest the existence of a compensatory mechanism for post-translational destruction/degradation of the protein itself. While the sealing function of CLDN-5 in BBB TJs is well established [83, 87], that of CLDN-3 and -12 are less understood. CLDN-1 and -3 sequences are highly homologous to CLDN-5, suggesting similar properties. Indeed, several studies strongly suggest that CLDN-3 contributes to BBB tightness [85, 88–90]. Conversely, CLDN-12 sequence is quite dissimilar from those of CLDN-1 and -3, and this might indicate a different function. Piontek et al. [91] showed that CLDN-12 cannot form homophilic trans-interactions or homopolymeric strands in vitro, suggesting that "heterophilic cis- and/or trans-interactions with another TJ-protein are necessary for the incorporation of CLDN-12 in strands." It may be hypothesized that the increased CLDN-5 we observed in ASD subjects might be compensatory to a decreased CLDN-12 in a heterophilic cis- and/or trans-interaction between the two claudins.

Our cohort of SCZ individuals did not show major changes in the genes analyzed compared to HC, except for an increased *IL-1b* in the CBL and significantly reduced levels of tPA and *IBA-1* in the cortex. Whereas we do not know the physiological relevance of downregulated IBA-1, our results are in agreement with data from other studies indicating activation of pro-inflammatory networks and reduced tPA activity in SCZ [92–102], this latter feature leading to a dysfunctional coagulation system and increased risk of thrombotic events in SCZ patients [101]. Other genes analyzed in SCZ appeared to follow a trend similar to ASD subjects (i.e., increased *CLDN-3* and reduced CLDN-12 protein level in the cortex). Furthermore, although non-statistically significant ($p = 0.07$), we did observe a trend toward reduced CLDN-5 protein level in the SCZ CBL as well, suggesting a possibly leaking BBB. Previous clinical and postmortem research in SCZ has suggested that an impaired BBB could be a contributing factor to the pathogenesis of the disease in only a subgroup of SCZ patients [103–105]. It is important to mention that the SCZ and ASD subjects studied were not selected on the basis of specific immune biomarkers and, therefore, may represent a mixed group of patients, which thereby limits the statistical significance of some of our findings. A sample stratification approach based on specific immunological features might be a better way of analyzing pathways of interest, and this may be particularly true for SCZ, a disorder characterized by marked clinical and neurobiological heterogeneity. Alternatively, SCZ physiopathology may lie in subtle changes that chronically affect brain function.

As for the intestine, due to the high heterogeneity intrinsic of ASD, our goal was to elucidate the TJ component profile from a functional perspective. Toward this aim, we have analyzed the expression level of TJ elements dividing them into two major functional groups: pore-forming (*CLDN-1, OCLN, TRIC*) and barrier-forming components (*CLDN-2, -10, -15*). These results, showing increased expression levels of pore-forming (66% of the ASD samples) and decreased levels of barrier-forming (75% of the ASD samples) TJ components in the duodenal samples, suggest an impaired gut barrier and serve as a proof of concept to support the hypothesis of a gut–brain axis dysfunction in a subgroup of ASD patients. According to this hypothesis, non-self antigens crossing a damaged intestinal barrier elicit a local and/or systemic inflammatory reaction that,

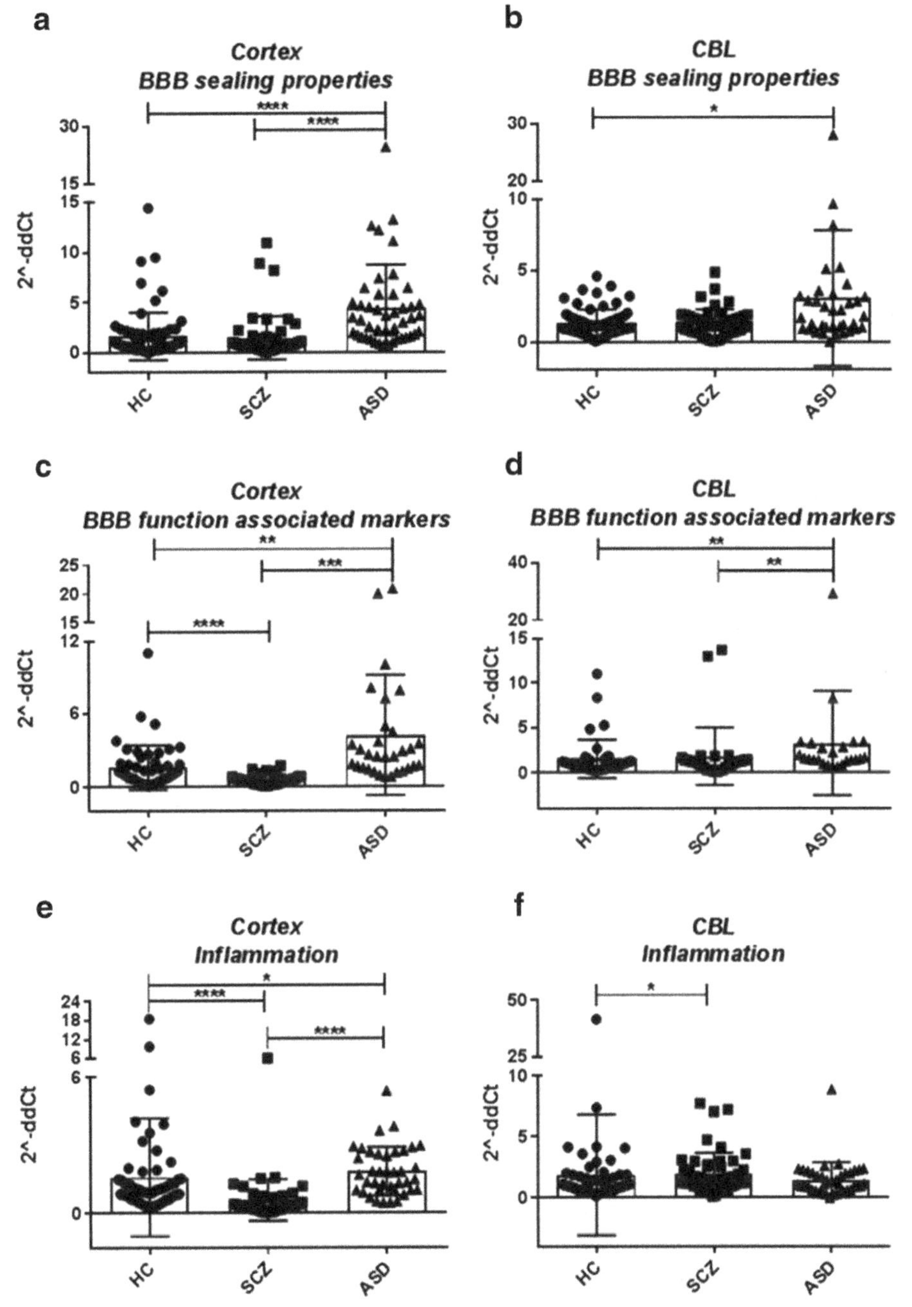

Fig. 8 Gene expression in the cortex and cerebellum (CBL) of HC, ASD, and SCZ subjects clustered by functional category. Results are represented as scatter plots where each *dot* represents data obtained from one subject sample. **a** Cortex *BBB sealing properties* group includes *CLDN-3, -5,* and *-12, TRIC,* and *OCLN*. **b** CBL "BBB sealing properties" group includes *CLDN-3, -5,* and *-12, TRIC,* and *OCLN*. **c** Cortex *BBB function associated markers* group includes *tPA, MMP2/9,* and *MSFD2A*. **d** CBL *BBB function associated markers* group includes *tPA* and *MMP-2/9*. **e** Cortex *Inflammation* group includes *IL-1b, IL-6,* and *IL-8; TSPO;* and *IBA-1*. **f** CBL *Inflammation* group includes *IL-1b, IL-6,* and *IL-8; TSPO; IBA-1*. Gene expression level is reported as 2^{-ddCT} with normalization of mRNA expression to the endogenous control *18S*. Mean ± SEM are reported for each group. One-way ANOVA test has been used to evaluate statistical significance. $^{*}p < 0.05$; $^{**}p < 0.01$; $^{***}p < 0.001$; $^{****}p < 0.0001$

associated with a breach of the BBB, may lead to ASD in genetically predisposed subjects.

This study addressed for the first time, at the molecular level, some relevant and still open questions regarding the gut–brain axis in neurobehavioral disorders and furthermore demonstrated that both the BBB and gut barrier may be affected in ASD. However, these findings present with a few limitations. The first lies in the postmortem nature of the samples with potential confounding factors deriving from tissue preservation and the personal history of each subject, including exposure to medications, health conditions, cause of death, and postmortem interval (PMI). Our statistical analysis of the PMI showed no differences among groups suggesting that PMI might not have affected our results. Similarly, data from medical records or postmortem toxicology analysis showed that about the same number of subjects in ASD and SCZ groups were on antipsychotics/antidepressants, so it is unlikely that the differences we observed among groups could be explained by the effects of the drugs. For clarity, a few studies addressing the impact of antipsychotics on the BBB function do suggest a disturbance effect on its sealing property [106, 107], whereas other studies on the blood–cerebrospinal (BCS) fluid barrier show divergent results [103, 108]. Furthermore, there are numerous studies reporting the suppressing effect of antipsychotics on the blood cytokine profile in SCZ and ASD [98, 109–118], as well as on microglia activation [119, 120], that could explain our data on *IBA-1* and the cytokine gene expression profiles. However, our *IBA*-1 results are well in agreement with the published studies on postmortem brain tissues showing no significant changes in its expression in ASD [121].

The second limitation of this study is represented by its descriptive nature that does not allow us to draw conclusions on the causality of a breach of the intestinal/BBB integrity supporting neuroinflammation and ASD and SCZ symptoms. However, our data is in line with animal studies suggesting causality between loss of barrier function and neurobehavioral changes compatible with ASD [122–124]. Finally, as already mentioned, a third limitation is represented by the small number of samples analyzed due to limited availability which might impact on the statistical significance of some of our results. However, given the complexity of the studies performed and the difficulty associated with the procurement of these samples, our study represents a solid foundation to justify a more robust sample collection and analysis to further investigate the gut–brain axis in ASD.

Conclusions

In conclusion, our results seem to point to a dysfunctional gut–brain axis associated with neuroinflammation in ASD. When clustered together by functional groups (barrier properties, pro-inflammatory markers, and enzymatic activity), our data support the notion that in ASD, there is a differential regulation of the pathways associated with our hypothesis of a gut–brain axis dysfunction involving the intestinal barrier, BBB integrity/function, and neuroinflammation (Fig. 8). Certainly, more in-depth molecular studies, possibly in animal or in vitro cell culture models, are necessary to understand the specific mechanisms behind the BBB disturbance we have herein reported. These studies will allow for patient stratification and personalized interventions (precision medicine) to target specific pathways involved in the pathogenesis of ASD.

Abbreviations

AJ: Adherens junction; ASD: Autism spectrum disorders; BBB: Blood–brain barrier; BCS: Blood–cerebrospinal; CBL: Cerebellum; CLDN: Claudin; CNS: Central nervous system; GBA: Gut–brain axis study; GI: Gastrointestinal; HC: Healthy controls; IBA-1: Ionized calcium-binding adaptor molecule 1; IL: Interleukin; INF: Interferon; MSFD2A: Major facilitator super family domain containing 2A; MMP: Matrix metalloprotease; NICHD: National Institute of Child Health and Human Development; OCLN: Occludin; PMI: Postmortem interval; SCZ: Schizophrenia; TJ: Tight junction; TNF: Tumor necrosis factor; tPA: Tissue plasminogen activator; tTG6: Tissue transglutaminase 6; TRIC: Tricellulin; TSPO: Translocator protein; VE-Cad: Vascular endothelial cadherin; ZO-1: Zonula occludens-1

Acknowledgements

The authors would like to thank the NICHD Brain and Tissue Bank for Developmental Disorders at the University of Maryland, Baltimore, MD, which is a Brain and Tissue Repository of the NIH NeuroBioBank, and the Maryland Brain Collection Steering Committee for their help in the brain acquisition and characterization. We would like to thank the tissue donors and their families for contributing to the advancement of brain research through the donation of tissue belonging to their self or their loved one.

Funding

The authors did not receive any funding for the study.

Authors' contributions

MF, AS, AF, and NC conceived the study. MF and AS conceived and designed the experiments. MF, AS, and SS performed the experiments. MF and AS analyzed the data. MF drafted the manuscript. AF, NC, AS, SS, and DLK helped with the interpretation of the data. AF, NC, DLK, SSC, and SS assisted in writing and/or editing the manuscript. SSC, SMK, and TMB actively contributed to the procurement of the duodenal biopsies and to the critical reading of the manuscript. All authors read and approved the final manuscript.

Competing interests

The authors declare that they have no competing interests.

Ethics approval and consent to participate

The human postmortem tissue collection, medical records, and family contact have been approved by the University of Maryland and Department of Health and Mental Hygiene Institutional Review Boards (IRBs). In addition, the specific collection was approved by the Maryland Psychiatric Research Center (MPRC), Maryland Brain Collection Steering Commitee, and the NIH NeuroBioBank Tissue Access Commitee. The specimens were collected under specific protocols, and the family consent was collected for the tissue to be used for scientific purposes including publication. Study procedures for the collection of the duodenal biopsies were reviewed and approved by the Partners Human Research Committee (PHRC) at Massachusetts General Hospital and performed in accordance with the Declaration of Helsinki.

The PHRC operates in full compliance with all applicable federal, state, and local laws and regulations to protect the rights and welfare of the human subjects. Written informed consent was obtained from all the subjects at the time of enrollment.

Author details

[1]Mucosal Immunology and Biology Research Center, Massachusetts General Hospital for Children, Boston, MA, USA. [2]Department of Medicine, Celiac Center, Division of Gastroenterology, Beth Israel Deaconess Medical Center and Harvard Medical School, Boston, MA, USA. [3]Center for Celiac Research and Division of Pediatric Gastroenterology and Nutrition, Massachusetts General Hospital for Children, Boston, MA, USA. [4]Department of Pediatrics, Harvard Medical School, Boston, MA, USA. [5]Maryland Psychiatric Research Center, University of Maryland School of Medicine, Baltimore, MD, USA. [6]Neuropsychiatry Program, Sheppard Pratt Health System, Baltimore, MD, USA.

References

1. Nelson KB, Grether JK, Croen LA, Dambrosia JM, Dickens BF, Jelliffe LL, Hansen RL, Phillips TM. Neuropeptides and neurotrophins in neonatal blood of children with autism or mental retardation. Ann Neurol. 2001;49(5):597–606.
2. Vargas DL, Nascimbene C, Krishnan C, Zimmerman AW, Pardo CA. Neuroglial activation and neuroinflammation in the brain of patients with autism. Ann Neurol. 2005;57(1):67–81.
3. Zimmerman AW, Connors SL, Matteson KJ, Lee LC, Singer HS, Castaneda JA, Pearce DA. Maternal antibrain antibodies in autism. Brain Behav Immun. 2007;21(3):351–7.
4. Zimmerman AW, Jyonouchi H, Comi AM, Connors SL, Milstien S, Varsou A, Heyes MP. Cerebrospinal fluid and serum markers of inflammation in autism. Pediatr Neurol. 2005;33(3):195–201.
5. Chez MG, Dowling T, Patel PB, Khanna P, Kominsky M. Elevation of tumor necrosis factor-alpha in cerebrospinal fluid of autistic children. Pediatr Neurol. 2007;36(6):361–5.
6. Pardo CA, Vargas DL, Zimmerman AW. Immunity, neuroglia and neuroinflammation in autism. Int Rev Psychiatry. 2005;17(6):485–95.
7. Kinney DK, Hintz K, Shearer EM, Barch DH, Riffin C, Whitley K, Butler R. A unifying hypothesis of schizophrenia: abnormal immune system development may help explain roles of prenatal hazards, post-pubertal onset, stress, genes, climate, infections, and brain dysfunction. Med Hypotheses. 2010;74(3):555–63.
8. Carter CJ. Schizophrenia: a pathogenetic autoimmune disease caused by viruses and pathogens and dependent on genes. J Pathog. 2011;2011:128318.
9. Barch DM, Carter CS. Amphetamine improves cognitive function in medicated individuals with schizophrenia and in healthy volunteers. Schizophr Res. 2005;77(1):43–58.
10. Eaton WW, Byrne M, Ewald H, Mors O, Chen CY, Agerbo E, Mortensen PB. Association of schizophrenia and autoimmune diseases: linkage of Danish national registers. Am J Psychiatry. 2006;163(3):521–8.
11. Avramopoulos D, Pearce BD, McGrath J, Wolyniec P, Wang R, Eckart N, Hatzimanolis A, Goes FS, Nestadt G, Mulle J, et al. Infection and inflammation in schizophrenia and bipolar disorder: a genome wide study for interactions with genetic variation. PLoS One. 2015;10(3):e0116696.
12. Gantert M, Kreczmanski P, Kuypers E, Jellema R, Strackx E, Bastian N, Gavilanes AW, Zimmermann LJ, Garnier Y, Schmitz C, et al. Effects of in utero endotoxemia on the ovine fetal brain: a model for schizophrenia? Front Biosci (Elite Ed). 2012;4:2845–53.
13. Hope S, Dieset I, Agartz I, Steen NE, Ueland T, Melle I, Aukrust P, Andreassen OA. Affective symptoms are associated with markers of inflammation and immune activation in bipolar disorders but not in schizophrenia. J Psychiatr Res. 2011;45(12):1608–16.
14. Yang Y, Wan C, Li H, Zhu H, La Y, Xi Z, Chen Y, Jiang L, Feng G, He L. Altered levels of acute phase proteins in the plasma of patients with schizophrenia. Anal Chem. 2006;78(11):3571–6.
15. Wan C, La Y, Zhu H, Yang Y, Jiang L, Chen Y, Feng G, Li H, Sang H, Hao X, et al. Abnormal changes of plasma acute phase proteins in schizophrenia and the relation between schizophrenia and haptoglobin (Hp) gene. Amino Acids. 2007;32(1):101–8.
16. Ashwood P, Wakefield AJ. Immune activation of peripheral blood and mucosal CD3+ lymphocyte cytokine profiles in children with autism and gastrointestinal symptoms. J Neuroimmunol. 2006;173(1–2):126–34.
17. Cascella NG, Santora D, Gregory P, Kelly DL, Fasano A, Eaton WW. Increased prevalence of transglutaminase 6 antibodies in sera from schizophrenia patients. Schizophr Bull. 2013;39(4):867–71.
18. Cohly HH, Panja A. Immunological findings in autism. Int Rev Neurobiol. 2005;71:317–41.
19. Singh VK. Phenotypic expression of autoimmune autistic disorder (AAD): a major subset of autism. Ann Clin Psychiatry. 2009;21(3):148–61.
20. Kliushnik TP, Androsova LV, Simashkova NV, Zozulia SA, Otman IN, Koval'-Zaitsev AA. [Innate and adaptive immunity in children with psychotic forms of autism-spectrum disorders]. Zh Nevrol Psikhiatr Im S S Korsakova. 2011;111(8 Pt 1):41–5.
21. Estes ML, McAllister AK. Immune mediators in the brain and peripheral tissues in autism spectrum disorder. Nat Rev Neurosci. 2015;16(8):469–86.
22. Chen SJ, Chao YL, Chen CY, Chang CM, Wu EC, Wu CS, Yeh HH, Chen CH, Tsai HJ. Prevalence of autoimmune diseases in in-patients with schizophrenia: nationwide population-based study. Br J Psychiatry. 2012;200(5):374–80.
23. Kalaydjian AE, Eaton W, Cascella N, Fasano A. The gluten connection: the association between schizophrenia and celiac disease. Acta Psychiatr Scand. 2006;113(2):82–90.
24. Wu S, Ding Y, Wu F, Li R, Xie G, Hou J, Mao P. Family history of autoimmune diseases is associated with an increased risk of autism in children: a systematic review and meta-analysis. Neurosci Biobehav Rev. 2015;55:322–32.
25. Billeci L, Tonacci A, Tartarisco G, Ruta L, Pioggia G, Gangemi S. Association between atopic dermatitis and autism spectrum disorders: a systematic review. Am J Clin Dermatol. 2015;16:371–88.
26. Kohane IS, McMurry A, Weber G, MacFadden D, Rappaport L, Kunkel L, Bickel J, Wattanasin N, Spence S, Murphy S, et al. The co-morbidity burden of children and young adults with autism spectrum disorders. PLoS One. 2012;7(4):e33224.
27. Zerbo O, Leong A, Barcellos L, Bernal P, Fireman B, Croen LA. Immune mediated conditions in autism spectrum disorders. Brain Behav Immun. 2015;46:232–6.
28. Magalhaes ES, Pinto-Mariz F, Bastos-Pinto S, Pontes AT, Prado AE, deAzevedo LC. Immune allergic response in Asperger syndrome. J Neuroimmunol. 2009; 216(1–2):108–12.
29. Gorrindo P, Williams KC, Lee EB, Walker LS, McGrew SG, Levitt P. Gastrointestinal dysfunction in autism: parental report, clinical evaluation, and associated factors. Autism Res. 2012;5(2):101–8.
30. Valicenti-McDermott MD, McVicar K, Cohen HJ, Wershil BK, Shinnar S. Gastrointestinal symptoms in children with an autism spectrum disorder and language regression. Pediatr Neurol. 2008;39(6):392–8.
31. Buie T, Campbell DB, Fuchs 3rd GJ, Furuta GT, Levy J, Vandewater J, Whitaker AH, Atkins D, Bauman ML, Beaudet AL, et al. Evaluation, diagnosis, and treatment of gastrointestinal disorders in individuals with ASDs: a consensus report. Pediatrics. 2010;125 Suppl 1:S1–18.
32. Lightdale JR, Hayer C, Duer A, Lind-White C, Jenkins S, Siegel B, Elliott GR, Heyman MB. Effects of intravenous secretin on language and behavior of children with autism and gastrointestinal symptoms: a single-blinded, open-label pilot study. Pediatrics. 2001;108(5), E90.
33. Horvath K, Papadimitriou JC, Rabsztyn A, Drachenberg C, Tildon JT. Gastrointestinal abnormalities in children with autistic disorder. J Pediatr. 1999;135(5):559–63.
34. Horvath K, Perman JA. Autism and gastrointestinal symptoms. Curr Gastroenterol Rep. 2002;4(3):251–8.
35. Horvath K, Perman JA. Autistic disorder and gastrointestinal disease. Curr Opin Pediatr. 2002;14(5):583–7.
36. Kang V, Wagner GC, Ming X. Gastrointestinal dysfunction in children with autism spectrum disorders. Autism Res. 2014;7(4):501–6.
37. Torrente F, Anthony A, Heuschkel RB, Thomson MA, Ashwood P, Murch SH. Focal-enhanced gastritis in regressive autism with features distinct from Crohn's and Helicobacter pylori gastritis. Am J Gastroenterol. 2004;99(4):598–605.
38. Torrente F, Ashwood P, Day R, Machado N, Furlano RI, Anthony A, Davies SE, Wakefield AJ, Thomson MA, Walker-Smith JA, et al. Small intestinal enteropathy with epithelial IgG and complement deposition in children with regressive autism. Mol Psychiatry. 2002;7(4):375–82. 334.
39. D'Eufemia P, Celli M, Finocchiaro R, Pacifico L, Viozzi L, Zaccagnini M, Cardi E, Giardini O. Abnormal intestinal permeability in children with autism. Acta Paediatr. 1996;85(9):1076–9.
40. de Magistris L, Familiari V, Pascotto A, Sapone A, Frolli A, Iardino P, Carteni M, De Rosa M, Francavilla R, Riegler G, et al. Alterations of the intestinal

barrier in patients with autism spectrum disorders and in their first-degree relatives. J Pediatr Gastroenterol Nutr. 2010;51(4):418–24.

41. de Magistris L, Picardi A, Siniscalco D, Riccio MP, Sapone A, Cariello R, Abbadessa S, Medici N, Lammers KM, Schiraldi C, et al. Antibodies against food antigens in patients with autistic spectrum disorders. Biomed Res Int. 2013;2013:729349.
42. Dalton N, Chandler S, Turner C, Charman T, Pickles A, Loucas T, Simonoff E, Sullivan P, Baird G. Gut permeability in autism spectrum disorders. Autism Res. 2014;7(3):305–13.
43. Niebuhr DW, Li Y, Cowan DN, Weber NS, Fisher JA, Ford GM, Yolken R. Association between bovine casein antibody and new onset schizophrenia among US military personnel. Schizophr Res. 2011;128(1–3):51–5.
44. Jackson J, Eaton W, Cascella N, Fasano A, Warfel D, Feldman S, Richardson C, Vyas G, Linthicum J, Santora D, et al. A gluten-free diet in people with schizophrenia and anti-tissue transglutaminase or anti-gliadin antibodies. Schizophr Res. 2012;140(1–3):262–3.
45. Severance EG, Dickerson FB, Halling M, Krivogorsky B, Haile L, Yang S, Stallings CR, Origoni AE, Bossis I, Xiao J, et al. Subunit and whole molecule specificity of the anti-bovine casein immune response in recent onset psychosis and schizophrenia. Schizophr Res. 2010;118(1–3):240–7.
46. Jackson J, Eaton W, Cascella N, Fasano A, Santora D, Sullivan K, Feldman S, Raley H, McMahon RP, Carpenter Jr WT, et al. Gluten sensitivity and relationship to psychiatric symptoms in people with schizophrenia. Schizophr Res. 2014;159(2–3):539–42.
47. Moor AC, de Vries HE, de Boer AG, Breimer DD. The blood–brain barrier and multiple sclerosis. Biochem Pharmacol. 1994;47(10):1717–24.
48. Hemmer B, Cepok S, Zhou D, Sommer N. Multiple sclerosis—a coordinated immune attack across the blood brain barrier. Curr Neurovasc Res. 2004;1(2):141–50.
49. Yang Y, Rosenberg GA. Blood–brain barrier breakdown in acute and chronic cerebrovascular disease. Stroke. 2011;42(11):3323–8.
50. Weissberg I, Reichert A, Heinemann U, Friedman A. Blood–brain barrier dysfunction in epileptogenesis of the temporal lobe. Epilepsy Res Treat. 2011;2011:143908.
51. de Vries HE, Kuiper J, de Boer AG, Van Berkel TJ, Breimer DD. The blood–brain barrier in neuroinflammatory diseases. Pharmacol Rev. 1997;49(2):143–55.
52. Heinemann U, Kaufer D, Friedman A. Blood–brain barrier dysfunction, TGFbeta signaling, and astrocyte dysfunction in epilepsy. Glia. 2012; 60(8):1251–7.
53. Seiffert E, Dreier JP, Ivens S, Bechmann I, Tomkins O, Heinemann U, Friedman A. Lasting blood–brain barrier disruption induces epileptic focus in the rat somatosensory cortex. J Neurosci. 2004;24(36):7829–36.
54. Gray MT, Woulfe JM. Striatal blood–brain barrier permeability in Parkinson's disease. J Cereb Blood Flow Metab. 2015;35(5):747–50.
55. Bell RD, Zlokovic BV. Neurovascular mechanisms and blood–brain barrier disorder in Alzheimer's disease. Acta Neuropathol. 2009;118(1):103–13.
56. Lee H, Pienaar IS. Disruption of the blood–brain barrier in Parkinson's disease: curse or route to a cure? Front Biosci (Landmark Ed). 2014;19:272–80.
57. Eaton W, Mortensen PB, Agerbo E, Byrne M, Mors O, Ewald H. Coeliac disease and schizophrenia: population based case control study with linkage of Danish national registers. BMJ. 2004;328(7437):438–9.
58. Hanson DR, Gottesman II. Theories of schizophrenia: a genetic-inflammatory-vascular synthesi. BMC Med Genet. 2005;6:7.
59. Schmittgen TD, Livak KJ. Analyzing real-time PCR data by the comparative C(T) method. Nat Protoc. 2008;3(6):1101–8.
60. Al Ahmad A, Gassmann M, Ogunshola OO. Involvement of oxidative stress in hypoxia-induced blood–brain barrier breakdown. Microvasc Res. 2012;84(2):222–5.
61. Engelhardt S, Al-Ahmad AJ, Gassmann M, Ogunshola OO. Hypoxia selectively disrupts brain microvascular endothelial tight junction complexes through a hypoxia-inducible factor-1 (HIF-1) dependent mechanism. J Cell Physiol. 2014;229(8):1096–105.
62. Amasheh S, Meiri N, Gitter AH, Schoneberg T, Mankertz J, Schulzke JD, Fromm M. Claudin-2 expression induces cation-selective channels in tight junctions of epithelial cells. J Cell Sci. 2002;115(Pt 24):4969–76.
63. Gunzel D, Stuiver M, Kausalya PJ, Haisch L, Krug SM, Rosenthal R, Meij IC, Hunziker W, Fromm M, Muller D. Claudin-10 exists in six alternatively spliced isoforms that exhibit distinct localization and function. J Cell Sci. 2009;122(Pt 10):1507–17.
64. Inai T, Kamimura T, Hirose E, Iida H, Shibata Y. The protoplasmic or exoplasmic face association of tight junction particles cannot predict paracellular permeability or heterotypic claudin compatibility. Eur J Cell Biol. 2010;89(7):547–56.
65. Tamura A, Hayashi H, Imasato M, Yamazaki Y, Hagiwara A, Wada M, Noda T, Watanabe M, Suzuki Y, Tsukita S. Loss of claudin-15, but not claudin-2, causes Na + deficiency and glucose malabsorption in mouse small intestine. Gastroenterology. 2011;140(3):913–23.
66. Leppert D, Ford J, Stabler G, Grygar C, Lienert C, Huber S, Miller KM, Hauser SL, Kappos L. Matrix metalloproteinase-9 (gelatinase B) is selectively elevated in CSF during relapses and stable phases of multiple sclerosis. Brain. 1998;121(Pt 12):2327–34.
67. Kandagaddala LD, Kang MJ, Chung BC, Patterson TA, Kwon OS. Expression and activation of matrix metalloproteinase-9 and NADPH oxidase in tissues and plasma of experimental autoimmune encephalomyelitis in mice. Exp Toxicol Pathol. 2012;64(1–2):109–14.
68. Minagar A, Alexander JS. Blood–brain barrier disruption in multiple sclerosis. Mult Scler. 2003;9(6):540–9.
69. Nygardas PT, Hinkkanen AE. Up-regulation of MMP-8 and MMP-9 activity in the BALB/c mouse spinal cord correlates with the severity of experimental autoimmune encephalomyelitis. Clin Exp Immunol. 2002;128(2):245–54.
70. Yong VW, Zabad RK, Agrawal S, Goncalves Dasilva A, Metz LM. Elevation of matrix metalloproteinases (MMPs) in multiple sclerosis and impact of immunomodulators. J Neurol Sci. 2007;259(1–2):79–84.
71. Chiu PS, Lai SC. Matrix metalloproteinase-9 leads to blood–brain barrier leakage in mice with eosinophilic meningoencephalitis caused by Angiostrongylus cantonensis. Acta Trop. 2014;140:141–50.
72. Dal-Pizzol F, Rojas HA, dos Santos EM, Vuolo F, Constantino L, Feier G, Pasquali M, Comim CM, Petronilho F, Gelain DP, et al. Matrix metalloproteinase-2 and metalloproteinase-9 activities are associated with blood–brain barrier dysfunction in an animal model of severe sepsis. Mol Neurobiol. 2013;48(1):62–70.
73. Lee MA, Palace J, Stabler G, Ford J, Gearing A, Miller K. Serum gelatinase B, TIMP-1 and TIMP-2 levels in multiple sclerosis. A longitudinal clinical and MRI study. Brain. 1999;122(Pt 2):191–7.
74. Waubant E. Biomarkers indicative of blood–brain barrier disruption in multiple sclerosis. Dis Markers. 2006;22(4):235–44.
75. Lavisse S, Guillermier M, Herard AS, Petit F, Delahaye M, Van Camp N, Ben Haim L, Lebon V, Remy P, Dolle F, et al. Reactive astrocytes overexpress TSPO and are detected by TSPO positron emission tomography imaging. J Neurosci. 2012;32(32):10809–18.
76. Wang M, Wang X, Zhao L, Ma W, Rodriguez IR, Fariss RN, Wong WT. Macroglia-microglia interactions via TSPO signaling regulates microglial activation in the mouse retina. J Neurosci. 2014;34(10):3793–806.
77. Rupprecht R, Papadopoulos V, Rammes G, Baghai TC, Fan J, Akula N, Groyer G, Adams D, Schumacher M. Translocator protein (18 kDa) (TSPO) as a therapeutic target for neurological and psychiatric disorders. Nat Rev Drug Discov. 2010;9(12):971–88.
78. Karlstetter M, Nothdurfter C, Aslanidis A, Moeller K, Horn F, Scholz R, Neumann H, Weber BH, Rupprecht R, Langmann T. Translocator protein (18 kDa) (TSPO) is expressed in reactive retinal microglia and modulates microglial inflammation and phagocytosis. J Neuroinflammation. 2014;11:3.
79. Chen MK, Guilarte TR. Translocator protein 18 kDa (TSPO): molecular sensor of brain injury and repair. Pharmacol Ther. 2008;118(1):1–17.
80. Cosenza-Nashat M, Zhao ML, Suh HS, Morgan J, Natividad R, Morgello S, Lee SC. Expression of the translocator protein of 18 kDa by microglia, macrophages and astrocytes based on immunohistochemical localization in abnormal human brain. Neuropathol Appl Neurobiol. 2009;35(3):306–28.
81. Vowinckel E, Reutens D, Becher B, Verge G, Evans A, Owens T, Antel JP. PK11195 binding to the peripheral benzodiazepine receptor as a marker of microglia activation in multiple sclerosis and experimental autoimmune encephalomyelitis. J Neurosci Res. 1997;50(2):345–53.
82. Morita K, Sasaki H, Furuse M, Tsukita S. Endothelial claudin: claudin-5/TMVCF constitutes tight junction strands in endothelial cells. J Cell Biol. 1999;147(1):185–94.
83. Nitta T, Hata M, Gotoh S, Seo Y, Sasaki H, Hashimoto N, Furuse M, Tsukita S. Size-selective loosening of the blood–brain barrier in claudin-5-deficient mice. J Cell Biol. 2003;161(3):653–60.
84. Liebner S, Fischmann A, Rascher G, Duffner F, Grote EH, Kalbacher H, Wolburg H. Claudin-1 and claudin-5 expression and tight junction morphology are altered in blood vessels of human glioblastoma multiforme. Acta Neuropathol. 2000;100(3):323–31.
85. Wolburg H, Wolburg-Buchholz K, Kraus J, Rascher-Eggstein G, Liebner S, Hamm S, Duffner F, Grote EH, Risau W, Engelhardt B. Localization of claudin-

3 in tight junctions of the blood–brain barrier is selectively lost during experimental autoimmune encephalomyelitis and human glioblastoma multiforme. Acta Neuropathol. 2003;105(6):586–92.

86. Krug SM, Amasheh S, Richter JF, Milatz S, Gunzel D, Westphal JK, Huber O, Schulzke JD, Fromm M. Tricellulin forms a barrier to macromolecules in tricellular tight junctions without affecting ion permeability. Mol Biol Cell. 2009;20(16):3713–24.
87. Ohtsuki S, Yamaguchi H, Katsukura Y, Asashima T, Terasaki T. mRNA expression levels of tight junction protein genes in mouse brain capillary endothelial cells highly purified by magnetic cell sorting. J Neurochem. 2008;104(1):147–54.
88. Liebner S, Corada M, Bangsow T, Babbage J, Taddei A, Czupalla CJ, Reis M, Felici A, Wolburg H, Fruttiger M, et al. Wnt/beta-catenin signaling controls development of the blood–brain barrier. J Cell Biol. 2008;183(3):409–17.
89. Schrade A, Sade H, Couraud PO, Romero IA, Weksler BB, Niewoehner J. Expression and localization of claudins-3 and -12 in transformed human brain endothelium. Fluids Barriers CNS. 2012;9:6.
90. Milatz S, Krug SM, Rosenthal R, Gunzel D, Muller D, Schulzke JD, Amasheh S, Fromm M. Claudin-3 acts as a sealing component of the tight junction for ions of either charge and uncharged solutes. Biochim Biophys Acta. 2010; 1798(11):2048–57.
91. Piontek J, Fritzsche S, Cording J, Richter S, Hartwig J, Walter M, Yu D, Turner JR, Gehring C, Rahn HP, et al. Elucidating the principles of the molecular organization of heteropolymeric tight junction strands. Cell Mol Life Sci. 2011;68(23):3903–18.
92. Theodoropoulou S, Spanakos G, Baxevanis CN, Economou M, Gritzapis AD, Papamichail MP, Stefanis CN. Cytokine serum levels, autologous mixed lymphocyte reaction and surface marker analysis in never medicated and chronically medicated schizophrenic patients. Schizophr Res. 2001;47(1):13–25.
93. Song XQ, Lv LX, Li WQ, Hao YH, Zhao JP. The interaction of nuclear factor-kappa B and cytokines is associated with schizophrenia. Biol Psychiatry. 2009;65(6):481–8.
94. Erbagci AB, Herken H, Koyluoglu O, Yilmaz N, Tarakcioglu M. Serum IL-1beta, sIL-2R, IL-6, IL-8 and TNF-alpha in schizophrenic patients, relation with symptomatology and responsiveness to risperidone treatment. Mediators Inflamm. 2001;10(3):109–15.
95. Coelho FM, Reis HJ, Nicolato R, Romano-Silva MA, Teixeira MM, Bauer ME, Teixeira AL. Increased serum levels of inflammatory markers in chronic institutionalized patients with schizophrenia. Neuroimmunomodulation. 2008;15(2):140–4.
96. Zakharyan R, Boyajyan A. Inflammatory cytokine network in schizophrenia. World J Biol Psychiatry. 2014;15(3):174–87.
97. Potvin S, Stip E, Sepehry AA, Gendron A, Bah R, Kouassi E. Inflammatory cytokine alterations in schizophrenia: a systematic quantitative review. Biol Psychiatry. 2008;63(8):801–8.
98. Miller BJ, Buckley P, Seabolt W, Mellor A, Kirkpatrick B. Meta-analysis of cytokine alterations in schizophrenia: clinical status and antipsychotic effects. Biol Psychiatry. 2011;70(7):663–71.
99. Goldsmith DR, Rapaport MH, Miller BJ. A meta-analysis of blood cytokine network alterations in psychiatric patients: comparisons between schizophrenia, bipolar disorder and depression. Mol Psychiatry. 2016;21(12):1696–709.
100. Al-Asmari AK, Khan MW. Inflammation and schizophrenia: alterations in cytokine levels and perturbation in antioxidative defense systems. Hum Exp Toxicol. 2014;33(2):115–22.
101. Hoirisch-Clapauch S, Nardi AE. Low activity of plasminogen activator: a common feature of non-iatrogenic comorbidities of schizophrenia. CNS Neurol Disord Drug Targets. 2015;14(3):325–30.
102. Hoirisch-Clapauch S, Nardi AE. Markers of low activity of tissue plasminogen activator/plasmin are prevalent in schizophrenia patients. Schizophr Res. 2014;159(1):118–23.
103. Kirch DG, Alexander RC, Suddath RL, Papadopoulos NM, Kaufmann CA, Daniel DG, Wyatt RJ. Blood-CSF barrier permeability and central nervous system immunoglobulin G in schizophrenia. J Neural Transm Gen Sect. 1992;89(3):219–32.
104. Uranova NA, Zimina IS, Vikhreva OV, Krukov NO, Rachmanova VI, Orlovskaya DD. Ultrastructural damage of capillaries in the neocortex in schizophrenia. World J Biol Psychiatry. 2010;11(3):567–78.
105. Bechter K, Benveniste H. Quinckes' pioneering 19th centuries CSF studies may inform 21th centuries research. Neurol Psychiatry Brain Res. 2015;21(2):79–81.
106. Muller N, Riedel M, Hadjamu M, Schwarz MJ, Ackenheil M, Gruber R. Increase in expression of adhesion molecule receptors on T helper cells during antipsychotic treatment and relationship to blood–brain barrier permeability in schizophrenia. Am J Psychiatry. 1999;156(4):634–6.
107. Elmorsy E, Smith PA. Bioenergetic disruption of human micro-vascular endothelial cells by antipsychotics. Biochem Biophys Res Commun. 2015;460(3):857–62.
108. Zetterberg H, Jakobsson J, Redsater M, Andreasson U, Palsson E, Ekman CJ, Sellgren C, Johansson AG, Blennow K, Landen M. Blood-cerebrospinal fluid barrier dysfunction in patients with bipolar disorder in relation to antipsychotic treatment. Psychiatry Res. 2014;217(3):143–6.
109. Al-Amin MM, Nasir Uddin MM, Mahmud Reza H. Effects of antipsychotics on the inflammatory response system of patients with schizophrenia in peripheral blood mononuclear cell cultures. Clin Psychopharmacol Neurosci. 2013;11(3):144–51.
110. Borovcanin M, Jovanovic I, Radosavljevic G, Djukic Dejanovic S, Stefanovic V, Arsenijevic N, Lukic ML. Antipsychotics can modulate the cytokine profile in schizophrenia: attenuation of the type-2 inflammatory response. Schizophr Res. 2013;147(1):103–9.
111. Tourjman V, Kouassi E, Koue ME, Rocchetti M, Fortin-Fournier S, Fusar-Poli P, Potvin S. Antipsychotics' effects on blood levels of cytokines in schizophrenia: a meta-analysis. Schizophr Res. 2013;151(1–3):43–7.
112. Song C, Lin A, Kenis G, Bosmans E, Maes M. Immunosuppressive effects of clozapine and haloperidol: enhanced production of the interleukin-1 receptor antagonist. Schizophr Res. 2000;42(2):157–64.
113. Ajami A, Abedian F, Hamzeh Hosseini S, Akbarian E, Alizadeh-Navaei R, Taghipour M. Serum TNF-alpha, IL-10 and IL-2 in schizophrenic patients before and after treatment with risperidone and clozapine. Iran J Immunol. 2014;11(3):200–9.
114. Cazzullo CL, Sacchetti E, Galluzzo A, Panariello A, Adorni A, Pegoraro M, Bosis S, Colombo F, Trabattoni D, Zagliani A, et al. Cytokine profiles in schizophrenic patients treated with risperidone: a 3-month follow-up study. Prog Neuropsychopharmacol Biol Psychiatry. 2002;26(1):33–9.
115. Noto C, Ota VK, Gouvea ES, Rizzo LB, Spindola LM, Honda PH, Cordeiro Q, Belangero SI, Bressan RA, Gadelha A et al. Effects of risperidone on cytokine profile in drug-naive first-episode psychosis. Int J Neuropsychopharmacol. 2015;18(4).
116. MacDowell KS, Garcia-Bueno B, Madrigal JL, Parellada M, Arango C, Mico JA, Leza JC. Risperidone normalizes increased inflammatory parameters and restores anti-inflammatory pathways in a model of neuroinflammation. Int J Neuropsychopharmacol. 2013;16(1):121–35.
117. Tobiasova Z, van der Lingen KH, Scahill L, Leckman JF, Zhang Y, Chae W, McCracken JT, McDougle CJ, Vitiello B, Tierney E, et al. Risperidone-related improvement of irritability in children with autism is not associated with changes in serum of epidermal growth factor and interleukin-13. J Child Adolesc Psychopharmacol. 2011;21(6):555–64.
118. Choi JE, Widjaja F, Careaga M, Bent S, Ashwood P, Hendren RL. Change in plasma cytokine levels during risperidone treatment in children with autism. J Child Adolesc Psychopharmacol. 2014;24(10):586–9.
119. Kato T, Monji A, Hashioka S, Kanba S. Risperidone significantly inhibits interferon-gamma-induced microglial activation in vitro. Schizophr Res. 2007;92(1–3):108–15.
120. Zhu F, Zheng Y, Ding YQ, Liu Y, Zhang X, Wu R, Guo X, Zhao J. Minocycline and risperidone prevent microglia activation and rescue behavioral deficits induced by neonatal intrahippocampal injection of lipopolysaccharide in rats. PLoS One. 2014;9(4):e93966.
121. Edmonson C, Ziats MN, Rennert OM. Altered glial marker expression in autistic post-mortem prefrontal cortex and cerebellum. Mol Autism. 2014;5(1):3.
122. de Theije CG, Koelink PJ, Korte-Bouws GA, Lopes da Silva S, Korte SM, Olivier B, Garssen J, Kraneveld AD. Intestinal inflammation in a murine model of autism spectrum disorders. Brain Behav Immun. 2014;37:240–7.
123. Hsiao EY, McBride SW, Hsien S, Sharon G, Hyde ER, McCue T, Codelli JA, Chow J, Reisman SE, Petrosino JF, et al. Microbiota modulate behavioral and physiological abnormalities associated with neurodevelopmental disorders. Cell. 2013;155(7):1451–63.
124. Braniste V, Al-Asmakh M, Kowal C, Anuar F, Abbaspour A, Toth M, Korecka A, Bakocevic N, Ng LG, Kundu P, et al. The gut microbiota influences blood–brain barrier permeability in mice. Sci Transl Med. 2014;6(263):263ra158.

Permissions

All chapters in this book were first published in MA, by BioMed Central; hereby published with permission under the Creative Commons Attribution License or equivalent. Every chapter published in this book has been scrutinized by our experts. Their significance has been extensively debated. The topics covered herein carry significant findings which will fuel the growth of the discipline. They may even be implemented as practical applications or may be referred to as a beginning point for another development.

The contributors of this book come from diverse backgrounds, making this book a truly international effort. This book will bring forth new frontiers with its revolutionizing research information and detailed analysis of the nascent developments around the world.

We would like to thank all the contributing authors for lending their expertise to make the book truly unique. They have played a crucial role in the development of this book. Without their invaluable contributions this book wouldn't have been possible. They have made vital efforts to compile up to date information on the varied aspects of this subject to make this book a valuable addition to the collection of many professionals and students.

This book was conceptualized with the vision of imparting up-to-date information and advanced data in this field. To ensure the same, a matchless editorial board was set up. Every individual on the board went through rigorous rounds of assessment to prove their worth. After which they invested a large part of their time researching and compiling the most relevant data for our readers.

The editorial board has been involved in producing this book since its inception. They have spent rigorous hours researching and exploring the diverse topics which have resulted in the successful publishing of this book. They have passed on their knowledge of decades through this book. To expedite this challenging task, the publisher supported the team at every step. A small team of assistant editors was also appointed to further simplify the editing procedure and attain best results for the readers.

Apart from the editorial board, the designing team has also invested a significant amount of their time in understanding the subject and creating the most relevant covers. They scrutinized every image to scout for the most suitable representation of the subject and create an appropriate cover for the book.

The publishing team has been an ardent support to the editorial, designing and production team. Their endless efforts to recruit the best for this project, has resulted in the accomplishment of this book. They are a veteran in the field of academics and their pool of knowledge is as vast as their experience in printing. Their expertise and guidance has proved useful at every step. Their uncompromising quality standards have made this book an exceptional effort. Their encouragement from time to time has been an inspiration for everyone.

The publisher and the editorial board hope that this book will prove to be a valuable piece of knowledge for researchers, students, practitioners and scholars across the globe.

List of Contributors

Philip J. Pell, Andrew J. Calder, Elisabeth A. H. von dem Hagen and Michael P. Ewban
Medical Research Council, Cognition and Brain Sciences Unit, Cambridge, UK

Isabelle Mareschal
School of Biological and Chemical Sciences, Psychology Department, Queen Mary University of London, London, UK

Simon Baron-Cohen
Autism Research Centre, Department of Psychiatry, University of Cambridge, Cambridge, UK

Elisabeth A. H. von dem Hagen
School of Psychology, Cardiff University, Cardiff, UK

Colin W. G. Clifford
School of Psychology, UNSW Australia, Sydney, NSW, Australia

Michael P. Ewbank
MRC Cognition and Brain Sciences Unit, 15 Chaucer Road, Cambridge CB2 7EF, UK

Anne Masi, Nicholas Glozier, Ian B. Hickie and Adam J. Guastella
Autism Clinic for Translational Research, Brain and Mind Centre, Central Clinical School, Sydney Medical School, University of Sydney, 100 Mallett Street, Camperdown, New South Wales 2050, Australia

Edmond J. Breen
Australian Proteome Analysis Facility, Macquarie University, Sydney, Australia.

Gail A. Alvares, Andrew J. O. Whitehouse and Anna Hunt
Telethon Kids Institute, University of Western Australia, Perth, Western Australia, Australia
Cooperative Research Centre for Living with Autism (Autism CRC), Long Pocket, Brisbane, Queensland, Australia

John Beilby and David Ravine
Pathwest Laboratory Medicine WA, Nedlands, Western Australia, Australia

Jennie Hui, John Beilby and David Ravine
School of Pathology and Laboratory Medicine, University of Western Australia, Perth, Western Australia, Australia

Jennie Hui
School of Population Health, University of Western Australia, Perth, Western Australia, Australia

John Wray
School of Pediatrics and Child Health, University of Western Australia, Perth, Western Australia, Australia

Anna May Kolesnik, Emily Jane Harrison Jones, and Mark Henry Johnson
Centre for Brain and Cognitive Development and Department of Psychology, Birkbeck, University of London, Malet Street, London WC1E 7HX, UK

Shruti Garg and Jonathan Green
Neuroscience & Experimental Psychology, Manchester Academic Health Science Centre, University of Manchester and Royal Manchester Children's Hospital, Central Manchester University Hospitals NHS Foundation, Manchester, UK

Tony Charman
Department of Psychology, Institute of Psychiatry, Psychology & Neuroscience, King's College London, London, UK

Kristin A. Bakke and Terje Nærlan
NevSom, Department of Rare Disorders, Oslo University Hospital, Oslo, Norway

Patricia Howlin
Institute of Psychiatry, Psychology and Neuroscience, King's College London, London, UK
Faculty of Health Sciences, University of Sydney, Sydney, NSW, Australia

Lars Retterstøl and Arvid Heiberg
Department of Medical Genetics, Oslo University Hospital, Oslo, Norway

Øivind J. Kanavin
Frambu National Resource Center for Rare Disorders, Siggerud, Norway

Terje Nærland
NORMENT, Institute of Clinical Medicine, University of Oslo, Oslo, Norway

E. Loth Sackler
Institute for Translational Neurodevelopment, Institute of Psychiatry, Psychology and Neuroscience, King's College London, De Crespigny Park, Denmark Hill, London SE5 8AF, UK

J. Ahmad, E. Watson, A. Duff and E. Loth
Department of Forensic and Neurodevelopmental Sciences, Institute of Psychiatry, Psychology and Neuroscience, King's College London, London, UK

L. Garrido
Division of Psychology, Department of Life Sciences, Brunel University, London, UK

B. Duchaine
Department of Psychological and Brain Sciences, Dartmouth College, Hanover, USA

Dorothea L. Floris, Tanmay Nath and Adriana Di Martino
Hassenfeld Children's Hospital at NYU Langone Health, Department of Child and Adolescent Psychiatry, Child Study Center, 1 Park Avenue, New York City, NY 10016, USA

Meng-Chuan Lai
Child and Youth Mental Health Collaborative at the Centre for Addiction and Mental Health and The Hospital for Sick Children, Department of Psychiatry, University of Toronto, Toronto, ON M6J 1H4, Canada
Autism Research Centre, Department of Psychiatry, University of Cambridge, Cambridge CB2 8AH, UK

Michael P. Milham
Center for the Developing Brain, Child Mind Institute, New York, NY 10022, USA
Nathan S Kline Institute for Psychiatric Research, Orangeburg, NY 10962, USA

Anneke de Boer, Karlijn Vermeulen and Nicolette S. Wouter Staal
Karakter Child and Adolescent Psychiatry University Centre, Nijmegen, the Netherlands

Tjitske Kleefstra, Hans van Bokhoven, Wouter Staal and Karlijn Vermeulen
Donders Institute for Brain, Cognition and Behavior, Centre for Neuroscience, Radboud University, Nijmegen, the Netherland

Joost G. E. Janzing, Wouter Staal, Karlijn Vermeulen and Anneke de Boer
Department of Psychiatry, Radboud University Medical Center, Nijmegen, the Netherlands

Jos I. M. Egger
Centre of Excellence for Neuropsychiatry, Vincent van Gogh Institute for Psychiatry, Venray, the Netherlands
Behavioural Science Institute, Radboud University, Nijmegen, the Netherlands
Donders Institute for Brain, Cognition and Behaviour, Centre for Cognition, Radboud University, Nijmegen, the Netherlands

Tjitske Kleefstra Nicole de Leeuw and Hans van Bokhoven
Department of Human Genetics, Radboud University Medical Center, 6500, HB, Nijmegen, the Netherlands

Hermine E. Veenstra-Knol
Department of Genetics, University Medical Centre Groningen, University of Groningen, Groningen, the Netherlands

den Hollander
Department of Clinical Genetics, Leiden University Medical Center, Leiden, the Netherlands

Wouter Staal
Faculty of Social Sciences, Leiden University, Leiden, the Netherlands
Leiden Institute for Brain and Cognition, Leiden University, Leiden, the Netherlands

Xi-Hong Zhou and Ya-Min Li
Clinical Nursing Teaching and Research Section, The Second Xiangya Hospital, Central South University, Changsha 410011, Hunan, China

Yong-Jiang Li
Department of Pharmacy, The Second Xiangya Hospital, Central South University, Changsha 410011, Hunan, China
Institute of Clinical Pharmacy, Central South University, Changsha 410011, Hunan, China

Jian-Jun Ou
Mental Health Institute, The Second Xiangya Hospital, Central South University, Changsha 410011, Hunan, China

Herwig Czech
Ethics, Collections, and History of Medicine, Medical University of Vienna, Währinger Straße 25, 1090 Vienna, Austria

Alain C. Burette, Benjamin D. Philpot and Matthew C. Judson
Department of Cell Biology and Physiology, University of North Carolina at Chapel Hill, 314 Taylor Hall, Campus, Chapel Hill, NC 27599-7545, USA

Richard J. Weinberg
Department of Cell Biology and Physiology and Neuroscience Center, University of North Carolina, Chapel Hill, NC 27599, USA

William W. Seeley
Department of Neurology, University of California, San Francisco, CA, USA

Alissa N. Li and William W. Seeley
Department of Pathology, UCSF Weill Institute for Neurosciences, University of California, San Francisco, CA, USA

Edward F. Chang
Department of Neurological Surgery, University of California, 505 Parnassus Avenue, San Francisco, CA 94143-0112, USA

Benjamin D. Philpot
Neuroscience Curriculum, Carolina Institute for Developmental Disabilities, University of North Carolina at Chapel Hill, Chapel Hill, NC 27599, USA

Sarah L. Barrett, Catherine R. G. Jones and Susan R. Leekam
Wales Autism Research Centre, School of Psychology, Cardiff University, Cardiff, UK

Mirko Uljarević
Department of Psychiatry and Behavioral Sciences, Stanford University School of Medicine, Stanford, California, USA

Maria Rosanna Bronzuoli, Roberta Facchinetti, Davide Ingrassia, Luca Steardo and Caterina Scuderi
Department of Physiology and Pharmacology, "Vittorio Erspamer" SAPIENZA University of Rome, 00185 Rome, Italy

Viviana Trezza, Michela Sarvadio and Sara Schiavi
Department of Science, Section of Biomedical Sciences and Technologies, University "Roma Tre", 00154 Rome, Italy

Alexei Verkhratsky
Faculty of Biology, Medicine and Health, The University of Manchester, Manchester M13 9PT, UK
Center for Basic and Translational Neuroscience, Faculty of Health and Medical Sciences, University of Copenhagen, 2200 Copenhagen, Denmark
Achucarro Center for Neuroscience, IKERBASQUE, Basque Foundation for Science, 48011 Bilbao, Spain

Rachel K. Earl, Caitlin M. Hudac, Jennifer Gerdts and Raphael A. Bernier
Department of Psychiatry and Behavioral Sciences, University of Washington, CHDD Seattle, WA 98195, USA

Tychele N. Turner and Evan E. Eichler
Department of Genome Sciences, University of Washington, Seattle, WA, USA

Heather C. Mefford
School of Medicine, University of Washington, Seattle, WA, USA

Evan E. Eichler
Howard Hughes Medical Institute, Seattle, WA, USA
Center on Human Development and Disability, University of Washington, Seattle, WA, USA

Shimrit Fridenson-Hayo, Shahar Tal and Ofer Golan
Department of Psychology, Bar-Ilan University, Ramat-Gan, Israel

Steve Berggren and Sven Bölte
Center of Neurodevelopmental Disorders (KIND), Department of Women's and Children's Health, Karolinska Institutet, Stockholm, Sweden

Simon Baron-Cohen, Delia Pigat and Amandine Lassalle
Autism Research Centre, Department of Psychiatry, University of Cambridge, Cambridge, UK

Amandine Lassalle
Athinoula A. Martinos Center for Biomedical Imaging, Massachusetts General Hospital, Harvard Medical School, Charlestown, MA, USA

Steve Berggren and Sven Bölte
Center of Psychiatry Research, Stockholm County Council, Stockholm, Sweden

Leila Bateman, Emily Ferguson and Juhi Pandey
Center for Autism Research, Children's Hospital of Philadelphia, Roberts
Center for Pediatric Research, 2716 South Street, Philadelphia, PA 19146, USA

Julia Parish-Morris, Mark Y. John D. Herrington, Benjamin E. Yerys and Robert T. Schultz
Center for Autism Research, Children's Hospital of Philadelphia, Roberts
Center for Pediatric Research, 2716 South Street, Philadelphia, PA 19146, USA Perelman School of Medicine, University of Pennsylvania, 3400 Civic Center Blvd, Philadelphia, PA 19104, USA

Liberman and Christopher Cieri
Linguistic Data Consortium, University of Pennsylvania, 3600 Market St #810, Philadelphia, PA 19104, USA

Joseph Donaher
Center for Childhood Communication, Buerger Center for Advanced Pediatric Care, Children's Hospital of Philadelphia, 3500 Civic Center Blvd, Philadelphia, PA 19104, USA

Federica Gevi and Lello Zolla
Department of Ecological and Biological Sciences, University of Tuscia, Viterbo, Italy

Caitlin C. Clements, Tara L. Wenger, Alisa R. Zoltowski, Jennifer R. Bertollo, Judith S. Miller, Ashley B. de Marchena, Benjamin E. Yerys and Beverly S. Schultz
Center for Autism Research, The Children's Hospital of Philadelphia, 2716 South Street, Philadelphia, PA 19104, USA

Caitlin C. Clements
Department of Psychology, University of Pennsylvania, 3720 Walnut Street, Philadelphia, PA 19104, USA

Tara L. Wenger
Department of Pediatrics, Seattle Children's Hospital, 4800 Sand Point Way NE, Seattle, WA 98105, USA

Alisa R. Zoltowski and Alisa R. Zoltowski
Vanderbilt Brain Institute, Vanderbilt University School of Medicine, 465 21st Avenue South, Nashville, TN 37232, USA

Judith S. Miller, Benjamin E. Yerys, Judith S. Miller and Beverly S. Schultz
Department of Psychiatry, University of Pennsylvania, 3400 Civic Center Boulevard, Philadelphia, PA 19104, USA

Ashley B. de Marchena
Department of Behavioral and Social Science, University of the Sciences, 600 South 43rd Street, Philadelphia, PA 19104, USA

Emanuel, Donna M. McDonald-McGinn, Robert T. Lauren M. Mitteer, Elaine H. Zackai and Beverly S. Schultz
Department of Pediatrics, The Children's Hospital of Philadelphia, 3400 Civic Center Boulevard, Philadelphia, PA 19104, USA

John C. Carey
Department of Pediatrics, University of Utah, Salt Lake City, UT 84108, USA

Stefano Gabriele
Unit of Child and Adolescent Neuropsychiatry, Laboratory of Molecular Psychiatry and Neurogenetics, University Campus Bio-Medico, Rome, Italy

Antonio M. Persico
Unit of Child and Adolescent Neuropsychiatry, Interdepartmental Program "Autism 0-90", "Gaetano Martino" University Hospital, University of Messina, Messina, Italy
Luce Center for Pervasive Developmental Disorders, Milan, Italy

Philip J. Pell and Andrew J. Calder
Medical Research Council, Cognition and Brain Sciences Unit, Cambridge, UK

Isabelle Mareschal
School of Biological and Chemical Sciences, Psychology Department, Queen Mary University of London, London, UK

Simon Baron-Cohen
Autism Research Centre, Department of Psychiatry, University of Cambridge, Cambridge, UK

Elisabeth A. H. von dem Hagen
Medical Research Council, Cognition and Brain Sciences Unit, Cambridge, UK
School of Psychology, Cardiff University, Cardiff, UK

Colin W. G. Clifford
School of Psychology, UNSW Australia, Sydney, NSW, Australia

Michael P. Ewbank
Medical Research Council, Cognition and Brain Sciences Unit, Cambridge, UK
MRC Cognition and Brain Sciences Unit, 15 Chaucer Road, Cambridge CB2 7EF, UK

Logan K. Wink, Ryan Adams and Craig A. Erickson
Cincinnati Children's Hospital Medical Center, University of Cincinnati College of Medicine, 3333 Burnet Avenue MLC 4002, Cincinnati, OH 45229, USA

Zemin Wang and James E. Klaunig
Investigative Toxicology and Pathology, School of Public Health, Indiana University, Bloomington, IN, USA

Martin H. Plawecki
Department of Psychiatry, Christian Sarkine Autism Treatment Center, Riley Hospital for Children at Indiana University Health, Indiana University School of Medicine, Indianapolis, IN, USA

David J. Posey
Indianapolis, IN, USA

Christopher J. McDougle
Lurie Center for Autism, Departments of Psychiatry and Pediatrics, Massachusetts General Hospital and MassGeneral Hospital for Children, Harvard Medical School, Boston, MA, USA

Takashi Itahashi, Hiromi Watanabe, Haruhisa Ohta, Chieko Kanai and Nobumasa Kato
Medical Institute of Developmental Disabilities Research, Showa University, 6-11-11 Kita-karasuyama, Setagaya-ku, Tokyo, Japan

Takashi Yamada
Medical Institute of Developmental Disabilities Research, Showa University, 6-11-11 Kita-karasuyama, Setagaya-ku, Tokyo, Japan
ATR Brain Information Communication Research Laboratory Group, 2-2-2 Hikaridai, Seika-cho, Sorakugun, Kyoto, Japan

Ryu-ichiro Hashimoto
Medical Institute of Developmental Disabilities Research, Showa University, 6-11-11 Kita-karasuyama, Setagaya-ku, Tokyo, Japan
ATR Brain Information Communication Research Laboratory Group, 2-2-2 Hikaridai, Seika-cho, Sorakugun, Kyoto, Japan
Department of Language Sciences, Graduate School of Humanities, Tokyo Metropolitan University, 1-1 Minami-Osawa, Hachioji-shi, Tokyo, Japan
Research Center for Language, Brain and Genetics, Tokyo Metropolitan University, 1-1 Minami-Osawa, Hachioji-shi, Tokyo, Japan

Motoaki Nakamura
Medical Institute of Developmental Disabilities Research, Showa University, 6-11-11 Kita-karasuyama, Setagaya-ku, Tokyo, Japan
Kinko Hospital, Kanagawa Psychiatric Center, 2-5-1 Serigaya, Yokohama, Kanagawa, Japan

Miho Kuroda
Medical Institute of Developmental Disabilities Research, Showa University, 6-11-11 Kita-karasuyama, Setagaya-ku, Tokyo, Japan
Child Mental Health-care Center, Fukushima University, 1 Kanayagawa, Fukusima-shi, Fukushima, Japan
Department of Child Neuropsychiatry, Graduate School of Medicine, The University of Tokyo, 7-3-1 Hongou, Bunkyo-ku, Tokyo, Japan

Anna Sapone
Mucosal Immunology and Biology Research Center, Massachusetts General Hospital for Children, Boston, MA, USA
Department of Medicine, Celiac Center, Division of Gastroenterology, Beth Israel Deaconess Medical Center and Harvard Medical School, Boston, MA, USA

Stephanie S. Camhi
Mucosal Immunology and Biology Research Center, Massachusetts General Hospital for Children, Boston, MA, USA
Center for Celiac Research and Division of Pediatric Gastroenterology and Nutrition, Massachusetts General Hospital for Children, Boston, MA, USA

Maria Fiorentino and Stefania Senger
Mucosal Immunology and Biology Research Center, Massachusetts General Hospital for Children, Boston, MA, USA
Department of Pediatrics, Harvard Medical School, Boston, MA, USA

Sarah M. Kadzielski and Timothy M. Buie
Department of Pediatrics, Harvard Medical School, Boston, MA, USA

Deanna L. Kelly
Maryland Psychiatric Research Center, University of Maryland School of Medicine, Baltimore, MD, USA

Nicola Cascella
Neuropsychiatry Program, Sheppard Pratt Health System, Baltimore, MD, USA

Index

O

P

Q

R

S

T

V

www.ingramcontent.com/pod-product-compliance
Lightning Source LLC
LaVergne TN
LVHW080737210926
848485LV00003B/569

* 9 7 8 1 6 3 9 2 7 2 8 1 5 *